The Yajurveda

The Vedas are the foundation on which the imposing Hindu religious edifice is built. The *Yajurveda* contains hymns taken from the older *Rigveda* and prose passages which are new. The hymns display considerable deviation from the original Rigvedic text. It can be called a priestly manual; for it lays down rules for the performance of various sacrifices. It has two Samhitas or a collection of hymns of mantras; these are *Taittiriya Samhita* and *Vajasaneya Samhita*, popularly known as *Black* and *White Yajur*, respectively. The subject-matter of both the Samhitas is almost the same, though the arrangement is somewhat different. Of the two the *Vajasaneya Samhita* is planned in a more systematic and orderly manner than the other. It also contains some texts which are not found in the *Taittiriya Samhita*. This translation of *Yajurveda* by Devi Chand is based upon Swami Dayanand's interpretation. The translator has provided references in the footnotes to the different views of other scholars. To bring home to the common man the message of the *Yajurveda*, he has spared no pains to remove all obscurities inherent in the old form of Sanskrit which was in vogue three thousand years ago. The introduction and the index are added to help the reader. Everyone interested in the Vedas will find this book indispensable.

Devi Chand had a closer understanding of Vedic literature and studied diverse interpretation of the Vedas. He has translated *Yajurveda*, *Samaveda*, and *Atharvaveda* which are standard editions. He was the founder of D.A.V. College, Hoshiarpur and a well-known educationist of Punjab.

The Yajurveda

Sanskrit text with English translation

Devi Chand

with *Introductory Remarks by*
M.C. Joshi

Munshiram Manoharlal
Publishers Pvt. Ltd.

ISBN 978-81-215-0294-8
Seventh Impression 2009

© Munshiram Manoharlal Publishers Pvt. Ltd.

All rights reserved, including those of translation into other languages.
No part of this book may be reproduced, stored in a retrieval system, or
transmitted in any form, or by any means, electronic, mechanical, photocopying,
recording, or otherwise, without the written permission of the publisher.

Published by
Munshiram Manoharlal Publishers Pvt. Ltd.
PO Box 5715, 54 Rani Jhansi Road, New Delhi 110 055, India

www.mrmlbooks.com

CONTENTS

Introductory Remarks — vii

Introduction — xi

Text and Translation — 1

Glossary and Index — 440

INTRODUCTORY REMARKS

THE traditional system of the Vedic learning in India is of a hoary antiquity and it has not yet died out totally. But such studies have remained primarily of ritualistic nature, and except for preserving the traditional contents and hymnal recitation these did not contribute much in the development of thought. There are on the other hand commentaries on the Vedas composed by traditional pundits containing their views and even interpretations on the subject. However, in these commentaries the treatment of the subject in general is not outside the frame of the orthodox tradition or the religious conservatism; none-the-less these are not totally devoid of scholarly brilliance.

The other side of the Vedic studies is represented by the works of European savants and their Indian counterparts who were guided by the western methodology and modern approach.

The growth of the western interest in Vedic researches and linguistic studies can be traced back to the last quarter of the sixteenth century AD when a Florentine merchant Fillipo Sassetti after five years' (1583-88) stay in Goa, proposed that there is a definite relation between Sanskrit and principal European languages which was subsequently proved by Sir William Jones in 1786 by establishing a common origin for Gothic, Greek, Latin, Celtic, Persian, Sanskrit, etc. However, the first notable contribution of a Westerner on Vedic literature was Calmette's work on *Rigveda* and *Aitareya Brahmana*. Later on, in the nineteenth and twentieth centuries great European scholars like Benfy, Max Muller, Roth, Whitney, Oldenberg, Weber, Burnell, Van Schroeder, Bloomfield, Griffith, Macdonell and many others, including Theme in recent times, contributed remarkably in the field of Vedic learning in diverse ways which unvieled many unknown aspects of our early literary heritage. Yet all the scholars from the west could not remain free of prejudices and could not always maintain objectivity in their writings. Some of them, it appears, aimed at perpetuating colonial rule in India while others expected to convert Indians to Christianity through their writings on Oriental subjects. This is indicated by the following statement of no less a person than the enlightened savant Monier-Williams: "....... I must draw attention to the fact that I am only the second occupant of the Boden Chair, and that its founder Colonel Boden, stated most explicitly in his will (dated August 15, 1811) that the special object of his munificent bequest was to promote translation of the scriptures into Sanskrit, so as to enable his countrymen to proceed in the conversion of the natives of India to the Christian Religion." Thus it is clear that the motive behind the establishment of the professorship of Sanskrit in the University of Oxford was something else than the promotion of Sanskrit learning. The ego of Roth was so much against Indian pundits that he considered himself to be a better authority than Yaska in the interpretation of the Vedas. In this respect even the great Max Muller was no exception. In a letter to his wife he exposed the purpose with which he translated the Vedas, as evidenced by the undernoted extract: ".... this edition of mine and the translation of the Vedas will hereafter tell to a great extent on the fate of India and on the growth of millions of souls in that country. It is the root of their religion and to show them what the root is, I feel sure, is the only way of uprooting all that has spring from it during the last three thousand years." Further in a letter dated the 16th December 1968 he wrote to the Secretary of State for India. "The ancient religion of India is doomed and if Christianity does not step in, whose fault will it be."

There are many more such instances but what we want to say is that European writings on Indological subjects and the western thought of the British Period, despite subjectivity, did make an impact on Indian mind in more than one way. Such intellectual developments gave Indians a vision different from the traditional one and enabled them to assess and compare ideas on the growth of religion and philosophy through the ages in the east and west. It has to be admitted that the western scholarship and knowledge in the early part of the colonial rule was certainly more advanced in relation to modernism than those of Indian traditionalists and it was impregnated with new thoughts, ideas and spirit of scientific investigation. It was this kind of academic development that was greatly responsible for influencing the course of higher learning and political, social and cultural ideas of Indian people in the ensuing period. In fact, India of today owes a lot to the intellectual growth of the nineteenth century. It seems that the Indian mind has received the Western intellectual impact in three different ways, viz., (i) full recognition and total acceptance of western knowledge, academic norms and concepts (ii) recognition of western systems and thoughts and modifying them wherever necessary according to Indian conditions and (iii) total rejection of the western knowledge and systems and creating conditions for self preservation.

The aforesaid trends served as the governing factors for almost all kinds of intellectual developments and other important activities in the last and present century, Indological studies including the present English translation of the *Yajurveda* by Devi Chand being no exception.

According to Devi Chand his translation of *Yajurveda* is mainly based on the commentary of Swami Dayananda Sarasvati (1824-83) whose ideas about the Vedas and their interpretations were different from those of traditionalists and modern writers on the subject. The Swami, a polyhistor with a strong background of Oriental learning, was one of the foremost social reformers of the last century. He founded Arya Samaj with a view to restoring the prestine purity of the Vedas and Aryan (noble) way of life. In his opinion only the *Samhita* portions (main text) of the Vedas are original and the *Śakhas* represent the explanations given by the Vedic sages. He regarded the original Vedas as the word of the God containing eternal and true knowledge. Swami Dayananda did not depend much on the traditional *commentors* of Vedas but explained the Vedic hymns on the basis of Yaska's *Nirukta*, Panini's and Patanjali's writings on Sanskrit grammar and other early texts. He stressed greatly on the etymological derivations of the Vedic terminology to understand the sacred texts and denied polytheism and history in the Vedas. Some, amongst the numerous followers of Dayananda, were good scholars who wrote commentaries on the Vedic literature. Of them those who deserve mention here include Yudhishthira Mimamsaka, Brahmadatta Jijnasu, Jayadeva Sharma Vidyalankara and many others. Unfortunately, they are little known outside the Arya Samaj fold, although their interpretations are, undoubtedly, thought provoking.

One may agree or disagree with the view of the Dayananda school of Vedic interpretation but some of the points raised by them are really interesting. For instance they cite the following hymns, to prove the divine origin of the Vedas, which certainly deserve serious consideration of scholars.

(i) तस्माद् यज्ञात् सर्वहुत ऋच: सामानि जज्ञिरे ।
छन्दाॅंसि जज्ञिरेतस्माद् यजुस्तस्मादनायत ॥

Yaju., XXXI. 7

(ii) सुपर्णोऽसि गरुत्मांस्त्रिवृत्ते शिरो गायत्रं चक्षुर्बृहद्रथन्तरे
पक्षौस्तोम् आत्मा छन्दांॅस्यङ्गानि यजूॅंषि नाम ।
साम ते तनूर्वामदेव्यं यज्ञायज्ञियं पुच्छद्धिष्ण्याशफा:
सुपर्णोऽसि गरुत्मान्दिवं गच्छ स्व:पत ॥

According to the former hymn, which records the Vedic belief, the Vedic *richas* (Rig.) Sama, Chhandas and Yaju emanated from Sarvahuta sacrifice. The latter one, however, refers to the Vedas as the part of the cosmic body of the mythical Suparna-Garutman representing the Sun or the solar aspect of the God according to generally accepted view.

However, the *Atharvaveda* (XIX 54.2) states that *richas* and Yaju are creations of Kala i.e. Time eternal.

कालादृच: समभवन् यजु: कालादजात् ॥

It is evident from these hymns that there was considerable time gap between the composition of earlier Vedic hymns and those of the later times, and it is because of this reason that the hymns cited above attributed the origin of Vedic *mantras* to Sarvahuta sacrifice, or the time eternal or located them in the body of Suparna. Besides the Vedic language itself may have taken a long time to evolve with cerebral sounds before composition of the earliest hymns. It is doubtful whether the process of such a development did take place outside the Rigvedic locale. This is further corroborated by the fact that the Vedas themselves do not preserve any memory of a pre-Vedic or of an early home of their composers in precise terms. It may not be out of context to point out here that so far neither the migration of the Vedic people or their ancestors nor their original home could be proved archaeologically. The linguistic evidence in this case too is very weak, for almost all the major languages of upper India including Bengal, Orissa and Maharashtra do not preserve a single layer of any verbal-structure of a non-Indo-Aryan speech, although the position regarding the four major languages of the south India is entirely different which to this date retain verbal-structure of early Dravidic speech in their entirety with sufficient number of Sanskritic nouns and adjectives. The expansion of the Indus valley culture in a vast area covering Sind, parts of Baluchistan, Gujarat, Punjab, Haryana, upper Rajasthan and border areas of western Uttar Pradesh has further posed problems in the identification of Vedic people. The Indus speech of yore is not known today, and there are scholars who believe it to be proto-Dravidian on the ground that it is pre-Vedic in its antiquity. Then the question arises as to what happened to its linguistic legacy in the subsequent periods? Keeping in view the regions occupied by Indus culture, it may be stated that it is difficult to assume that the language of the Indus Valley people died without leaving any cognizable traces of it in such a vast area while their other cultural traits could survive for a long time. It is also unlikely that the Vedic (Aryan) invaders/migrants outnumbered pre-Vedic local people of India and imposed their own speech on them, for this has never happened in Indian history in spite of numerous invasions of powerful conquerors.

The question then arises as to why the process of lingual development in north and south India was different from each other. Scholars, who believe in the theory of Aryan invasion, have not been able to answer this point properly as this questions the very basis of their thesis. The logical inference of such a type of lingual growth is that from earliest times language/speech of the bulk of population in north and south India were, respectively, Sanskritic and Dravidic in character and the area covered by Indus culture could not have been an exception. However, one is not in a position to say in positive terms that the Indus Valley culture is of Vedic affinity, although it appears to be almost certain that the earliest Vedic hymns belong to a pre-1500 BC date.

So far as the commentaries of the Dayananda school are concerned it may be mentioned that they are somewhat different in contents from those of the traditionalists and modern scholars and are not without value for they are based on logical inferences and etymological derivations although they may not be totally free of the elements of subjectivity.

Devichand's translation is first of its kind in English and, I am sure, it would enrich the knowledge of modern readers and will be useful in the analysis of the modern Indian thought to a great extent.

New Delhi
3 Sept. 1980

M.C. Joshi

OM

INTRODUCTION

GENESIS OF THE VEDAS

VEDAS are the Word of God, revealed in the beginning of creation for the moral, spiritual and physical guidance and uplift of humanity. They are replete with eternal truths and throw a flood of light on the various aspects of life to make a man perfect and ideal. God out of His infinite source of knowledge reveals in the beginning of creation a part of it adequate for the requirements of the soul, its spiritual satisfaction, fulfilment of its thirst for truth and making its journey of life successful.

God is infinite, the soul is finite. The finite soul cannot contain the infinite knowledge of God. God creates, sustains and dissolves the world. Whenever the world is created God reveals the Vedas. The process is going on since eternity and will go on for ever.

Rigveda Mandal 10, Sukta 90, Mantra 9; Yajurveda chapter 31, verse 7; Atharvaveda Kand 10, Sukta 7, Mantra 20 speak of the revelation of the four Vedas—Rig, Yajur, Sama and Atharva.

Swami Dayananda, whose commentary I have mainly followed in my translation, has discussed the subject more thoroughly in his Introduction to the translation of the Vedas.

Maharshi Patanjali writes in the Mahabhashya, that there are 101 Shakhas (schools of thought) of the Yajurveda. All of these commentaries are not available at present except the Kanva, Madhyandini, Taittriya, Maitrayani, Kathak, and Kapishthala. On this point Maharshi Dayananda agrees with Patanjali.

There are 20358 verses in all the four Vedas, as given below:

Rigveda	10522
Yajurveda	1984
Samveda	1875
Atharvaveda	5977

There was a time when the learned Pundits memorised one or more Vedas, could recite or reproduce them from memory, but alas this system is no longer in vogue due to lack of public and state patronage.

The names of the Rishis attached to the Mantras are the names of those research scholars and seers, who expounded the meanings of the verses and commented upon them. They are not the authors or writers of those verses as the western scholars say. Devata is the subject-matter of a verse, the topic discussed in it. All good men and beneficent forces of nature like air, fire, water, electricity, months, sun, moon, breaths, lightning, father, mother, teacher, preacher, and soul, which are beneficial to humanity are called devatas. They are not all living, personified beings as some erroneously believe them to be.

For correct interpretation of the Vedas, the words should be taken in their derivative, analytical sense, i.e., root-meanings should be given to the Vedic words, and not the traditional, customary, conventional, and generally accepted ones. The word पुरीष in the conventional sense is faeces, whereas in the Veda it signifies water. The Brahmanas and Upanishadas do not form a part of the Veda. They are compositions of man of a much later date. The Veda contains only the संहिता (the real text of the Vedas) as revealed by God in the beginning of Creation on Agni, Vayu, Aditya and Angiras, the four Rishis most competent to receive God's Revelation.

The teachings of the Vedas are universal. Yajurveda 26-2 clearly enjoins all learned persons to preach the Vedic truths to all, the Brahmanas, the Kshatriyas, the Vaishyas, the Shudras, the Chandals, the degraded and the forlorn. Dwijas, the twice-born alone are not entitled to study the Vedas. The shudras and even women are equally entitled to read the Vedas. Persons like Kavish Aylush (the seer of *RV*. X. 30) a Shudra by birth, vide Aitareya Brahmana 11-19 and women like Lopa Mudra were the seers of the meanings of Vedic texts and their names are from times immemorial attached to the Vedic verses. God is not expected to be partial to one portion of mankind, and antagonistic to the other by depriving them of their birth-right to study the Veda. In the eyes of God all men, high or low, are equally entitled to God's gifts and bounties, say air, water, sunshine and His Knowledge. In the Vedic church none is religiously great or small. All are brothers who should co-operate to conduce to the prosperity and amelioration of mankind.

According to Swami Bhoomananda Sarasvati, the Vedic seer is a poet and prophet but his poetry is not imaginary and his prophecy is not a mystery unless by that term we mean something beyond our comprehension and not something entirely opposed to the order of Nature. A seer of 'second sight' in the spiritist parlance is not a Vedic seer or Rishi. A person who voices out a number of incoherent statements void of any clear, rational significance like the "Revelation" of John in the New Testament is also no Rishi. A Vedic seer is the inspired recipient or medium of Divine Revelation—a person who, by his righteous, pure and holy life is able to grasp higher and Divine things which are far above the ken of the generality of mankind, Sir Oliver Lodge calls such seers as 'peaks of humanity.'

AUROBINDO GHOSH ON SWAMI DAYANANDA AND HIS VEDIC INTERPRETATION

Among the great company of remarkable figures that will appear to the eye of posterity at the head of the Indian Ranaissance, one stands out by himself with peculiar and solitary distinctness, one unique in his type as he is unique in his work. Such is the impression created on my mind by Dayananda.

It was Kathiawar that gave birth to this puissant renovator and new-creator. And something of the very soul and temperament of that particular land entered into his spirit, something of that humanity which seems to be made of the virgin and unspoilt stuff of Nature, fair and robust in body, instinct with a fresh and primal vigour, crude but in a developed nature capable of becoming a great force of genial creation.

When I seek to give an account to myself of my sentiment and put into precise form the impression, I have received, I find myself starting from two great characteristics of this man's life and work which mark him off from his contemporaries and compeers. Other great Indians have helped to make India of today by a sort of self-pouring into the psychological material of the race, a spiritual infusion of themselves into the fluent and indeterminate mass which will one day settle into consistency and appear as a great formal birth of Nature. One remembers them as great souls and great influences who live on, in the soul of India. They are in us and we would not be what we are without them. But of no precise form can we say that this was what the man meant, still less that this form was the very body of the spirit.

The example of Mahadeva Govinda Ranade presents itself to my mind as the very type of this peculiar action so necessary to a period of large and complex formation. Vivekananda was a soul of puissance if ever there was one, a very lion among men, but the definite work he has left behind is quite incommensurate with our impression of his creative might and energy. So it is with all. Not only are the men greater than their definite works, but their influence is so wide and formless that it has little relation of any formal work that they have left behind them.

Very different was the manner of working of Dayananda. Here was one who did not infuse himself informally into the indeterminate soul of things, but stamped his figure indelibly as in bronze on men and things. Here was one whose formal works are the very children of his iritua body, children fair and robust and full of vitality, the image of their creator. Here was one who knew definitely and clearly the work he was sent to do, chose his materials, determined his condition with a sovereign clairvoyance of the spirit, and executed his conception with the puissant mastery of the born worker. As I regard the figure of this formidable artisan in God's workshop images crowd on me which are all of battle and work and conquest and triumphant labour. Here, I say to myself, was a very soldier of Light, a warrior in God's world, a sculptor of men and institutions, a bold and rugged victor of the difficulties which matter presents to spirit. And the whole sums itself up to me in a powerful impression of spiritual practicality. The combination of these two words, usually so divorced from each other in our conceptions, seems to me the very definition of Dayananda.

He brings back an old Aryan element into the national character. Dayananda seized on all that entered into him, held it in himself, masterfully shaped into the form that he saw to be right and threw it out again into the forms he saw to be right. That which strikes us in him as militant and aggressive, was a part of his strength of self-definition.

He was not only plastic to the great hand of Nature, but asserted his own right and power to use Life and Nature as plastic material. We can imagine his soul crying still to us with our insufficient spring of manhood and action. "Be a thinker but be also a doer, be a soul, but be also a man; be a servant of God, but be also a master of Nature."

In Dayananda's life we see always the puissant jet of this spiritual practicality. A spontaneous power and decisiveness is stamped every-where on his work. And to begin with, what a master-glance of practical intuition was this to go back trenchantly to the very root of Indian life and culture, to derive from the flower of its birth the seed for a radical new birth. And what an act of grandiose intellectual courage to lay hold upon this scripture defaced by ignorant comment and oblivion of its spirit, degraded by misunderstanding to the level of an ancient document of barbarism and to perceive in it its real worth as a scripture which conceals in itself the deep and energetic spirit of the forefathers who made this country and nation, a scripture of divine Knowledge, divine worship and divine action. I know not whether Dayananda's powerful and original commentary will be widely accepted as the definite word on the Veda. The essential is that he seized justly on the Veda as India's Rock of Ages and had the daring conception to build on what his penetrating glance perceived in it a whole education of youth, a whole manhood, a whole nationhood. Ramamohan Roy stopped short at the Upanishadas. Dayananda looked beyond and perceived that our true original seed was the Veda.

And in the work as in the man we find that faculty of spontaneous definite labour and vigorous formation which proceeds, from an inner principle of perfect clearness, truth and sincerity. To be clear in one's own mind, entirely true and plain with one's self and with others, wholly honest with the conditions and materials of one's labour, is a rare gift in our crooked, complex and faltering humanity. It is the spirit of the Aryan worker and sure secret of vigorous success. It is good that the spirit of the Master should leave its trace in his followers, that somewhere in India there should be a body of whom it can be said that when a work is seen to be necessary and right, the men will be forthcoming, the means forthcoming, and that work will surely be done.

Truth seems a simple thing and is yet most difficult. Truth was the master-word of the Vedic teaching, truth in the soul, truth in vision, truth in the intention, truth in the act. Practical truth, Aryatva, an inner candour and a strong sincerity, clearness and open honour in the word and deed, was the temperament of the old Aryan morals. This was the stamp that Dayananda left behind him and it should be the mark and effigy of himself by which the parentage of his work can be recognised. May his spirit act in India pure, unspoilt, unmodified and help to give us back that of which our life stands specially in need, pure energy, high clearness, the penetrating eye, the masterful hand, the noble and dominant sincerity.

Dayananda accepted the Veda as the rock of firm foundation, he took it for his guiding view of life, his rule of inner existence and his inspiration for external work, but he regarded it as even more, the word of eternal. Truth on which man's knowledge of God and his relations with the Divine Being and with fellows can be rightly and securely founded.

But among all the materials of our past the Veda is the most venerable and has been directly and indirectly the most potent. Even when its sense was no longer understood, even when its traditions were lost behind Pauranic forms, it was still held in honour, though without knowledge, as authoritative revelation, and inspired Book of Knowledge, the source of all sanctions and standard of all truth.

While Western scholarship extending the hints of Sayana seemed to have classed the Veda for ever as a ritual liturgy to Nature Gods, the genius of the race looking through the eyes of Dayananda pierced behind the error of many centuries and again the intuition of a timeless revelation and a divine truth given to humanity. In any case we have to make one choice or another. Either the Veda is what Sayana says it is, and then we have to leave it behind for ever as the document of a mythology and ritual which have no longer any living truth or force for thinking minds, or it is what the European scholars say it is, and then we have to put it away among the relics of the past as an antique record of semibarbarous worship or else it is indeed Veda, a book of divine knowledge, and then it becomes of supreme importance to us to know and to hear its message.

It is objected to the sense Dayananda gave to the Veda that it is no true sense, but an arbitrary fabrication of imaginative learning and ingenuity, to his method that it is fantastic and unacceptable to the critical reason, to his teaching of a revealed scripture that the very idea is a rejected superstition impossible for any enlightened mind to admit or to announce sincerely. I will not examine the solidity of Dayananda's interpretation of Vedic texts, nor anticipate the verdict of the future on his commentary, nor discuss his theory of revelation. I shall only state his broad principles underlying his thought about the Veda they present themselves to me.

To start with the negation of his work by his critics, in whose mouth does it lie to accuse Dayananda's dealings with the Veda of a fantastic or arbitrary ingenuity? Nor in the mouth of those who accept Sayana's traditional interpretation. For if ever there was a monument of arbitrarily erudite ingenuity, of great learning divorced, as great learning too often is from sound judgement and sure taste and a faithful critical and comparative observation; from direct seeing and often even from plainest common sense or of a constant fitting to the text into the Procrustean bed of preconceived theory. It is surely this commentary, otherwise so imposing, so useful as first crude material, so erudite and laborious, left to us by the Acharya Sayana. Nor does the reproach lie in the mouth of those who take as final the recent labours of European scholarship. For if ever there was a tor of interpretation in which the loosest vein has been given to an ingenius speculation, in which doubtful indications have been snatched at, as certain proofs, in which the boldest conclusions have been insisted upon with the scantiest justification, the most enormous difficulties ignored and preconceived prejudice maintained in face of the clear and often admitted suggestions of the text, it is surely this labour, so eminently respectable otherwise for its industry, goodwill and power of research, performed through a long century by European Vedic scholarship.

An interpretation of Veda must stand or fall by its central conception of the Vedic religion and the amount of support given to it by intrinsic evidence of Veda itself. Here Dayananda's view is quite clear, its foundation unexpugnable. Vedic hymns are chanted to the One Deity under many names, names which are used and even designed to express His qualities and powers. Was this conception of Dayananda's arbitrary conceit fetched out of his own too ingenius imagination? Not at all; it is the explicit statement of the Veda itself; "One existent sages" not the ignorant, mind you, but the seers, the men of knowledge,—"speak of many ways, as Indra, as Yama, as Matriswan, as Agni." The Vedic Rishis ought surely to have known something about their own religion, more, let us hope than Roth or Max Muller, and this is what they knew.

Immediately the whole character of the Veda is fixed in the sense Dayananda gave to it; the merely ritual, mythological, polytheistic interpretation of Sayana collapses, the merely meteorological and naturalistic European interpretation collapses. We have instead a real scripture, one of the world's sacred books and the divine word of lofty and noble religion.

Dayananda asserts the presence of an ethical element, he finds in the Veda the law of life given by God to the human being. And if the Vedic godheads express the powers of a supreme Deity who is Creator, Ruler and Father of the universe then there must inevitably be in the Veda a large part, cosmology the Law of creation and cosmos. Dayananda asserts the presence of such a cosmic element, he finds in the Veda the secrets of creation and law of Nature by which the Omniscient governs the world.

Neither western scholarship nor ritualistic learning has succeeded in eliminating the psychological and ethical value of the hymns, but they have both tended in different degrees to minimise it. Western scholars minimise because they feel uneasy whenever ideas that are not primitive seem to insist on their presence in these primeval utterances; they do not hesitate openly to abandon in certain passages interpretations which they adopt in others and which are admittedly necessitated by their own philological and critical reasoning because, if admitted always they would often involve deep and subtle psychological conceptions which cannot have occurred to primitive minds! Sayana minimises because his theory of Vedic discipline was not ethical righteousness with a moral and spiritual result but mechanical performance of ritual with a material reward. The Veda is as much and more a book of divine law as Bible or Zoroastrian Avesta.

Dayananda affirms that the truths of modern physical science are discoverable in the hymns. There is nothing fantastic in Dayananda's idea that Veda contains truth of science as well as truth of religion. I will even add my own conviction that Veda contains the other truths of science the modern world does not at all possess, and in that case Dayananda has rather understated than overstated the depth and range of the Vedic wisdom. Objection has also been made to the philological and etymological method by which he arrived at his results, especially in his dealings with the names of god-heads. But this objection, I feel certain is an error. In early language the word was a living thing with essential powers of signification; its root meanings were remembered because they were still in use, its wealth of force was vividly present to the mind of the speaker. The Nirukta bears evidence to this capacity and in the Brahmanas and Upanishadas we find the memory of this free and symbolic use of words still subsisting.

Interpretation in detail is a work of intelligence and scholarship and in matter of intelligent opinion and scholarship men seem likely to differ to the end of the chapter, but in all the basic principles, in those great and fundamental decisions where the eye of intuition has to aid the workings of the intellect, Dayananda stands justified by the substance of Veda itself, by logic and reason and by our growing knowledge of the past of mankind. The Veda does hymn the one Deity of many names and powers; it does celebrate the divine Law and man's aspiration to fulfil it; it does purport to give us the Law of the cosmos.

On the question of revelation I have left myself no space to write. Suffice it to say that here too Dayananda was perfectly logical and it is quite grotesque to charge him with insincerity because he held to and proclaimed the doctrine. There are always three fundamental entities which we have to admit and whose relations we have to know if we would understand existence of all, God, Nature and the Soul. If as Dayananda held on strong enough grounds, the Veda reveals to us God, reveals to us the Law of Nature, reveals to us the relations of the soul to God and Nature, what is it but a revelation of divine Truth? And if, as Dayananda held, it reveals them to us with a perfect truth, flawlessly, he might well hold it for an infallible scripture. The rest is a question of the method of revelation, of the divine dealings with our race, of man's psychology and possibilities. Modern thought, affirming Nature and Law but denying God, denied also the possibility of revelation, but so also has it denied many things which a more modern thought is very busy, reaffirming.

We cannot demand of a great mind that it shall make itself a slave to vulgarly received opinion or the transient dogmas of the hour; the very essence of its greatness is this, that it looks beyond, that it sees deeper.

In the matter of Vedic interpretation I am convinced that whatever may be the final complete interpretation, Dayananda will be honoured as the first discoverer of the right clues. Amidst the chaos and obscurity of old ignorance and age-long misunderstanding his was the eye of direct vision that pierced to the truth and fastened on that which was essential. He has found the keys of the doors that time had closed and rent asunder the seals of the imprisoned fountains.

History in the Vedas

Swami Dayananda does not believe in history in the Vedas. Western scholar like Griffith, Max-Muller, Monier-Williams, Macdonnel, Bloomfield, and Eastern scholars like Sayana, Mahidhar, Ubbat and Damodar Satavalekar, believe in history in the Vedas. History in the Vedas militates against its eternity and revelation from God, and reduces it to a man-made composition.

The interpretation put by Pandit Satavalekar on the 22nd, 23rd verses of Sukta 28, Mandal 7 of the Rigveda, clearly shows that he does not believe in the infallibility of the Vedas. Yaska Acharya, the author of the Nirukta does not believe in history in the Vedas, but there were scholars in his time also who believed in history in the Vedas. According to the etymological formation of the Nirukta, all so-called historical names denote ordinary things according to the science of rhetoric.

In ordinary usage लङ् लुङ् लिट् three tenses are used to denote the past. Wherever these tenses are used in the Vedas, the interpreters of history nourish tradition in the Vedas, taking these tenses to denote the past. This is their error.

Panini says in his Ashtadhyayi छन्दसि लुङ् लङ् लिट्: 3-4-6. Kashika interprets it like this. "छन्दसि विषये धातुसम्बन्धे सर्वकालेषु लुङ् लङ् लिट: प्रत्यया: भवन्ति ।" In the Vedas लुङ् लङ् लिट् are used in all the three tenses in connection with verbal roots. Taking their use limited only to the past and deduce history therefrom is incorrect. The Vedas are eternal, hence in their sight all tenses are like the ever present, and there arises no question in the Vedas about the past tense. On this support all the tenses generally denoting the past denote ordinarily the present. Similarly the Vedic words being derivatives are not traditional or personal names. Scholars, when they give up grammar and Nirukta, the two important limbs of Vedic interpretation, begin to import history in the Vedas, and trace therein the unfounded traditions of Babylonia.

Patanjali, the author of Mahabhashya, commenting on this exposition of Kashika, writes that to interpret these three Lakaras as denoting the past tense when used in the Vedas, is contradictory to the science of grammar, their main limb. As long as Panini's Vyakaran is extent, to interpret the Vedic texts as historical, is a clear sacrilege on the Vedic verses.

Having failed to understand the derivative significance of Vedic words, scholars have misinterpreted them as names of historical personages. Below I give the true significance of certain Vedic words which the commentators, mistaking for historical names, have uselessly attempted to prove history in the Vedas.

1. Sita. This word used in the Veda does not signify the wife of Shri Ram Chandra. It means the furrow traced in a field by the plough.

2. Babara is not the name of a King or person. It denotes the air that hums, thunders and flows.

3. Sudas is not the name of a king. A charitably disposed person is called Sudas.

सुदा: कल्याणदान: । Nirukta 2-25.

4. Paijwan is not the name of a King. An individual whose impetuosity is

INTRODUCTION

constant, whose speed or force is unending is called Paijwan, vide Nirukta 2-24.

5. Devas is not the name of a king. It is the name of a learned priest who officiates at a sacrifice.

6. Agu (अगु) does not denote any historical personage. An ignorant person devoid of knowledge and Vedic speech is called Agu अ=not, गु=Vedic speech.

7. Devapi in the Veda is not the name of any historical person. Devapi is a person who admires and befriends the learned. It is also the name of lightning or thunderbolt.

8. Shantanu is not the name of a king. According to Yaska, a man of tranquillity with mental peace is called Shantanu. Water is also called Shantanu as it grants peace and conduces to the good of humanity.

9. Angiras is not the name of any special person. Blazing fire is called Angiras. God is also called Angiras, as God is Fire (अग्नि) God engulfs the earth as we do the breaths, hence. He is Angiras. A learned person is also called Angiras. Rishi Dayananda writes (अंगिरः) अंगति जानाति यो विद्वान्. He who knows is Angiras.

10. In the 13th chapter of the Yajurveda the word Vasishtha occurs in the 54th verse, Bharadwaja in the 55th, Jamdagni in the 56th, Vishvamitra in the 57th, and Vishwakarma in the 58th. Historical school of thought interprets these words as names of Rishis, but the Shatpatha Brahmana interprets them thus,

(a) प्राणो वै वसिष्ठ ऋषिः ।
Prana is called Vasishtha, as it is excellent of all breaths.

(b) मनोवै भरद्वाज ऋषिः ।
Mind is called Bharadwaja, as it strengthens by food.

(c) चक्षुर्वै जमदग्निर् ऋषिः ।
Eye is called Jamadagni, as it sees the world.

(d) श्रोत्रं वै विश्वामित्र ऋषिः ।
Ear is called Vishwamitra, as it hears all things, and all directions befriend it.

(e) वाग् वै विश्वकर्मा ऋषिः ।
Speech is Vishwakarma as it manifests and illuminates all topics.

In the Brahman Granthas Vasishtha is described as Prajapati, God, King, and household lord. Jamdagni is also spoken of as such. Vishvamitra is described as speech. Vishvakarma, the master of all deeds, is spoken of as God, King, Prajapati and household lord.

Rishi Yajnavalkya speaks of the right ear as Gautama, and the left ear as Bharadwaja. He describes the right eye as Vishwamitra and the left as Jamdagni, the right nose as Vasishtha and the left as Kashyap. Speech is described as Attri, as food is taken by the tongue. Being the eater, one is अत्रि, अत्रि is अत्ति from the root अद् to eat.

11. Urvashi is not a historical name. उरु वशे यस्याः । Lightning is Urvashi, which controls all things. उरु बहु अश्नुते. That which eats much. Lightning is Urvashi the fall of which consumes many objects.

12. Pururava is not the name of a person. It is the name of a cloud, which roars, thunders and makes noise, vide Nirukta 5-46.

13. Apsara does not denote celestial dancing nymphs. In the Upanishads they are called Pranas. In Shilpa Samhita they mean the China-clay basins. In Astrology they are spoken of as directions and sub-directions. In bacteriology they mean watery germs. In Alchemy they denote electric currents.

14. Bhrigu is not a proper Noun. They who exert for self maintenance are Bhrigus. भृ for self-maintenance गु exert themselves. They are Bhrigus who continue their exertions to the extreme.

15. Sayana considers Bheda, Tritsu, Yamuna, Ajasa, Shigru and Yakshu to be historical names. This is an erroneous view. The right interpretation of these words is given below.

(1) Bheda:—An enemy's emissary who creates parties in the society.
(2) Tritsu is a hero who overcomes all afflictions.
(3) Yamuna is a ruler, an administrator who maintains law and discipline.
(4) Ajasa is a hero who exerts and agitates.
(5) Shigru:—He who possesses beauty, excellence in action.
(6) Yakshu:—A sacrificer, who performs the Yajna.

16. Bharata is he, who wants to advance and progress, being wellfed. Bharata, the brother of Shri Ram Chandra has no place in the Veda. Tritsu is he who is thirsty for self-amelioration.

Vasishtha is he, who is expert in settling his subjects; or a teacher or preceptor who is most exalted amongst the Vasu Brahmchari disciples of his.

Pratrida is he, whose ears have been opened by the preceptor through the knowledge of God and the Veda. Bharatas are disciples who are reared and looked after by their teacher.

17. Parashara is not a historical person.

A farsighted learned person, the arrows of whose intellect can reach far and pierce through the subtle topic and unravel the mysteries of Nature is a Parashara. Such calm, judicious, self-abnegating souls, who abandon the captivating, carnal enjoyments of the world are called Parasharas.

18. Saraswati is not the name of a river in the Veda. In the Brahman Granthas Saraswati has got thirteen meanings. In the Nighantu 57 synonyms have been given for Saraswati. वाक् सरस्वती। शत० 7-5-1-31. Maharshi Dayananda interprets Saraswati as God out of His one hundred names enumerated in the first chapter of the Satyartha Prakash. He has interpreted Saraswati as wife while discussing marriage. In the Rigveda Mandal 7 Sukta 9 Mantra 5 Swami Dayananda translates Saraswati as instructive speech. Pt. Satavalekar agrees with Rishi Dayananda and translates Saraswati as knowledge and learning.

19. Jamdagni (जमत् अग्नि) is the name of blazing fire, and not of a particular person.

RIVERS IN THE VEDA

In fifteen places in the Rigveda, there is a mention of seven rivers according

INTRODUCTION

to Sayana. He has interpreted them as the names of rivers the Ganges, the Yamuna etc. Pt. Satavalekar has thus nicely interpreted them.

In the centre is the soul force. From that original place there flow seven streams of (1) Egotism (2) Mind (3) Ear (4) Touch (5) Eye (6) Taste (7) Smell. The stream of egotism is flowing in the field of arrogance. The stream of mind waters the field of contemplation. The stream of ear coursing through ears is flowing in the field of words. The stream of touch, through skin is flowing in the field of touch. The stream of eye, through eyesight, is flowing in the field of sight. The stream of taste is flowing from the tongue in the field of relish. Similarly the stream of smell is flowing through breath in the nostrils. These seven streams coming out of the soul, in a state of profound sleep सुषुप्ति begin to flow inside and are absorbed in the soul. In a waking state, they begin to flow out of the soul and work in the world. These seven streams are the seven rays and the seven hands of the soul.

Patanjali Rishi puts the following exposition on this subject in the Mahabhashya. Commenting upon the Rigveda 8, 69, 12 he writes O' Varuna, noble, talented soul thou art Sudeva (सुदेव) a true divinity, the seven streams, the seven case-terminations (विभक्ति) are thy seven forces, which flow towards the palate, wherein the tongue speaks. Just as fire shines entering an iron bar through its pores, so do the main breaths come out of the soul through its gates. Like the division of the force of breath, there are in a grammar seven case-terminations, which express the significance of words. The same case-terminations, being the seven streams of speech convey knowledge. He who uses them properly is really the knower of speech, Sudeva, a divine deity.

In Vedic literature Indra is soul, which makes the seven streams flow. In the Rigveda 4, 28, it is clearly written, that Indra the soul set in motion the seven streams, i.e., opened the clogged organs of sense. It is clear that in the Veda, the names of so-called rivers do not denote any historical, temporary or transient objects. These names have got spiritual significance. Saraswati is speech. The smell conveying current flowing out of the nostril is the Ganges. The current flowing out of the ear is Yamuna. The organ of touch is Shatadru. The current flowing towards the head is Vipasha. Aurobindo Ghosh also does not believe in सप्तनद्य: to signify geographical non-eternal substances.

इमं मे गङ्गे यमुने सरस्वती शुतुद्रि स्तोमं सचता परुष्ण्या ।
असिक्न्या मरुद्वृधे वितस्तयार्जीकीये श्रृणुह्या सुषोमया ॥

Rigveda Mandal 10, Sukta 75, Mantra 5.

O Ganga, Yamuna, Saraswati, Shutudri, Parushni enjoy my praise. O Marudvridha along with Asakni, and Arjikiya with Vatista and Sushoma, listen to my praise.

Really speaking these are not the names of rivers. In metaphysics they are the names of arteries in the body. They are called नदी as they (नन्दति) make sound. Their voice is heard even when the ears are shut.

The real purport of the verse is given below. 'O Ganga, Ida (इडा) artery, O Yamuna, Pingala artery, Shutudri, Parushni, Saraswati, i.e., Sushumna artery, enjoy my praise sung in the verse about the arteries. O Marudvridha, Sushumna, with Asikriya, i.e., Pingala; O Arjikiya, Ida, with Vitasta the Sushumna listen to my praise.

In this connection Maharshi Dayananda writes thus in the Rigveda Adi Bhashya Bhumika. Ida, Pingala, Sushumna and Kurma arteries are appellations for Ganga, Yamuna etc. In Yoga philosophy these names are used for God as well, Whose contemplation alleviates miseries and grants salvation. These Ida etc. arteries are used for abstraction of the mind and its steadfastness. In this verse there is repetition of God from the previous verse.

Shri Pt. Pali Ratna describes Ganga as an artery instrumental in the circulation of blood. Yamuna is the artery which guides the motion of all parts of the body. The weakening of this artery results in paralysis. Saraswati is that artery which brings knowledge. We call it Sushumna as well. Shutudri is a part of Sushumna which quickly brings knowledge. Purushni is an artery which maintains heat in all parts of the body and helps in the fine blood circulation. Asiknis are ductless glands. Marudvridha is Pran (breath) that strengthens the body. Vitasta is an artery pervading throughout the flesh. Arjikipa or Vipush is an artery that works without any restriction.

Sushoma is an artery which remains wet.

Scholars, by believing in history in the Vedas have undermined their grandeur and put a stain upon them. Rishi Dayananda by refuting the doctrine of history in the Vedas, has established their eternity, and enhanced their excellence.

SCIENTIFIC GLEANINGS FROM THE VEDAS

Hymn, second of the tenth Kāṇḍa of the Atharvaveda, is a basic text on anatomy, vide verses 1, 31, 32, 33. Having failed to understand its main tenor Winternitz in his "History of Indian Literature" in writing about some portions of the Atharvaveda has used language quite unbecoming of a scholar. On the basis of human anatomy this hymn (Sukta) teaches great moral and spiritual truths. Similar texts are found in the Yajurveda also where long lists of animals etc. are given for the instruction of humanity.

"What is it that has fitted man with two heels, who has padded him with flesh, who has made his two ankles, who has formed his fingers with beautiful joints, who has provided him with his sense-organs, who fitted soles to his feet and put firmness in his waist?

Atharva 10-2-1

"There is an impregnable city (in the shape of the human body) with nine portals (with seven apertures in the head and two below) and eight circles in which dwell celestial (very powerful) beings (the mind, the will, the ego, the five senses) and in which there is a golden (very powerful) celestial (advancing towards final beatitude) treasure-chest (the human soul) surrounded by Light (God the self-effulgent)."

Atharva 10-2-31

INTRODUCTION

"Possessors of divine knowledge know that most Holy and Powerful Being to be God Almighty Who resides in that treasure-chest with three spokes (birth, name and place) established in three diverse ways (works=karma, worship of God=upasana and right knowledge of things=Jnana) Atharva 10-2-32 "Almighty God has entered from all sides that unconquered golden city, lustrous, giving relief from all fatigue, and surrounded by glory from all round" Atharva 10-2-33.

(Translation of these Mantras is taken from Swami Bhumananda's Introduction to Ecclesia Divina).

Agriculture and cloth-weaving also are treated of in the Vedas. Shri Aurobindo Ghosh, the great Yogi, Rishi and Seer of Pondichery, is of opinion that there are truths of science in the Vedas, which the present science has not yet been able to discover.

In the Yajurveda 22-26 the formation of clouds is discussed. In the Yajurveda 24-20 six seasons are spoken of. In the Yajurveda 17-2 the science of Arithmetic is discussed. Digits are numbered from the unit to billions and trillions.

Pt. Guru Dutt Vidyarthi, M.A. translates Mitra and Varuna, as oxygen and hydrogen, whose synthesis results in water H_2O. In the Yajurveda Chapter 33, Verse Seven, there is a mention of aeroplanes, and their non-stop flight for thousands of miles.

In Atharvaveda 4-37 and 19-36-6 the words 'Apsaras' and 'Gandharva' mean the germs of epidemic disease, which have the power to spread, pervade or get diffused quickly over a wide area. Their forms and shapes, their habitat are described and herbal remedies to check or forestall their spread, are prescribed.

In Atharvaveda 6-111-4 and 6-130-1 Apsara means vitality, electricity or energy, and in 6-118-1 it means the sun's rays.

In Atharvaveda 2-2-4 the word Gandharva is used to denote the sun. In Atharvaveda 12-1-23 'Ghandharva' means some terrigenous product endowed with fragrance. In Rigveda 8-77-5 Gandharva means a cloud.

There is a mention of Astronomy, Geography, Geology, Hydrostatics, Medicine, and air-flight in the Yajurveda, Chapter Six, verse twenty-one.

SCHOOLS OF VEDIC INTERPRETATION

1. The Nirukta. This method was pre-eminently philological as in its attempt to interpret Vedic words it invariably insisted upon enquiring into the origins of Vedic speech. This was the most fastidious, thorough-going and perfectly critical method. It has come down to us in Yaska's Nirukta and is known to consist in a full enquiry into the etymology and history of words and expressions it has to interpret. In Vedic interpretation this is the only faultless and at the same time intelligible method.

2. The Aitihasika or historic method. This is the Aitihasika method as Yaska calls it. It consisted in elucidating a Vedic passage by referring parti-

cular events in known history. The names of king and great men in India have, from the earliest ages, conformed to Vedic words. It has never been difficult therefore to find some king, or wise man having a name occurring in one of the four Vedas and their innumerable Schools. Hence it was easy for teachers to refer to events in the lives of such men to illustrate and explain Vedic statements. In course of time, however this method lost its force as people were thereby, often led astray into, attaching greater importance to the historical illustration than to the Vedic truth itself. The Saayanic commentator has made use of the first as well as the second method.

3. The mythological. It was not possible to find historical examples for every Vedic statement, hence to make up for the deficiency, scholars were often led to refer to folklore or to invent stories to exemplify Vedic truths. The available "grand-mothers' tales" or "old wives' fables" as they might be called, were collected together and utilised from time to time to explain Vedic statements to the commonalty. Like the historical, this method was very attractive and appealing, but it was more advantageous as it hardly left any Vedic statement unillustrated. Besides it was quite easy to frame a tale just at the nick of time to explain things to the audience. Yaska calls this also as 'itihaasa.' Whenever he criticises these or other methods which seem faulty to him, he uses language that very often savours of assent, but it is not so; he is really criticising the advocates of mythology but his style is so charming and gentle that he often seems to agree with his opponents.

4. The scientific. After the Nirukta method this is most difficult. It consists in identifying Vedic truths with natural phenomena and explaining them as physical-scientific truths. This method though difficult and abstruse is very frequently resorted to by all scholars as in many cases it is the only process that yields the right meaning. Besides there are certain portions in the Vedas which clearly treat of Scientific truths.

5. The esoteric or intuitional. This is an extremely abstract and abstruse method of interpretation and is possible only for those who are given to yogic spiritual discipline. It deals with God, the soul, and the human body taking account of the 'outside' world only as an external phenomenon. Yaska used this method in the fourteenth chapter of his book. There are some Vedic texts which cannot be explained in any other way but this, e.g. Rigveda 10-119. When other methods are employed they yield faulty results.

6. The ritualistic method. Perhaps this is the easiest and the most direct way of interpreting Vedic texts. A Vedic passage, for example, embodies a scientific truth or a prayer to God but at the time of the child's tonsure it is used with reference to the barber or the razor. Here in interpreting the statement it may be supposed, for the time being, to concern only with the barber or the razor, and the vocative, if any rendered accordingly.

Of all these methods, it will be seen at a glance, the second historical, the third mythological and the 6th ritualistic are only shabby time-serving devices and cannot be depended upon. They are, at best, rough processes, intended to bring home to the less deliberative, vedic truths in tentative and attractive, though not enduring and correct forms. The Saayanic[1] commentator has committed a great fault in utilising these methods in season and out of season to explain the texts of Rigveda.

Max Muller's Sole Object

Max Muller's sole object in pursuing Sanskrit studies as he himself often expressed, was to convert India to Christianity. A letter written to him by E. B. Pussey reads thus.—"Your work will form a new era in the efforts for the conversion of India, and Oxford will have reason to be thankful that, by giving you a home, it will have facilitated a work of such primary and lasting importance for the conversion of India, and which by enabling us to compare that early false religion with the true illustrates the more than blessedness of what we enjoy."

In 1886 Max Muller thus wrote to his wife:—".........I hope I shall finish the work, and I feel convinced though I shall not live to see it, yet this edition of mine and the translation of the Veda will hereafter tell to a great extent on the fate of India and on the growth of millions of souls in that country. It is the root of their religion and to show them what the root is, I feel sure, is the only way of uprooting all that has sprung from it during the last three thousand years."

To the then Secretary of State for India, the Duke of Argyl, he writes thus in his letter of 16th December 1868:—"......The ancient religion of India is doomed and if Christianity does not step in, whose fault will it be."

To Byranjee Malabari. he wrote thus on 29th January 1882:—"As I told you on a former occasion, my thoughts while writing the lectures (the Hibbert) were with the people of India. I wanted to tell to those few at least whom I might hope to reach in English what the true historical value of this ancient religion is, as looked upon, not from an exclusively European or Christian, but from a historical point of view. I wished to warn against two dangers, that of undervaluing and despising the ancient national religion, as is often done by your half-Europeanised youths and that of overvaluing it and interpreting it as it was never meant to be interpreted of which you may see a painful source in Dayananda Saraswati's labour on the Veda. Accept the Veda as an ancient historical document, containing thoughts in accordance with the character of an ancient and simple-minded race of men, and you will be able to admire it, and to retain some of it, particularly the teachings of the Upanishads even in these modern days. But discover in it "steam engines and electricity and European philosophy and morality," and you deprive it of its

---

[1]It is a mistake to speak of certain books as the work of Sayana. He was not the author of all the works that go under his non-de-plume Mahamahopadhyaya Pt. Shivdatta, Shastri, in his introduction to the Mahabhashya mentions the name of 103 works. All these could not have been written by Sayana, especially when we know that the commentary on the Rigveda itself can be a man's life work.

(From Introduction to Ecclesia Divina by Swami Bhumananda Saraswati, pp. 149-151).

true character, you destroy its real value, and you break the historical continuity that ought to bind the present with the past. Accept the past as a reality, study it, and try to understand it and you will then have less difficulty in finding the right way towards the future.

'Tis pity Max Muller pooh-poohs the eternal truth and teachings, and belittles the etymological and scientific method employed by Rishi Dayananda in interpreting the Vedas, which Max Muller, the follower of Sayana's historical method, hopelessly failed to understand.

The following is from a letter to his son:

"Would you say that any one sacred book is superior to all others in the world? It may sound prejudiced, but, taking all in all, I say the New Testament. After that I should place the Koran, which, in its moral teachings, is hardly more than a later edition of the New Testament. Then would follow the Old Testament, the Southern Buddhist Tripataka, the Taote King of Laotize, the Kings of Confucius, the Veda and the Avesta. There is no doubt, however, that the ethical teaching is far more prominent in the Old and New Testament than in any other sacred book. Therein lies the distinctiveness of the Bible. Other sacred books are generally collections of whatever was remembered of ancient times."

What a pity Max Muller ranks the Veda as inferior to the Bible and the Koran, whereas in the Lofty ethical teachings these books stand in no comparison with the Veda. To me the disparaging remarks of the scholar are based on ignorance or misunderstanding of the true purport of the Vedas. It would be rather harsh and unjust to say that the scholar has made these remarks intentionally to degrade the Vedas in the eyes of the civilized world.

To N. K. Majumdar, a Brahmo Samajist, he wrote as follows in 1899:

".........You know for how many years I have watched your efforts to purify the popular religion in India and thereby to bring it nearer to the purity and perfection of other religions, particularly of Christianity. The first thing you have to do is to settle how much of your ancient religion you are willing to give up, if not as utterly false, still as antiquated; You have given up a great deal, polytheism, idolatry, and your eleborate sacrificial worship.

Take then the New Testament and read it for yourselves, and judge for yourselves, whether the words of Christ as contained in it satisfy you or not. Christ comes to you as he comes to us in the only trustworthy records preserved of him in the Gospels. We have not even the right to dictate our interpretation of these Gospels to you, particularly if we consider how differently we interpret them ourselves. If you accept his teachings as there recorded, you are a Christian.

Tell me some of your chief difficulties that prevent you and your countrymen from openly following Christ, and when I write to you I shall do my best to explain how I and many who agree with me have met them, and solved them. From my point of view, India, at least the best part of it, is already converted to Christianity. You want no persuasion to become a follower of Christ. Then make up your mind to work for yourselves. The bridge has been built for you by those who came before you. Step boldly forward, it will not break under you, and you will find many friends to welcome you on the other shore, and among them none more delighted than your old friend and fellow labourer, F. Max Muller." (From "Life and Letters of Frederick Max Muller").

These letters clearly prove that the real aim of Western scholars, under the garb of research, is to let down the Vedas, and establish the superiority of the Bible. Research scholars in their quest for truth, should proceed without bias, without pre-conceived notions and prejudiced minds. 'Tis pity the Western scholars have miserably failed to follow the requisites of true research, and some of them have in their religious frenzy and bigotry remarked, the Vedas are "mad-man's raving and child's prattle." Their poor knowledge of the Vedic literature, their lack of a thorough unbiassed study of our scriptures, their zealous missionary spirit that blurred their vision, their antipathy towards Non-Christian religions, and their convictions of the superiority of the ethical teachings of the Bible have resulted in arriving at wrong and poor notions of the Vedas, the encyclopaedia of knowledge, and the repository of eternal, lofty, moral teachings.

Concluding Remarks

Since long I was contemplating to undertake the stupendous task of translating in English the Commentary of Maharshi Dayananda on the Yajurveda. My circumstances and multifarious engagements spared me no time for the task. My iron determination and unflagging resolve, however, helped me in the long run, to fulfil my ambition. Constant labour for some years has enabled me to complete the translation. I am not a scholar, nor do I possess thorough knowledge of Sanskrit. I am a mere devotee of the Vedas. I am a fallible human being and claim no perfection to my work. Errors might have crept into my translation, which, if pointed out by learned scholars, will be acknowledged and rectified. The readers should appreciate my sincerity and faith and overlook my shortcomings. I feel obliged to Pt. Jaidev Vidyalankar, and Swami Bhumananda Saraswati, M.A., whose works I copiously consulted and wherefrom derived help and information. My sincere thanks are due to Shri Dina Nath, B.A., LL.B., Ex. Public Prosecutor and Ex. Official Receiver, Gurdaspur, who lent me valuable help in going through the manuscript with me, and making useful suggestions for improving the language of this translation. But for this help, the publication of the work would have inordinately been delayed.

DEVI CHAND
Ex-President,
All India Dayanand Salvation Mission.

Hoshiarpur.
16th April, 1964.

CHAPTER I

१. इषे त्वोर्जे त्वा वायव स्थ देवो व: सविता प्रार्पयतु श्रेष्ठतमाय कर्मण आप्यायध्वमघ्न्या इन्द्राय भागं प्रजावतीरनमीवा अयक्ष्मा मा व स्तेन ईशत माघशँ'सो ध्रुवा अस्मिन् गोपतौ स्यात् बह्वीर्यजमानस्य पशून्पाहि ॥

1. O Lord, we resort to Thee for the supply of foodstuffs and vigour. May the Creator, the fountain of happiness and knowledge, inspire us for the performance of noblest deeds with our organs. May the cows, which should never be killed, be healthy and strong. For the attainment of prosperity and wealth, may the cows be full of calves, free from consumption and other diseases. May a thief and a sinner be never born amongst us. May the lord of land and cattle be in constant and full possession of these. May Ye protect the cattle, wealth and progeny of the virtuous soul!

२. वसो: पवित्रमसि द्यौरसि पृथिव्यसि मातरिश्वनो घर्मोऽसि विश्वधा असि । परमेण धाम्ना दृँ'हस्व मा ह्वार्मा ते यज्ञपतिर्ह्वार्षीत् ॥

2. Yajna acts as purifier, makes explicit, true and perfect knowledge, spread in space through the rays, of the sun, purifies the air, is the mainstay of the universe, and also adds to our comfort through its exalted office. It behoves us all the learned and their followers not to give up the performance of yajnas.

३. वसो: पवित्रमसि शतधारं वसो: पवित्रमसि सहस्रधारम् । देवस्त्वा सविता पुनातु वसो: पवित्रेण शतधारेण सुप्वा कामधुक्ष: ॥

3. The yajna of the Great Lord is the supporter of innumerable worlds and purifies us all. May the Self-Effulgent Lord, lead us aright on the path of virtue. May He purify us through the store of true knowledge and all sciences contained in the Vedas, and elevating selfless deeds. O ye men which branches of true knowledge do ye want to comprehend?

४. सा विश्वायु: सा विश्वकर्मा सा विश्वधाया: । इन्द्रस्य त्वा भागँ'सोमेनातनच्मि विष्णो सत्यँ'रक्ष ॥

4. Vedas are the true source of knowledge and their study enables us to enjoy the full span of life. They contain the detailed instructions concerning various duties. May we through His Grace be firmly convinced of the utility of industrial achievements, and may He, the Omnipresent Lord protect our yajnas and the knowledge and means thereof.

५. अग्ने व्रतपते व्रतं चरिष्यामि तच्छकेयं तन्मे राध्यताम् । इदमहमनृतात्सत्यमुपैमि ॥

5. O God, the Lord of Vows, I will observe the vow. May I have strength for that. Pray grant me success in the fulfilment of my vow. I take the vow of renouncing untruth and embracing truth!

६. कस्त्वा युनक्ति स त्वा युनक्ति कस्मै त्वा युनक्ति तस्मै त्वा युनक्ति ।
कर्मणे वां वेषाय वाम् ॥

6. Who prompts you to do good deeds? It is He, the Great Lord Who guides us on the path of virtue. Why does He do so? For the performance of noble, virtuous deeds and the fulfilment of the vow of leading a truthful life. The Lord enjoins the workers and their organisers, the teacher and the taught to be constantly engaged in doing good deeds and achieving fine qualities and true knowledge.

७. प्रत्युष्टꣳ रक्ष: प्रत्युष्टा अरातयो निष्टप्तꣳ रक्षो निष्टप्ता अरातय: ।
उर्वन्तरिक्षमन्वेमि ॥

7. May we root out the evil tendencies of the wicked, the unsympathetic and uncharitable exploiters of humanity. May we take to task the disturbers of peace, and expose the wicked.

May we thus get many an opportunity of attaining to prosperity and bliss.

८. धूरसि धूर्व धूर्वन्तं धूर्व तं योऽस्मान्धूर्वति तं धूर्व यं वयं धूर्वाम: ।
देवानामसि वह्नितमꣳ सस्नितमं पप्रितमं जुष्टतमं देवहूतमम् ॥

8. O Lord, Thou art the dispeller of vices. May Thou punish the wicked. May Thou deal with the vicious that put the sages to trouble. May Thou inspire the sinful with noble thought, whom we, too, exhort to do noble deeds. We worship Thee, the Giver of happiness and knowledge to the learned, purifier of them, the Promulgator of learning and joy in the universe, and worthy of adoration by the religious minded devotees and the wise!

९. अह॒नुतमसि हविर्धानं दृꣳहस्व मा ह्वार्मा ते यज्ञपतिर्हर्षीत् ।
विष्णुस्त्वा क्रमतामुरु वातायापहतꣳ रक्षो यच्छन्तां पञ्च ॥

9. O Ye men, increase the store of goods acquired by honest and fair means to be used in the service of humanity. May your life, be constantly dedicated to this principle. May the spiritually minded people, also, not give up this humanitarian work. May your lives be constantly consecrated to the performance of five daily duties. The heat of the sun destroys dirt and odour, and draws substances consigned to fire, in their atomic form for the purification of air!

१०. देवस्य त्वा सवितु: प्रसवेऽश्विनोर्बाहुभ्यां पूष्णो हस्ताभ्याम् ।
अग्नये जुष्टंगृह्णाम्यग्नीषोमाभ्यां जुष्टंगृह्णामि ॥

10. In this universe created by the All Effulgent God, I realize the power and influence of the sun and moon, feel the inhalation and exhalation of

lifegiving breath, appreciate the efforts made by the votaries of knowledge for mastering the science of electricity. I follow the researches made by the learned in the application of water and fire.

११. भूताय त्वा नारातये स्वरभिविख्येषं दृ🕉हन्तां दुर्याः पृथिव्यामुर्वन्तरिक्षमन्वेमि । पृथिव्यास्त्वा नाभौ सादयाम्यदित्या उपस्थेऽग्ने हव्य🕉 रक्ष ॥

11. I resort to agriculture and craft for removing poverty and ministering happiness to all. May I feel joy in my domestic life. May our houses be sufficiently commodious, airy, fully comfortable, and built in the middle of an open space. May our life be in conformity with Vedic teachings. O Lord we pray unto Thee to preserve and protect whatever gives us happiness.

१२. पवित्रे स्थो वैष्णव्यौ सवितुर्वः प्रसव उत्पुनाम्यच्छिद्रेण पवित्रेण सूर्यस्य रश्मिभिः । देवीरापो अग्रेगुवो अग्रेपुवोऽग्र इममद्य यज्ञं नयताग्रे यज्ञपति🕉 सुधातुं यज्ञपति देवयुवम् ।

12. O learned persons, just as in this world created by God, inhaling and exhaling breaths are purified by the faultless and pure rays of the sun, just as charming and beautiful waters, which run to the ocean and go up in the atmosphere and nourish medicines are purified by these rays, so do ye perform Homa with pure substances. I always promote this yajna, and sanctify the worshipper with pure mind and strong body, the worshipper full of learning and noble qualities.

१३. युष्मा इन्द्रोऽवृणीत वृत्रतूर्ये यूयमिन्द्रमवृणीध्वं वृत्रतूर्ये प्रोक्षिता स्थ । अग्नये त्वा जुष्टं प्रोक्षाम्यग्नीषोमाभ्यां त्वा जुष्टं प्रोक्षामि । दैव्याय कर्मणे शुन्धध्वं देवयज्यायै यद्वोऽशुद्धाः पराजघ्नुरिदं वस्तच्छुन्धामि ॥

13. O performers of yajnas, as the sun receives the aforesaid waters and the air to dispel clouds, and absorbs them for the fast moving clouds, hence ye should always perform yajnas!

We all should perform agreeable yajnas, for the attainment of God, for noble acts, for the acquisition of fine virtues and for temporal and spiritual advancement. With the aid of yajnas purify all substances and human beings. Yajnas will remove all your physical and mental defects. I, the Revealer of the Veda, advance this purificatory act of yours.

१४. शमास्यवधूत🕉 रक्षोऽवधूता अरातयो अदित्यास्त्वगसि प्रति त्वादितिर्वेत्तु । अद्रिरसि वानस्पत्यो ग्रावासि पृथुबुध्नः प्रति त्वादित्यास्त्वग्वेत्तु ॥

14. May your house be comfortable. It should afford no shelter to the wicked and the uncharitable. May your house serve on as skin of the Earth.

[13]I refers to God.
[14]Just as skin protects and beautifies the body, so should our houses beautify the plot on which they are built.

May all persons acquire such a house through the grace of God. Clouds receive moisture from forests, reside in the vast space, and receive water from air. May God impart you this knowledge of clouds and building houses. May the learned understand the building of houses, which serve as skin of the earth.

१५. अग्नेस्तनूरसि वाचो विसर्जनंदेववीतये त्वा गृह्णामि बृहद्ग्रावाऽसि वानस्पत्यः स इदं देवेभ्यो हविः शमीष्व सुशमि शमीष्व । हविष्कृदेहि हविष्कृदेहि ॥

15. O yajna, thou art the body of the fire. Thou art performed with the recitation of vedic verses, I perform thee for the acquisition of noble qualities. Thou art a great cloud, the fosterer of herbs. Cleanse this oblation, the assuager of mental pain, for the happiness of the learned Cleanse it well. Those who read and teach the Vedas, become acquainted with the Vedic lore, inspiring us for the performance of yajnas!

१६. कुक्कुटोऽसि मधुजिह्व इषमूर्जमावद त्वया वयꣳ संघातꣳ संघातं जेष्म वर्षवृद्धमसि प्रति त्वा वर्षवृद्धं वेत्तु परापूतꣳ रक्षः परापूता अरातयो ऽपहतꣳ रक्षो वायुर्वो विविनक्तु देवो वः सविता हिरण्यपाणिः प्रतिगृभ्णात्वच्छिद्रेण पाणिना ॥

16. The yajna keeps away the thieves, refines and sweetens the speech, is productive of foodstuffs and is the bestower of knowledge and vigour. Let the performance of such yajnas be inculcated. May we through the aid of heroic persons win battles again and again.

The yajna is instrumental in producing rain, may we know thee as rain producer. We should try to efface the dacoits and exploiters of impure minds who lead an impious life.

Just as the air with its strong hands of definite motion to and fro receives the oblations and just as the bright Sun full of luminous beams, with his faultless rays resolves into atoms the substances put into the fire, so do God and the scholars preach all sciences for the good of humanity.

१७. घृष्टिरस्यपाऽग्ने अग्निमामादं जहि निष्क्रव्यादꣳ सेधा देवयजं वह । ध्रुवमसि पृथिवीं दृꣳह ब्रह्मवनि त्वा क्षत्रवनि सजातवन्युपदधामि भ्रातृव्यस्य बधाय ॥

17. O Lord, dauntless art Thou. Let us avoid in a yajna the use of fire that burns the corpses, and use the fire, that ripens the raw commodities, and endows us with nobler qualities. Through thy teachings remove our miseries and confer bliss on us!

O Lord, Thou art the Bestower of permanent happiness. May the Earth and the beings living on it advance through high merits. We realise in our hearts for the removal of the wicked, Thee, Who bestoweth happiness upon the learned, the heroic and all sentient beings!

१८. अग्ने ब्रह्म गृभ्णीष्व धरुणमस्यन्तरिक्षं दृꣳह ब्रह्मवनि त्वा क्षत्रवनि सजातवन्युपदधामि भ्रातृव्यस्य बधाय ।

धर्मासि दिवं दृꣳह ब्रह्मवनि त्वा क्षत्रवनि सजातवन्युपदधामि भ्रातृव्यस्य बधाय । विश्वाभ्यस्त्वाशाभ्य उपदधामि चित् स्थोर्ध्वचितो भृगुणामङ्गिरसां तपसा तप्यध्वम् ॥

18. O' Lord, Thou art the sustainer of the universe. Accept our adoration offered through Vedic verses and develop our inexhaustible mental knowledge. For the destruction of internal foes I realise Thee in my heart as the Supporter of the learned, the Statesman and the Guide on the path of duty of different classes. Thou art the Supporter of the universe, we pray unto Thee to increase our knowledge. For the destruction of our internal foes, we realise Thee in our hearts as the Supporter of the learned, the Statesman and the Guide on the path of duty of different classes. I imbibe in my heart Thee, the All pervader, the Giver of happiness from all directions!

O Ye men, lead a life of penance by controlling your breath, and following the wise, the scientists and the learned!

१६. शर्मास्यवधूतꣳ रक्षोऽवधूता अरातयोऽदित्यास्त्वगसि प्रति त्वादितिर्वेत्तु । धिषणासि पर्वती प्रति त्वादित्यास्त्वभ्वेत्तु दिवस्कम्भनीरसि धिषणासि पार्वतेयी प्रति त्वा पर्वती वेत्तु ॥

19. The yajna is the giver of happiness, puts an end to the selfish and miserly habits and protects the mid-regions as skin protects the body. May the performer of the yajna realise its significance. The proper recitation of the vedic hymns is the yajna in itself. The yajna performed on special occasions also protects the truth as skin protects the body. The yajna is the sustainer of the illustrious sun, the embodiment of Vedic lore. May we realise the yajna as the bringer of rain, and the giver of spiritual knowledge.

२०. धान्यमसि धिनुहि देवान् प्राणाय त्वो दानाय त्वा व्यानाय त्वा । दीर्घामनु प्रसितिमायुषे धां देवो व: सविता हिरण्यपाणि: प्रतिगृभ्णात्वच्छिद्रेण पाणिना चक्षुषे त्वा महीनां पयोऽसि ॥

20. The foodstuffs and water purified by the performance of yajna strengthen the body and sense organs. May we resort to yajna for sound health, for activities, for vitality, for long life full of happiness and prosperity. The glorious Creator and Emancipator of the universe, through His perfect Omnipresence, blesses us for the dissemination of true sublime knowledge.

२१. देवस्य त्वा सवितु: प्रसवेऽश्विनोर्बाह्वयां पूष्णो हस्ताभ्याम् । सं वपामि समाप ओषधीभि: समोषधयो रसेन । सꣳ रेवतीर्जगतीभि: पृच्यन्ताꣳ सं मधुमतीर्मधुमतीभि: पृच्यन्ताम् ॥

21. O men, just as I the Lord, propagate the knowledge of this yajna in the world created by Me, and perform it through the bright sun, stable Earth, vitalizing air and various kinds of breaths in the human organism, so do ye. May you prepare, for your benefit, mixtures of different medicines with water and with juices and dilute the same again with distilled water. May you, thus, effect useful combinations of the beneficial medicines, with refined tinctures!

२२. जनयत्यै त्वा संयौमीदमग्नेरिदमग्नीषोमयोरिषे त्वा घर्मोऽसि विश्वायुरुरुप्रथा उरु प्रथस्वोरु ते यज्ञपति: प्रथताम्निष्टे त्वचं मा हिꣳसीद्देवस्त्वा सविता श्रपयतु वर्षिष्ठेऽधि नाके ॥

22. I fully harness the yajna for the attainment of happiness and material prosperity. This oblation is put into the fire, which expands, reaches in the middle region of the sun and moon and produces food-stuff. The yajna confers fuller life and happiness. May this yajna be performed everywhere. May the performer of the yajna spread its knowledge. May the sacrificial Agni keep us free from diseases. May the indwelling Effulgent God, make our yajna perfect for the attainment of complete joys.

२३. मा भेर्मा संविक्थाः व्रतमेरुर्यज्ञोऽतमेरुर्यजमानस्य प्रजा भूयात् त्रिताय त्वा द्विताय त्वैकताय त्वा ॥

23. Be fearless and do not waver as to the performance of yajna. Let the offspring of the performer of this yajna be excellent, faithful and free from weakness. We whole-heartedly take recourse to yajnas for the realisation of the one Lord, for the purification of air and water and for getting the blessings of mother, father and preceptor.

२४. देवस्य त्वा सवितुः प्रसवऽश्विनोर्बाहुभ्यां पूष्णो हस्ताभ्याम् । आददेऽध्वरकृतं देवेभ्य इन्द्रस्य बाहुरसि दक्षिणः सहस्रभृष्टिः शततेजा वायुरसि तिग्मतेजा द्विषतो वधः ॥

24. By the impulse of God, the Giver of bliss, I perform the yajna free from Hinsa (violence), for the attainment of noble qualities and association of the learned, through the aid of life-giving-breath, vitalising air, and through the rejuvenating rays of the sun and moon. A yajna is the recipient of the rays of the sun that ripens a large variety of objects and is full of immense lustre, and innumerable rays. A yajna is the illuminating source of rain. With the aid of the yajna we should remove our miseries.

२५. पृथिवि देवयजन्योषध्यास्ते मूलं मा हिꣳसिषं व्रजं गच्छ गोष्ठानं वर्षतु ते द्यौर्बधान देव सवितः परमस्यां पृथिव्याꣳ शतेन पाशैर्योऽस्मान्द्वेष्टि यं च वयं द्विष्मस्तमतो मा मौक् ॥

25. O God, the Creator of the solar and bright regions we implore Thee that through Thy grace, may we not destroy the medicinal herbs of the earth, on which the learned perform the yajnas. May the yajna reach the clouds. Let the sun pour rain on the earth through its rays. O heroic persons bind by various fetters a wicked man in this world, who is opposed to us and is opposed by us, and release him not!

२६. अपाररुꣳ पृथिव्यै देवयजनाद्ध्यासं व्रजं गच्छ गोष्ठानं वर्षतु ते द्यौर्बधान देव सवितः परमस्यां पृथिव्याꣳ शतेन पाशैर्योऽस्मान्द्वेष्टि यं च वयं द्विष्मस्तमतो मा मौक् ।

---

[33] Shri Jai Dev Vidyalankar, interprets the last portion of the Mantra as for the mastery of the three Vedas, the two Vedas and One Veda. Recitation of Vedic hymns in the performance of a yajna is essential, as by their constant repetitions, one masters them.

[34] For the maintenance of peace and order in the society, it is essential to punish the wicked. The Veda generally inculcates the spirit of non-hatred and mutual love, but where this law is violated the violators have to be punished to bring them on the right path.

अररो दिवं मा पप्तो द्रप्सस्ते द्यां मा स्कन् व्रजं गच्छ गोष्ठानं वर्षन्तु ते द्यौर्बंधान देव
सवित: परमस्यां-पृथिव्याꣳ शतेन पार्शैर्योस्मान्द्रेष्टि यं च वयं द्विष्मस्तमतो मा
मौक् ॥

26. O' Omnipresent Lord, the Giver of happiness, may we subjugate the wicked folk on this earth where the sages perform yajnas. May we associate with the learned and, thus spread freely the system of education as propounded in the Vedic hymns. Just as My light of knowledge is valued by all, so should yours. The ignorant moving in the dark who are opposed to the learned, and whom the learned disapprove for their antagonism to knowledge, should be brought round to the path of virtue by hundreds of means available and let the restriction on them be not removed till their enlightenment. May the wicked be not blessed with prosperity, and the pleasure of knowledge. O' Ye dutiful may ye persistently follow the path of virtue!

Just as the light of the sun brightens up the mid region, so does God fulfil our desires. The sun controls the earth by the force of gravitation, attracts it towards him, and maintains it in its proper place.

The cruel who are opposed to the just, and are opposed by the peace-loving, be bound by all the means possible and be never let loose till they have been brought to their senses.

२७. गायत्रेण त्वा छन्दसा परिगृह्णामि त्रैष्टुभेन त्वा छन्दसा परिगृह्णामि जागतेन त्वा छन्दसा
परिगृह्णामि ।
सुक्ष्मा चासि शिवा चासि स्योना चासि सुषदा चास्यूर्जस्वती चासि पयस्वती च ॥

27. I perform the yajna with the recitation of vedic verses in Gayatri, Trishtup, and Jagati metres. O Earth, thou art beautiful, a source of prosperity, and happiness, a fit place to dwell upon comfortably, full of corn, milk, sweet juices and fruits!

२८. पुरा क्रूरस्य विसृपो विरप्शिन्नुदादाय पृथिवीं जीवदानुम् ।
यामैरयँश्चन्द्रमसि स्वधाभिस्तामु धीरासो अनुदिश्य यजन्ते ।
प्रोक्षणीरासादय द्विषतो वधोऽसि ।

28. O Almighty Lord Thou hast suspended in space near Moon, this Earth, full of foodstuffs, and producer of all the life-giving substances for the living creatures. May the learned of refined intellect, full of happiness, residing upon it, the well-wisher of all, abiding by Thy eternal laws, conquer all foes waging severe fight with the aid of warriors and arms, and thus attain to

---

[27]According to some interpreters, Gayatri Chhand is synonymous with a Brahman, Trishtup with a Kshatriya, and Jatati with a Vaishya. Some interpret these words as earth, midregion, and sun. Some interpret Gayatri as fire. Trishtup as air, and Jagati as sun. Some interpret them as head, chest and loins, some as Vasu, Rudra and Aditya, and some as Pran, Apan and Vyan. In prosody Gayatri metre consists of 24, Trishtup of 44 and Jagati of 48 syllables just as a Vasu Brahmachari observes celibacy for 24 years, a Rudra for 44, and an Aditya for 48 years.

power. O learned person, just as from times immemorial the dutiful have been acquiring wealth, so do thou full of wealth worship God. Let evil be eradicated!

२९. प्रत्युष्ट ँ रक्ष: प्रत्युष्टा अरातयो निष्टप्त ँ रक्षो निष्टप्ता अरातय: ।
अनिशितोऽसि सपत्नक्षिद्राजिनं त्वा वाजेध्यायै सम्माज्मि ।
प्रत्युष्ट ँ रक्ष: प्रत्युष्टा अरातयो निष्टप्त ँ रक्षो निष्टप्ता अरातय: ।
अनिशिताऽसि सपत्नक्षिद्राजिनीं त्वा वाजेध्यायै सम्माज्मि ॥

29. The wicked should be removed, the enemies of truth should be punished, those fit to be shackled should be cast aside and those opposed to knowledge should come to grief. Oh destroyer of foes, Thou art not wrathful, I prepare thee full of virility for battle!

Those who can't tolerate the good of others must be chastised, and openly condemned. Those who cause harm to others should be humiliated. I duly instruct the army to be strong for weakening the foe, and waging war.

३०. अदित्यै रास्नासि विष्णोर्वेष्पोऽस्यूर्जे त्वाऽदब्धेन त्वा चक्षुषावपश्यामि । अग्नेर्जिह्वासि
सुहूर्देवेभ्यो धाम्ने धाम्ने मे भव यजुषे यजुषे ॥

30. O' Lord Thou art the Creator of juices in the soil. Thou art the Omnipresent, the Pervader of all. Like the flame of fire Thou art inextinguishable. Thou art worthy of worship by the sages at all places, meant for it, through the recitation of the vedic texts. May we realise Thee through our peaceful spiritual vision, for our advancement !

३१. सवितुस्त्वा प्रसव उत्पुनाम्यच्छिद्रेण पवित्रेण सूर्यस्य रश्मिभि: ।
सवितुर्व: प्रसव उत्पुनाम्यच्छिद्रेण पवित्रेण सूर्यस्य रश्मिभि: ।
तेजोऽसि शुक्रमस्यमृतमसि धाम नामासि प्रियं देवानामनाधृष्टं देवयजनमसि ॥

31. I consecrate the yajna, which purifies all objects with the flawless, pure rays of the sun. In this world created by the Great Lord, I sanctify the hearts and souls of the people by the pure and ever soul-illuminating knowledge. O' Lord Thou art the source of all light, Pure, Giver of the bliss of emancipation, the final resort of the universe; fit to be adored by the learned, loved by the sincere, fearless devotees, Invincible and worshipped by the sages!

---

[31] I denotes the priest.

CHAPTER II

१. कृष्णोऽस्याखरेप्ठोऽग्नये त्वा जुष्टं प्रोक्षामि वेदिरसि बर्हिषे त्वा जुष्टां प्रोक्षामि बर्हिरसि स्रुग्भ्यस्त्वा जुष्टं प्रोक्षामि ॥

1. Oh yajna, thou art being performed in a well dug place, thou art rarefied by fire and attracted by the air. For the sake of Havan I consecrate the oblation agreeably rectified by ghee. Thou art an altar for taking the oblations high up into the space; I erect thee and consecrate thee with ghee. Just as water in the space contributes to the purification of the material objects, so do I carefully cleanse the oblations to be put into the fire ladles!

२. अदित्यै व्युन्दनमसि विष्णो स्तुपोऽस्यूर्णंम्रदसं त्वा स्तृणामि स्वासस्थं देवेभ्यो भुवपतये स्वाहा भुवनपतये स्वाहा भूतानां पतये स्वाहा ॥

2. Yajna showers water on the Earth. Mortar is the chief receptacle of the yajna. I prepare the altar for the learned to sit on. May those scholars sing the praises of God, the Earth's Lord, the World's Lord, the Lord of Kings.

३. गन्धर्वस्त्वा विश्वावसुः परिदधातु विश्वस्यारिष्टयै यजमानस्य परिधिरस्यग्निरिड ईडितः ।
इन्द्रस्य बाहूरसि दक्षिणो विश्वस्यारिष्टयै यजमानस्य परिधिरस्यग्निरिड ईडितः ।
मित्रावरुणौ त्वोत्तरतः परिधत्तां ध्रुवेण धर्मणा विश्वस्यारिष्टयै यजमानस्य परिधिरस्य-ग्निरिड ईडितः ॥

3. The sun, the sustainer of the world and the holder of the earth, spreads the yajna far and wide for the happiness of the universe. Adorable fire, being adored in the yajna, thou art the guardian of the worshipper. O yajna

---

[1]Adhvaryu, the priest speaks.
Thee refers to altar.

[2]Mortar उलूखल is the crown of yajna, for हवि for oblations is prepared through it. By preparing the altar is meant spreading Asanas on it after washing and cleansing it, so that the learned Pandits may sit on them, for participation in the performance of the yajna. I refers to the worshipper the यजमान. Griffith following Mahidhar and Ubbat interprets Bhuvpati, Bhuvanpati, and Bhutanampati, as three brothers of Agni; which is manifestly absurd. Rishi Dayananda interprets them as three manifestations of God.

[3]Griffith in the wake of Ubbat and Mahidhara considers Gandharva and Vishvavasu as two Vedic deities. Rishi Dayananda interprets these words as meaning Sun, that holds the Earth, and sustains the universe. (गन्धर्वः) यो गां पृथिबीं धरति गन्धर्वः सूर्यलोकः । (विश्वावसुः) विश्वं वासयति यः सः । (दक्षिणा) वृष्टे प्रापकः that which brings rain (Dayananda). Griffith and others interpret it as right arm of Indra. (बाहुः) has been interpreted by Dayananda as बलकारी powerful. Mitra and Varuna mean Pran and Apana according to Dayananda, but two gods according to Mahidhar etc. प्राणो वै मित्रः अपानो वरुणः ।
Shatapata 8—4—2—6.
Adoring of the fire means the throwing of the oblations into it in accompaniment with the recital of the Vedic mantras.

thou art the inducer of rain through the power of sun for the happiness of the universe. Adorable fire, being adored in the yajna, thou art the guardian of the worshipper. Inhalation and exhalation, for the happiness of the universe, protect thee (yajna) with firm strength every now and then. Adorable fire, being adored in the yajna, thou art the protector of the worshipper!

४. वीतिहोत्रंत्वा कवे द्युमन्तꣳ समिधीमहि । अग्ने बृहन्तमध्वरे ॥

4. May we, in a friendly spirit, manifest Thy glory Oh Omniscient, All-illumining God, the Giver of great happiness to all, the Embodiment of effulgence, and the Preacher of the yajnas!

५. समिदसि सूर्यस्त्वा पुरस्तात् पातु कस्याश्चिदभिशस्त्यै । सवितुर्बाहू स्थऊर्णम्रदसंत्वा स्तृणामि स्वासस्थं देवेभ्य आ त्वा वसवो रुद्रा आदित्याः सदन्तु ॥

5. Oh yajna, Thou art beautiful like the spring. The sun protects thee from time immemorial, for unfolding all objects. Thou art diffused through the power and potency (the two arms) of the sun. Just as Vasus, Rudras, and Adityas promote the yajna, the giver of happiness, pervaded in space, so do I for the acquisition of divine qualities, perform the yajna!

६. घृताच्यसि जुहूर्नाम्ना सेदं प्रियेण धाम्ना प्रियꣳ सद आसीद घृताच्यस्युपभृन्नाम्ना सेदं प्रियेण धाम्ना प्रियꣳ सद आसीद घृताच्यसि ध्रुवा नाम्ना सेदं प्रियेण धाम्ना प्रियꣳ सद आसीद । प्रियेण धाम्ना प्रियꣳ सद आसीद । ध्रुवा असदन्नृतस्य योनौ ता विष्णो पाहि पाहि यज्ञं पाहि यज्ञपतिं पाहि मां यज्ञन्यम् ॥

6. Oh Yajna, thy name is sky, thou art full of butter, be confirmed in this decorated place with thy lovely glory. Oh yajna thy name is space, thou art full of water, be confirmed in this decorated space with thy lovely glory. Oh Yajna thy name is Earth, thou art the giver of longevity, be confirmed in this decorated place with thy lovely glory. May necessary articles be placed in the holy yajna. O God, may Thou protect those articles, may Thou protect the

⁴Swami Dayananda has put two interpretations upon this mantra. Agni has been taken to mean God and physical fire. I have accepted the first interpretation, the second one referring to fire also holds good.
⁵The power and potency (बल and वीर्य) are spoken of as the two arms of the sun. They help in the diffusion of the yajna. Vasus, Rudras and Adityas have been translated by some commentators as deities and by others as learned persons, who take part in the yajna. Swami Dayananda translates Vasus as Agni, Prithvi, Vayu, Antriksha, Aditya, Dyau, Chandrama and Nakshatra, as all living objects dwell and reside in these eight Vasus. Rudras he translates as Pran, Apan, Vyan, Udan, Saman, Nag, Kurma, Krikal, Devadutta, Dhananjay and Jeeva (Soul).
These eleven vital Breaths are called Rudras, as they make all relatives weep when they leave the body at the time of death. The twelve months of the year are called Adityas. The Vasus, Rudras and Adityas are helpful in the performance and promotion of the Yajna. 'I' refers to the worshipper the performer of the Yajna.

Yajna, may Thou protect the worshipper, may Thou protect me the conductor of the Yajna!

७. अग्ने वाजजिद्वाजं त्वा सरिष्यन्त वाजजितॐ सम्माजि॑म ।
नमो देवेभ्यः स्वधा पितृभ्यः सुयमे मे भूयास्तम् ॥

7. I kindle the fire, the giver of corn, full of intensity, the carrier of all oblations to the sky, and the bringer of victory in war. The fire properly used in the Yajna brings water through the forces of nature, and food through the seasons that protect us. May these (water and food) the givers of strength and power be for my use.

८. अस्कन्नमद्य देवेभ्य आज्यंॐ संभ्रियासमङ्घ्रणा विष्णो मा त्वावक्रमिषं वसुमतीमग्ने ते छायामुपस्थेषं विष्णो स्थानमसीत इन्द्रो वीर्यमकृणोदूर्ध्वोऽध्वर आस्थात् ॥

8. May I today for the acquisition of comforts collect through Yajna butter and other articles which contribute to happiness.

O God may I never violate it (Yajna). O Lord may I obtain Thy refuge, abounding in store of riches. This fire is the abode of yajna. Through it (*yajna*) sun and air gain strength. This yajna resides in space and fire!

९. अग्ने वेहोर्त्रं वेदूर्त्यमवतान्त्वां द्यावापृथिवी अव त्वं द्यावापृथिवी स्विष्टकृद्देभ्यः इन्द्र आज्येन हविषा भूत्स्नाहा सं ज्योतिषा ज्योतिः ॥

9. Oh God protect the sun and earth, which protect the yajna. Just as fire acquiring the yajna and acting as an envoy, protects the sun and earth, so protect us, Oh Lord, the doer of the noble deeds for the learned. Just as the sun combining light with light through the oblations put into fire, protects the heaven and earth so God guard us with the light of spiritual knowledge. This is thus ordained the Veda!

१०. मयीदमिन्द्र इन्द्रियं दधात्वस्मान् रायो मघवानः सचन्ताम् ।
अस्माकॐ सन्त्वाशिषः सत्या नः सन्त्वाशिष उपहूता पृथिवी मातोप मां पृथिवी माता ह्वयतामग्निराग्नीध्रात्स्वाहा ॥

10. May God bestow on me spiritual power. May we obtain wealth full of various kinds of splendour, and earthly power. May our desires be fulfilled,

---

[6]In Yajna there are three ladles, named Juhu, Upabhrit and Dhruva. These three are named in the universe as Dyau, Antriksha and Prithvi. In this mantra Juhu, means sky, upabhrit means space, and Dhruva means Earth. All these three names are used for the Yajna, with which they are connected

चौर्जुंहू:	Satapatha 1. 3. 2. 4.
अन्तरिक्षमुपभृत्	Satapatha 1. 3. 2. 4.
इयं पृथ्वी एव ध्रुवा	Satapatha 1. 3. 2. 4.

Me refers to any of the Hota, Adhwaryu, Udgata or Brahma, the participating priets of the Yajna.

[8]Articles, necessary for the performance of yajna.

[9]Agni is the messenger of the forces of nature, as it takes to sky, air, sun, etc, in a rarefied form the oblations put into it.

may they attain to fruition, Men use this Earth and knowledge (whereby salvation is attained) for the pleasures of kingship. May these Earth and knowledge advise me. May God, as my last Refuge and resort instruct me. This is thus ordained in the Veda.

११. उपहूतो द्यौष्पितोप मां द्यौष्पिता ह्वयतामग्निराग्नीध्रात्स्वाहा ।
देवस्य त्वा सवितुः प्रसवेऽश्विनोर्बाहुभ्यां पूष्णो हस्ताभ्याम् ।
प्रतिगृह्णाम्यग्नेष्ट्वास्येन प्राश्नामि ॥

11. I have prayed to the Effulgent, All sustaining God, May the Lord Father accept my prayer. Our digestive faculty digests by means of gastric juice the food put into the stomach. In this universe created by the All-Blissful God, I take that food through the qualities of attraction and retention, of inhalation and exhalation; and the forces of purification and permeation of the invigorating air, throughout the body. Cooking my food in the burnt fire I eat it with my mouth.

१२. एतं ते देव सवितर्यज्ञं प्राहुर्बृहस्पतये ब्रह्मणे ।
तेन यज्ञमव तेन यज्ञपतिं तेन मामव ॥

12. Oh Lord, the Creator of the universe, the Vedas and the learned proclaim this fore-mentioned yajna of Thine for Brihaspati and Brahma. Through that great sacrifice protect my yajna, protect the performer of the yajna, protect Thou me!

१३. मनो जूतिर्जुषतामाज्यस्य बृहस्पतिर्यज्ञमिमं तनोत्वरिष्टं यज्ञ ७ समिमं दधातु ।
विश्वे देवास इह मादयन्तामोऽम्प्रतिष्ठ ॥

13. May my active mind enjoy the yajna's provisions. May God expand and preserve this unabandonable acquisition of knowledge, which is a kind of yajna. May all the learned persons in the world rejoice. May Om be seated in our hearts.

१४. एषा ते अग्ने समित्तया वर्धस्व चा च प्यायस्व ।
वर्धिषीमहि च वयमा च प्यासिषीमहि ।
अग्ने वाजजिद्वाजं त्वा ससृवा ७ सं वाजजित ७ सम्मार्ज्मि ॥

[10] माता and पृथिवी have not been translated by Swami Dayananda as mother and Earth, but as knowledge whereby we attain to salvation, and earth that gives us various sorts of pleasures.

[11] अश्विनौ has been translated by some commentators as sun and moon, and by others as vedic deities, but Swami Dayananda translates it as Pran and Apan. He considers Ashwin to mean Pran and Apan, i.e. inhalation and exhalation the breaths we take in and out. Their qualities of attraction and retention are their two arms. Pushan is not a god but invigorating air, whose two hands are its forces of purification and permeation and of the food taken.

[12] Brihaspati is one who protects and guards the vedic verses. Brahma is one who has read and mastered all the four vedas. Yajnapati is the yajman, the worshipper.

[13] Om is the most sacred name of God.

14. Oh God, may Thou be glorified by our praises sung through Thy Vedas. May Thou promote our knowledge. Oh God, may we advance our soul. O God Thou controllest the activities of all. Thou art the embodiment of knowledge. Thou art Omniscient and the Bringer of victory in battles. May we prosper and sing Thy praises. I become pure and holy by following Thy commands!

१५. अग्नीषोमयोरुज्जितिमनूज्जेषं वाजस्य मा प्रसवेन प्रोहामि ।
अग्नीषोमौ तमपनुदतां योऽस्मान्द्वेष्टि यं च वयं द्विष्मो वाजस्यैनं प्रसवेनापोहामि ।
इन्द्राग्न्योरुज्जितिमनूज्जेषं वाजस्य मा प्रसवेन प्रोहामि ।
इन्द्राग्नी तमपनुदतां योऽस्मान्द्वेष्टि यं च वयं द्विष्मो वाजस्यैनं प्रसवेनापोहामि ॥

15. May I achieve victory like the victory of Fire and Moon. May I speed onward with the materials of war. May Fire and Moon, drive off him who hates us, drive off the man whom we detest. May I remove that sinful enemy by warlike, military skill and equipment. May I achieve victory like the victory of Air and Lightning. May I achieve happiness through the impulse of knowledge, used for the acquisition of supremacy. May air and lightning properly employed, drive off him who hates us, drive off the man whom we dislike. I purify this ignorant person by the light of knowledge.

१६. वसुभ्यस्त्वा रुद्रेभ्यस्त्वाऽऽदित्येभ्यस्त्वा संजानाथां द्यावापृथिवी मित्रावरुणौ त्वा वृष्ट्यावताम् ।
व्यन्तु वयोक्तँ रिहाणा मरुतां पृष्तीर्गच्छ वशा पृश्निर्भूत्वा दिवं गच्छ ततो नो वृष्टिमावह । चक्षुष्पा अग्नेऽसि चक्षुर्मे पाहि ॥

16. We perform the yajna for Vasus, Rudras and Adityas. The light of the sun and earth bring thee (yajna) to light. The Pran (external air) and Udan (internal air) protect thee through rain. Just as birds go to their nests, so let us daily go to the yajna reciting Gayatri Mantras.

The desired oblation (Ahuti) reaches the space, comes in contact with air and the light of the sun. It thence brings down rain for us, which fills

---

[15] Fire means a commander of the army and moon means a calm and considerate king. तम may refer to the enemy or the disease which is the enemy of our body. the disease that attacks us, and which we try to throw off, must be removed.

इन्द्राग्नी may mean बल and तेज i.e., power and lustre vide गो० 1-22 or ब्रह्म and क्षत्र vide कौ० 12-8 or Pran and Udan vide Shatapata 4-3-1-22. The victory of Agni and Som is their rightful use in the universe, whereby victory is achieved in a battle. I may refer to the king or the worshipper.

[16] As for Vasus, Rudras and Adityas see foot-note to 2-5. Prishni has been translated by Ubbat and Mahidhar as cow that goes to heaven. The word means, oblation staying in the space in its rarefied form.

The mantra merely explains the scientific process how rain is caused, but some commentators have failed to grasp its real sense.

streams and stalks of plants and flowers. Oh Fire thou protectest the eye from darkness, may thou protect my physical and spiritual eye!

१७. यं परिधि पर्यधत्था अग्ने देव पणिभिर्गुंह्यमान: ।
तं त एतमनु जोषं भराम्येष नेत्त्वदपचेतयाता अग्ने: प्रियं पाथोऽपीतम् ॥

17. Oh Omnipresent God, extolled by the praises of the learned, Thou attainest to greatness through those lovely panegyrics. I realise that greatness of Thine in my heart. May I never disobey Thee. May I, Oh God, never abuse the pleasant and invigorating food, I have secured in thy creation!

१८. सूस्त्ववभागा स्थेषा बृहन्त: प्रस्तरेष्ठा: परिधेयाश्च देवा: ।
इमां वाचमभि विश्वे गृणन्त आसद्यास्मिन् बर्हिषि मादयध्वूं स्वाहा वाट् ॥

18. May ye thriving, justice loving, wise, learned persons, preachers of the knowledge of the Vedas, become supreme through knowledge. Let all seekers after truth, devotees of learning and action, attain to happiness. Preach My noble word, that brings all kinds of joys.

१९. घृताची स्थो धुर्यौं पातूं सुम्ने स्थ: सुम्ने मा धत्तम् ।
यज्ञ नमश्च त उप च यज्ञस्य शिवे सन्तिष्ठस्व स्विष्टे मे सन्तिष्ठस्व ॥

19. Oh fire and air, ye are the bringers of rain. Ye protect the yajna, and conduce to our comfort, bring comfort to me. God and humility are near me for my good, as they are for thine. Just as I derive happiness by the performance of yajna, so should you.

२०. अग्नेऽद्ब्धायोऽशीतम पाहि मा दिद्यो: पाहि प्रसित्यै पाहि दुरिष्टच्यै पाहि दुरद्मन्या अविषं न: पितुं कृणु सुषदा योनौ स्वाहा वाङग्नये संवेशपतये स्वाहा सरस्वत्यै यशोभगिन्यै स्वाहा ॥

20. Oh Immortal, Omnipresent God, protect me from intense pain, protect me from the bondages of sin and ignorance, protect me from the company of evil-minded persons, protect me from food injurious to health. Make Thou our food free from poison. Let me live in a comfortable house; praying to Thee and doing noble needs. This is our prayer to the Lord of the Universe, may we get pure knowledge through the vedas, the givers of glory and prosperity!

---

[17]Griffith translates पणिभि: as demons of darkness who steal the gods' cows, the rays of light, and hide them in caverns. Swami Dayananda translates the word as 'praises' sung by the learned unto God. Paridhi has been translated by Griffith, Mahidhar and Ubbat as the stick, which is put into the fire. Dayananda translates it as greatness.

[19]Me:—the sacrificer (Yajman)............

[20]संवेश has been translated by Griffith as cohabitation by the husband and wife, sleeping on the same couch. Rishi Dayananda translates it as Earth, and संवेशपति as God Who is the Lord of earth, sun and other worlds.

CHAPTER II

२१. वेदोऽसि येन त्वं देव वेद देवेभ्यो वेदोऽभवस्तेन मह्यं वेदो भूयाः ।
देवा गातुविदो गातुं वित्त्वा गातुमित । मनसस्पत इमं देव यज्ञ~ स्वाहा वाते धाः ॥

21. Oh God, Thou knowest the animate and the inanimate creation. Thou knowest everything in the universe. Just as Thou art the expounder of knowledge for the learned, so dost Thou expound knowledge unto me. Ye learned people, who know how to sing praises unto God, knowing the veda that shows the right path, should master knowledge!
Oh God, the Master of learning, rightfully fix this yajna like world in the air!

२२. संबर्हिरङ्क्तां~ हविषा घृतेन समादित्यैर्वसुभिः सम्मरुद्भिः ।
समिन्द्रो विश्वदेवेभिरङ्क्तां दिव्यं नभो गच्छतु यत् स्वाहा ॥

22. May the mighty space unite with oblation and butter. May it unite with the twelve months of the year, and eight lifegiving agencies and vital breaths, May the sun be harnessed with all its rays. May pure water rain whenever duly consecrated oblations are offered.

२३. कस्त्वा विमुञ्चति स त्वा विमुञ्चति कस्मै त्वा विमुञ्चति तस्मै त्वा विमुञ्चति ।
पोषाय रक्षसां भागोऽसि ॥

23. Does anybody abandon the sacrifice? He who abandons it, is abandoned by God. For what purpose does the worshipper put the oblations into the fire? He does it for the happiness of all. He does it for gaining strength, health and vigour. The inferior articles not used in the sacrifice are the allotted portion of the fiends.

२४. सं वर्चसा पयसा सं तनूभिरगन्महि मनसा स~ शिवेन ।
त्वष्टा सुदत्रो विदधातु रायोऽनुमार्ष्टु तन्वो यद्विलिष्टम् ॥

24. May we be endowed with the study of the Vedas, knowledge, stout bodies, peaceful and devoted minds. May God, the Giver of happiness grant us riches, and banish each blemish from our body.

२५. दिवि विष्णुर्व्य~स्त जागतेन छन्दसा ततो निर्भक्तो योऽस्मान्द्वेष्टि यं च वयं द्विष्मो
ऽन्तरिक्षे विष्णुर्व्यक्र~स्त त्रैष्टुभेन छन्दसा ततो निर्भक्तो योऽस्मान्द्वेष्टि यं च वयं द्विष्मः ।

---

²¹ बर्हि: does not mean grass here as interpreted by Ubbat and Mahidhar. It means Antriksha, the space, in which all things grow, increase and expand.
Swami Dayananda has translated the word as Antriksha. All the oblations mixed with ghee, rise heavenwards in the space, when they are put into the fire. Adityas mean the twelve months and Vasus, the eight lifegiving agencies explained in foot-note to 2.5. Space is intimately connected with these, विश्वदेवाः means rays of the sun, and not certain gods as explained by Griffith. रश्मयो ह्यास्य विश्वदेवाः Satapatha 3—7—3—6 vishvedevas according to SatapathaBrahman means rays. Swami Dayananda has translated the word as rays.

²³Rakhshasas means the evil minded persons, who do not perform yajna. They eat the inferior articles rejected in the yajna.

पृथिव्यां विष्णुर्व्यक्र॒ꣳस्त गायत्रेण छन्दसा ततो निर्भक्तो योऽस्मान्द्वेष्टि यं च वयं द्विष्मो
ऽस्मादन्नादस्यै प्रतिष्ठाया अगन्म स्वः सं ज्योतिषाभूम ॥

25. The yajna performed by us in Jagati metre goes up to the sky. From there it is sent back and pleases the world. By means of this Yajna, may we ward off the man who hates us, and him whom we detest.

The yajna performed by us in Trishtup metre goes up in the air. From there it is released and affords happiness to the world by the purification of air and water. By means of this yajna, we keep away the man who hates us, and him whom we dislike. The yajna performed by us in Gayatri metre spreads on the Earth; and being released from there goes up to heaven, and purifies the objects of the Earth. By means of this yajna we remove the man who hates us, and him whom we despise. By the use of food purified through yajna, may we get happiness, for the accomplishment of the yajna, and be combined with lustre.

२६. स्वयंभूरसि श्रेष्ठो रश्मिवर्चोदा असि वर्चो मे देहि । सूर्यस्यावृतमन्वावर्तं ।

26. Oh God, Thou art Self-Existent, Most Excellent, and Self-Effulgent, Giver art thou of knowledge. Give me knowledge, I follow the command of God!

२७. अग्ने गृहपते सुगृहपतिस्त्वायाऽग्नेह गृहपतिना भूयासꣳ सुगृहपतिस्त्वं मयाऽग्ने गृह-पतिना भूयाः । अस्थूरि नौ गार्हपत्यानि सन्तु शतꣳ हिमाः सूर्यस्यावृतमन्वावर्तं ॥

27. Oh Lord of the universe, Oh God, may I become a good householder through Thee, the Protector of the universe. Oh Lord may Thou protect my house, being adored by me, the guardian of my house. May our domestic duties be performed free from idleness. May I live for a hundred years day and night in the presence of God !

२८. अग्ने व्रतपते व्रतमचारिषं तदशकं तन्मेऽराधी दमहं य एवास्मि सोऽस्मि ॥

28. Oh God, the Lord of vows, pray grant me success in the performance

---

²⁵The performance of the yajna by means of Gayatri. Trishtup and Jagati metres means the recitation of the Veda Mantras in these metres throughout the yajna. We should keep our enemies away from us through the strength and vigour we derive from the Yajnas. Vishnu has been translated as God by Pt. Jai Dev Vidyalankar. God pervades the sky, the air and earth, nay throughout the universe, by means his Jagati Chhand, the power of creating the world. His Trishtup Chhand, the operation of protecting the three worlds, and His Gayatri Chhand, the power of guarding the vital breaths.

²⁷Our :— Husband and wife. अस्थूरि means, according to Pt. Jai Dev Vidyalankar, not स्थूरि. A cart drawn by only one ox is called स्थूरि. It can't work well. Just as the cart drawn by two bullocks goes well without interruption, so should the household affairs be performed through the joint deliberations of both the husband and wife, and not singly and independently. Swami Dayananda interprets the word as free from idleness.

of the vows, which I have undertaken, and which I find myself confident to discharge. I reap as I sow!

२९. अग्नये कव्यवाहनाय स्वाहा सोमाय पितृमते स्वाहा ।
अपहता असुरा रक्षांसि वेदिषद: ॥

29. Speak reverentially to the learned, the repository of knowledge. Speak sweetly and gently to your father, mother, teacher and the Brahmchari. Exterminate all fiends and evil-minded persons in the world.

३०. ये रूपाणि प्रतिमुञ्चमाना असुरा: सन्त: स्वधया चरन्ति ।
परापुरो निपुरो ये भरन्त्यनिष्टाँल्लोकात्प्रणुदात्यस्मात् ॥

30. Oh God remove from this world the demoniacal beings who walk on the earth, dissembling their real intentions, who are immersed in the attainment of their selfish aims, and are filled with evil ambitions!

३१. अत्र पितरो मादयध्वं यथाभागमावृषायध्वम् ।
अमीमदन्त पितरो यथाभागमावृषायिषत ।

31. In this world, let the wise and the learned enjoy, let them be strong. healthy and pleased, according to their capacity. Let them be happy, hale and hearty according to their resources.

३२. नमो व: पितरो रसाय नमो व: पितर: शोषाय नमो व: पितरो जीवाय नमो व: पितर: स्वधायै नमो व: पितरो घोरायै नमो व: पितरो मन्यवे नमो व: पितर: पितरो नमो वो गृहान्न: पितरो दत्त सतो व: पितरो देष्मैतद्व: पितरो वास आधत्त ॥

32. Obeisance unto Yee, O Fathers, for the acquisition of happiness and knowledge. Obeisance unto Yee, O Fathers for the removal of misery and enemies. Obeisance unto Yee, O Fathers for longevity, Obeisance unto Yee, O Fathers, for sovereignty, and display of justice. Obeisance unto Yee, O Fathers, for the cessation of manifold calamities, obeisance unto yee, O Fathers, for righteous indignation. Fathers, know our desire to acquire knowledge. Fathers, know our reverence unto Ye is for your respect. Fathers, come daily to our houses, and give us instructions.

Fathers we always give unto yee, whatever we have.
We give yee these clothes, pray accept them!

[28]God is the fulfiller of our vows. Whatever good or bad action a man performs, he reaps accordingly the fruit thereof, and consequently becomes good or bad according to the nature of his deeds. A man is the architect of his fate, as he sows so does he reap.

[32]Fathers means, the wise, the learned, the high souled, just, religious-minded, philanthropic persons, who work for humanity, and are free from ignoble passions, selfishness, and sordid motives.

The repetition of the words नम: is meant to indicate the different qualities of the fathers. For fuller explanation see Swami Dayananda's Commentary, Ubbat, Mahidhar and Griffith have interpreted पितर; as six seasons of the year.

३३. आधत्त पितरो गर्भं कुमारं पुष्करस्रजम् ।
यथेह पुरुषोऽसत् ॥

33. Accept thou teacher, in the womb of thy discipleship, the youth, with a garland of flowers in hand, eager for knowledge, so that he may attain to full manhood.

३४. ऊर्जं वहन्तीरमृतं घृतं पयः कीलालं परिस्रुतम् ।
स्वधा स्थ तर्पयत मे पितॄन् ॥

34. Oh sons, please my parents and teachers by offering them various juices, sweet waters, disease-dissipation articles, milk, clarified butter, well-cooked food, and juicy fruits. Enjoy your own wealth, and covet not the wealth of others.

---

³³Just as mother keeps the child in her womb, and slowly and gradually develops its body by the use of proper diet and taking necessary precautions, so does a teacher, who accepts a student in his discipleship, acting like a mother, develop the student physically, intellectually, morally and spiritually by his teachings.

CHAPTER III

१. समिधाऽग्निं दुवस्यत घृतैर्बोधयतातिथिम् ।
आस्मिन् हव्या जुहोतन ॥

1. Oh learned persons, kindle the fire with the wood sticks, with butter, set ablaze the fire, which is worthy of respect like a Sanyasi. Put oblations in this fire of the yajna!

२. सुसमिद्धाय शोचिषे घृतं तीव्रं जुहोतन ।
अग्नये जातवेदसे ॥

2. Put the oblations of ghee that removes physical infirmities, into this well ablaze, disease-killing fire present in all objects.

३. तं त्वा समिद्भिरङ्गिरो घृतेन वर्धयामसि ।
बृहच्छोचा यविष्ठ्य ॥

3. We fan with sticks of wood and ghee the fire, that is powerful in splitting all things, and burns intensely.

४. उप त्वाऽग्ने हविष्मतीर्घृताचीर्यन्तु हर्यत ।
जुषस्व समिधो मम ॥

4. O beautiful fire, wood sticks soaked with ghee go unto thee along with oblations. May thou accept my fuel put into thee!

५. भूर्भुवः स्वर्द्यौरिव भूम्ना पृथिवीव वरिम्णा ।
तस्यास्ते पृथिवि देवयजनि पृष्ठेऽग्निमन्नादमन्नाद्यायादधे ॥

5. I lay upon the back of the Earth upon which the learned perform yajna, which is like Heaven in plenty, and like Earth in grandeur, for gain of eatable food, this food-eating fire, that pervades the Earth, Ether, and Sky.

---

²Ghee is clarified butter. Agni is called जातवेदस् as it is present in every object created.

³Agni may mean God as well. In that case, the verse will be interpreted thus. O God, we glorify Thee through yoga and spiritual force. O Omnipotent God, Thou art Great and Resplendent. Here समिद्ध: is yoga, and घृत is the spiritual force; यविष्ठय means the powerful God, Who unites and disunites all things in the world.

⁴In this verse also अग्नि may mean God. The verse would then be interpreted thus. O God, may my austerity, knowledge, worship and yoga, which contribute to my learning, splendour and beauty, be accepted by Thee.

⁵भूर्भुवः स्वः mean (1) Earth, Ether, Sky or (2) Brahman, Kshatriya, Vaish or (3) Subjects, offspring, cattle, or (4) Rig, Yaju, Sama, Mahidhara and Ubbat have ascribed these meanings to these vayahritis. May I become plentiful like Heaven. As heaven is full of stars, so I may be endowed with progeny and cattle. May I spread like the earth. As earth gives shelter to many, so I may afford shelter to the distressed.

६. आयं गौः पृश्निरक्रमीदसदन् मातरं पुरः ।
पितरं च प्रयन्त्स्वः ॥

6. This Earth revolves in the space, it revolves with its mother water in its orbit. It moves round its father, the Sun.

७. अन्तश्चरति रोचनास्य प्राणादपानती ।
व्यख्यन् महिषो दिवम् ॥

7. The lustre of this fire, goes up and comes down in the space like exhalation and inhalation in the body. This great fire displays the Sun.

८. त्रिँ॒शद्धाम विराजति वाक् पतङ्गाय धीयते ।
प्रति वस्तोरह द्युभिः ॥

8. God's word rules supreme throughout the world. The Vedas are recited for acquiring the knowledge of God. We should resolutely recite and understand the Vedas everyday with their illuminating sayings.

९. अग्निर्ज्योतिर्ज्योतिरग्निः स्वाहा सूर्यो ज्योतिर्ज्योतिः सूर्यः स्वाहा ।
अग्निर्वर्चो ज्योतिर्वर्चः स्वाहा सूर्यो वर्चो ज्योतिर्वर्चः स्वाहा ॥
ज्योतिः सूर्यः सूर्यो ज्योतिः स्वाहा ॥

9. Just as God gives the light of truthful speech to all human beings, so does physical fire give light that illumines all substances. Just as God inculcates knowledge in the souls of all, that man should speak, as he feels in his heart, so does the Sun bring to light all physical objects. Just as God reveals for humanity all the four Vedas, the storehouse of knowledge, so does fire in the shape of lightning exist in the space, and become the source of rain and knowledge.

Just as God, through the Vedas displays all sciences, fire, and lightning, so does the Sun develop our physical and spiritual forces. Sun illumines all objects. God is self-Resplendent. This is the manifestation of His Glory.

१०. सजूर्देवेन सवित्रा सजू राज्ञेन्द्रवत्या ।
जुषाणो अग्निर्वेतु स्वाहा ।
सजूर्देवेन सवित्रा सजूरुषसेन्द्रवत्या ।
जुषाणः सूर्यो वेतु स्वाहा ॥

⁶Water is the mother of Earth, as Earth is produced by the mixture of the particles of water with its own particles, and remains pregnant with water. Sun is the father of the Earth, as from the Sun, it derives all light and sustenance.

⁷Lightning is the lustre of fire. Just as Pran and Apan go up and down in the body, so does fire rise in the sky and then it comes down.

⁸त्रिंशद्धाम according to Ubbat means the thirty parts मुहूर्त of the day. According to Mahidhar, it means the thirty days of the month. According to Swami Dayananda it means the thirty three devatas, excluding the space (Antriksha), Sun, and Fire. The word 'thirty realms' means all the parts of the world. The number thirty is used indefinitely. पतंग means physical fire and God. वाक् may mean speech and the word of God.

⁹These are Agni Hotra Mantras for morning and evening.

CHAPTER III

10. This enjoyable fire, in accompaniment with the recital of Vedic texts, mixed with God's creation and dark night, with flashes of lightning pervades all objects.

This sun, mixed with God's creation and brilliant dawn, receives the oblations put into the fire, and carries them to places far and wide.

११. उपप्रयन्तो अध्वरं मन्त्रं वोचेमाग्नये ।
आरे अस्मे च शृण्वते ॥

11. Performing sacrifice, may we pronounce vedic texts, in praise of God, Who hears us from far and near.

१२. अग्निर्मूर्धा दिवः ककुत्पतिः पृथिव्या अयम् ।
अपाꣳ रेताꣳसि जिन्वति ॥

12. Men should worship God alone, Who is the Great and Supreme Lord, Who sustains the luminous Sun, and the non-luminous Earth, Who knows the formation of the vitality of waters.

१३. उभा वामिन्द्राग्नी आहुवध्या उभा राधसः सह मादयध्यै ।
उभा दातारविषाꣳ रयीणामुभा वाजस्य सातये हुवे वाम् ॥

13. Oh Electricity and Fire, I invoke Ye both for knowing your attributes, for enjoying the pleasures of riches. Ye both are the givers of desired sovereignty. Ye twain I invoke for consuming excellent food.

१४. अयं ते योनिर्ऋत्वियो यतो जातो अरोचथाः ।
तं जानन्नग्न आरोहाथा नो वर्धया रयिम् ॥

14. Oh God, in Thy creation, sacrificial fire, whose cause of birth is air, burns in different seasons, and develops in all directions. Knowing this, cause our riches increase!

१५. अयमिह प्रथमो धायि धातृभिर्होता यजिष्ठो अध्वरेष्वीड्यः ।
यमप्नवानो भृगवो विरुरुचुर्वनेषु चित्रं विभ्वं विशेविशे ॥

15. In this world the instructors and the learned kindle in serviceable yajnas, for mankind, the ubiquitous fire of extra-ordinary qualities.

[12] अग्नि means physical fire as well. Rishi Dayananda has given both the spiritual and physical interpretations of this mantra. I have chosen the former where Agni means God.

[13] The proper application of fire and electricity in industries and machines, and full knowledge of their attributes lead to the acquisition of wealth, enjoyment, worldly happiness and greatness.

[15] Apnawana (अप्नवान) has been translated by Mahidhar, as a Rishi, belonging to the Bhrigu family. There is no history in the Veda, hence his interpretation is inadmissible. Swami Dayananda translates Apnavana as a learned instructor who teaches his sons, and Bhrigu as a wise person who knows how to perform a yajna.

That fire is recognised by the regulators of sacrifice as worthy of adoration, as the first means of the performance of a yajna, as the receiver of sacrifice and giver of happiness and scientific knowledge.

१६. अस्य प्रत्नामनु द्युतꣳ शुक्रं दुदुहे॑ अह्रय: ।
पय: सहस्रसामृषिम् ॥

16. The learned, knowing the eternity, lustre, thousandfold service, and usefulness of fire, get pure water from it.

१७. तनूपा अग्नेऽसि तन्वं मे पाह्यायुर्दा अग्नेऽस्यायुर्मे देहि वर्चोदा अग्नेऽसि वर्चो मे देहि ।
अग्ने यन्मे तन्वा ऊनं तन्म आपृण ॥

17. Thou, God, art our bodies' Protector. Protect Thou my body.
Giver of longevity art Thou, O God, Give me longevity.
Giver of splendour art Thou, O God, Give me splendour.
Remove, O God, all the defects of my body and soul!

१८. इन्धानास्त्वा शतꣳ हिमा द्युमन्तꣳ समिधीमहि। वयस्वन्तो वयस्कृतꣳ सहस्वत: सहस्कृतम् ।
अग्ने सपत्नदम्भनमदब्धासो अदाभ्यम् ।
चित्रावसो स्वस्ति ते पारमशीय ॥

18. O God, the Lord of manifold riches, may we, being free from pride, enjoying long life, and practising forbearance, live for a hundred years, praising Thee the Effulgent, the Eternal, the Forbearing, the Unconquerable, and the Killer of foes!
Through Thy kindness, being free from woes, may we attain to happiness.

१९. सं त्वमग्ने सूर्यस्य वर्चसागथा: समृषीणाꣳ स्तुतेन ।
सं प्रियेण धाम्ना समहमायुषा सं वर्चसा सं प्रजया सꣳ रायस्पोषेण गमिषीय ॥

19. Oh God, Thou art full of splendour like the Sun, sung by the sages with vedic verses, and O Thou full of power for protection. May I attain to long life, to splendour, to offspring, and abundant riches!

२०. अन्ध स्थान्धो वो भक्षीय मह स्थ महो वो भक्षीयोर्जं स्थोर्जं वो भक्षीय रायस्पोष स्थ रायस्पोषं वो भक्षीय ॥

20. May I enjoy the life-bestowing food through the plants and medicines that contribute to health and vigour. May I utilise the science of air and water for the accomplishment of my deeds. May I get the essence of food from milk, honey and fruits. May I enjoy the abundance of good articles through objects full of manifold qualities.

[16] When Havan is performed in the fire, the result is the raining of pure water on the Earth
[18] Ubbat and Mahidhar translate चित्रावसो as night, in which shine different stars and darkness resides. Maharshi Dayananda translates it as God, in Whom reside the manifold riche of the world, and Who is the source of all wealth.

२१. रेवती रमध्वमस्मिन्योनावस्मिन् गोष्ठेऽस्मिँल्लोकेऽस्मिन् श्रये ।
इहैव स्त मापगात ॥

21. Oh Vedic speech, may thou remain in this altar, in this yajna, in this spot and in this house. Remain here, and go not far from hence!

२२. सँहितासि विश्वरूप्यूर्जा माविश गौपत्येन ।
उप त्वाग्ने दिवेदिवे दोषावस्तर्द्धिया वयम् ।
नमो भरन्त एमसि ॥

22. Oh universal vedic text, thou art full of vigour and valour, may we attain unto thee, the master of the yajna. O God, may we be in communion with Thee, everyday, morning and evening, bowing unto Thee through our intellect!

२३. राजन्तमध्वराणां गोपामृतस्य दीदिविम् ।
वर्द्धमानँ स्वे दमे ॥

23. May we worship God, Who is the Guardian of sacrifices Radiant, the Revealer of the vedas, and attained to complete redemption.

२४. स नः पितेव सूनवेऽग्ने सूपायनो भव ।
सचस्वा नः स्वस्तये ॥

24. Oh God, Thou givest unto us knowledge, as a father to his son. Unite us perpetually with pleasure!

२५. अग्ने त्वं नो अन्तम उत त्राता शिवो भवा वरूथ्यः ।
वसुरग्निर्वसुश्रवा अच्छा नक्षि द्युम्त्तमँ रयिं दाः ॥

25. Oh God, Thou art the Bestower on us of ears to hear goodness, the Shelter of mankind, the Embodiment of lustre of knowledge, and real Omnipresence. Thou pervadest our soul. Thou art our Protector, Our Benefactor, and possessest excellent nature, attributes and deeds. Give us wealth most splendidly renowned!

२६. तं त्वा शोचिष्ठ दीदिवः सुम्नाय नूनमीमहे सखिभ्यः ।
स नो बोधि श्रुधी हवमुरुष्या णो अघायतः समस्मात् ॥

26. O most pure, O radiant God, verily do we pray to Thee for the happiness of our friends. Give us knowledge, listen to our praises and prayers, and keep us far from every evil!

२७. इड एह्यदिति एहि काम्या एत ।
मयि वः कामघरण भूयात् ॥

---

[1]Revati has been translated as wise policy by Swami Dayanandji. According to this interpretation the Mantra may mean 'Oh wise policy, 'Oh Statesmanship, may thou remain in this abode, this fold, this spot and this dwelling. 'Remain just here and go not thence.' वाग्वै रेवती । Satapatha 3-8-1-121.

27. O God, may I get land for ruling over it, may I be endowed with statesmanship. May noble desires reside in me. May I be the centre of the fulfilment of all ambitions!

२८. सोमान्ँ॒ स्वरणं॑ कृणुहि ब्रह्मणस्पते ।
कक्षीवन्तं य औशिजः ॥

28. O God, the Guardian of the primordial vedas, make me, like the son of a learned person, endowed with different capacities for the acquisition of knowledge, an imparter of instruction, and a fulfiller of the aim of education!

२९. यो रेवान्यो अमीवहा वसुवित्पुष्टिवर्द्ध॑नः ।
स नः सिषक्तु यस्तुरः ॥

29. God is rich and the Dispeller of ignorance. He knows the true nature of all things, and grants us physical and spiritual strength. He is prompt. May he goad us to noble deeds.

३०. मा नः शँ॒सो अ॒ररु॒षो धू॒र्तिः प्रण॒ङ् मर्त्य॑स्य ।
रक्षा णो ब्रह्मणस्पते ॥

30. O God, may not our knowledge of the Vedas ever perish. May Thou preserve us from the violence of the uncharitable person!

३१. महि त्रीणामवोऽस्तु द्युक्षं मित्रस्यार्यम्णः ।
दुराधर्षं वरुणस्य ॥

31. O God, may we get the great, wise and unassailable protection of the three forces of nature, the water, the sun and the air!

३२. नहि तेषाममा चन नाधवसु वारणेषु ।
ईशे रिपुरघशँ॒सः ॥

32. Those who worship God are not molested by evil-minded foes neither at home, nor upon pathways and battlefields. I become capable of acquiring God and the sages.

३३. ते हि पुत्रासो अदितेः प्र जीवसे मर्त्याय ।
ज्योतिर्यच्छन्त्यजस्रम् ॥

33. They, the sons of indestructible matter, bestow eternal light upon man for his life and death.

---

[28] Ubbat and Mahidhar tanslate Kakshivant as a Rishi, whose mother was Ushik, and father Dirghatama. This interpretation involving history is not apt, as the vedas are free from historical references, due to their primordiality and eternity. Swami Dayananda translates Ushik as the son of a learned person and Kakshivant as full of different capabilities, modes and methods for the acquisition of knowledge.

[33] Aditi has been interpreted differently. It means (1) Earth (2) Matter (3) Veda (4) Forces of Nature.

३४. कदा चन स्तरीरसि नेन्द्र सश्चसि दाशुषे ।
उपोपेन्नु मघवन् भूय इन्नु ते दानं देवस्य पृच्यते ॥

34. O God, Thou art the Giver of happiness. If Thou dost not bestow knowledge promptly on a charitable person, he again, O Liberal Lord, does not attain to Thy bounty!

३५. तत्सवितुर्वरेण्यं भर्गो देवस्य धीमहि ।
धियो यो नः प्रचोदयात् ॥

35. O Creator of the Universe! O All holy and worthy of adoration! May we meditate on Thy adorable self. May Thou guide our understanding!

३६. परि ते दूड़भो रथोऽस्मान्र अश्नोतु विश्वतः ।
येन रक्षसि दाशुषः ॥

36. Oh God, may Thine immortal knowledge, wherewith Thou guardest the learned in all directions, come close from all sides!

३७. भूर्भुवः स्वः सुप्रजाः प्रजाभिः स्याँ सुवीरै वीरैः सुपोषः पोषैः ।
नर्य प्रजां मे पाहि शँस्य पशून्मे पाह्यर्थ्य पितुं मे पाहि ॥

37. O God, friendly to the wise, do Thou protect my offspring. O worthy of praise do Thou protect my cattle. O God, above all suspicion, protect my food. O God, through Thy grace, in unison with the three life-winds, Pran, Apan and Vyan, may I be rich in offspring, well-manned with men, a hero with the heroes, and strong with wise and invigorating deeds.

३८. आ गन्म विश्ववेदसमस्मभ्यं वसुवित्तमम् ।
अग्ने सम्राडभि द्युम्नमभि सह आ यच्छस्व ॥

अदितिरिति वाड्नाम । निघं० 1–11.
वाग्वा अदिति । श० 6-5-2-5.

So according to Nighantu and Shatapath Aditi means वेदविद्या
'They' refers to Mitra, Aryama and Varuna, i.e., the air, the sun and the water. They are the sons of Matter, as they protect mankind from misery. पुत्र is one who helps his parents in crossing the ocean of worldly miseries. As air, sun, and water help mankind to overcome difficulties and physical infirmities, they are hence named as sons of Nature.

[34]God is the giver of the fruits of our actions. If this be not so, man will never systematically and according to Law, reap the fruits of his actions.

[35]This is the Gayatri Mantra, the Lord's Prayer of the Aryans. This is considered to be the best and most perfect form of prayer, as in it we pray not for one's selfish advancement, but for the betterment of humanity. We pray not for things mundane, which we can acquire through our intellect and understanding, but for the purification of our loftiest and noblest gift, the wise understanding. We don't pray for bread, and physical objects and comforts. Highest form of prayer is offered to God, the highest Authority. This prayer is perfect as it contains all the three elements of prayer, i.e., laudation, स्तुति supplication प्रार्थना and meditation उपासना

38. O, Ocean of Light, the Omniscient, the best knower of all the worlds, and enjoyments may we well approach Thee. May Thou spread for us splendour and strength in all directions!

३८. अयमग्निगृ॑हपतिर्गार्हपत्यः प्रजाया वसुवित्तमः ।
अग्ने गृहपतेऽभि द्युम्नमभि सह आ यच्छस्व ॥

39. Lord of our houses, O God, Thou art the best Finder of riches for our children, Thou art the Protector of our hearths, and the Companion of the householders. Bestow splendour and strength on us!

४०. अयमग्निः पुरीष्यो रयिमान् पुष्टिवर्द्धनः ।
अग्ने पुरीष्याभि द्युम्नमभि सह आ यच्छस्व ॥

40. This fire assists us in the accomplishment of our deeds. It is rich, and furtherer of plenty. O God, the Giver of our comforts, bestow splendour and strength upon us!

४१. गृहा मा बिभीत मा वेपध्वमूर्जं बिभ्रत एमसि ।
ऊर्जं बिभ्रद्भः सुमनाः सुमेधा गृहानैमि मनसा मोदमानः ॥

41. Fear not, nor tremble Ye, O householers. We, bearing strength, come to Ye. May I bearing strength, intelligent and happy, rejoicing in my mind, enjoy all pleasures and approach the householders!

४२. येषामध्येति प्रवसन्येषु सौमनसो बहुः ।
गृहानुपह्वयामहे ते नो जानन्तु जानतः ॥

42. We praise the householders, whom the guest staying far from home remembers and whom he loves much. The loving householders welcome us, the religious guests.

४३. उपहूता इह गाव उपहूता अजावयः ।
अथो अन्नस्य कीलाल उपहूतो गृहेषु नः ।
क्षेमाय वः शान्त्यै प्रपद्ये शिवं शर्मं शंयोः शंयाः ॥

43. May we in this world get cows, goats, sheep and abundant food in our houses. I come to you for safety and quietude. May I acquire mundane and celestial joy and felicity.

४४. प्रघासिनो हवामहे मरुतश्च रिशादसः ।
करम्भेण सजोषसः ॥

---

[40](Pureeshya) पुरीष्य has been translated by Ubbat and Mahidhar, as Master of the cattle. Swami Dayananda translates it as helper in the doing of deeds, and giver of comforts. It means water as well.
vide Nighantu 1-12.
It also means earth; vide Satapatha 12-5-2-5.
[41]We and I refer to the learned persons.
[42]We and you refer to householders, and I to a learned person शंयोः used twice refers to earthly happiness, and happiness after death.

44. We invocate the guests, who are delightful, free from ignorance, removers of sins, eaters of the food well cooked, and full of knowledge.

४५. यद्ग्रामे यदरण्ये यत्सभायां यदिन्द्रिये ।
यदेनश्चक्रमा वयमिदं तदवयजामहे स्वाहा ॥

45. May we forsake each sinful act that we have committed in village or solitude, in an assembly or corporeal sense. Let every man so resolve.

४६. मो षू ण इन्द्रात्र पृत्सु देवैरस्ति हि ष्मा ते शुष्मिन्नवया: ।
महश्चिद्यस्य मीढुषो यव्या हविष्मतो मरुतो वन्दते गी: ॥

46. O God, protect us in battles, in this world, with the help of heroes and destroy us not. O mighty hero, verily, as the vedic voice, replete with noble virtues, offering oblations, displays the qualities of the learned worshippers, so does the worshipper, put oblations into the fire, which contribute to the happiness of mankind.

४७. अक्रन् कर्म कर्मकृत: सह वाचा मयोभुवा । देवेभ्य: कर्म कृत्वास्तं प्रेत सचाभुव: ।

47. They, who with delightful vedic voice, working in cooperation, perform their desired deeds, go to their comfortable house, after the completion of their task for the acquisition of noble virtues.

४८. अवभृथ निचुम्पुण निचेरुरसि निचुम्पुण: ।
अव देवैर्देवकृतमेनोऽयासिषमव मर्त्यैर्मर्त्यकृतं पुरुराग्णो देव रिषस्पाहि ॥

48. O purified through knowledge and righteousness, O patient teacher of grammar, just as I a seeker after knowledge, and a firm gleaner of wisdom, wash out the sin that I have committed through my senses and the mortal body, so do thou O God, preserve me from tortuous sin!

४९. पूर्णा दर्वि परा पत सुपूर्णा पुनरा पत ।
वस्नेव विक्रीणावहा इषमूर्जं शतक्रतो ॥

49. The oblation full of cooked articles put into the fire, goes up to the sky, and returns therefrom full of rain.
O God, Let us twain, like traders, barter our food and strength !

⁴⁴"The householders should always serve the learned, delightful, and pious guests who are Atithis, i.e., whose date of coming is not fixed. Griffith following Mahidhar, puts this mantra in the mouth of the sacrificer's wife, who is first called upon to confess her infidelities, if she has been guilty of any and to declare the name or names of her lover or lovers. After confession or declaration of innocence, she is made to recite the text." This is humbug and sheer nonsense.

⁴⁵Corporeal sense means by abuse of the mind, tongue, eye, ear or any other sensual organ.

⁴⁹When we perform Homa, the oblation put into the fire, being rarefied goes up to the sky, wherefrom, it comes back in the shape of rain. We two, the worshipper who performs the Yajna, and the priest who officiates, barter our food and strength-giving articles, i.e., we put these into the fire, and get, in return, rain, which gives us happiness,

५०. देहि मे ददामि ते नि मे धेहि नि ते दधे ।
निहारं च हरासि मे निहारं नि हराणि ते स्वाहा ॥

50. Give me this article and I will give you that in return. Keep this as my deposit, I keep this as your deposit. Give me the cash price for it. I give you the price demanded. Let people thus transact business truthfully.

५१. प्रक्षन्नमीमदन्त ह्व पिया अधूषत ।
अस्तोषत स्वभानवो विप्रा नविष्ठया मती योजा न्विन्द्र ते हरी ॥

51. Thou chairman, just as comrades, luminous in themselves, pleasing others, advanced in knowledge, with their sharpest intellect, do verily praise God, and being regaled with nutritious diet, overcome miseries, so do thou yoke thy vigour and prowess with them.

५२. सुसंदृशं त्वा वयं मघवन्वन्दिषीमहि ।
प्र नूनं पूर्णबन्धुर स्तुतो यासि वशाँर२ अनु योजा न्विन्द्र ते हरी ॥

52. We revere Thee, O God of Bounty, Who art fair to see. Being praised by us, O best Companion, Thou fulfillest all our desires. O Lord, yoke Thy vigour and prowess for us!

५३. मनो न्वाह्वामहे नाराशँसेन स्तोमेन ।
पितॄणां च मन्मभिः ॥

53. By reflecting on the merits of the learned, and following the high principles of the elders, we strengthen our mind through non-attachment.

५४. आ न एतु मनः पुनः क्रत्वे दक्षाय जीवसे ।
ज्योक् च सूर्यं दृशे ॥

54. May we get in future births again and again the mind, for doing virtuous deeds, for acquiring strength, for longevity, and contemplation of God for long.

५५. पुनर्नः पितरो मनो ददातु दैव्यो जनः ।
जीवं व्रातँ सचेमहि ॥

ripens our harvest of grain and helps the growth of medicinal herbs. This process of giving and taking has been described as a kind of bartering, as does a trader who gives articles, and takes cash in return.

[50] In this verse, it is stated that all borrowing and lending, all sales and purchases, all mortgages and deposits should be carried on in strict compliance with the principle of truth. There should be no fraud and falsehood exercised in business. All dealings should be plain, straightforward and true.

[51] There ought to be full cooperation between the president of a society and its members.

[53] Lives of great-men teach us many lessons. We should learn from and profit by the experiences of great souls, and try to emulate them.

[54-55] Both the verses preach the transmigration of soul.

CHAPTER III

55. O venerable elders, may this man endowed with godly qualities, give us in this and the next life, intellect whereby we may enjoy a long life and perform noble deeds!

५६. वयंꣳ सोम व्रते तव मनस्तनूषु बिभ्रत: ।
प्रजावन्त: सचेमहि ॥

56. O God, acting upon Thy Law, possessing mental self-consciousness in healthy bodies, blest with progeny, let us enjoy happiness!

५७. एष ते रुद्र भाग: सह स्वस्राम्बिकया तं जुषस्व स्वाहैष ते रुद्र भाग आखुस्ते पशु: ॥

57. O learned person, the chastiser of the sinful and the unrighteous, all these eatable things are for thee. Accept them with thy knowledge and vedic lore. O learned man, follow the Veda and the law of Dharma. O learned person, accept the food worth eating which uproots all diseases!

५८. अव रुद्रमदीमह्यव देवं त्र्यम्बकम् ।
यथा नो वस्यसस्करद्यथा न: श्रेयसस्करद्यथा नो व्यवसाययात् ॥

58. May we ward off all calamities by worshipping God, Who is unchangeable in the past, present and future, chastises the sinners, and is highly benevolent. Just as God makes us better housed, more prosperous, and determined so may we adore Him.

५९. भेषजमसि भेषजं गवेऽश्वाय पुरुषाय भेषजम् ।
सुखं मेषाय मेष्यै ॥

59. O God, Thou art the healer of the physical, mental and spiritual maladies. Heal, Thou the sufferings of cow, horse and all mankind. Grant happiness to ram and ewe.

६०. त्र्यम्बकं यजामहे सुगन्धि पुष्टिवर्धनम् ।
उर्वारुकमिव बन्धनान्मृत्योर्मुक्षीय मामृतात् ।
त्र्यम्बकं यजामहे सुगन्धि पतिवेदनम् ।
उर्वारुकमिव बन्धनादितो मुक्षीय मामुत: ॥

[57]Ambika has been translated by Ubbat and Mahidhar as the sister of god Rudra. Swami Dayananda translates it as vedic text. आखु has been interpreted by Ubbat and Mahidhar as a mouse, on whose hole, a pudding is to be put. Maharshi Dayananda translates it as a remover of diseases.

[58]Triyambaka has been translated differently by various commentators, e.g., free from the threefold sufferings, i.e. physical, elemental and spiritual, and beyond the reach of time, i.e., Past, Present and Future, or ruling over the three worlds.
Triyambaka is interpreted by Griffith as a name of Rudra as having three wives, sisters or mothers, or Triocular, the Three Eyed God. Rishi Dayananda's interpretation is more rational and significant. He interprets the word as God Who remains unchanged in the Past, Present and Future.

[59]The enumeration of a few animals like cow, horse, ram and ewe, is symbolic of the animal kingdom. Prayer is offered for the happiness of mankind and animal world.

60. We worship the Omnipresent, Pure God, Who augments our physical, spiritual and social forces. Through His Grace may we be released from this mortal coil without the agony of death, as naturally as a ripe cucumber is from its stem. Let us not be bereft of immortality. We worship the Omnipresent, Pure God, Who grants us wisdom. Through His Grace, may we be released easily from this world, as a ripe cucumber is from its stem, but not from immortality.

६१. एतत्ते रुद्रावसं तेन परो मूजवतोऽतीहि ।
अवततधन्वा पिनाकावस: कृत्तिवासा अहिꣳ सन्न: शिवोऽतीहि ॥

61. O hero, the chastiser of enemies, and expert in the art of war, with bow extended, with self-protecting trident, with full armour, with grace and power, meet thy foes on the other side of the mountain. With thy this power of protection, come to us, without causing us any harm.

६२. ꣳयायुषं जमदग्ने: कश्यपस्य ꣳयायुषम् ।
यद्देवेषु ꣳयायुषं तन्नो अस्तु ꣳयायुषम् ॥

62. May we be endowed with triple life, as a truth-seer sage, or the custodian of knowledge through the grace of God, is endowed with, or as the learned persons enjoy triple life.

६३. शिवो नामासि स्वधितिस्ते पिता नमस्ते अस्तु मा मा हिꣳसी: ।
नि वर्तयाम्यायुषेऽन्नाद्याय प्रजननाय रायस्पोषाय सुप्रजास्त्वाय सुवीर्याय ॥

63. O God, Thou art certainly the Embodiment of grace, self-Existent, our Father, obeisance be to Thee. Harm me not. I approach Thee for long life, for nice food, for progeny, for riches in abundance, for noble children, and for heroic vigour.

---

[60] Just as a cucumber, when ripe, falls, full of sweetness, of its own accord, to the ground, so should we die when we have spent our full age of at least one hundred years. Our death should be easy, and natural, free from the protracted, and excruciating agonies of death, to which several persons are subjected. We should in no case be deprived of our immortal life through salvation, which is the aim of this worldly life.

[62] ꣳयायुषम् means three times the ordinary span of life, i.e., three times a hundred years. May we live for 300 years or more, like the sages of yore. ꣳयायुषम् may also mean the three stages of life, boyhood, youth and old age, or Brahmacharya, Grihastha and Vanaprastha Ashramas.

CHAPTER IV

१. एदमगन्म देवयजनंपृथिव्या यत्र देवासो अजुषन्त विश्वे ।
ऋक्सामाभ्याꣽ सन्तरन्तो यजुर्भी रायस्पोषेण समिषा मदेम ।
इमा आप: शमु मे सन्तु देवी: । ओषधे त्रायस्व स्वधिते मैनꣽ हिꣽसी: ॥

1. May we, on this earth, where reside happily all the learned persons, be able to revere the sages.
May we acting on the teachings of the Rig, Sam and Yajur Vedas, end all our miseries. May we rejoice in food and growth of riches. These pure, disease-killing waters be gracious to me. May the herbs protect me. Thou armed king, harm not the worshipper.

२. आपो अस्मान्मातर: शुन्धयन्तु घृतेन नो घृतप्व: पुनन्तु ।
विश्वꣽ हि रिप्रं प्रवहन्ति देवी: । उदिदाभ्य: शुचिरा पूत एमि ।
दीक्षातपसोस्तनूरसि तां त्वा शिवाꣽशग्मां परि दधे भद्रं वर्ण पुष्यन् ॥

2. May waters, like mother, purify our bodies. May the waters purified by clarified butter, purify us through rain. Pure waters remove all our physical imperfections.
May I advance in life, being bright and pure through waters. Through celibacy and abstemiousness may I possess a body, healthy, comfortable, excellent, beautiful and strong.

३. महीनां पयोऽसि वर्चोदा असि वर्चो मे देहि ।
वृत्रस्यासि कनीनकश्चक्षुर्दा असि चक्षुर्मे देहि ॥

3. O Sun, thou bringest rain on different parts of the earth. Giver of splendour art thou; bestow on me the gift of splendour. The disperser of cloud art thou with thy brilliance. The giver of eye art thou. Give me the gift of vision!

४. चित्पतिर्मा पुनातु वाक्पतिर्मा पुनातु देवो मा सविता पुनात्वच्छिद्रेण पवित्रेण सूर्यस्य रश्मिभि: ।
तस्य ते पवित्रपते पवित्रपूतस्य यत्काम: पुने तच्छकेयम् ॥

4. Purify me, the Lord of Purity. Purify me, the Lord of knowledge. Purify me, the Lord of the Vedas.

---

[1] Ghee when used in Havan, purifies the rain, and water, which in turn purifies our bodies, and removes our physical infirmities and defects.
[2] Sun gives light to the eyes, so he is addressed as giver of eyes.

O Lord, Creator of the universe, purify me, through sun-beams and thy immortal purifying knowledge.

O Master of the purified souls, may I full of lofty sentiments accomplish the desire actuated by which, through your grace, I purify myself!

५. आ वो देवास ईमहे वामं प्रयत्यध्वरे ।
आ वो देवास आशिषो यज्ञियासो हवामहे ॥

5. O sages, we admire your praiseworthy qualities, during the performance of this happy sacrifice. O sages, we beg of you the fulfilment of our desires pertaining to the sacrifice!

६. स्वाहा यज्ञं मनसः स्वाहोरोरन्तरिक्षात् स्वाहा । द्यावापृथिवीभ्याᳪ स्वाहा वातादारभे स्वाहा ॥

6. O men, just as I actively and wisely commence performing the sacrifice, with vedic texts, with cultured tongue, with wisdom-teaching voice, with a tongue full of sweetness and truth, in an orderly and well-directed way, with the help of the extended firmament, Earth, sky and air, so do Ye!

७. आकूत्यै प्रयुजेऽग्नये स्वाहा मेधायै मनसेऽग्नये स्वाहा दीक्षायै तपसेऽग्नये स्वाहा सरस्वत्यै पूष्णेऽग्नये स्वाहा ।
आपो देवीर्बृहतीर्विश्वशम्भुवो द्यावापृथिवी उरो अन्तरिक्ष । बृहस्पतये हविषा विधेम स्वाहा ॥

7. We perform the yajna for resolution, for good religious acts, for kindling fire, for the propagation of the Vedas, for the development of wisdom, for the enhancement of knowledge, for utilizing lightning, for philanthropy, for following the laws of Dharma, for austerity, for digestive faculty, for learning and teaching, for eloquent and weighty speech, for worshipping rightly God, for purifying gastric juice, and for practising Truth.

Ye, meritorious, all-beneficial divine waters, Ye Heaven and Earth and spacious air between them, we serve with Oblation!

८. विश्वो देवस्य नेतुर्मर्तो वुरीत सख्यम् ।
विश्वो राय इषुध्यति द्युम्नं वृणीत पुष्यसे स्वाहा ॥

8. May every mortal man seek the friendship of the Guiding God. May we all have recourse to the use of arms for the acquisition of due wealth. May every man acquire riches and become strong through wise deeds.

९. ऋक्सामयोः शिल्पे स्थस्ते वामारभे ते मा पातमास्य यज्ञस्योदृचः ।
शर्मासि शर्म मे यच्छ नमस्ते अस्तु मा मा हिᳪसीः ॥

---

*A sage or a learned person says this to ordinary house-holders and men of the world.

9. After the study of the Rig and Yajur Vedas, I commence using their scientific aspects, *i.e.*, theoretical and practical. They protect me in this yajna, in which vedic texts are recited. O yajna, thou art happiness, give me happiness; here are these oblations of corn for thee; forbear to harm me!

१०. उर्गस्याङ्गिरस्यूर्णम्रदा ऊर्जं मयि धेहि ।
सोमस्य नीविरसि विष्णो: शर्मासि शर्म यजमानस्येन्द्रस्य योनिरसि सुसस्या: कृषीस्कृधि ।
उच्छ्रयस्व वनस्पत ऊर्ध्वो मा पाह्ँहस आस्य यज्ञस्योदृच: ॥

10. O learned person, may mechanical science, perfected by the application of fire, the giver of light, bestow strength on me. It is the guardian of manifold objects, giver of happiness to the learned, the mechanic, and the source of prosperity, make the crops produce abundant grain through its aid. O learned person, depend on thyself for advancement. Protect me from the misery of sin. Accomplish this yajna with the recitation of vedic texts!

११. व्रतं कृणुताग्निब्रह्माग्निर्यज्ञो वनस्पतिर्यज्ञिय: ।
देवी धिय मनामहे सुमृडीकामभिष्टये वर्चोधां यज्ञवाहस्ँ सुतीर्थां नो असद्दशे । ये देवा मनोजाता मनोयुजो दक्षक्रतवस्ते नोऽवन्तु ते न: पान्तु तेभ्य: स्वाहा ।

11. Take a vow. God is Agni. Yajna is Agni. God, the Guardian of our soul, is fit for worship. For the attainment of an ideal, I long for divine, pleasant, radiant intelligence that unites me with God. May that intelligence, that makes me happily cross the ocean of this mundane existence, be within my control.

May the philosophic, meditative and energetic sages urge us on to noble deeds, may they be our protectors. We invoke them from the inmost recesses of our heart.

१२. श्वात्रा: पीता भवत यूयमापो अस्माकमन्तरुदरे सुशेवा: ।
ता अस्मभ्यमयक्ष्मा अनमीवा अनागस: स्वदन्तु देवीरमृता ऋतावृध: ॥

12. O men, the waters that we have drunk, staying within our belly, give us peace, riches, freedom from consumption, disease, and pangs of hunger and thirst. They are the strengtheners of our true knowledge, full of divine qualities, and undying flavours. May they be pleasant to your taste!

१३. इयं ते यज्ञिया तनूरपो मुञ्चामि न प्रजाम् ।
अर्ँहोमुच: स्वाहाकृता: पृथिवीमा विशत पृथिव्या सम्भव ॥

---

⁹The two aspects of the vedas may be Karma and Jnan Kand, the practical and theoretical sides.

* God may also be addressed as yajna, then नम will mean obeisance; and शर्म will mean shelter. God affords shelter to all.

¹¹श्वात्रा: may be translated as givers of peace, vide Shatapath 3-9-4-16. Swami Dayananda has translated it as givers of knowledge and wealth.

13. O learned man, just as this sacrificial body of thine, protects the vital breaths and the people, and thou forsakest it not, so do I not forsake it without enjoying the full span of life. Just as disease-curing and pure waters flow on the earth, so shouldst thou live in the world wisely; and so do I!

१४. अग्ने त्वꣳसु जागृहि वयꣳसु मन्दिषीमहि ।
रक्षा णो अप्रयुच्छन् प्रबुधे न: पुनस्कृधि ॥

14. The fire, which keeps us active in our wakeful state, makes us take joy in most refreshing sleep. It protects us free from idleness and casts away the idlers. We should use this fire properly which deals with us again and again.

१५. पुनर्मन: पुनरायुर्म आगन् पुन: प्राण: पुनरात्मा म आगन् पुनश्चक्षु: पुन: श्रोत्रं म आगन् ।
वैश्वानरो अदब्धस्तनूपा अग्निर्न: पातु दूरितादवद्यात् ॥

15. I get back after rebirth mind, life, breath, soul, eyes and ears.
May God the Leader of all, Non-violent, Omniscient, Guardian of our souls, save us from misfortune and sin.

१६. त्वमग्ने व्रतपा असि देव आ मर्त्येष्वा ।
त्वं यज्ञेष्वीड्यः रास्वेयत्सोमा भूयो भर देवो न: सविता वसोर्दाता वस्वदात् ॥

16. O God, Thou art the Guardian of sacred vows among mankind. Thou art meet for praise at holy rites. O Giver of Splendour, Come unto us, grant us wealth, give us more. God, the Creator, the Giver of wealth, gives us riches!

१७. एषा ते शुक्र तनूरेतद्वर्चस्तया सम्भव भ्राजं गच्छ ।
जूरसि धृता मनसा जुष्टा विष्णवे ॥

17. O learned person, this body thou hast got and reared is for the meditation of God and sacrifice. Through this body, being vigorous, gain splendour and lustre. Be active through knowledge!

---

[14] Agni may mean God as well. The mantra will then be interpreted thus. O God, Thou art ever wakeful, but we are sleeping in ignorance. Protect us unceasingly, Awake us again and again for the acquisition of true knowledge. Agni may mean Pran i.e., vital breaths. Pran also is wakeful while all other senses go to sleep. These vital breaths protect us, and restore us consciousness after sleep.

[15] Man regets after rebirth and the creation of the universe; his physical and mental faculties. This mantra clearly demonstrates the doctrine of the Transmigration of soul, and the creation of the universe after each cycle, Kalpa.

[16] Agni can be interpreted as fire as well. The second interpretation with Agni meaning fire has been given by Swami Dayananda in his commentary. The mantra is clear, with Agni substituted for fire in place of God.

CHAPTER IV

१८. तस्यास्ते सत्यसवसः प्रसवे तन्वो यन्त्रमशीय स्वाहा ।
शुक्रमसि चन्द्रमस्यमृतमसि वैश्वदेवमसि ॥

18. O resplendent God, in this world created by Thee, may I obtain mastery over the vast power of speech. O Speech, thou art pure, pleasant and dear to the sages!

१९. चिदसि मनासि धीरसि दक्षिणासि क्षत्रियासि यज्ञियास्यदितिरस्युभयतःशीर्ष्णी ।
सा नः सुप्राची सुप्रतीच्येधि मित्रस्त्वा पदि बध्नीतां पूषाऽध्वनस्पात्विन्द्रायाध्यक्षाय ॥

19. O Speech, thou art thought, mind, intelligence, giver of knowledge and victory; thou art power, worthy of worship, immortal, and double-headed. May thou give us comfort in the past and future. May breath, the strength giving friend of time advance thee in knowledge, and guard thy pathways for God, Whose eye is over all!

२०. अनु त्वा माता मन्यतामनु पिताऽनु भ्राता सगर्भ्योऽनु सखा सयूथ्यः ।
सा देवि देवमच्छेहीन्द्राय सोम ॐ रुद्रस्त्वा वर्तयतु स्वस्ति सोमसखा पुनरेहि ॥

20. O man, may thy mother, thy father, thy own brother, and thy friend of the same society grant thee leave to tread on the path ordained by God. O speech, for the acquisition of splendour, may thou unite with God, the Prompter of all. May the Celibate student choose thee.

May thou, O man, happily acquire again and again this speech, the friend of the learned!

२१. वस्व्यस्यदितिरस्यादित्यासि रुद्रासि चन्द्रासि ।
बृहस्पतिष्ट्वा सुम्ने रमतु रुद्रो वसुभिरा चके ॥

21. O speech, thou art all-pervading, eternal, lustrous, sublime and pleasant. The learned person uses thee for happiness. The sage, the chastiser of the wicked longs for thee along with other educated persons!

२२. अदित्यास्त्वा मूर्धन्नाजिघर्मि देवयजने पृथिव्या इडायास्पदमसि घृतवत् स्वाहा ।
अस्मे रमस्वास्मे ते बन्धुस्त्वे रायो मे रायो मा वय ॐ रायस्पोषेण विगौषम ततो रायः ।

---

[18]Swaha means both speech and lightning.

[19]Speech has been spoken of as double-headed, as its one part gives us the knowledge of external objects, and the other part of internal ones; or speech makes us cognisant of internal pain and pleasure and external occurences; or the external organs like eyes etc. represent its one face, and the internal organ, the mind, the other.

सुप्राची and सुप्रतीची may also mean that speech helps us in mastering the external problems that come before us, and solving the subtle questionings of the soul.

Mitra may also mean the soul, which binds the speech to God, (पदि) as it is through the persuasion of our soul, that we sing the glory and praises of God. अध्वनः means the path of knowledge and yoga which leads us to God. There is another interpretation as well of this mantra, with lightning विद्युत् instead of speech वाणी as its devata.

22. O speech, I use thee in the heights of sky and the sacrificial places on the Earth. Thou art the preserver of vedic verses. May thou be enriched with high knowledge. May thou rest in us. May thou be united to us. Thou art rich. May I be full of riches. Let us not be deprived of abundant riches. May splendour reside in thee full of understanding!

२३. समर्च्ये देव्या धिया सं दक्षिणयोरुचक्षसा ।
मा म आयु: प्रमोषीर्मो अहं तव वीरं विदेय तव देवि संदृशि ॥

23. O speech, I praise thee with divine, ignorance-removing and penetrating intelligence. End not my life. I will not through ignorance spoil thee. O vedic text, in thy protection, may I be blessed with heroism!

२४. एष ते गायत्रो भाग इति मे सोमाय ब्रूतादेष ते त्रैष्टुभो भाग इति मे सोमाय ब्रूतादेष ते जागतो भाग इति मे सोमाय ब्रूताच्छन्दोनामान‍ँ साम्राज्यं गच्छेति मे सोमाय ब्रूतात् ।
ब्रूतादास्माकोऽसि शुक्रस्ते ग्रह्यो विचितस्त्वा वि चिन्वन्तु ॥

24. O learned person "This is thy share of the sacrifice allied with Gayatri verses" so may he say unto me a student of science. This is thy share of the sacrifice allied with Trishtup verses, so may he say unto me, the seeker of the essence of things. "This is thy share of the sacrifice allied with verses in Jagati metre,' so may he say unto me a student of science. 'May thou attain to sovereignty detailed in vedic verses in all other metres.' May he thus preach the art of kingship unto me, full of affluence. O learned persons, just as ye are our purifying preachers, so am I your worthy disciple, endowed with virtues and wealth. May ye develop me and this sacrifice (yajna) as well!

२५. अभि त्यं देव‍ँ सवितारमोण्यो: कविक्रतुमर्चामि सत्यसव‍ँ रत्नधामभि प्रियं मति कविम् ।
ऊर्ध्वा यस्यामतिर्भा अदिद्युतत्सवीमनि हिरण्यपाणिरमिमीत । सुक्रतु: कृपा स्व:
प्रजाभ्यस्त्वा प्रजास्त्वा ऽनुप्राणन्तु प्रजास्त्वमनुप्राणिहि ॥

[22]The sacrificial places mean the places where the wise and the learned perform yajnas on this earth by the recitation of vedic verses.
Speech is the protector and preserver of the vedic verses, as by their recitation and memorisation they are preserved.
[23]A king prays for strength.
[24]A learned person asks another learned person 'What is the share of the sacrifice allied with vedic verses in Gayatri, Trishtup and Jagati metres. His answer is embodied in this mantra 'He' refers to the learned person. Vedic verses in different metres like Gayatri, Trishtup, Jagati and Ushnik etc. are recited during the performance of a yajna.
Pt. Jai Dev Vidyalankar of Ajmere, has in his commentary translated Gayatri as alluding to the Brahmanas, Trishtupa to the Kshatriyas and Jagati to the Vaishas.

25. I adore God, the Creator of the Earth and Sky, the Source of all Knowledge, the Embodiment of Splendour, the Sustainer of all the beautiful planets, the Centre of love, object of praise by the Vedas, and their Revealer. His lofty effulgent Self is divulged in the created world. He has fixed the bright sun and the moon in their conduct. He is the wisest Actor. His mercy grants us happiness. O God I worship Thee as Bestower of happiness on mankind. May all mortals enjoy life, through Thee. May Thou grant life to all human beings!

२६. शुक्रं त्वा शुक्रेण क्रीणामि चन्द्रं चन्द्रेणामृतममृतेन ।
सग्मे ते गोरस्मे ते चन्द्राणि तपस्तनूरसि प्रजापतेर्वर्ण: परमेण पशुना क्रीयसे सहस्रपोषं पुषेयम् ॥

26. In the yajna, we should please the learned performer by offering him cash and kind. May the praiseworthy brilliance of the sun make me strong through its thousandfold abundance. O wise person, may we also obtain the riches, which thou hast secured through thy rule over the earth. Just as I accomplish the sacrifice through noble, pure sentiments, earn gold with gold, attain to salvation through immortal knowledge, so may thou!

२७. मित्रो न एहि सुमित्रध इन्द्रस्योह्मा विश दक्षिणमुशन्नुशन्त्ँ स्योन: स्योनम् ।
स्वान भ्राजाङ्घारे बम्भारे हस्त सुहस्त कृशानवेते व: सोमक्रयणास्तानक्षध्वं मावा दभन् ॥

27. O king, famous for eloquence, brilliance, enmity to fraud, antagonism to the thoughtless, pleasing manners, dexterity, defeating the designs of the ill-minded, friendship, and the art of befriending others, with longing for delight, come unto us!
May thou, with a beautiful and healthy body, and endowed with all cherished objects, enjoy, enviable happiness. These intelligent and faithful subjects and servants, who all-round protect you, should be protected by you to ward off your enemy from doing injury unto you.

२८. परि माऽग्ने दुश्चरिताद्बाधस्वा मा सुचरिते भज ।
उदायुषा स्वायुषोदस्थाममृताँ२ अनु ॥

28. Oh God, dissuade me from sin, and establish me firmly in righteousness. May I enjoy the pleasures of final beatitude by leading a long and virtuous life!

२९. प्रति पन्थामपद्महि स्वस्तिगामनेहसम् ।
येन विश्वा: परि द्विषो वृणक्ति विन्दते वसु ॥

29. May we tread the path free from sin, and full of delight, by which a wise man overcomes all carnal pleasures, and gathers wealth.

३०. अदितिरस्तवगस्यदित्यै सद आसीद् ।
अस्तभ्नाद्द्यां वृषभो अन्तरिक्षममिमीत वरिमाणं पृथिव्या: ।
आसीदद्विश्वा भुवनानि सम्राडिश्वेतानि वरुणस्य व्रतानि ॥

30. O God, Thou art the protector of the Earth. O Mighty Lord, Thou fixest the Earth in its Orbit. Thou Controllest the Sun. Thou hast created the beautiful sky. O Lord of all, thou fixest in space all the worlds. All these are the works of Him alone, so do we know!

३१. वनेषु व्यन्तरिक्षं ततान वाजमर्वत्सु पय उस्त्रियासु ।
हृत्सु क्रतुं वरुणो विश्वग्निं दिवि सूर्यमदधात् सोममद्रौ ॥

31. We should worship God, Who hast created the sky over the forests, put speed in horses, milk in cows, intellect in hearts, gastric juice in men, sun in heaven, and medicinal plants like Soma in the mountains!

३२. सूर्यस्य चक्षुरारोहान्नेरक्षण: कनीनकम् ।
यत्रैतशेभिरीयसे आजमानो विपश्चिता ॥

32. O God, where resplendent through Thy qualities of knowledge, Thou art known by the learned, and where Thou createst lustrous eyes, the intruments for seeing the sun and fire, there we worship Thee!

३३. उस्रावेतं धूर्षाहौ युज्येथामनश्रू अवीरहणौ ब्रह्मचोदनौ ।
स्वस्ति यजमानस्य गृहान् गच्छतम् ॥

33. Let man and woman, who study the vedas kill not their heroes, are limited in resources, be ever joyous, who live together and are fit to bear the burden of domestic life, be united together in married life. May such couples visit the houses of religious persons and give them happiness.

३४. भद्रो मेअसि प्रच्यवस्य भुवस्पते विश्वान्यभि धामानि ।
मा त्वा परिपरिणो विदन् मा त्वा परिपन्थिनो विदन् मा त्वा वृका अघायवो विदन् ।
श्येनो भूत्वा परा पत यजमानस्य गृहान् गच्छ तन्नौ सँस्कृतम् ॥

---

[30] The Mantra can similarly be interpreted for sun and air instead of God. Maharshi Dayananda has given two interpretations to this verse, one for God, and the other for the sun and air.

[31] The creation of the sky over mountains means the pouring of rain over them for their growth.

[32] God is universal and ubiquitous so He should be worshipped everywhere. He has created everywhere the sun, fire, and eyes, and so He is adorable by us at all places.

[33] Mahidhar and Ubbat have referred this mantra to a pair of oxen. Maharshi Dayananda uses अनश्रू in place of अनश्रू the usual text as observed in all editions. अनश्रू has been translated by Rishi Dayananda अव्यापिन i.e., limited. Mahidhar translates अनश्रू as those who weep not.

CHAPTER IV

34. O learned man, the Lord of Earth, thou art my gracious helper. Fly happily to all the stations in our well overhauled aeroplane. Doing so, let not thieves, robbers, and malignant opponents meet thee. Fall like a falcon upon such foes. Go to the houses of religious persons, situated in distant parts of the world.

३५. नमो मित्रस्य वरुणस्य चक्षसे महो देवाय तदृतꣳ सपर्यत ।
दूरेदृशे देवजाताय केतवे दिवस्पुत्राय सूर्याय शꣳसत ॥

35. Do homage unto God, the Friend of all, Ever Pure, and Resplendent. Worship the true nature of the Mighty God. Sing praises unto God, the Purifier of all radiant objects, the Omniscient, the Embodiment of virtues, and the Exhibitor of distant objects.

३६. वरुणस्योत्तम्भनमसि वरुणस्य स्कम्भसर्जनी स्थो वरुणस्य ऋतसदन्यसि । वरुणस्य ऋतसदनमसि वरुणस्य ऋतसदनमा सीद ॥

36. O God, Thou art the Director of this fine world; the Creator of objects dependable on air, and the Force inherent in the sun for the motion of waters, the stay and support of all excellent objects. O Lord, Thou makest us reach the destination of true and high knowledge!

३७. या ते धामानि हविषा यजन्ति ता ते विश्वा परिभूरस्तु यज्ञम् ।
गयस्फान: प्रतरण: सुवीरोऽवीरहा प्र चरा सोम दुर्यान् ॥

37. O God, just as learned persons, utilize Thy created objects by Oblations, so should we utilize all of them. Thy Yajna is the advancer of our progeny, wealth and houses, dispeller of diseases, bestower of heroes, remover of the idlers and cowards from amongst us, and giver of happiness in manifold ways, may that conduce to our benefit. O learned persons, may ye perform this yajna, and live happily in your houses!

---

[34]In this verse, we are instructed to construct aeroplanes, and visit thereby the distant places of the world, add to our wealth by commerce, keep our foes away, and lead a happy and comfortable life.

CHAPTER V

१. अग्नेस्तनूरसि विष्णवे त्वा सोमस्य तनूरसि विष्णवे त्वा ऽतिथेरातिथ्यमसि विष्णवे त्वा श्येनाय त्वा सोमभृते विष्णवे त्वाऽग्ने त्वा रायस्पोषदे विष्णवे त्वा ॥

1. Oh oblation, thou art the body of fire, I accept thee for the completion of sacrifice. Thou art the material of all the created objects in the universe, I use thee for the purification of air. Thou art the source of reception of the unexpected guest. I accept thee for the acquisition of knowledge. Thou art fast in speed like the falcon, I put thee into the fire, I accept thee, the source of happiness for the learned and active worshipper. I accept thee as giver of wealth, knowledge, action and all noble qualities.

२. अग्नेर्जनित्रमसि वृषणौ स्थ उर्वश्यस्यायुरसि पुरूरवा असि । गायत्रेण त्वा छन्दसा मन्थामि त्रैष्टुभेन त्वा छन्दसा मन्थामि जागतेन त्वा छन्दसा मन्थामि ॥

2. O Yajna, thou art the creator of fire. Ye (sun and air) are the cause of rain. Thou art the source of manifold comforts, the giver of life, and the instrument for preaching the shastras!
O fire I kindle thee with the verses in Gayatri metre, with the verses in Trishtup metre, and with the verses in Jagati metre!

३. भवतं नः समनसौ सचेतसावरेपसौ । मा यज्ञ ँ हिँसिष्टं मा यज्ञपतिं जातवेदसौ शिवौ भवतमद्य नः ॥

3. O teacher and disciple, be ye for us of the same one thought, free from sin, and conversant with the knowledge of the vedas. Harm not the sacrifice, harm not the sacrifice's lord, the worshipper. Be kind to us this day!

४. अग्नावग्निश्चरति प्रविष्टऋषीणां पुत्रो अभिशस्तिपावा ।
स नः स्योनः सुयजा यजेह देवेभ्यो हव्य ँ सदमप्रयुच्छन्त्स्वाहा ॥

4. The learned disciple of the experts in vedic lore, the protector against violence, the master of the science of electricity, the giver of pleasure, the expositor of the different branches of knowledge, and the enemy of indolence, enjoys life happily. He, endowed with noble qualities, grants us in this world knowledge and provisions for performing Havan. Let us go to such a man.

---

[1]The performance of Havan, by means of हवि: 'oblation'of clarified butter and सामग्री 'provisions' contributes to our wisdom, knowledge, activity and good qualities.
[2]verses in Gayatri Trishtup and Jagati metres are recited when fire is ignited in a yajna.

५. आपतये त्वा परिपतये गृह्णामि तनूनप्त्रे शाक्वराय शक्वन ओजिष्ठाय । अनाधृष्टमस्यनाधृष्यं देवानामोजोऽनभिशस्त्यभिशस्तिपा अनभिशस्तेन्यमञ्जसा सत्यमुपगेषꣳ स्विते मा धाः ॥

5. O God, Thou art my Protector against violence. I take Thee as my Sovereign Lord, as the Guardian in all directions, as the Giver of sound body, as the Embodiment of strength, and the Securer of valiant soldiers!

Through God's grace, may I easily attain to truth and invincible, irresistible, inviolate and invulnerable strength of the learned. Set me O God on the path of virtue.

६. अग्ने व्रतपास्त्वे व्रतपा या तव तनूरियꣳ सा मयि यो मम तनूरेषा सा त्वयि । सह नौ व्रतपते व्रतान्यनु मे दीक्षां दीक्षापतिर्मन्यतामनु तपस्तपस्पतिः ॥

6. O God, Thou art the Guardian of religious vows, may I be competent to fulfil my vows under Thy guidance. May Thy vast power rule over me, and may my power remain under Thee. O Protector of the vedas, may our pledge of continence be fulfilled in toto. May the Lord of Consecration, persuade me for initiation. May the Lord of penance induce me to take a vow of austerity.

७. अꣳशुꣳ शुष्टे देव सोमाप्यायतामिन्द्रायैकधनविदे ।
आ तुभ्यमिन्द्रः प्यायतामा त्वमिन्द्राय प्यायस्व ।
आप्याययास्मान्त्सखीन्त्सन्या मेधया स्वस्ति ते देव सोम सुत्यामशीय ।
एष्टा रायः प्रेषे भगाय ऋतमृतवादिभ्यो नमो द्यावापृथिवीभ्याम् ॥

7. O resplendent God, may Thy each pervading force advance the glorious soul, that longs for the sole wealth of knowledge. May the soul glorify Thee, may Thou advance the soul. May Thou, Friend to all, advance us by means of God-reaching intelligence. O Mighty God, May I attain with pleasure to Thy beatitude!

May we obtain the longed-for wealth for food and success. Let us receive truth from whose speech is truthful. Let us receive food from Heaven and Earth.

८. या ते अग्नेऽयःशया तनूर्वर्षिष्ठा गह्वरेष्ठा ।
उग्रं वचो अपावधीत्त्वेषं वचो अपावधीत्स्वाहा ।
या ते अग्ने रजःशया तनूर्वर्षिष्ठा गह्वरेष्ठा ।
उग्रं वचो अपावधीत्त्वेषं वचो अपावधीत्स्वाहा ।
या ते अग्ने हरिशया तनूर्वर्षिष्ठा गह्वरेष्ठा ।
उग्रं वचो अपावधीत्त्वेषं वचो अपावधीत्स्वाहा ॥

---

[5]This mantra has been interpreted by Swami Dayananda Saraswati for lightning as well.

[6]नौ (Our) refers to the vows of celibacy and continence taken by the teacher and the disciple. दीक्षा means initiation into a sacred vow.

8. O fire, thy force which is present in metals like gold, in all the spheres like the sun and in lightning: is vast and deep. It creates an awful and formidable sound; and is powerful to emit invigorating utterances. That force is present in every object!

९. तप्तायनी मेऽसि वित्तायनी मेऽस्यवतान्मा नाथितादवतान्मा व्यथितात् । विदेदग्निर्नभोनामा ग्ने्ऽङ्गिर आयुना नाम्नेहि योऽस्यां पृथिव्यामसि यत्तेऽज्ञाधृष्टं नाम यज्ञियं तेन त्वा दधे विदेदग्निर्नभो नामाऽग्ने अङ्गिर आयुना नाम्नेहि यो द्वितीयस्यां पृथि- व्यामसि यत्तेऽज्ञाधृष्टं नाम यज्ञियं तेन त्वा दधे विदेदग्निर्नभो नामा अग्ने अङ्गिर आयुना नाम्नेहि यस्तृतीयस्यां पृथिव्यामसि यत्तेऽज्ञाधृष्टं नाम यज्ञि यं तेन त्वा दधे । अनु त्वा देववीतये ॥

9. O fire, for me thou art the home of all fixed objects. For me thou art the gathering place of wealth. Protect me from dictatorship. Protect me from fear!

May physical fire attain to water in the space. May fire with the names of Angira and Ayu approach us. The fire which is in the Earth, I kindle with its inviolate, holy lustre in the yajna.

May physical fire attain to water in the space. May fire with the names of Angira and Ayu approach us. The fire which is in the space, I kindle with its inviolate, holy lustre in the yajna.

May physical fire attain to water in the space. May fire with the names of Angira and Ayu approach us. The fire which is in the sky, I kindle with its inviolate, holy lustre in the yajna.

May we utilize the sacrificial fire for the acquisition of good qualities.

१०. सिँह्यसि सपत्नसाही देवेभ्य: कल्पस्व सिँह्यसि सपत्नसाही देवेभ्य: । शुन्धस्व सिँह्यसि सपत्नसाही देवेभ्य: शुम्भस्व ॥

10. O speech, thou pronouncest words and overawest foes, attain to the learned. O speech, thou art the dispeller of ignorance, and remover of evils, purify the religious-minded people. O speech, thou art the destroyer of ignoble character and the subduer of mean demeanour, adorn thyself for the well-behaved learned persons!

११. इन्द्रघोषस्त्वा वसुभि: पुरस्तात्पातु प्रचेतास्त्वा रुद्रै: पश्चात्पातु मनोजवास्त्वा पितृभिर्द- क्षिणत: पातु विश्वकर्मा त्वाऽऽदित्यैरुत्तरत: पातिवदमहं तप्तं वार्बर्हिर्घा यज्ञात्रि: सृजामि ॥

11. O speech, may the teaching of God's revealed vedas, protect thee in the east with Vasu Brahmcharis, may the highly intellectual people guard thee in the west with the Rudra Brahmcharis; may the deep thinkers protect thee in the south with the wise, may the learned persons guard thee in the north with Aditya Brahmcharis!

---

⁹Five is named Angira, as it pervades all the organs of the body. It is named Ayu, as it is the giver of heat and life. Without it there can be no life or existence.

Let us banish from our sacrifice, *i.e.*, soul and body, the hot unhealthy water, anger, anxiety and anguish.

१२. सिꣳह्यसि स्वाहा सिꣳह्यस्यादित्यवनि: स्वाहा सिꣳह्यसि ब्रह्मवनि: क्षत्रवनि: सिꣳह्यसि सुप्रजावनी रायस्पोषवनि: स्वाहा सिꣳह्यस्या वह देवान् यजमानाय स्वाहा भूतेभ्यस्त्वा ॥

12. O speech, thou art the dispeller of ignorance. O speech, hallowed by astronomy, remover of the weakness of ferocity, thou describest the twelve months of the year. Thou, attained to by the seekers after God and the vedas, by the heroes expert in military science, art the remover of unwisdom. Thou art the remover of thieves and robbers, and the giver of noble offspring, and abundant wealth. Thou art the killer of all miseries. Endowed with knowledge, thou makest the worshipper obtain good qualities!

I utilise thee through sacrifice (yajna) for the good of humanity.

१३. ध्रुवोसि पृथिवीं दृꣳह ध्रुवक्षिदस्यन्तरिक्षं दृꣳहाच्युतक्षिदसि दिवं दृꣳहाग्ने: पुरीषमसि ॥

13. Oh learned people ye should develop the yajna, which is firm and develops the objects residing on the earth, which confers happiness and imparts the knowledge of sacred lore and develops the dwellers in the air, which affords shelter to indestructible objects, and diffuses knowledge; which replenishes lightning and the beasts!

१४. युञ्जते मन उत युञ्जते धियो विप्रा विप्रस्य बृहतो विपश्चित: । वि होत्रा दधे वयुनाविदेक इन्मही देवस्य सवितु: परिष्टुति: स्वाहा ॥

14. The sages, who consecrate their soul to Him, concentrate their mind and intellect upon God, Who is Omnipresent, Omnipotent, and Omniscient. They sing His praises in various ways. He is the sole Knower of all good acts, and self-existing. Great is the praise of Him, the Creator and Seer of all. He is the preacher of Truth.

१५. इदं विष्णुर्वि चक्रमे त्रेधा नि दधे पदम् । समूढमस्य पाꣳसुरे स्वाहा ॥

15. He Who pervades the animate and the inanimate worlds, has created the visible and invisible worlds, and has established His dignity in three ways. His invisible form is hidden in the space. He is worthy of worship by all.

[11]Speech means vedic text वेदवाणी ।

[12]Just as the science of astronomy explains the creation of the twelve months of the year by the motion of heavenly bodies, so does speech describe the creation, and climatic nature of these twelve months.

[13]The yajna contributes to the growth of inmates of the earth and air. by purifying the air and water and growing corns and grass for the use of men and animals. It adds to our kn₀wledge by the recitation of the Vedic texts which accompany it.

[15] त्रेधा may refer to Satva, Rajas and Tamas. God exhibits His might in the world in these three forms. It may also refer to earth, air and sky. It may also refer to sun full of brightness, to earth devoid of light, and minute atoms.

१६. इरावती धेनुमती हि भूतᳮ सूयवसिनी मनवे दशस्या ।
व्यस्कभ्ना रोदसी विष्णवेते दाधर्थ पृथिवीमभितो मयूखैः स्वाहा ॥

16. O, Omnipresent God, Thou preservest on all sides, with knowledge, this earth, rich in nice food, rich in good milch-kine, and full of elements and compounds. Thou preservest the vedic speech and the created-world. We all implore for the whole world to Him, Who is All-knowing and Chastiser!

१७. देवश्रुतौ देवेष्वा घोषतं प्राची प्रेतमध्वरं कल्पयन्तीऊर्ध्वं यज्ञं नयतं मा जिह्वरतम् ।
स्वं गोष्ठमा वदतं देवि दुर्ये आयुर्मा निर्वादिष्टं प्रजां मा निर्वादिष्टमत्र रमेथां वर्ष्मन् पृथिव्याः ॥

17. O man and woman, having acquired knowledge from the learned, proclaim amongst the wise the fact of your intention of entering the married life. Attain to fame, observing the noble virtue of non-violence, and uplift your soul. Shun crookedness. Converse together happily. Living in a peaceful home, spoil not your life; spoil not your progeny. In this world, pass your life happily, on this wide earth full of enjoyment!

१८. विष्णोर्नु᳭कं वीर्याणि प्र वोचं यः पार्थिवानि विममे रजाᳮसि ।
यो अस्कभायदुत्तरᳮ सधस्थं विचक्रमाणस्त्रेधोरुगायो विष्णवे त्वा ।

18. I describe the mighty deeds of Omnipresent God, Who unifies the different parts of the physical cause of the universe, Who preaches all truths through the Vedas, Who creates the three-fold worlds in the space, Who keeps under His control matter, the highest cause, and Who is resorted to for worship. O God, I hastily seek Thy shelter, Who is Ever-Blissful.

१९. दिवो वा विष्ण उत वा पृथिव्या महो वा विष्ण उरोरन्तरिक्षात् ।
उभा हि हस्ता वसुना पृणस्वा प्र यच्छ दक्षिणादोत सव्याद्विष्णवे त्वा ॥

19. O Omnipresent God, fill both of our hands with riches from all sources like electricity, earth, and vast wide air's mid-region. Grant us pleasures from the right and the left. We worship Thee for the knowledge of yoga.

२०. प्र तद्विष्णु स्तवते वीर्येण मृगो न भीमः कुचरो गिरिष्ठाः ।
यस्योरुषु त्रिषु विक्रमणेष्वधिक्षियन्ति भुवनानि विश्वा ॥

20. God, in whose three-fold world reside all created objects, is praised for His power, like a dreadful, mountain-roaming tiger, that kills the despicable beings. He punishes the sinners, and preaches to all the vedic knowledge.

[20]This verse means, just as a lion keeps under his control other beasts, so does God regulate all the created worlds. The adjectives used in the verse are applicable to God as well. He is मृग: as He controls all living beings. He is भीम: as all men are afraid of Him. He is कुचर: as He chastises all the sinful and wicked people. He is गिरिष्ठ: as He is sung and praised in the vedas. सत्व, रजस and तामस are the three-fold varieties of creation, or Earth, Sky and Space, constitute the three-fold world in which all living creatures have their habitation.

२१. विष्णो रराटमसि विष्णो: श्नप्त्रे स्थो विष्णो: स्यूरसि विष्णोर्ध्रुवोऽसि ।
वैष्णवमसि विष्णवे त्वा ॥

21. O World, thou art created by God, O animate and inanimate objects, ye are the two-fold pure powers of God, O Air, thou art wide-spread through God's strength. O soul, thou art ever immortal through God's grace. O complete universe, thou art created by God. O man I ordain thee to worship the All-pervading God!

२२. देवस्य त्वा सवितु: प्रसवेऽश्विनोर्बाहुभ्यां पूष्णो हस्ताभ्याम् ।
आ ददे नार्य॑सीदमहँ रक्षसां ग्रीवा अपि कृन्तामि ।
बृहन्नसि बृहद्रवा बृहतीमिन्द्राय वाचं वद ।

22. O man, just as I perform the sacrifice (yajna) in this world of God, the Creator of the universe, by the force and strength of vital breaths, and the earth's power of attraction and retention, so do thou. Just as I observe the details of the performance of the sacrifice, so do thou. Just as I cut the necks of the sinners and punish them, so do thou. Just as I through this yajna, attain to eminence, and become a big preacher of the vedas, so do thou. Just as I preach to the king the lofty teachings of the vedas, so do thou!

२३. रक्षोहणं वलगहनं वैष्णवीमिदमहं तं बलगमुत्किरामि यं मे निष्ट्यो निच-
खानेदमहं तं बलगमुत्किरामि यं मे समानो यमसमानो निचखानेदमहं तं बलगमुत्किरामि
यं मे सबन्धुर्यमसबन्धुनिचखानेदमहं तं बलगमुत्किरामि यं मे सजातो यमसजातो
निचखानोत्कृत्यां किरामि ॥

23. O learned man, just as I with the aid of vedic speech, the Killer of fiends and infuser of strength, perform the invigorating sacrifice, so do thou. Just as my wise, and able man, expert in the science of yajna, performs the sacrifice or unearths this place to test it geologically, so shouldst do thy man!
Just as I a geologist resort to strength-giving agriculture and the science of geology, so do thou. Just as my equal and unequal man geologically digs a place, so shouldst do thy man. Just as I a learner and teacher, perform the sacrifice, the giver of soul-force or practise this act of reading and teaching, so do thou. Just as my similar or dissimilar companion regularly performs this sacrifice so shouldst do thine.

[21]In this verse a learned man speaks to an ordinary person to follow him, and do as he does.

[23]Swami Dayananda translates बलगहनम् as infuser of strength, Ubbat and Mahidhar translate the word as the killer or remover of बलग । बलग is translated as bones, hair, and nails buried in the ground as magic to do injury to an opponent. This verse is interpreted for digging out and removing that magical charm. A story has been coined by Mahidhar, that the Rakshsas were defeated by Indra, and they buried the magical charm i.e., बलग underneath the ground one hand deep. To me this interpretation appears irrational, as the vedas are free from historical references, being the eternal word of God, given to mankind in the beginning of creation.

Just as I, the friend of all, perform this yajna, the giver of kindly power, or have recourse to the science of geology, so do thou.

Just as my contemporary or non-contemporary performs this noble deed, so shouldst ever do thine.

Just as I perform noble and virtuous deeds, so do thou.

२४. स्वराडसि सपत्नहा सत्रराडस्यभिमातिहा जनराडसि रक्षोहा सर्वराडस्यमित्रहा ॥

24. O king, thou art self-effulgent, hence thou art the conqueror of foes. Thou art renowned in sacrifices, hence thou art the subduer of the proud enemies. Man's ruler art thou, hence thou art the slayer of fiends. All ruler art thou, hence thou art the killer of foes!

२५. रक्षोहणो वो बलगहनः प्रोक्षामि वैष्णवान् रक्षोहणो वो बलगहनोऽवनयामि वैष्णवान् रक्षहणो वो बलगहनोऽवस्तृणामि वैष्णवान् रक्षोहणौ वां बलगहनौ उप दधामि वैष्णवी रक्षोहणौ वां बलगहनौ पर्यूहामि वैष्णवी वैष्णवमसि वैष्णवा स्थ ॥

25. O members of an Assembly, just as ye are the removers of miseries, so I, the diffuser of the force of foes, having paid my homage to ye, devoted people, set right these proud people by arms in the battle. Just as ye are the killers of the sinners, so I, the scanner of the forces of the enemy, having made ye, devoted people, comfortable, turn aside the ignoble people. Just as I, the arranger of the troops in different orders, fill with ease, ye, the destroyers of foes and performers of sacrifices, so do ye. Just as ye the killers of foes and acquirers of strength, receive the worshipper and the learned priest, so do I. Just as ye the destroyers of foes, and acquirers of strength, know through reasoning the ways of the learned, and the knowledge pertaining to God, so should I. Just as ye all are worshippers of All pervading God, so am I !

२६. देवस्य त्वा सवितुः प्रसवेऽश्विनोर्बाहुभ्यां पूष्णो हस्ताभ्याम् । आ ददे नार्यसीदमहꣳ रक्षसां ग्रीवा अपि कृन्तामि । यवोऽसि यवयास्मद्द्वेषो यवयारातीर्दिवे त्वान्तरिक्षाय त्वा पृथिव्यै त्वा शुन्धन्तांल्लोकाः पितृषदनाः पितृषदनमसि ॥

26. O learned man, in this world created by the happiness-bestowing God, I receive thee with the force and strength of vital breaths, and the arm and power of punishment of a fully developed hero!

Swami Dayananda rightly interprets बलगहनम् as forceful vedic speech. The underlying spirit of the verse is that one should follow the rule of conduct of the learned and not the ignorant.

समान: means equal in wealth, position and knowledge and असमान: are those who differ in these things.

[25]In this verse a learned man addresses the members of an assembly or Parliament. The gist of this verse is that through the worship of God, having acquired physical and spiritual strength, and subduing our foes, we should rule peacefully and calmly.

CHAPTER V

Protecting this world, I behead the sinners, Thou hast the power of imparting virtue and removing vice. Remove from us our haters and enemies. For the exposition of Truth, for flying in air, for consolidating our material forces, we seek thy refuge.

This is the abode of the learned. May all who reside near them make themselves pure. O woman thou also behave likewise!

२७. उद्दिवꣳ स्तभानान्तरिक्षं पृण दृꣳहस्व पृथिव्यां द्युतानस्त्वा मारुतो मिनोतु मित्रावरुणौ ध्रुवेण धर्मणा ।
ब्रह्मवनि त्वा क्षत्रवनि रायस्पोषवनि पर्यूहामि ।
ब्रह्म दृꣳह क्षत्रं दृꣳहायुर्दꣳह प्रजां दृꣳह ॥

27. O highly learned man, just as air with its definite strength, and vital breaths moves thee, so kindly discriminate for us the light of knowledge from ignorance; fill full the space, and preaching noble virtues on Earth, strengthen delights. Strengthen the knowledge of the Vedas, strengthen our kingdom, strengthen our age, and strengthen our offspring. I consider thee as the source of spiritual knowledge, earthly power, and vast riches!

२८. ध्रुवासि ध्रुवोऽयं यजमानोऽस्मिन्नायतने प्रजया पशुभिर्भूयात् ।
घृतेन द्यावापृथिवी पूर्येथामिन्द्रस्य छदिरसि विश्वजनस्य छाया ॥

28. O wife of the worshipper, just as thou with thy offspring and cattle, art firm in thy resolution, in this world; so should this husband of thine be determined in his purpose. Both of you should fill the Heaven and Earth with fragrance of clarified butter!

Thou art the guardian of glory, and the shelter of all people.

२९. परि त्वा गिर्वणो गिर इमा भवन्तु विश्वतः ।
वृद्धायुमनु वृद्धयो जुष्टा भवन्तु जुष्टयः ॥

29. O Adorable God, may all my praises be directed unto Thee. O God, Wise like the aged, may my lovable ever increasing praises be soft and sweet!

३०. इन्द्रस्य स्यूरसीन्द्रस्य ध्रुवोऽसि । ऐन्द्रमसि वैश्वदेवमसि ॥

30. O God, Thou unitest the soul with Thee, Thou art the refuge of the soul. Thou art the friend of the soul. Thou art the receptacle of all noble virtues!

[26] A king addresses a learned man in this verse. We should purify ourselves in the company of the learned.
[27] Here too a king addresses the learned person.
To fill the space full means to enable us to fly freely in the air.
[28] Husband and wife are asked to perform the yajna daily, and fill the heaven and earth with the fragrant smell of ghee used in it.

३१. विभूरसि प्रवाहणो वह्निरसि हव्यवाहनः ।
श्वात्रोऽसि प्रचेतास्तुथोऽसि विश्ववेदाः ॥

31. O God, Thou art Omnipresent, and fit to take the burden of the world. Just as fire carries up in a rarefied form the articles put into it, so dost Thou diffuse all knowledge. Thou art All-knowing, and Thou Teacher of all, Thou art Omniscient, and Developer of wisdom!

३२. उशिगसि कविरङ्घारिरसि बम्भारिरवस्यूरसि दुवस्वाञ्छन्द्यूरसि मार्जालीयः ।
सम्राडसि कृशानुः परिषद्योऽसि पवमानो नभोऽसि प्रतक्वा मृष्टोऽसि हव्यसूदन ऋत-
धामासि स्वर्ज्योतिः ॥

32. O God, Thou art Effulgent, Wise, Hostile to the sinners, Enemy of thraldom, the Unifier and Protector of all. Thou art fit for service by us. Thou art Pure and Purifier. Thou art a Just Ruler; and the Prop. of the weak. Thou art adored in Assemblies. Thou art the Giver of holiness, the Chastiser of thieves and robbers and Bestower of joy. Thou givest us strength to endure pleasure and pain; and grantest us splendour. Thou art the abode of Truth, and the Giver of lustre to the sky!

३३. समुद्रोऽसि विश्वव्यचा अजोऽस्येकपादहिरसि बुध्न्यो वागस्यैन्द्रमसि सदोऽस्यृतस्य द्वारौ
मा मा सन्तात्प्तमध्वनामध्वपते प्र मा तिर स्वस्ति मेऽस्मिन्पथि देवयाने भूयात् ॥

33. O God, Thy knowledge is fathomless. Thou art Omnipresent, and Unborn. Thou holdest the universe with a part of Thy Energy. Thou art the Master of all forms of knowledge; and the Source of Universe. Thou art the highest Teacher; and full of splendour, Thou art the Asylum of all. Ye two gates of knowledge do not distress me. O Lord of religious paths, lead me onward, through religious ways. May I be happy in this God-reaching path!

३४. मित्रस्य मा चक्षुषेक्षध्वमग्नयः सगराः सगरा स्थ सगरेण नाम्ना रौद्रेणानीकेन पात माऽग्नयः पिपृत माऽग्नयो गोपायत मा नमो वोऽस्तु मा मा हिꣳसिष्ट ॥

34. O learned persons full of knowledge and inculcations, look upon me with the eye of a friend. May ye preach knowledge. O learned people protect me with your air-force and renowned army, that make the enemy weep. O learned person fill me with wisdom and virtues, and guard me on all sides. Unto thee be my adoration. Do not injure me!

*एकपात् may also mean, the one and sole protector. The two gates of knowledge are external and internal happiness, i.e., physical and mental ease. If one's physical health is lost, he can't advance his knowledge, and same is the case when one's mental peace is disturbed. These are the two sources for the acquisition of knowledge. A devotee prays for physical and mental health. Lord of religious path is the learned person who shows the true path. God-reaching path is the path of salvation, on which the wise and the learned tread.

३५. ज्योतिरसि विश्वरूपं विश्वेषां देवानाᳪ᳴समित् । त्वᳪ᳴ सोम तनूकृद्भ्यो द्वेषोभ्योऽन्य-
कृतेभ्य उरु यन्तासि वरुथᳪ᳴स्वाहा ।
जुषाणो अप्तुराज्यस्य वेतु स्वाहा ॥

35. O Splendid God, Thou art the light and fine illuminator of all the learned persons. Thou art the controller of the sins committed by us and others, and those who practise hatred. Let the man possessing a fine home, good speech and vast knowledge know the vedas!

३६. अग्ने नय सुपथा राये अस्मान्विश्वानि देव वयुनानि विद्वान् ।
यूयोध्यस्मज्जुहुराणमेनो भूयिष्ठां ते नम उक्तिं विधेम ॥

36. O God, the Master of all, and the Giver of all kinds of happiness, and the Knower of all of our actions and thoughts, lead us to salvation through the path of virtue. Keep away from us all crooked sins. We offer Thee most ample obeisance!

३७. अयं नो अग्निर्वरिवस्कृणोत्वयं मृधः पुर एतु प्रभिन्दन् ।
अयं वाजाञ्जयतु वाजसातावयᳪ᳴ शत्रूञ्जयतु जह्‌षाणः स्वाहा ॥

37. May this General, the queller of the sinners like fire, give us protection. This General, expert in military skill, should in the battle first attack and subdue the wicked foes. May he win all wars. May he conquer foes. May he come out successful in combats, issuing necessary administrative orders?

३८. उरु विष्णो वि क्रमस्वोरु क्षयाय नस्कृधि ।
घृतं घृतयोने पिब प्र प्र यज्ञपतिं तिर स्वाहा ॥

38. O General, attack the enemy with full force, and make ample room for our abode. O learned General, just as fire assimilates ghee and burns brightly; so shouldst thou develop thy virtues and shine in battles. Just as priests protecting the worshipper make him overcome all calamities, so shouldst thou with thy oratory win battles!

३९. देव सवितरेष ते सोमस्तᳪ᳴ रक्षस्व मा त्वा दभन् ।
एतत्त्वं देव सोम देवो देवाᳪ᳴
उपागा इदमहं मनुष्यान्त्सह रायस्पोषेण स्वाहा निर्वरुणस्य पाशान्मुच्ये ॥

39. O learned person, the propagator of all kinds of knowledge and full of splendour, this is thy glory, protect it, let none harm thee. O king, the giver of happiness, and leader of men on the path of virtue, and hence well established in the diffusion of knowledge, go thou to the sages. Abiding by this advice, just as I deliver the wise persons from the noose of the despicable knaves; so shouldst thou!

---

[39]The verse is a kind of dialogue between a learned person and a king. The learned person advises a king to seek the company of the learned, and the king replies that he protects the wise and the learned from the baneful influence of the wicked persons.

४०. अग्ने व्रतपास्त्वे व्रतपा या तव तनूर्मय्यभूदेषा सा त्वयि यो मम तनूस्त्वय्यभूदियँ सा मयि ।
यथायथं नौ व्रतपते व्रतान्यनु मे दीक्षां दीक्षापतिरमँस्तानु तपस्तपस्पति: ॥

40. O learned teacher, thou art the guardian of my vow. Let thy vast knowledge be mine. Let my learning be subordinate to thee. Let my wisdom depend upon thine. O Lord of vows, let our vows of noble conduct be accomplished friendly. O lord of initiation, teach me truth. O lord of austerity, teach me to lead an austere life!

४१. उरु विष्णो वि क्रमस्वोरु क्षयाय नस्कृधि ।
घृतं घृतयोने पिब प्रप्र यज्ञपतिं तिर स्वाहा ॥

41. O learned person, mayest thou be conversant with all branches of knowledge, for the vast development of learning. Give us happiness. Drink thou the water, the precursor of which is lightning. Just as I make the worshipper overcome all obstacles, so shouldst thou be totally free from all ills, by the regular performance of Havan!

४२. व्रतयन्याँर् अगां नान्याँर् उपागामवर्किं त्वा परेभ्योऽविदं परोऽवरेभ्य: ।
तं त्वा जुषामहे देव वनस्पते देवयज्यायै देवास्त्वा देवयज्यायै जुषन्तां विष्णवे त्वा ।
श्रोषधे त्रायस्व स्वधिते मैनँ हिँसी: ॥

42. O learned botanist, just as thou shunnest the foolish and seekest the company of the wise, so may I avoid the company of the enemies of the wise, and go to the wise. May I approach thee more learned among the learned but the humblest among the humble. Just as the learned long for the acquisition of good qualities, so do I. Just as medicinal herbs, rendered fit for the yajana protect all, so do we for sacrifice hail thee, the remover of diseases, and the assuager of affliction!

O learned person, just as I do not want to spoil this yajna, so shouldst thou not!

४३. द्यां मा लेखीरन्तरिक्षं मा हिँसी: पृथिव्या सम्भव ।
अयँ हि त्वा स्वधितिस्तेतिजान: प्रणिनाय महते सौभगाय ।
व्रतस्त्वं देव वनस्पते शतवल्शो वि रोह सहस्रवल्शो वि वयँ रुहेम ॥

43. Just as I gaze not at the sun, so shouldst thou not. Just as I disturb not the proper arrangement of things, so shouldst thou not. Just as I live on the

---

[40] The disciple addresses the teacher. Our refers to the disciple and the Guru.

[41] A priest addresses a learned person. Lightning flashes before it begins to rain. It is the precursor of rain. Rain-water is the purest form of water. This verse is identical with verse thirtyeight of this chapter. The charge of repetition is unfounded as both the verses have different meanings.

[42] A disciple addresses a teacher; or a seeker after knowledge addresses a learned person.

CHAPTER V

earth in a spirit of friendliness towards all, so shouldst thou.

As a well-sharpened axe, gives splendour by the removal of enemies, so may this grant thee glory.

O happy learned person, the master of forests, may thy dynasty increase, just as a tree does with its hundred roots. May our progeny increase in numbers, just as a tree does with its manifold boughs.

---

[48]This is a dialogue between a learned person and a worshipper.

CHAPTER VI

१. देवस्य त्वा सवितुः प्रसवेऽश्विनोर्बाहुभ्यां पूष्णो हस्ताभ्याम् । आददे नार्यंसीदमहꣳ रक्षसां ग्रीवा अपि कृन्तामि ।
यवोऽसि यवयास्मद् द्वेषो यवयारातीर्दिवे त्वान्तरिक्षाय त्वा पृथिव्यै त्वा शुन्धन्तां लोकाः पितृषदनाः पितृषदनमसि ॥

1. O king, just as the wise and aged persons, in this world, created by the Effulgent God, accept thee, with the force and strength of vital breaths, and attraction and retention of breath, the source of strength; so do I!
Just as I cut the throats of the sinners, so shouldst thou.
O king, thou hast the power of imparting virtue and removing vice, remove from us our despisers and foes!
Just as I sanctify thee, the exponent of justice, for the display of knowledge, thee, the embodiment of truth, for spiritual advancement; thee, the administrator, for rule over the Earth; so should these justice-loving people do.
O king thou art a father unto thine subjects, rear them up!
O Queen, thou also shouldst behave similarly!

२. अग्रेणीरसि स्ववेश उन्नेतृणामेतस्य वित्तादधि त्वा स्थास्यति देवस्त्वा सविता मध्वानक्तु सुपिप्पलाभ्यस्त्वौषधीभ्यः ।
द्यामग्रेणास्पृक्ष आन्तरिक्षं मध्येनाप्राः पृथिवीमुपरेणादृꣳही: ॥

2. O king, thou art our leader; thou putteth upon the path of rectitude, even the leaders of a high order. Know thou this art of government!
God, the Creator will rule over thee. Just as the state officials anoint thee with sweet juices and flower-laden herbs, so should the subjects do.
Thy first duty is to undertake the spread of knowledge and the administration of justice.
Thy second duty is to propagate religious truths. Thy foremost duty is to strengthen thy rule over the Earth.

३. या ते धामान्युश्मसि गमध्यै यत्र गावो भूरिशृङ्गा अयासः ।
अत्राह तदुरुगायस्य विष्णोः परमं पदमव भारि भूरि ।
ब्रह्मवनि त्वा क्षत्रवनि रायस्पोषवनि पर्यूहामि । ब्रह्म दृꣳह क्षत्रं दृꣳहायुर्दृꣳह प्रजां दृꣳह ॥

---

[1] This verse is exactly similar to 5.26. The objection of repetition does not arise, as the Devatas and meanings of both the verses are different. The former is addressed to a general, the latter describes the qualities, an Acharya ought to preach to a king at the time of his coronation.

3. O king, we desire to reach all thy abodes, where the resplendent beams of adorable God's knowledge spread far and wide!

In those very places, have the sages attained to the highest bliss of God.

I consider thee as the source of spiritual knowledge, earthly power, and vast riches.

Advance the knowledge of the vedas, improve thy rule and military experts, prolong thy life, and advance thy progeny.

४. विष्णो: कर्माणि पश्यत यतो व्रतानि पस्पशे ।
इन्द्रस्य युज्य: सखा ॥

4. O men study God's works of Creation, preservation and dissolution of the universe; whereby He determines His laws!
Each one of us is His close-allied friend.

५. तद्विष्णो: परमं पदꣳ सदा पश्यन्ति सूरय: ।
दिवीव चक्षुराततम् ॥

5. The learned scholars of the vedas realise the lofty attributes of God, as the extended eye gazes at the sun.

६. परिवीरसि परि त्वा दैवीर्विशो व्ययन्तां परीमं यजमानꣳ रायो मनुष्याणाम् ।
दिव: सूनुरस्येष ते पृथिव्याँल्लोक आरण्यस्ते पशु: ॥

6. O king, thou art the repository of knowledge like a sage!

The learned subjects obey thee in all directions. May riches fit for men be secured by this intelligent devotee. Thou art lustrous like the beams of the sun. May all people on the earth and all beasts of the forest be under thy control.

७. उपावीरस्युप देवान्दैवीर्विश: प्रागुरुशिजो वह्नितमान् ।
देव त्वष्टर्वसु रम हव्या ते स्वदन्ताम् ॥

7. O king, thou art the embodiment of noble qualities, and remover of the miseries of thy subjects. Thou protectest those who take refuge under thy shelter. May thy noble subjects be associated with learned persons, full of splendour and efficient to undertake the responsibility of government. Feel pleasure, and let thy subjects enjoy thy pleasurable precious riches!

८. रेवती रमध्वं बृहस्पते धारया वसूनि ।
ऋतस्य त्वा देवहवि: पाशेन प्रति मुञ्चामि धर्षा मानुष: ॥

---

[a]A learned person preaches to a king. The king should arrange for such calm, quiet, healthy and comfortable places, where the learned may resort to for peaceful meditation of God.

8. O rich sons, roam in knowledge and good training. O highly learned teacher, please accept the honestly earned money, we offer thee. O prince, thou art liked by the learned, I, a scholar of scriptures, release thee from the bondage of ignorance, be steadfast and firm in the acquisition of knowledge!

९. देवस्य त्वा सवितु: प्रसवेऽश्विनोर्बाहुभ्यां पूष्णो हस्ताभ्याम् ।
अग्नीषोमाभ्यां जुष्टं नि युनज्मि ।
अद्रुचस्त्वौषधीभिर्योऽनु त्वा माता मन्यतामनु पिताऽनु भ्राता सगर्भ्योऽनु सखा सयूथ्य: ।
अग्नीषोमाभ्यां त्वा जुष्टं प्रोक्षामि ॥

9. O disciple, in this world—created by God, full of splendour, and the Revealer of the Vedas, with the attributes of the Sun and moon, and with the retention and gravitation of the Earth, namely its hands I welcome thee. I lovingly initiate thee endowed with prosperity and peace in the Brahmcharya Ashram sprinkling thee with water and corn!

May thy mother, father, brother, friend and fellow students grant thee permission for my discipleship.

For observing the vow of celibacy, I lovingly anoint thee in peace and prosperity.

१०. अपां पेरुरस्यापो देवी: स्वदन्तु स्वात्तं चित्सद्देवहवि: ।
सं ते प्राणो वातेन गच्छताꣳ समज्ञानि यजत्रै: सं यज्ञपतिराशिषा ॥

10. O pupil, thou art the purifier of water through yajna. May people purified by thy sacrifice enjoy pleasant waters, and substances obtained by virtuous means, as do the sages!

Through my benediction, may all thy organs be devoted to the performance of the yajna along with the learned priests.

May thy breath roam freely with the wind, and may thou be the performer of the yajna of the spread of knowledge.

११. घृतेनाक्तौ पशूꣳस्त्रायेथाꣳ रेवति यजमाने प्रियं धा आ विश ।
उरोरन्तरिक्षात्सजूर्देवेन वातेनास्य हविस्तमना यज समस्य तन्वा भव ।
वर्षो वर्षीयसि यज्ञे यज्ञपति धा: स्वाहा देवेभ्यो देवेभ्य: स्वाहा ॥

[8]In the first part of the verse the father addresses the sons and the teacher. In the latter part the teacher addresses the disciple.

[9]अश्विनो: means the sun and moon. बाहुभ्याम् means with qualities that work like arms. This is a figurative use of the word. The qualities of lustre and prevention of evil of the sun and moon are referred to. Both give light, and conduce to our health and ward off diseases. पूषेति पृथिवीनामसु पठितम् निघं० १-१. The qualities of retention and gravitation are figuratively spoken of as earth's hands. In this verse the teacher addresses the pupil at the time of the ceremony of investiture of the sacred thread (yajnopavit).

[10]Roaming freely of the breath with wind means, your breath should be full of force and strength like the wind.

CHAPTER VI

11. O performers of yajna and its supervisor fond of ghee as ye are, rear cows. Let each one of you regulate by purifying all pervading air the worshipper full of splendour, pleasure, born of wide space; and understand his primary aim. Perform duly yourself the yajna with all its materials, and be one with the full observance of the details of the yajna!

O giver of happiness through yajna, welcome with sweet words all the religious minded and learned persons who visit the yajna again and again, and establish the worshipper in the pleasure-giving yajna!

१२. माहिर्भूर्मा पृदाकुनमस्त्रातानानर्वा प्रेहि ।
घृतस्य कुल्या उप ऋतस्य पथ्या अनु ॥

12. O learned person, the diffuser of delight, behave not crookedly like a serpent, or proudly like a fool, or ferociously like a tiger. Food is ready for thee everywhere. Tread on the paths of truth and rectitude. just as shelterless persons without any conveyance feel happy when they reach a stream of water!

१३. देवीराप: शुद्धा वोढ्वꣳ सुपरिविष्टा देवेषु सुपरिविष्टा वयं परिवेष्टारो भूयास्म ॥

13. O girls, just as women, endowed with noble qualities, pure, and highly educated are married to their deserving husbands, and serve them faithfully; and educated husbands are married to worthy wives, so should ye be married; and so shall we be joined in wedlock!

१४. वाचं ते शुन्धामि प्राणं ते शुन्धामि चक्षुस्ते शुन्धामि श्रोत्रं ते शुन्धामि नाभिं ते शुन्धामि मेढ्रं ते शुन्धामि पायुं ते शुन्धामि चरित्राँ स्ते शुन्धामि ॥

14. O disciple, through various sermons, I enjoin upon thee to purify thy voice, thy breath, thy eye, thy ear, thy navel, thy penis, thy anus; and all thy dealings!

१५. मनस्त आ प्यायतां वाक्त आ प्यायतां प्राणस्त आ प्यायतां चक्षुस्त आ प्यायताꣳ
श्रोत्रं त आ प्यायताम् ।
यत्ते क्रूरं यदास्थितं तत्त आ प्यायतां निष्टचायतां तत्ते शुध्यतु शमहोभ्यँ: ।
ओषधे त्रायस्व स्वधिते मैनꣳ हिꣳसी: ॥

15. O disciple, through my teaching, let thy mind be filled with noble qualities, thy voice and breath be strong, thy eye clear in vision, thy ear quick of hearing. Let thy evil designs be removed, and thy intentions fulfilled. Let all thy doings be pure, and may thou daily derive happiness!

O exalted teacher, guard this disciple, and spoil him not through fondness and wrong teaching. O noble mistress, protect this girl, and chastise her not uselessly!

[14]The teacher addresses the student, advising him to keep all the organs of his body and mind pure, healthy, and free from evil desires.
[15]In the last portion of the verse the wife of the teacher addresses her husband and he addresses her.

१६. रक्षसां भागोऽसि निरस्तꣳ रक्ष इदमहꣳ रक्षोऽभि तिष्ठामीदमहꣳ रक्षोऽव बाध इदमहꣳ रक्षोऽधमं तमो नयामि ।
घृतेन द्यावापृथिवी प्रोर्णुवाथां वायो वे स्तोकानामग्निराज्यस्य वेतु स्वाहा स्वाहा-
कृते ऊर्ध्वनभसं मारुतं गच्छतम् ॥

16. O sinner, demons pay homage unto thee. Get out ye evil spirited. I stand before such a devil for dishonouring him, rather I chastise such a despicable fellow with great disgust. I carry such a satan to the lowest depth of distress. O disciple, the discriminator between virtue and vice, and cultivator of goodness, understand all the intricate problems, fill the Earth and Sun with water rendered pure through thy yajna. Let the learned person know thy yajna performed with clarified butter. Let the Earth and Sun filled with the greasy substance of Homa attain to the air which carries up the water purified by thy yajna!

१७. इदमाप: प्र वहतावद्यं च मलं च यत् ।
यच्चाभिदुद्रोहानृतं यच्च शेपे अभीरुणम् ।
आपो मा तस्मादेनस: पवमानश्च मुञ्चतु ॥

17. Ye masters of knowledge, just as waters purify us, so do ye wash away this indescribable sin and ignorance of mine. O learned persons keep me away from the vice of false malice, and accusation of the innocent. May noble, virtuous deed save me from sin!

१८. सं ते मनो मनसा सं प्राण: प्राणेन गच्छताम् ।
रेडस्यग्निष्ट्वा श्रीणात्वा पस्त्वा समरिणन्वातस्य त्वा ध्राज्यै पूष्णो रꣳह्या ऊष्मणो
व्यथिषत् प्रयुतं द्वेष: ॥

18. O warlike hero, may thy mind in battle be filled with knowledge, and thy breath be united to life's force. O hero, thou art the killer of foes. May the fire of righteous indignation created by battle mature thee. Facing millions of the army of enemies, let not the heat generated by battle disturb thee!

May thou get refreshing drinks to fight in war with the velocity of wind, and speed of the sun.

१९. घृतं घृतपावान: पिबत वसां वसापावान: पिबतान्तरिक्षस्य हविरसि स्वाहा ।
दिश: प्रदिश आदिशो विदिश उद्दिशो दिग्भ्य: स्वाहा ॥

19. Oh warriors, drinkers of water, drink refreshing water. O warriors expert in statesmanship, follow the policy of heroic action. O general, thou shouldst stop the foes in the air. With thy martial and commanding voice

---

[16]This verse condemns vice and upholds virtue. The disciple is advised by the preceptor to purify water and air through the daily performance of yajna, spread them over the Earth and send them up to the Sun.

२०. ऐन्द्रः प्राणो अङ्गे अङ्गे नि दीध्यदैन्द्र उदानो अङ्गे अङ्गे निधीतः ।
देव त्वष्टर्भूरि ते सꣳ समेतु सलक्ष्मा यद्विषुरूपं भवाति ।
देवत्रा यन्तमवसे सखायोऽनु त्वा माता पितरो मदन्तु ॥

20. O destroyer of the strength of the enemy, O general endowed with beautiful knowledge, shine forth in the battle-field subduing all thy foes, as the in-going breath pertaining to our soul, overcomes all other breaths in every part of the body!
Just as Udan breath permeates all our organs, so do thou O general shine forth in the battle leading all your warriors. Let thy diverse forces in uniform gather together in large numbers. O general, may all warriors behave friendly towards thee for thy protection. May thy mother, father and relatives be pleased to see thee moving in the midst of warriors.

२१. समुद्रं गच्छ स्वाहा ऽन्तरिक्षं गच्छ स्वाहा देवꣳ सवितारं गच्छ स्वाहा ।
मित्रावरुणौ गच्छ स्वाहा ऽहोरात्रे गच्छ स्वाहा छन्दाꣳसि गच्छ स्वाहा द्यावापृथिवी गच्छ स्वाहा यज्ञं गच्छ स्वाहा सोमं गच्छ स्वाहा दिव्यं नभो गच्छ स्वाहा ऽग्निं वैश्वानरं गच्छ स्वाहा मनो मे हार्दि यच्छ दिवं ते धूमो गच्छतु स्वज्योतिः पृथिवीं भस्मनाऽऽपृण स्वाहा ॥

21. O disciple, a student in the science of government, sail in oceans in steamers, fly in the air in aeroplanes, know God the Creator through the vedas, control thy breath through yoga, through astronomy know the functions of day and night, know all the Vedas, Rig, Yajur, Sama, and Atharva, by means of their constituent parts!
Through astronomy, geography, and geology go thou to all the different countries of the world under the sun. Mayest thou attain through good preaching to statesmanship, and artisanship, through medical science obtain knowledge of all medicinal plants, through hydrostatics, learn the different uses of water, through electricity understand the working of ever-lustrous lightning. Carry out my instructions willingly. May the smoke of thy yajna and military machines reach the sun, and may their flames go up to heaven; and may thou cover the earth with the ashes, the residue of thy yajna.

२२. माऽपो मौषधीहिꣳसीर्धाम्नो धाम्नो राजँस्ततो वरुण नो मुञ्च ।
यदाहुरध्या इति वरुणेति शपामहे ततो वरुण नो मुञ्च ।

---

[21] Angas are the constituent parts of the vedas. They are six in number—sciences of pronunciation. शिक्षा, rituals कल्प grammar व्याकरण, etymology निरूक्त astronomy ज्योतिष, prosody छन्दस्. Their study helps in the correct pronunciation and interpretation of the vedas. भस्मना may also mean with thy splendour, prestige, and agony caused in the heart of a foe.

सुमित्रिया न आप ओषधय: सन्तु दुर्मित्रियास्तस्मै सन्तु योऽस्मान्द्वेष्टि यं च वयं द्विष्म: ॥

22. O praiseworthy king, do not destroy canals, wells, tanks, corn fields and forests. Protect us at every place. O Justice-loving king, we take a solemn vow that cows and learned Brahmans whom thou declarest to be unworthy of destruction, will not be killed by us. We will stick to this resolve and so shouldst thou!

O king, in thy rule, may waters and medicines be friendly to us, and unfriendly to him who dislikes us or whom we dislike!

२३. हविष्मतीरिमा आपो हविष्माँ२ आं विवासति ।
हविष्मान् देवो अध्वरो हविष्माँ२ अस्तु सूर्य: ॥

23. O learned persons, see that these waters contribute to your purity, comfort and usefulness. Air can be used and abused. May pleasure-promoting yajna grant us happiness, may the sun give us health and comfort!

२४. अग्नेर्वोऽपन्नगृहस्य सदसि सादयामीन्द्राग्न्योर्भागधेयी स्थ मित्रावरुणयोर्भागधेयी स्थ विश्वेषां देवानां भागधेयी स्थ ।
अमूर्या उप सूर्ये याभिर्वा सूर्य: सह । ता नो हिन्वन्त्वध्वरम् ॥

24. O virgins, I set ye down in the assembly of learned bachelors. Ye are cognisant of the diverse qualities of sun and lighting, ye know fully well the science of the control of breath, ye can make selection of learned husbands!

Those of you, who after marriage live with husbands brilliant like the sun, and with you whom, live brilliant husbands, should both advance our domestic dealings.

२५. हृदे त्वा मनसे त्वा दिवे त्वा सूर्याय त्वा ।
ऊर्ध्वमिममध्वरं दिवि देवेषु होत्रा यच्छ ॥

25. O virgins, just as we live with our husbands and perform the Havan, so do ye. Just as we impart instruction unto ye for mental peace, for discriminating between virtue and vice, for spreading happiness, and acquiring brilliance like the sun, so do ye uplift the domestic life for the diffusion of all kinds of happiness!

२६. सोम राजन् विश्वास्तवं प्रजा उपावरोह विश्वास्तवां प्रजा उपावरोहन्तु ।
शृणोत्वग्नि: समिधा हवं मे शृण्वन्त्वापो धिषणाश्च देवी: ।
श्रोता ग्रावाणो विदुषो न यज्ञं शृणोतु देव: सविता हवं मे स्वाहा ॥

---

[24]The mistress addresses the girl pupils.

[25]The mistress addresses her girl students. अध्वरम् is the domestic life, the household yajna, which the newly married wife is asked to advance and uplift through her devotion, piety and sagacity.

26. O noble king, like a father go near thy subjects, and let the subjects like sons come near thee to seek protection. Just as fire is kindled with woodsticks, so hear my complaint and kindle justice. Let versatile, learned and noble-minded queens, like mothers, hear the complaints of women, and do justice unto them!

You magistrates who distinguish justice from injustice, listen to our grievances!

O supreme king, endowed with knowledge, hear like sacrificing learned persons, our requests made in an humble, laudatory tone!

२७. देवीरापो अ्रपां नपाद्यो व ऊर्मिहंविष्य इन्द्रियावान् मदिन्तमः ।
तं देवेभ्यो देवत्रा दत्त शुक्रपेभ्यो येषां भाग स्थ स्वाहा ॥

27. O noble and virtuous subjects, select as your king for the benefit of the learned persons and Brahmcharis who preserve their semen, one, born out of you, who is high like the flood in water, fit for service with food, endowed with strength, capable of subduing his foes, and completely capable of adding to the happiness of his kingdom. Ye too constitute a part of those learned persons!

२८. कार्षिरसि समुद्रस्य त्वा क्षित्या उन्नयामि ।
समापो अद्भिरग्मत समोषधीभिरोषधीः ॥

28. O farmer, thou art fit to cultivate the land, I uplift thee for the purification of space. Get waters from waters, and medicinal plants from plants!

२९. यमग्ने पृत्स्तु मर्त्यमवा वाजेषु यं जुनाः ।
स यन्ता शश्वतीरिष: स्वाहा ॥

29. O king, whomsoever thou protectest in the battle and appointest for the supervision of food supply, deserves the award of a permanent pension for his maintenance. This is a proper rule!

३० देवस्य त्वा सवितुः प्रसवेऽश्विनोर्बाहुभ्यां पूष्णो हस्ताभ्याम् ।
श्रा ददे रावाऽसि गभीरमिममध्वरं कृधीन्द्राय सुषूतमम् ।
उत्तमेन पविनोर्जस्वन्तं मधुमन्तं पयस्वन्तं निग्राभ्या स्थ देवश्रुतस्तर्पयत मा ॥

²⁸A learned teacher addresses a cultivator. A farmer tills the land, and grows the plants. Those plants श्रोषध्यः are used for performing Agnihotra. The oblations being rarefied rise up to heaven, fill the space Antriksha with vapours, purify the air, and descend down to earth in the form of pure rainy water, which again grows the plants. This is a natural process going on in nature; aided by our yajna. Farmer is the main source of the growth of plants, whereby Yajnas are performed, which fill the space with vapours, which bring down pure rain, which again helps in the growth of plants.

²⁹He who succeeds in the battle, rules over many persons whom he subjugates. Similarly one who is in charge of food-supply is the master of the destinies of thousands of persons who depend upon him for the supply of necessaries of life.

30. O my subjects, in this world created by God, the Giver of happiness and the Source of all splendour, I receive ye with the strength and coolness of the sun and moon, and the disease-killing, and bodily humours—equilibrium maintaining qualities of the herbs!

For me full of splendour, in a civilised manner, pay open-heartedly the tax which is highly useful, is levied on all your products, which conduces to efficient administration, which is utilized for the advancement of industries and improving the cattle breed. O my subjects, ye who take interest in the welfare of your king, deserve to be welcomed by me! Please me by paying your taxes.

३१. मनो मे तर्पयत वाचं मे तर्पयत प्राणं मे तर्पयत चक्षुर्मे तर्पयत श्रोत्रं मे तर्पयता-त्मानं मे तर्पयत प्रजां मे तर्पयत पशून्मे तर्पयत गणान्मे तर्पयत गणा मे मा वि तृषन् ॥

31. O subjects and legislators, satisfy my mind, satisfy my speech, satisfy my breath, satisfy my eye, satisfy my ear, satisfy my soul, satisfy my progeny, satisfy my cattle, satisfy my subordinate officers, so that my officers may not feel sad!

३२. इन्द्राय त्वा वसुमते रुद्रवत इन्द्राय त्वाऽऽदित्यवत इन्द्राय त्वा अभिमातिघ्ने । श्येनाय त्वा सोमभृते अग्नये त्वा रायस्पोषदे ॥

32. O Lord, we appoint thee as a king, as thou possessest the vigour of a Vasu Brahmchari, as thou hast got the strength of a Rudra Brahmchari, as thou art full of splendour, full of knowledge like an Aditya Brahmchari, as thou hast the power of killing the proud foes, as thou art full of dignity, and art quick in attacking in the battle-field like a falcon, as thou strengthenest our finances, and advancest the knowledge of science!

३३. यत्ते सोम दिवि ज्योतिर्यत्पृथिव्यां यदुरावन्तरिक्षे । तेनास्मै यजमानायोरु राये कृध्यधि दात्रे वोच: ॥

---

[30] A king addresses his subjects. He is described to possess the strength and coolness of the sun and moon, spoken of as arms, and the healing properties of the herbs spoken of as hands. Just as medicinal plants remove our diseases, so does a king arrange for the maintenance of the health of his subjects by spending liberally on sanitation, and medical institutions.

There are three affections or humours धातव: in our body; *i.e.*, वात, पित्त, कफ, *i.e.* flatulence, bile and phlegm. The harmonious equilibrium of these maintains the body in a healthy state. The king advises the subjects to pay gladly the taxes imposed, which will be utilised for their advancement.

[31] The king addresses the subjects.

[32] A Vasu Brahmchari is one who observes the vow of celibacy for twentyfour years, one who remains celibate for 36 years and acquires knowledge is Rudra Brahmchari, and he who continues his studies observing celibacy for 48 years is called an Aditya Brahmchari. The verse means the king selected should not be voluptuous and slave to passions. but one who has duly observed the vow of celibacy and acquired knowledge.

33. O king thy rule extends over Heaven, Earth and mid-air wide region. With that power show obligation to this worshipper who performs the yajna, and has recourse to measures conducive to the propagation of national wealth!

३४. श्वात्रा स्थ वृत्रतुरो राधो गूर्त्ता अमृतस्य पत्नी: ।
ता देवीर्देवत्रेमं यज्ञं नयतोपहूता: सोमस्य पिबत ॥

34. O ladies, ye are the possessors of practical wisdom, removers of all impediments, augmenters of wealth, helpers in the yajna, and lovers of your virtuous husbands. Fulfil this sacrifice of domestic life. Being invited taste with your husbands the sweet juice of the plants like Soma!

३५. मा भेर्मा सं विक्था ऊर्जं धत्स्व धिषणे वीड्वी सती वीड्येथामूर्जं दधाथाम् ।
पाप्मा हतो न सोम: ॥

35. O woman, full of physical and spiritual strength, be not afraid of thy husband, shake not with terror, cultivate the strength of your body and soul. O man, thou also shouldst behave similarly towards thy wife, Ye both, like the sun and earth should become strong and resolute; whereby the shortcomings of ye both be removed, and ye become happy like the moon!

३६. प्रागपागुदगधराक्सर्वतस्त्वा दिश आ धावन्तु ।
अम्ब निष्पर समरीविदाम् ॥

36. O mother, love thy children, who run unto thee from east, west, north, south and all other directions; and they too should love thee!

३७. त्वमङ्ग प्रशंसिषो देव: शविष्ठ मर्त्यम् ।
न त्वदन्यो मघवन्नस्ति मङितेन्द्र ब्रवीमि ते वच: ॥

37. O mighty, glorious king, render thy subjects praiseworthy. Thou art the conqueror of foes. None but thee is the giver of pleasure. I say this unto thee!

CHAPTER VII

१. वाचस्पतये पवस्व वृष्णोऽꣳशुभ्यां गभस्तिपूतः ।
देवो देवेभ्यः पवस्व येषां भागोऽसि ॥

1. O man, for realising God, the Lord of Speech, purify thy mind. Just as objects are purified by the rays of the sun, so purify thyself with the outward and inward powers of a strong king. Be a learned man, work pure-heartedly for the sages, who are adorable by thee!

२. मधुमतीनं इषस्कृधि यत्ते सोमादाभ्यं नाम जागृवि तस्मै ते सोम सोमाय स्वाहा स्वाहोर्वन्तरिक्षमन्वेमि ॥

2. O superb man of knowledge, sweeten our foods. O learned preacher of virtuous deeds, whatever well-known name free from harm, thou hast, for the acquisition of power and carrying out thy instructions, I attain to true deed, truthful speech and wide atmosphere of prosperity!

३. स्वाङ्कृतोऽसि विश्वेभ्यो इन्द्रियेभ्यो दिव्येभ्यः पार्थिवेभ्यो मनस्त्वाष्टु स्वाहा त्वा सुभ्वे सूर्याय देवेभ्यस्त्वा मरीचिपेभ्यो देवाꣳशो यस्मै त्वेडे तत्सत्यमुपरिप्रुता भङ्क्तेन हतोऽसौ फट् प्राणाय त्वा व्यानाय त्वा ॥

3. O brilliant soul, self-made art thou, for all subtle and gross bodily organs, and for the learned who purify us like the beams of the sun. May knowledge and vedic lore be acquired by thee!
O virtuous soul, I praise thee for thy nearness to God. Attain to that Adorable, Truthful God. Thou hast promptly crushed and killed the demon of ignorance. I extol thee for longevity and the acquisition of happiness!

४. उपयामगृहीतोऽस्यन्तर्यच्छ मधवन् पाहि सोमम् ।
उरुष्य राय एषो यजस्व ॥

4. O aspirant after yoga, thou art the master of yamas and niyamas. Control thou the internal vital breaths, mind and organs!
O rich lord, guard the supremacy emanating from yoga. Remove through the power of yoga all ills arising from ignorance, whereby thou mayest obtain supernatural power and the fulfilment of desires!

५. अन्तस्ते द्यावापृथिवी दधाम्यन्तर्दधाम्युर्वन्तरिक्षम् ।
सजूर्देवेभिरवरैः परैश्चान्तर्यामे मधवन् मादयस्व ॥

¹Through the grace and instructions of learned persons, one attains to the height of prosperity, truthful speech and true deed. Free from harm means fit to afford protection.

CHAPTER VII

5. O Yogi, I place in thy heart knowledge spacious like the sun and moon and mid-air's wide region. Like a friend, acquiring learning from the sages, and practising internal austerities, gladden others with the preliminary and advanced usages of Yoga!

६. स्वाङ्‌कृतोऽसि विश्वेभ्य इन्द्रियेभ्यो दिव्येभ्यः पार्थिवेभ्यो मनस्त्वाष्टु स्वाहा त्वा सुभव सूर्याय देवेभ्यस्त्वा मरीचिपेभ्यः उदानाय त्वा ॥

6. O supreme yogi, thy soul is self-made and eternal. Thou art competent to cultivate all spiritual, mundane and physical forces. I instruct thee to follow the lustrous usages of yoga, for exhibiting the practices of yoga like the sun, and for leading a pure and noble life by controlling breath!

May thou an aspirant after yoga attain to a mind full of yogic concentration, and know the best course for the observance of truth.

७. आ वायो भूष शुचिपा उप नः सहस्रं ते नियुतो विश्ववार ।
उपो ते अन्धो मद्मयामि यस्य देव दधिषे पूर्वपेयं वायवे त्वा ॥

7. O yogi, the cultivator of purity, and expert in the practices of yoga, adorn thyself with the manifold definite virtues of mental peace and contentment. O yogi, the possessor of diverse qualities, I send unto thee the hunger-allaying food. O elevator of the soul through yoga, thou possessest the yogic power to protect the pure yogis. I instruct thee to practice such a yoga!

८. इन्द्रवायू इमे सुता उप प्रयोभिरागतम् ।
इन्दवो वामुशन्ति हि ।
उपयामगृहीतोऽसि वायव इन्द्रवायुभ्यां त्वैष ते योनिः सजोषोभ्यां त्वा ॥

8. O student and teacher of yoga, these created pleasant objects like water etc. long for ye both. Come with them. O aspirant after yoga, thou hast been accepted with yogic yamas and niyamas, by the teacher of yoga, for acquiring the knowledge of the animate and inanimate objects through the power of yoga!

O teacher of yoga, this yoga is like your pain-dispelling house. I long for thee, well versed in the practice of yogic concentration, and the student of yoga, full of qualities necessary for yoga!

९. अयं वां मित्रावरुणा सुतः सोम ऋतावृधा ।
ममेदिह श्रुतꣳ हवम् ।
उपयामगृहीतोऽसि मित्रावरुणाभ्यां त्वा ॥

---

[5] God addresses a yogi. I means God.

[6] In this verse also God addresses a yogi. Just as the sun spreads lustre on the globe, so should a yogi teach the practices and systems of yoga to others.

[7] In this verse God addresses a yogi. A yogi ought to be very careful in his diet. He should take little but nourishing diet to satisfy his hunger.

9. O student and teacher of yoga, the augmenters of true knowledge, living in unison like the vital breaths, the Prana and Udana, here is this your accomplished supremacy of yoga. Listen to my praise. O worshipper, thou art endowed with noble traits, I welcome thee, who controls the vital breaths, the Prana and Udana!

१०. राया वयꣳ ससवाꣳसो मदेम हव्येन देवा यवसेन गाव: ।
तां धेनुं मित्रावरुणा युवं नो विश्वाहा धत्तमनपस्फुरन्तीमेष ते योनिर्ऋतायुभ्यां त्वा ॥

10. O learned persons, the discriminators between right and wrong, ye and we, should be delighted with acquirable riches, just as cows are with grass. O noble and friendly souls, ye both give us daily the speech that rightly teaches us the knowledge of yoga. O worshipper, this knowledge of yours is thy shelter like a house. We welcome thee along with the observers of Truth!

११. या वां कशा मधुमत्यश्विना सूनृतावती ।
तया यज्ञं मिमिक्षतम् ।
उपयामगृहीतोऽस्यश्विभ्यां त्वेष ते योनिर्माध्वीभ्यां त्वा ॥

11. O student and teacher of yoga, resplendent like the sun and the moon, desire to develop yoga by your sweet and dawn-like pleasant speech. O student of yoga, thou hast been welcomed for thy noble traits. This yoga of yours is a house unto thee for comfort!
We approach thee, well versed in yogic laws of the control of breath, and thy teacher, expert in the sweet practices and methods of yoga.

१२. तं प्रत्नथा पूर्वथा विश्वथेमथा ज्येष्ठतार्ति बर्हिषदꣳ स्वर्विदम् ।
प्रतीचीनं वृजनं दोहसे धुनिमाशुं जयन्तमनु यासु वर्धसे ।
उपयामगृहीतोऽसि शण्डाय त्वेष ते योनिर्वीरितां पाह्यपमृष्ट: शण्डो देवास्त्वा शुक्रपा:
प्र णयन्त्वनाधृष्टाऽसि ॥

12. O yogi, thou art the master of all the branches of yoga. This yogic propensity of thine conduces to thy happiness. Through yoga, freed from the shackles of ignorance, thou art full of peace. Thou elevatest thy soul through various yogic practices!

---

[9] Mitra and Varuna are the disciple and teacher. The disciple is spoken of as मित्र and the teacher as वरुण as he dispels the deficiencies and drawbacks of the disciple; or the teacher may be considered as मित्र being friendly and affectionate to his pupils, and the disciple as वरुण who cultivates virtues and shuns vices.

[10] मित्रावरुणा are the student and the teacher of yoga; ऋतायुभ्याम् also means the teacher and the disciple who aspire after Truth.

CHAPTER VII

Like all the ancient sages and yogis and modern yogis, thou perfectest the yoga, which is highly commendable, deeply seated in the soul, pleasure-giving, inimical to nescience, quick at success, elevating, victory-giving, and quiverer of bodily organs.

Let the guardians of yogic force, and yogis resplendent with the power of yoga, instruct thee in yoga. Mayest thou be invincible througn that yoga. Proect thou the manly power, which in turn will protect thee.

१३. सुवीरो वीरान् प्रजनयन् परीह्यभि रायस्पोषेण यजमानम् ।
सञ्जग्मानो दिवा पृथिव्या शुक्र: शुक्रशोचिषा निरस्त: शण्ड: शुक्रस्याधिष्ठानमसि ॥

13. O yogi, endowed with yogic force, cultivate noble traits, like an exalted hero. Go to all places. Be friendly towards the charitably disposed person, who perfects his riches through charity!

Thou art the mainstay of yoga, being full of mental peace, free from desire for passions, full of strength like the sun and earth, and purifier of all like the sun.

१४. अच्छिन्नस्य ते देव सोम सुवीर्यस्य रायस्पोषस्य ददितार: स्याम् ।
सा प्रथमा संस्कृतिर्विश्ववारा स प्रथमो वरुणो मित्रो अग्नि: ॥

14. O well mannered disciple desiring to learn yoga, we your teachers, are the givers for you of uninterrupted, chivalrous strength of the knowledge of yoga!

May our preliminary method of teaching, acceptable to all, be accomodating to thee. May he, who is spiritually advanced and highly learned amongst us, be first of all friendly to thee.

१५. स प्रथमो बृहस्पतिश्चिकित्वांस्तस्मा इन्द्राय सुतमा जुहोत स्वाहा ॥
तृम्पन्तु होत्रा मध्वो या: स्विष्टा या: सुप्रीता: सुहुता यत्स्वाहा स्याद्‌ग्नीत् ।

15. O pupils, just as a learned teacher, the protector of knowledge tries for advancement, so should ye, to be great, resort to truth and virtuous deeds!

Just as affable, sweet, high-minded, happy ladies, well versed in yoga, and a learned yogi, remain contented, so should ye, like them.

[12]This verse clearly describes the qualities and characteristics of a yogi. There is no ambiguity about its meaning. Mr. Griffith remarks, "The text taken with a variation from Rgveda 5.44.1 is hopelessly obscure." I find no obscurity in it. Mr. Griffith, interprets Shanda as a demon for whom the cup is drawn, and then offered to a deity, whereas Maharshi Dayananda interprets the word as 'full of peace.' A yogi is spoken of as invincible, but Mr. Griffith remarks: the right hip of the high altar, on which the Adhvaryu-deposits his cup is addressed and secured from the attacks of demons.' What sense is there in calling the hip of the altar as invincible. The interpretation of vedic mantras by Mr. Griffith is a meaningless jargon, the perusal of which shakens one's faith in the revelation of the vedas. God does not utter nonsense in the vedas, which are full of sense, wisdom, knowledge and truth. A biased interpreter cannot arrive at the correct significance of vedic hymns. To him the plainest verse seems to be hopelessly obscure, which is highly regrettable.

१६. अयं वेनश्चोदयत्पृश्निगर्भा ज्योतिर्जरायू रजसो विमाने ।
इममपाᳪ᳭ सङ्गमे सूर्यस्य शिशुं न विप्रा मतिभीरिहन्ति उपयामगृहीतोऽसि मर्काय त्वा ॥

16. O' skilful ruler, thou art equipped with army, the essential mainstay of kingship. I fix in its orbit, in the midst of spacious regions, this beautiful moon that covers the luminous stars, and is linked with the sun and the waters that it attracts. Just as learned persons wisely and respectfully accept a young pupil, so do I accept thee for curbing the sinful and establishing the code of morality!

१७. मनो न येषु हवनेषु तिग्मं विपः शच्या वनुथो द्रवन्ता ।
आ यः शर्याभिस्तुविनृम्णो अस्याश्रीणीतादिशं गमस्तावेष ते योनिः प्रजाः पाह्यपमृष्टो मर्कों देवास्त्वा मन्थिपाः प्र णयन्त्वनाधृष्टासि ॥

17. O' skilful ruler, this art of government is thy mainstay. Just as thou, master of wealth, and protector of thy subjects, and the wise people of thine, both perform Havan with alertness, and determined mind, and acting wisely contribute to tne welfare of the state, so should each subordinate of thine, on the signal of thy finger, remove enemies from all sides. Let the wicked and agonising foe be cast aside. Protect thy subjects!
Let the learned, who quell the foes, add to thy happiness. O people protect the ruler that grants ye independence and fearlessness!

१८. सुप्रजाः प्रजाः प्रजनयन् परीहृच्चभि रायस्योषेण यजमानम् ।
सञ्जग्मानो दिवा पृथिव्या मन्थी मन्थिशोचिषा निरस्तो मर्कों मन्थिनोऽधिष्ठानमसि ॥

18. O' ruler, having loyal subjects, whose maker art thou, fill with profuse wealth him who does noble deeds. Be thou patient like the Sun and Earth. Thou art the support of the just. With the moral power of thy justice, may the unjust be suppressed!

१९. ये देवासो दिव्येकादश स्थ पृथिव्यामध्येकादश स्थ ।
अप्सुक्षितो महिनैकादश स्थ ते देवासो यज्ञमिमं जुषध्वम् ॥

19. In their majesty, eleven mighty substances reside in heaven, on the earth and in respiration. Just as they perform their functions faithfully, so should you the members of the House of the People, carry on the administration of the State with zeal and devotion.

[19](a) The eleven substances in heaven are, Pran, Apan, Udan, Vyan, Saman, Nag, Kurma, Krikla, Dev Dutt, Dhananjya and soul. The first ten are the names of different breaths.
(b) The eleven substances on the earth are Earth, Water, Fire, Air, Space, Sun, Moon, Stars, Ego (अहंकार), and Mahat Tatva (महत्तत्व), Intellect, the second of the 25 principles of the Sankhyas and matter.
(c) The eleven substances in respiration are, Ear, Skin, Eye. Tongue, Nose, Speech, Hands, Feet, Anus, penis and mind.

२०. उपयामगृहीतोऽस्याग्रयणोऽसि स्वाग्रयण: ।
पाहि यज्ञं पाहि यज्ञपतिं विष्णुस्त्वामिन्द्रियेण पातु विष्णुं त्वम् पाह्यभि सवनानि पाहि ॥

20. O' ruler, thou art an embodiment of humility and vedic lore, thou art the doer of laudable deeds, and worthy of respect. Protect the administration of justice. May the virtuous, and the learned protect thee. May thou fully protect the learned, and all works that contribute to prosperity!

२१. सोम: पवते सोम: पवतेऽस्मै ब्रह्मणेऽस्मै क्षत्रायास्मै सुन्वते यजमानाय पवत एष ऊर्जे पवतेऽद्भ्य: श्रोषधीभ्य: पवते द्यावापृथिवीभ्यां पवते सुभूताय पवते विश्वेभ्यस्त्वा देवेभ्य एष ते योनिर्विश्वेभ्यस्त्वा देवेभ्य: ॥

21. O' learned people, just as the amiable ruler purifies himself for knowing God and the veda, tries to acquire military knowledge, makes strenuous efforts for the advancement of scholars and friends of learning, is eager to produce foodstuffs which add to our vitality, exerts for the collection of medicines and canalizing waters, desires for the light of the sun and improvement of all material objects, avoids vice to acquire virtue, so should ye and other citizens do. O ruler, successful administration is thy aim. We honour thee for the betterment of the learned, and noble qualities of thine!

२२. उपयामगृहीतोऽसीन्द्राय त्वा बृहद्वते वयस्वत उक्थाव्यं गृह्णामि ।
यत्त इन्द्र बहद्व्रयस्तस्मै त्वा विष्णवे त्वैष ते योनिरुक्थेभ्यस्त्वा देवेभ्यस्त्वा देवाव्यं यज्ञस्यायुषे गृह्णामि ॥

22. O General, I appoint thee, well versed in knowledge, the doer of valorous deeds, advanced in age, full of dignity, expert in the knowledge of arms, as Commander-in-chief of the forces. I direct thee to lead a grand life. I advise thee to be God-fearing. The command of the army is thy foremost duty. I enjoin thee to preserve the interests of the state, to perform praiseworthy vedic acts, cultivate and preserve noble qualities!

२३. मित्रावरुणाभ्यां त्वा देवाव्यं यज्ञस्यायुषे गृह्णामीन्द्राय त्वा देवाव्यं यज्ञस्यायुषे गृह्णामी-न्द्राग्निभ्यां त्वा देवाव्यं यज्ञस्यायुषे गृह्णामीन्द्रावरुणाभ्यां त्वा देवाव्यं यज्ञस्यायुषे गृह्णामीन्द्राबृहस्पतिभ्यां त्वा देवाव्यं यज्ञस्यायुषे गृह्णामीन्द्राविष्णुभ्यां त्वा देवाव्यं यज्ञस्यायुषे गृह्णामि ॥

23. We elect thee as head of the state, for the betterment of our country's administration, for the protection of the learned, the friendly and noble souls.
We elect thee, for the promotion of political conferences, for the encouragement of the learned and lofty souls.
We elect thee, for the promotion of engineering works, for establishing electrical power-houses, and for the advancement of knowledge.

[12]In this mantra the head of the state is advised to appoint a man as Commander-in-Chief who is the embodiment of knowledge, spirituality and valour. I refers to the head of the state.

We elect thee for making full use of electricity and water, for promoting industrial works, and spreading their knowledge. We elect thee, the master of the science of yoga, for the spread of literacy, and encouragement of the sages who preach religious truths.

We elect thee, the gratifier of those who know God, for the promotion of scientific knowledge, for the spread of theism and vedic lore.

२४. मूर्धानं दिवो अरति पृथिव्या वैश्वानरमृत आ जातमग्निम् ।
कविँ सम्राजमतिथिं जनानामासन्ना पात्रं जनयन्त देवाः ॥

24. Just as masters of the science of archery, who are at the top of the learned, like the sun that stands highest in the atmosphere, know the qualities of ores inside the earth, are well known for their good behaviour in the path of righteousness, afford delight to all, and are respected by all like a guest, protect mechanical arts through their selfless life, establish the qualities of lustrous fire as a king establishes the greatness of his country in the world, so should all do.

२५. उपयामगृहीतोऽसि ध्रुवोऽसि ध्रुवक्षितिर्ध्रुवाणां ध्रुवतमोऽच्युतानामच्युतक्षित्तम एष ते योनिर्वैश्वानराय त्वा ।
ध्रुवं ध्रुवेण मनसा वाचा सोममव नयामि ।
अथा न इन्द्र इद्विशोऽसपत्नाः समनसस्करत् ॥

25. O' God, Thou art realised through spiritual knowledge. Thou art unchangeable, the earth rests in Thee, Thou art firmest amongst the firm substances like sound and space, Thou art most Immortal amongst the immortal, Thou art the Fountain of the light of truth. I constantly, with a determined mind and voice accept Thee, as leader of humanity on the path of righteousness, and Creator of the universe. So now may Thou, the Dispeller of all miseries, make our people all of one heart and mind, and free from foes!

२६. यस्ते द्रप्स स्कन्दति यस्ते अँ शुग्र्वाच्युतो धिषणयोरुपस्थात् ।
अध्वर्योर्वा परि वा यः पवित्रात्तं ते जुहोमि मनसा वषट्कृतँ स्वाहा देवानामुत्क्रमणमसि ॥

26. O' performer of yajna, thy substances collected for the yajna, go forth in air everywhere. The substances offered in the yajna, being purified are let loose from the clouds in the sky, and come down to the earth. I ask thee to perform that yajna, which is conducted by Adhvaryu, Hota, Udgata and Brahma, and carry out thy resolution with a stout heart and truthful speech! Thou art the exalted light for the learned.

---

[23]In this mantra the subjects have been asked to elect their own ruler, who should be imbued with knowledge and noble qualities, and devoted to improve the country industrially and mechanically. This mantra is a clear proof that the vedas preach democracy, and are against autocracy.

[24]Swami Dayananda gives the purport of this mantra as follows:
Just as those who have the knowledge of the Dhanur Veda gain victory over their enemies by the use of fire in arms and planes, so should all others do.

[26]In this mantra God inculcates the yajman to perform the yajnas. Adhvaryu, Hota,

२७. प्राणाय मे वर्चोदा वर्चसे पवस्व व्यानाय मे वर्चोदा वर्चसे पवस्वो दानाय मे वर्चोदा वर्चसे पवस्व वाचे मे वर्चोदा वर्चसे पवस्व क्रतूदक्षाभ्यां मे वर्चोदा वर्चसे पवस्व श्रोत्राय मे वर्चोदा वर्चसे पवस्व चक्षुर्भ्यां मे वर्चोदसौ वर्चसे पवेथाम् ॥

27. O' teacher, grow thou pure for my outward breath, and impart knowledge to me. O' giver of spirituality, grow thou pure for my spreading breath, and supply food to me. O imparter of knowledge grow thou pure for my upward breath and grant me prowess. O' preacher of truth, be attentive to my speech and eminence. O educator teach me as how to improve my soul-force and intellect, and how to acquire sound knowledge. O teacher of grammar, teach for my ear that catches sound, the relation of the words with their meanings and their use. O' learned guest and teacher teach me true principles!

२८. आत्मने मे वर्चोदा वर्चसे पवस्वौजसे मे वर्चोदा वर्चसे पवस्वायुषे मे वर्चोदा वर्चसे पवस्व विश्वाभ्यो मे प्रजाभ्यो वर्चोदसौ वर्चसे पवेथाम् ॥

28. O teacher of yoga and knowledge of God, reveal thy soul-force for my soul. O giver of knowledge, teach me yoga, for the amelioration of my soul. O' giver of strength, for my long life, give me the disease-killing medicine. O' learner and teacher of yoga, ye both strive for imparting noble qualities to my descendants!

२९. कोऽसि कतमोऽसि कस्यासि को नामासि ।
यस्य ते नामामन्महि यं त्वा सोमेनातीतृपाम ।
भूर्भुवः स्वः सुप्रजाः प्रजाभिः स्याॐ सुवीरो वीरैः सुपोषैः पोषैः ॥

29. O' king, who art thou? Who amongst us all art thou? Whose son art thou? What is thy name? We want to have thy knowledge, and satisfy thee with wealth!
I like the majesty of the Earth, the Space, and the Sun, desirous of my betterment, wish to have good subjects like you; be possessed of warlike soldiers like you, be vigorous by the use of life-giving substances.

३०. उपयामगृहीतोऽसि मधवे त्वोपयामगृहीतोऽसि माधवाय त्वोपयामगृहीतोऽसि शुक्राय त्वोपयामगृहीतोऽसि शुचये त्वोपयामगृहीतोऽसि नभसे त्वोपयामगृहीतोऽसि नभस्याय त्वोपयामगृहीतोऽसीषे त्वोपयामगृहीतोऽस्यूर्जे त्वोपयामगृहीतोऽसि सहसे त्वोपयाम-गृहीतोऽसि सहस्याय त्वोपयामगृहीतोऽसि तपसे त्वोपयामगृहीतोऽसि तपस्याय त्वो-पयामगृहीतोऽस्यॐ हससपतये त्वा ॥

Udgata, and Brahma are the custodians and conductors of the yajna with separate duties alloted to them.

²⁹This mantra is a dialogue between the king and his subjects. In the first part of the text the subjects question the ruler to know his identity. In the second half, the ruler replies identifying himself completely with the men placed in his charge.

30. O King, thou art the master of the art of administration, we accept thee as our Lord, in all the twelve months of Chaitra, Vaisakha, Jyaishtha, Ashadha, Sravana, Bhadra, Asvin, Kartika, Margashirsha, Pausha, Magha, Phalguna months, and for the protection of us all!

३१. इन्द्राग्नी आ गत ॐ सुतं गीर्भिर्नभो वरेण्यम् ।
अस्य पातं धियेषिता ।
उपयामगृहीतोऽसीन्द्राग्निभ्यां त्वैष ते योनिरिन्द्राग्निभ्यां त्वा ॥

31. O Speaker and members of the Assembly, shining like the sun and fire, assemble together, and add to our immense pleasure through didactic discussions. Protect our welfare with your trained intellect!

You have been initiated in the rules and duties of government. We realise your relation towards us. The art of administration is your shelter. We explain this to you.

३२. आ घा ये अग्निमिन्धते स्तृणन्ति बर्हिरानुषक् ।
येषामिन्द्रो युवा सखा ।
उपयामगृहीतोऽस्यग्नीन्द्राभ्यां त्वैष ते योनिरग्नीन्द्राभ्यां त्वा ॥

32. The members of the Parliament, well versed in vedic lore, throw light on learning and science; and overcast the sky uninterruptedly with planes. The President of the Republic is ever young, stout in body, friendly and imposing. Those brilliant and illustrious members take you as loyal subjects. Justice is your shelter. We teach you the above mentioned arts.

३३. आ मासश्चर्षणीधृतो विश्वे देवास आ गत ।
दाश्वा ॐ सो दाशुषः सुतम् ।
उपयामगृहीतोऽसि विश्वेभ्यस्त्वा देवेभ्य एष ते योनिर्विश्वेभ्यस्त्वा देवेभ्यः ॥

33. O' ye all learned people, the nourishers and preservers of humanity with noble qualities; the imparters of knowledge, accept this son of a charitably disposed person as your pupil!

O pupil, I accept thee as a seeker after knowledge. I instruct thee to serve all the learned persons, whereby thou mayest enlarge thy store of knowledge. I move the learned to impart good instructions to thee!

---

[30] The subjects accept the king as their ruler throughout the year, and the king accepts the subjects as his advisers for the whole year. This is the ideal of democracy. The ruler is elected vide vedic teaching. There is no vestige of autocracy, despotism or totalitarianism. The king is made and unmade. Chaitra is Mid March to Mid April. Vaisakh is April-May, Jyaishtha is May-June, Ashadh June-July, Sravana, July-August. Bhadra, August-September, Aswin, September-October, Kartika, October-November, Margashirsha, November-December, Pausha, December-January. Magha, January-February. Phalguna, February-March.

[31] We means the Speaker and members of the Parliament, and you the subjects. The text is a dialogue. In the first half, the people request the Speaker and members of the House of the People, and in the latter half of the text they reply.

३४. विश्वे देवास आ गत शृणुता म इमꣳ हवम् ।
एदं बर्हिनिषीदत ।
उपयामगृहीतोऽसि विश्वेभ्यस्त्वा देवेभ्य एष ते योनिर्विश्वेभ्यस्त्वा देवेभ्यः ॥

34. O ye all learned people, come near us, hear our invocations. Seat yourselves upon this seat. O son, thou hast been accepted as a pupil by the learned, we hand thee over to them for acquiring knowledge. Let the attainment of learning be thy aim. We desire thee to receive knowledge from them!

३५. इन्द्र मरुत्व इह पाहि सोमं यथा शार्याते अपिबः सुतस्य ।
तव प्रणीती तव शूर शर्मन्ना विवासन्ति कवयः सुयज्ञाः ।
उपयामगृहीतोऽसीन्द्राय त्वा मरुत्वत एष ते योनिरिन्द्राय त्वा मरुत्वते ॥

35. O' ruler, the remover of our difficulties, worthy of praise, and guardian of the subjects, advance the cause of education in the universe, as thou hast drunk deep the essence of knowledge with thy efforts!

O valiant king, under thy just rule, the wise and the learned, carry out thy sound policy!

O king, thou hast been recognised for the protection of the subjects. We like thee for thy good relations with the subjects and thy august personality. The spread of education is thy foremost duty. We recognise thee as our ruler for thy good relations with the subjects and thy august personality!

३६. मरुत्वन्तं वृषभं वावृधानमकवारिं दिव्यꣳ शासमिन्द्रम् ।
विश्वासाहमवसे नूतनायोग्रꣳ सहोदामिह तꣳ हुवेम ।
उपयामगृहीतोऽसीन्द्राय त्वा मरुत्वत एष ते योनिरिन्द्राय त्वा मरुत्वते ।
उपयामगृहीतोऽसि मरुतां त्वौजसे ॥

36. We learned persons accept as our ruler, thee, the introducer of new plans for our advancement, the master of loyal subjects, the embodiment of virtue, the most advanced in noble qualities and acts, the queller of the irreligious, the pure, the specimen of endurance, the master of prowess, and the helper and educator of all.

As thou art the master of all laws big or small; we accept thee, for having good subjects, and possessing supremacy. The administration of justice is thy duty. As thou art the master of all laws big or small, we accept thee for having good subjects and possessing supremacy. We accept thee as our head for enhancing the might of the people.

---

[34]"We refers to the parents.

[35]Mahidhar and Griffith have wrongly interpreted शार्याते as the grandson of Manu and the son of Sharyati, as there is no mention to this effect in the Shatapath Brahman, and the Vedas are free from historical references. Rishi Dayananda translates it as through the exertion of hands and feet.

३७. सजोषा इन्द्र सगणो मरुद्भिः सोमं पिब वृत्रहा शूर विद्वान् ।
जहि शत्रूँ२ रप मृधो नुदस्वाथाभयं कृणुहि विश्वतो नः ।
उपयामगृहीतोऽसीन्द्राय त्वा मरुत्वतं एष ते योनिरिन्द्राय त्वा मरुत्वते ॥

37. O' Commander of the army, fearless in the extirpation of foes, thou art accepted as head according to military laws. This exalted position is a source of inspiration for thee.

I enjoin thee to prepare for war embodying the use of shooting weapons. I acknowledge thee as exerting utmost for the battle. Be thou friendly unto all, and lead thy soldiers. Just as the sun, imbibes the essence of all objects through air, so should'st thou realise the significance of all objects. Acquire knowledge, and suppress the opponents of truth and justice. Be victorious in the battle-field. Make all free from fear everywhere.

३८. मरुत्वाँ२ इन्द्र वृषभो रणाय पिबा सोममनुष्वधं मदाय ।
आ सिञ्चस्व जठरे मध्व ऊर्मिं त्वँ राजासि प्रतिपत्सुतानाम् ।
उपयामगृहीतोऽसीन्द्राय त्वा मरुत्वत एष ते योनिरिन्द्राय त्वा मरुत्वते ॥

38. Thou, head of the state, the conqueror of enemies, the lord of five classes of subjects under thy sway, and armies, strong in body and soul, take with thy meals, invigorating herbs, for pleasure and conquest. Fill thy belly with the sweet flow of well-cooked meals. Thou art the sovereign of all great deeds and requiring deep thought. Thou hast been initiated in the rules of administration; we harness thee for battle involving the use of arms and weapons. This battle is the source of thy prosperity; hence we goad thee to that battle.

३६. महाँ२ इन्द्रो नृवदा चर्षणिप्रा उत द्विबर्हा अमिनः सहोभिः ।
अस्मद्रघ्चवावृधे वीर्यायोः पृथुः सुकृतः कर्तृभिर्भूत् ।
उपयामगृहीतोऽसि महेन्द्राय त्वेष ते योनिमंहेन्द्राय त्वा ॥

39. O' God, Thou art attainable through yoga. Thy worship contributes to our good and advancement. We serve Thee to become great. Thou art Supreme. Come like a just leader. Thou impartest pleasure to humanity. Thou art coupled with temporal and spiritual knowledge. Through omniscience Thou knowest us all. Unlimited is Thy might. Thou art vast and Great. Noble souls take Thee as the doer of great deeds and full of splendour. Depending upon Thee, we are encouraged to be great through acts of prowess!

४०. महाँ२ इन्द्रो य ओजसा पर्जन्यो वृष्टिमाँ२ इव ।
स्तोमैर्वत्सस्य वावृधे ।
उपयामगृहीतोऽसि महेन्द्राय त्वेष ते योनिमंहेन्द्राय त्वा ॥

[37] I means God. In this text God asks the Commander of the army to do his duty faithfully and energetically.

[38] Five subjects:—Brahmanas, Kshatriyas, Vaishas, Sudras and Dasyus. We refers to learned persons expert in military arts.

CHAPTER VII

40. O' Eternal, Omnipresent God, Thou art attainable through yoga, we resort to Thee for supremacy that results from yoga. This yoga performed for Thine attainments conduces to our welfare. Hence we worship Thee for emancipation. Thou art Great. Like the raining cloud, Thou art famous with the praises of the worshipper. Knowing Thee, the yogi attains to spiritual advancement!

४१. उदु त्यं जातवेदसं देवं वहन्ति केतवः ।
दृशे विश्वाय सूर्यꣳ स्वाहा ॥

41. Just as rays exhibit the shining all-penetrating sun to the whole world, so do the learned, with truthful speech expatiate on God, All knowing, the light of all, for the benefit of humanity.

४२. चित्रं देवानामुदगादनीकं चक्षुर्मित्रस्य वरुणस्याग्नेः ।
आप्रा द्यावापृथिवी अन्तरिक्षꣳ सूर्य आत्मा जगतस्तस्थुषश्च स्वाहा ॥

42. God is wonderful, mightier than all the forces of nature and learned persons. He is the Displayer of air, water and fire. He is the Protector of the Sun, Earth and Atmosphere. He is Resplendent, and Soul of all that moves and all that moves not. Always worship Him alone.

४३. अग्ने नय सुपथा राये अस्मान्विश्वानि देव वयुनानि विद्वान् ।
युयोध्यस्मज्जुहुराणमेनो भूयिष्ठां ते नम उक्तिं विधेम स्वाहा ॥

43. O' God, for the attainment of yoga, lead us on, through the path of yoga, to all the secrets of yoga. Whereby, we may offer Thee ample adoration through vedic texts. Thou, the Giver and Knower of Yoga, remove from us the sin resulting from the crookedness of our heart!

४४. अयं नो अग्निर्वरिवस्कृणोत्वयं मृधः पुर एतु प्रभिन्दन् ॥
अयं वाजाञ्जयतु वाजसातावयꣳ शत्रूञ्जयतु जह्ऱ्षाणः स्वाहा ॥

44. This first warrior, the master of medical science, keeps us free from disease on the battle-field. This second warrior, the destroyer of foes, marches forth on the battle-field. This third warrior, the preacher, should encourage the fast moving brave soldiers. This fourth warrior, full of delight, should subdue the irreligious foes.

४५. रूपेण वो रूपमभ्यागां तुथो वो विश्ववेदा वि भजतु ।
ऋतस्य पथा प्रेत चन्द्रदक्षिणा वि स्वः पश्य व्यन्तरिक्षं यतस्व सदस्यः ॥

⁴³This verse is identical with 5.36. but has a different interpretation.
⁴⁴In this text four kinds of warriors have been mentioned as necessary in war. One who is a medical man, and looks to the health of the soldiers. The other is a preacher, who with his eloquence keeps up the drooping spirits of the soldiers. The third scolds, chides and rebukes the foes. The fourth defeats the foes. Victory is won by the concerted action of all the four. This verse is identical with 5.37, but has a different interpretation.

45. O' people, just as I have attained to your beauty through my beauty; so like the Omniscient God, the President of the State should fix ye in your respective duty!

O head of the State, the encyclopaedia of knowledge, like the lustrous sun, through the path of righteousness, settle thy mature policy, and exert in unison with the members of the House of the People. O' ye rich persons, the givers of gold as remuneration lead a religious life!

४६. ब्राह्मणमद्य विदेयं पितृमन्तं पैतृमत्यमृषिमार्षेय꣱ सुधातुदक्षिणम् । अस्मद्द्राता देवत्रा गच्छत प्रदातारमा विशत ॥

46. May I honour the Brahman, who knows God and the Vedas, is sprung from a laudable father and grandfather, is a sage himself, knows the knowledge imparted by the sages, is the fit recipient of rich guerdon, and is charitably disposed; so should you approach the learned who possess noble qualities, acts, and attributes, are the bestowers of virtue on us, and learn good traits from them.

४७. अग्नये त्वा मह्यां वरुणो ददातु सोऽमृतत्त्वमशीयायुर्दात्र एधि मयो मह्यां प्रतिग्रहीत्रे रुद्राय त्वा मह्यां वरुणो ददातु सोऽमृतत्त्वमशीय प्राणो दात्र एधि वयो मह्यां प्रतिग्रहीत्रे वृहस्पतये त्वा मह्यां वरुणो ददातु सोऽमृतत्त्वमशीय त्वग्दात्र एधि मयो मह्यां प्रतिग्रहीत्रे यमाय त्वा मह्यां वरुणो ददातु सोऽमृतत्त्वमशीय हयो दात्र एधि वयो मह्यां प्रतिग्रहीत्रे ॥

47. O' teacher, I, thy pupil anxious to lead a life of Brahmcharya for 24 years have been handed over to thee by the learned. May I acquire knowledge. May the learned live long. Grant happiness to me, the seeker after knowledge.

O' teacher, the subduer of the wicked, I thy pupil, desirous of leading a life of Brahmcharya for fortyfour years, have been handed over to thee by the learned. May I learn the ways of achieving salvation, and my teacher the science of yoga. Grant me, the seeker after knowledge, the pleasure of the three stages of life. O illustrious teacher, I, thy pupil, desirous of leading a life of celibacy for forty-eight years, have been handed over to thee by the learned. May I enjoy the pleasure of knowledge; and my teacher feel comfortable both in heat and cold. Grant the pleasure of full knowledge to me, the seeker after knowledge, O' self-controlled, sinless, learned teacher, I, thy pupil, free from the pleasures of a married life, have been handed over to thee by the learned. May I attain to the pleasure of salvation; and my learned

---

[45]Rishi Dayananda writes in the purport of this mantra, that a king should organise three societies for effective administration of his rule, Raj Sabha, which should deal with the political affairs of the state, Vidya Sabha, which should spread education, and Dharam Sabha, which should administer to the spiritual requirements of the people.

[46]I means the ruler, the head of the state, and you the people, the subjects.

[47]Three stages of life are childhood, manhood and old age.

CHAPTER VII
75

teacher acquire the knowledge of God and the vedas.
Grant me, a student of thine the pleasure of a long life.

४८. कोऽदात्कस्मा अदात्कामोऽदात्कामायादात् ।
कामो दाता काम: प्रतिग्रहीता कामैतत्ते ॥

48. Who bestows. Upon whom does he bestow? God bestows. To soul is bestowed the fruit of its actions.

God is the giver and soul the receiver. O' soul, for thy benefit, do I give this vedic instruction.

CHAPTER VIII

१. उपयामगृहीतोऽस्यादित्येभ्यस्त्वा । विष्णु उरुगायैष ते सोमस्तꣳ रक्षस्व मा त्वा दभन् ॥

1. O' Brahmchari, who hast observed celibacy upto forty eight years, I who hast led a life of celibacy for twenty-four years, select thee as my husband. Thou knowest the details of religious lore, dost possess an august personality. This domestic life contributes to thy prosperity. Protect it. May the arrows of Cupid never torment thee!

२. कदा चन स्तरीरसि नेन्द्र सश्चसि दाशुषे ।
उपोपेन्नु मधवन् भूय इन्नु ते दानं देवस्य पृच्यत आदित्येभ्यस्त्वा ॥

2. O' glorious husband, thou never keepest anything secret from me, thou befriendest the charitably disposed person. O' laudable wealthy husband thou art learned. May thy gift of knowledge and riches reach me soon. I select thee as my husband, as thou art always a source of comfort for me!

३. कदा चन प्र युच्छस्युभे नि पासि जन्मनी ।
तुरीयादित्य सवनं त इन्द्रियमातस्थावमृतं दिव्यादित्येभ्यस्त्वा ॥

3. O' husband, thou art never neglectful, thou guardest both the present life, and the life to come. Thou, shining like the sun in knowledge, if thou controllest thy organ of procreation, wilt derive perpetual pleasure in thy affairs. O' finisher of the fourth Ashrama (stage of life) I select thee as my husband for my perpetual happiness!

४. यज्ञो देवानां प्रत्येति सुम्नमादित्यासो भवता मृडयन्तः ।
आ वोऽर्वाची सुमतिर्ववृत्याद्ꣳ होश्चिद्या वरिवोवित्तरासदादित्येभ्यस्त्वा ॥

4. Marriage of the learned couple is a source of pleasure. O noble persons may your fine intellect, that understands the significance of married life, make you well versed in knowledge after the completion of student life; and teach you how to conduct truthful dealings, and tread on the path of virtue. May you conduce to the pleasure of the newly married couple, through the knowledge and teaching you receive from the learned.

५. विवस्वन्नादित्यैष ते सोमपीथस्तस्मिन् मत्स्व ।
श्रदस्मै नरो वचसे दधातन यदाशीर्दा दम्पती वाममश्नुत ।
पुमान् पुत्रो जायते विन्दते वसुधा विश्वाहारप एधते गृहे ॥

5. O' husband, the master of different sciences, may this married life, in which thou drinkest the juices of different medicinal herbs, always give thee pleasure. O entrants into married life, stick to truth, honouring the vows taken at the time of marriage. In a home, where the husband and wife fulfil honestly the duties of married life, is born a son, who fulfils your desires, is sinless, enterprising, earns riches and prospers!

६. वाममद्य सवितर्वाममु श्वो दिवे दिवे वाममस्मभ्यꣳ सावी: ।
वामस्य हि क्षयस्य देव भूरेरया धिया वामभाज: स्याम ॥

6. O' God, the Fountain of happiness, give us happiness, today, tomorrow and on each day that passes; whereby, with our refined intellect, we may perform noble deeds in our married life, full of beauty and manifold aspirations!

७. उपयामगृहीतोऽसि सावित्रोऽसि चनोधाश्चनोधा असि चनो मयि धेहि ।
जिन्व यज्ञं जिन्व यज्ञपतिं भगाय देवाय त्वा सवित्रे ।

7. O' husband, thou hast been united with me through the ties of marriage. Thou art the worshipper of God. Thou art the master of foodstuffs; grant them to me. Safeguard your married life. I accept thee as the preserver of the yajna of our domestic life, the lord of riches, the pattern of beauty, and the progenitor of offspring!

८. उपयामगृहीतोऽसि सुशर्माऽसि सुप्रतिष्ठानो बृहदुक्षाय नम: ।
विश्वेभ्यस्त्वा देवेभ्य एष ते योनिर्विश्वेभ्यस्त्वा देवेभ्य: ॥

8. O husband, thou hast been united with me through the ties of wedlock. Thou art the master of fine houses, and a man of position. I give well cooked food to thee, full of vitality. This is thy comfortable edifice. I accept thee as the giver of different kinds of comforts, I place thee in the company of the learned !

९. उपयामगृहीतोऽसि बृहस्पतिसुतस्य देव सोम त इन्दोरिन्द्रियावत: ।
पत्नीवतो ग्रहाꣳ ऋध्यासम् ।
अहं परस्तादहमवस्तादन्तरिक्षं तदु मे पिताऽभूत् ।
अहꣳ सूर्यमुभयतो ददर्शाहं देवानां परमं गुहा यत् ॥

9. O prosperous and handsome husband, thou hast been united with me through ties of marriage. Thou art the embodiment of gentlemanliness, the lord of wealth, the master of a loyal wife, and the son of a father, having the knowledge of the Vedas. May I prosper on all sides following the teachings received at the time of marriage. May I obtain the imperishable knowledge that resides in the inmost recesses of the hearts of the learned. May I, receiving complete instruction from my teacher, a father unto me, realise on all sides the existence of God!

१०. अग्ना३इ पत्नीवन्त्सजूर्देवेन त्वष्ट्रा सोमं पिब स्वाहा ।
प्रजापतिर्वृषाऽसि रेतोधा रेतो मयि धेहि प्रजापतेस्ते वृष्णो रेतोधसो रेतोधामशीय ॥

10. O' husband, full of affection for me, the supplier of excellent comforts for me, the dispeller of all of my miseries, truthful in speech, drink the juice of medicinal herbs. O' master of a devoted wife, full of prowess and semen, thou art the progenitor of offspring. Impregnate semen in me. May I give birth to a valorous son, in connection with thee, the impregnator, the lord of vigour, and the guardian of the children!

११. उपयामगृहीतोऽसि हरिरसि हार्योयोजनो हरिभ्यां त्वा ।
हर्योधाना स्थ सहसोमा इन्द्राय ॥

11. O' husband, thou hast been accepted by me for married life. Just as a charioteer yokes the horses, so art thou fully competent to carry on the duties of a married man. May I serve thee seated in a war chariot yoked with disciplined horses. Ye members of my family, full of noble qualities, for acquiring prosperity, protect me and my husband, working together like horses for pulling on this chariot of our married life!

१२. यस्ते अश्वसनिर्भक्षो यो गोसनिस्तस्य त इष्टयजुष स्तुतस्तोमस्य शस्तोक्थस्योपहू-
तस्योपहूतो भक्षयामि ॥

12. O' affectionate and heroic husband, thou art the giver of scientific knowledge, polished speech, land and good instruction. Thou art conversant with the Yajur-veda, the Sama Veda, and the Rig Veda. Thou art invited and honoured by the learned. Invited by thee I eat the delicious meal prepared by thee!

१३. देवकृतस्यैनसोऽवयजनमसि मनुष्यकृतस्यैनसोऽवयजनमसि पितृकृतस्यैनसोऽवयजनमस्या-
त्मकृतस्यैनसोऽवयजनमस्येनस एनसोऽवयजनमसि ।
यच्चाहमेनो विद्वाँश्चकार यच्चाविद्वाँस्तस्य सर्वस्यैनसोऽवयजनमसि ॥

13. O' philanthropic husband, thou removest the sins of the donors. Thou removest the sins committed by ordinary human beings. Thou removest the sins committed by the parents. Thou removest the sins committed by yourself. Thou removest every sort of sin. The sin that I have knowingly committed, and the sin that unawares I have committed, of all that sin, thou art the remover!

१४. सं वर्चसा पयसा सं तनूभिरगन्महि मनसा सꣳ शिवेन ।
त्वष्टा सुदत्रो वि दधातु रायोऽनुमार्ष्टु तन्वो यद्विलिष्टम् ॥

14. O teacher, the giver of boons, the instructor of all doings, with noble intentions, water and food, remove thou our physical deficiency, and give us wealth. May we strengthen our bodies by the vow of celibacy!

१५. समिन्द्र णो मनसा नेषि गोभि: सꣳ सूरिभिर्मघवन्त्सꣳ स्वस्त्या ।
सं ब्रह्मणा देवकृतं यदस्ति सं देवानाꣳ सुमतौ यज्ञियानाꣳ स्वाहा ॥

15. O' adorable and learned teacher and preacher, as thou leadest us on the right path with the nobility of thy mind, teachest us exertion, with thy

---

[12] Naming three vedas means Karma, Jnana and Upasana, and not that the vedas are three and not four. Thee in both places means wife.

[13] Charity covers a multitude of sins. The husband is asked to remove the flaws of the donors by asking them to make the proper use of their wealth which will make them pure and noble by giving it in charity for the good of humanity. Sins can be avoided by didactic teachings by a selfless, learned husband.

sweet and joyful words, givest us knowledge through the learned and the teachings of the vedas, layest before us for example, the noble acts performed by the sages through wisdom and truthful speech, hence thou art worthy of respect by us!

१६. सं वर्चसा पयसा सं तनूभिरगन्महि मनसा सꣳ शिवेन ।
त्वष्टा सुदत्रो वि दधातु रायोऽनुमाष्टुं तन्वो यद्विलिष्टम् ॥

16. O highly learned persons, acting upon your judgment, may we approach amongst ye, him, who gives us good knowledge, removes the ills of ignorance, imparts knowledge to us day and night out of his vast store, and removes the ills of our body!

१७. धाता रातिः सविता दं जुषन्तां प्रजापतिर्निधिपा देवो अग्निः ।
त्वष्टा विष्णुः प्रजया सꣳ ररणा यजमानाय द्रविणं दधात स्वाहा ॥

17. O householder, thou art the source of happiness to all, the begetter of prosperity, the bringer-up of children. the guardian of the treasure of knowledge, the controller of vices, the extinguisher of the darkness of ignorance, the enlarger of pleasure, the pervader in all noble qualities and acts, being charitably disposed towards thy offspring, fulfil thou rightly the duties of married life, and grant stores of riches to the sacrificer!

१८. सुगा वो देवाः सदना अकर्म य आजग्मेदꣳ सवनं जुषाणाः
भरमाणा वहमाना हवीꣳ ष्यस्मे धत वसवो वसूनि स्वाहा ॥

18. O noble-minded learned people, earnestly have we acquired this wealth, retain it by self-effort and preserve it with the help of others. We prepare these comfortable houses for ye and amass wealth for mutual use. May ye also grant us abundant riches!

१९. याँꣳ२ आऽवह उशतो देव देवाँस्तान् प्रेरय स्वे अग्ने सधस्थे ।
जक्षिवाꣳ सः पपिवाꣳ सश्च विश्वेऽस्मिन् धर्मेꣳ स्वरातिष्ठतानु स्वाहा ॥

19. O good-natured teacher, persuade them to br religious-minded, who have gathered round thee to acquire knowledge. O, married people, lead ye all a life of happiness, taking nutritious diet, drinking pure water, rightly performing yajnas, and sharpening your intellect.

२०. वयꣳ हि त्वा प्रयति यज्ञे अस्मिन्नग्ने होतारमवृणीमहीह ।
ऋधगया ऋधगुताशमिष्ठाः प्रजानन् यज्ञमुप याहि विद्वान्त्स्वाहा ॥

20. O learned person, we married people, have, in this world, accepted thee as Hota in this yajna which is fulfilled through ceaseless effort!

[16]This verse has not been translated by Griffith and Pt. Jaidev Vidayalankar, as being a repetition of Yajur 2.24 and 8.14. No doubt all these three verses are the same in wording, but different in meaning. Readers can see for themselves the different interpretations put by Maharshi Dayananda on them.
[17]Sacrificer: the yajman, who perform, the yajna faithfully.
[20]Hota: one of the watchers and helpers of a yajna.

O' learned person, thou knowest the details of the yajna; come unto us, perform according to vedic rites, the yajna that leads us to prosperity, and grants us peace of mind through its performance!

२१. देवा गातुविदो गातुं विस्त्वा गातुमित ।
मनसस्पत इमं देव यज्ञ ❁ स्वाहा वाते धाः ॥

21. Ye, married people, who know the laws of gravitation, having known the science of geology, know ye the art of government. O' self-controlled, married learned people, let each one of ye, perform in a truly religious spirit this yajna of married life for pure dealings!

२२. यज्ञ यज्ञं गच्छ यज्ञपतिं गच्छ स्वां योनिं गच्छ स्वाहा ।
एष ते यज्ञो यज्ञपते सहसूक्तवाकः सर्ववीरस्तं जुषस्व स्वाहा ॥

22. O noble householder, perform rightly thy duties of married life: serve thy king, fully understand thy nature. O performer of yajna, perform truly and justly this yajna of domestic life, full of vedic texts, and giver of physically fit and spiritually advanced offspring!

२३. माहिर्भूर्मा पृदाकुः । उरु ❁ हि राजा वरुणश्चकार सूर्याय पन्थामन्वेतवा उ ।
अपदे पादा प्रतिधातवेऽकरुतापवक्ता हृदयाविधश्चत् ।
नमो वरुणायाभिष्ठितो वरुणस्य पाशः ॥

23. O ruler, be just progress. For easy walk make the inaccessible paths fit for journey. Establish the path of justice, so that people being God-fearing lead a religious life!

Never tell a lie. Don't use abusive language like him who hurts the feelings of noble souls.

Be not angry like a venomous serpent. Thou, full of valour, shouldst always try to keep ever ready thy fetters and sharp instruments.

२४. अग्नेरनीकमप आ विवेशापां नपात् प्रतिरक्षन्नसुर्यम् ।
दमेदमे समिधं यक्ष्यग्ने प्रति ते जिह्वा घृतमुच्चरण्यत् स्वाहा ॥

24. O married man, understand thou fully, the significance of water and the lustrous fire!

With full knowledge of the qualities that lead to success, unfaltering in nature, keeping thy gold in safety, preach thou in each house, the deeds that lead to the fulfilment of aims. Let thy tongue taste clarified butter and mayest thou duly protect thy body.

२५. समुद्रे ते हृदयमप्स्वन्तः सं त्वा विशन्त्वोषधीरुतापः ।
यज्ञस्य त्वा यज्ञपते सूक्तोक्तौ नमो वाके विधेम यत् स्वाहा ॥

25. O householder, let thy heart devoted to the study of the vedas, full of reverential words, controlled by vital breaths, be engaged in virtuous acts. May thou enjoy food, fruit and water. In affectionate accents, we urge thee to discharge faithfully thy duties of married life!

[25]We: Other learned householders.

CHAPTER VIII

२६. देवीराप एष वो गर्भस्त꣱ सुप्रीत꣱ सुभृतं बिभृत ।
देव सोमँष ते लोकस्तस्मिञ्छ च वक्ष्व परि च वक्ष्व ॥

26. O good tempered, lovely women, retain carefully, dearly loved, and well nurtured child in the womb.
O nice, dignified husband, this is thy domestic life, make it resplendent with pleasure and instruction, and guard it in every possible way!

२७. अवभृथ निचुम्पुण निचेरुरसि निचुम्पुण: ।
अब देवैर्देवकृतमेनोऽयासिषभव मर्त्यैर्मर्त्यकृतं पुरुरावणो देवं रिषस्पाहि देवाना꣱ समिदसि ॥

27. O husband, thou art the guardian of my pregnancy, a slow walker, a captivator of the heart, an accumulator of wealth in a righteous way; and supreme among the learned!
Thou enjoying the company of the wise and ordinary mortals, guard me against the ignoble and impious sin, I may be tempted to commit towards lascivious and ordinary people.

२८. एजतु दशमास्यो गर्भो जरायुणा सह ।
यथायं वायुरेजति यथा समुद्र एजति ।
एवायं दशमास्यो अस्रञ्जरायुणा सह ॥

28. Let, still unborn, the ten-month old child move with the secundines. Just as the wind moves, as the ocean moves, uninterruptedly, so may this ten-month child come forth together with the secundines.

२९. यस्यै ते यज्ञियो गर्भो यस्यै योनिहिरण्ययी ।
अङ्गान्यहुता यस्य तं मात्रा समजीगम꣱ स्वाहा ॥

29. O wife, thou hast a womb free from disease and offspring meet for adoration. May I graciously receive thee with the child undeformed; after cohabitation with thee desirous of pregnancy!

३०. पुरुदस्मो विषुरूप इन्दुरन्तर्महिमानमानञ्ज धीर: ।
एकपदीं द्विपदीं त्रिपदीं चतुष्पदीमष्टापदीं भुवनानु प्रथन्ता꣱ स्वाहा ।

30. A husband, the dispeller of miseries, handsome in appearance, full of dignity, and strong in mind should wish for successful pregnancy in his life.
He should preach to mankind the one footed, two-footed, three-footed, four-footed and eight-footed knowledge of the vedas.

[28]Secundines: After-birth Jrayu.
[30]One-footed: that teaches the significance of Om alone. Two-footed: that tells of the pleasures of this world and the next world.
Three-footed: that preaches the delights of speech, mind and body.
Four-footed: That tells us of Dharma (religion) Artha. (worldly prosperity).
Kama (Desire) and Moksha (Salvation, final beatitude).
Eight-footed that dilates on four Ashramas and four Varunas.
Pt. Jaidev Vidyalankar, interprets two-footed as words and their significance.
Three-footed as Rig, Yaju, and Sam.

३१. मरुतो यस्य हि क्षये पाथा दिवो विमहसः ।
स सुगोपातमो जनः ॥

31. O adorable, learned married persons, in whomsoever's house ye go, and observe therein the display of wealth and fine qualities, he is truly the cultivator of earth, and master of speech!

३२. मही द्यौः पृथिवी च न इमं यज्ञं मिमिक्षताम् ।
पिपृतां नो भरीमभिः ॥

32. O praiseworthy and well-built husband and forbearing wife. desire to fulfil with pleasure, and perform this domestic yajna. May ye both provide us with food and clothes!

३३. आ तिष्ठ वृत्रहन्रथं युक्ता ते ब्रह्मणा हरी ।
अर्वाचीनँ सु ते मनो ग्रावा कृणोतु वग्नुना ।
उपयामगृहीतोऽसीन्द्राय त्वा षोडशिन एष ते योनिरिन्द्राय त्वा षोडशिने ॥

33. O married man, thou art the dispeller of foes, and sprinkler of happiness like a cloud. In this chariot of thy life of a house-holder, possessing water and riches, are yoked two horses of restraint and attraction. Take a vow to lead the life of a householder. Appease thy drooping mind with the sayings of the vedas. Thou art fully equipped with the requisites of married life. I order thee to lead married life full of prosperity and sixteen traits. This is thy home. I order thee to lead married life full of prosperity and sixteen traits!

३४. युक्ष्वा हि केशिना हरी वृषणा कक्ष्यप्रा ।
अथा न इन्द्र सोमपा गिरामुपश्रुतिं चर ।
उपयामगृहीतोऽसीन्द्राय त्वा षोडशिन एष ते योनिरिन्द्राय त्वा षोडशिने ॥

34. O protector of riches, and dispeller of foes, harness in the chariot thy pair of studs, long-maned, stout in body, and fast to lead thee to destination. Know thou the requests made in our applications!

Thou art fully equipped with the requisites of married life. I order thee to lead married life full of prosperity and sixteen traits. This is thy home. I order thee to lead a married life full of prosperity and sixteen traits.

---

[32]Yajna: Grihastha, i.e., married life.
[33]Sixteen kalas or parts in the life of a householder.
1. Pran (Breath), 2. Shradha (Faith), 3. Kham (Happiness), 4. Vayu (Activity), 5. Jyoti (Brilliance), 6. Apa (water) 7. Prithvi (Forbearance), 8. Indriya (organ), 9. Manas (mind), 10. Anna (food), 11. Virya (Semen), 12. Tapa (Penance, religious austerity), 13. Mantra (understanding), 14. Ichha (Ambition), 15. Loka (Mankind), 16. Nam (Anger or censure) vide Prashnopanishad A Grihasthi should cultivate these sixteen qualities. Pt. Jaidev Vidyalankar, mentions sixteen ministers of a country as 16 kalas of a ruler.

I: God.
[34]In this verse reference is made to a married ruler. First portion refers to the subjects, and the second to God.

३५. इन्द्रमिद्धरी वहतोऽप्रतिधृष्टशवसम् ।
ऋषीणां च स्तुतीरुप यज्ञं च मानुषाणाम् ।
उपयामगृहीतोऽसीन्द्राय त्वा षोडशिन एष ते योनिरिन्द्राय त्वा षोडशिने ॥

35. Pair of trained horses, carry the commander of forces, whose strength is unconquerable.

O brave king, accept thou the praises of the seers of the purport of the vedas, of the warriors, and the homage of ordinary mortals. I order thee to lead a married life full of prosperity and sixteen traits. This is thy duty as a ruler. I order thee to lead a married life full of prosperity and sixteen traits, so that thy subjects and soldiers may seek thy protection!

३६. यस्मान्न जातः परो अन्यो अस्ति य आविवेश भुवनानि विश्वा ।
प्रजापतिः प्रजया संरराणस्त्रीणि ज्योतींषि सचते स षोडशी ॥

36. Than Whom there is none other born more mighty, Who hast pervaded all places. God, the giver of blessings to the whole world, maintains the three lustres in all substances. He is the giver of sixteen qualities.

३७. इन्द्रश्च सम्राड् वरुणश्च राजा तौ ते भक्षं चक्रतुरग्र एतम् ।
तयोरहमनु भक्षं भक्षयामि वाग्देवी जुषाणा सोमस्य तृप्यतु सह प्राणेन स्वाहा ॥

37. O people, the powerful central ruler, and the noble provincial ruler, serve and protect ye first. I serve ye after them!

For the attainment of knowledge and progress, may we all be contented with strength, truthful speech, and divine vedic lore.

३८. अग्ने पवस्व स्वपा अस्मे वर्चः सुवीर्यम् ।
दधद्रयिं मयि पोषम् ।
उपयामगृहीतोऽस्यग्नये त्वा वर्चसे एष ते योनिरग्नये त्वा वर्चसे ।
अग्ने वर्चस्विन्वर्चस्वांस्त्वं देवेष्वसि वर्चस्वानहं मनुष्येषु भूयासम् ॥

38. O ruler, the doer of noble deeds, and a student of the vedas, be thou pure. Grant us strength, and the study of the Vedas. Grant me wealth and affluence. We have chosen thee for administrative purposes. We accept thee for the grant of strength and the attainment of God. This country is thy home. We accept thee for the grant of strength, and the attainment of God. O' lustrous ruler, thou art splendid amid the sages. May I among mankind be bright with lustre!

३९. उत्तिष्ठन्नोजसा सह पीत्वी शिप्रे अवेपयः । सोममिन्द्र चमू सुतम् ।
उपयामगृहीतोऽसीन्द्राय त्वौजस एष ते योनिरिन्द्राय त्वौजसे ।
इन्द्रौजिष्ठौजिष्ठस्त्वं देवेष्वस्योजिष्ठोऽहं मनुष्येषु भूयासम् ॥

---

[36] Three lustres: sun, lightning, and fire. Shodashi:-the sixteen kalas mentioned in the Prashnopanishad. He does not possess all these qualities in Him, but is their Giver and Author. A Grihasthi should worship Him alone.

[37] I : A learned public-spirited person.

39. O powerful ruler, having attained to strength through thy army, and arising in thy physical and spiritual strength, thou shockest thy jaws!

We have chosen thee for administrative purposes. We accept thee for the grant of strength and the attainment of God. This country is thy home. We accept thee for the grant of strength and the attainment of God. O' most lustrous ruler, thou art the mightiest amongst the kings fighting for victory! Among mankind I fain would be most mighty.

४०. अदृश्रमस्य केतवो वि रश्मयो जनाँ२ अनु । भ्राजन्तो अग्नयो यथा ।
उपयामगृहीतोऽसि सूर्याय त्वा भ्राजायैष ते योनि: सूर्याय त्वा भ्राजाय ।
सूर्ये भ्राजिष्ठ भ्राजिष्ठस्त्वं देवेष्वसि भ्राजिष्ठोऽहं मनुष्येषु भूयासम् ॥

40. Just as resplendent rays and fires make known the objects of this earth, so do I make known men.

We have chosen thee for administrative purposes.

We accept thee for the grant of strength and the attainment of God. This duty of administration conduces to thy prosperity. I remind thee to spread the light of knowledge and lead a pure life. I urge thee to follow the Self-Effulgent God in administering justice and spreading learning.

O brightest ruler, thou art brightest among the sages. Among mankind I fain would be the brightest!

४१. उदु त्यं जातवेदसं देवं वहन्ति केतव: ।
दृशे विश्वाय सूर्यम् । उपयामगहीतोऽसि सूर्याय त्वा भ्राजायैष ते योनि: सूर्याय त्वा भ्राजाय ॥

41. The learned as seers, verily dilate upon God, the Creator of the vedas, the Embodiment of purity and effulgence; for the good of humanity. May we realise that God. We accept thee for the control of highly active breath, through yoga and laws of austerity.

Thy universal pervasion through the union of cause and effect is an unsurpassed authority. We accept Thee as the Giver of resplendent knowledge.

४२. आ जिघ्र कलशं मह्या त्वा विशन्त्विन्दव: ।
पुनरूर्जा नि वर्तस्व सा न: सहस्रं धुक्ष्वोरुधारा पयस्वती पुनर्मा विशताद्रयि: ॥

42. O exalted wife, possessing vast knowledge, eatable and drinkable articles, smell thou the jar. Mayest thou obtain thousands of juices of medicinal herbs, whereby thou mayest be free from sorrow. Fill us again with prosperity. Let riches come again to me!

४३. इडे रन्ते हव्ये काम्ये चन्द्रे ज्योतेऽदिते सरस्वति महि विश्रुति ।
एता ते अद्य्ने नामानि देवेभ्यो मा सुकृतं ब्रूतात् ॥

---

[39] Shocking the jaws indicates readiness for battle.

[42] The jars in which the wife keeps eatables should be smelt and examined by her if they are fit for consumption and have not become rotten and decayed.

43. Praiseworthy, delightful, worshipful, lovable, pleasuregiving, well known for good behaviour, Inviolable, full of knowledge, Adorable, Knower of the vedas, worthy of respect. These are thy names O wife! Teach me the good lesson of acquiring noble qualities.

४४. वि न इन्द्र मृधो जहि नीचा यच्छ पृतन्यतः ।
यो अस्माँर् अभिदासत्यधरं गमया तमः ।
उपयामगृहीतोऽसीन्द्राय त्वा विमृध एष ते योनिर्न्द्राय त्वा विमृधे ॥

44. O general, beat our foes away, humble the men who challenge us. As the sun removes darkness, so send down to a degraded position, him who seeks to do us injury!

We accept thee equipped with forces for the grant of happiness and dispelling our foes. This action of thine is the secret of thy rule. We urge thee to grant us happiness and remove our enemies.

४५. वाचस्पतिं विश्वं कर्मणमूतये मनोजुवं वाजे अद्या हुवेम ।
स नो विश्वानि हवनानि जोषद्विश्वशम्भूरवसे साधुकर्मा ।
उपयामगृहीतोऽसीन्द्राय त्वा विश्वकर्मण एष ते योनिरिन्द्राय त्वा विश्वकर्मणे ॥

45. Let us invoke to-day, to aid our struggle for existence, the Lord of the Vedas, the Doer of all noble deeds, and the Knower of what passes in our minds. May He hear kindly all our invocations, Who gives us all bliss, Whose works are righteous.

This act of God is due to His love. We pray unto Thee for prosperity and success in all actions. We adore Thee for success in all actions and for prosperity.

४६. विश्वकर्मन् हविषा वर्धनेन त्रातारमिन्द्रमकृणोरवध्यम् ।
तस्मै विशः समनमन्त पूर्वीरयमुग्रो विहव्यो यथासत् ।
उपयामगृहीतोऽसीन्द्राय त्वा विश्वकर्मण एष ते योनिरिन्द्राय त्वा विश्वकर्मणे ॥

46. O doer of all good deeds, with ever-growing knowledge, thou selectest as a ruler one who is free from vice and irreligion, the giver of prosperity and protection. The educated subjects bow unto him. Exert that he becomes the suppressor of the wicked and the master of all resources. This act of thine is due to your love. We invoke thy aid for prosperity and success in all actions. We pray to thee for success in all actions, and for prosperity!

४७. उपयामगृहीतोऽस्यग्नये त्वा गायत्रच्छन्दसं गृह्णामीन्द्राय त्वा त्रिष्टुप्छन्दसं गृह्णामि
विश्वेभ्यस्त्वा देवेभ्यो जगच्छन्दसं गृह्णाम्यनुष्टप्तेऽभिगरः ॥

---

[43] In this verse eleven names of a wife have been enumerated, e.g., Ida, Ratna, Havya, Kamya, Chandra, Jyoti, Aditi, Saraswati, Mahi, Vishruti and Aghanya. How beautiful and splendid this verse is, which gives eleven qualities a woman should possess.

[46] Vedas preach the doctrine of democracy. A ruler is selected by election and not succession.

47. O noble king, thy praiseworthy speech dispels our ignorance. I accept thee, the knower of Gayatri metre verses, for knowing the attributes of fire and electricity. I accept thee, the preacher of the significance of vedic verses in Trishtup metre!

I accept thee, the expounder of the Jagati verses, for acquiring all good qualities, actions and attributes. Anushtap verses are thy preceptor. We have accepted thee for all these qualities.

४८. ब्रशीनाँ त्वा पत्मन्ना धूनोमि ।
कुकूननानां त्वा पत्मन्ना धूनोमि ।
भन्दनानां त्वा पत्मन्ना धूनोमि ।
मदिन्तमानां त्वा पत्मन्ना धूनोमि ।
मधुन्तमानां त्वा पत्मन्ना धूनोमि ।
"शुक्रं त्वा शुक्र आ धूनोभ्यह्ने रूपे सूर्यस्य रश्मिषु ॥

48. O irreligious husband, I warn thee against cohabitation with the pure and noble wives of others. O' evil-minded husband, I desist thee from approaching the tender-hearted wives of others. O' ill-intentioned husband I keep thee away from going near the philanthropic wives of others. O' unsteady husband, I censure thee again and again for teasing the delightful wives of others. O' stone-hearted husband, I separate thee from the company of sweet-tongued wives of others. O' ignorant husband, full of virility, I prohibit thee from sexual intercourse in day's light and sun's beams!

४६. ककुभं रूपं वृषभस्य रोचते बृहच्छुक्रः शुक्रस्य पुरोगाः सोमः सोमस्य पुरोगाः ।
यत्ते सोमादाभ्यं नाम जागृवि तस्मै त्वा गृह्लामि तस्मै ते सोम सोमाय स्वाहा ॥

49. O learned and educated King, the giver of pleasures, thy beauty shines pure like vast space. Be thou the undefiled leader of holy religion. Be thou the excellent leader of thy advancing country. Whatever invincible and stimulating popularity is thine, for that popularity I take thee. O king, as our stimulator for noble deeds, may I utter true words for thee, the doer of noble deeds!

५०. उशिक् त्वं देव सोमाग्नेः प्रियं पाथोऽपीहि वशी त्वं देव सोमेन्द्रस्य प्रियं पाथोऽपीह्यस्मत्सखा त्वं देव सोम विश्वेषां देवानां प्रियं पाथोऽपीहि ॥

50. O virtuous and prosperous King, eagerly know thou the lovable and protective conduct of a learned person. O charitable King, our impeller towards progress and affluence, controlling the passions, know thou the conduct of a religious person. O learned and wealthy King, being friend unto us, know thou, the beautiful conduct of all sages!

[47]Gayatri, Trishtup, Jagati and Anushtup are metres in which the vedic verses are revealed.
[48]This is a beautiful verse in which the wife is described as the saviour of her husband from moral degradation.

CHAPTER VIII

५१. इह रतिरिह रमध्वमिह धृतिरिह स्वधृतिः स्वाहा ।
उपसृजन् धरुणं मात्रे धरुणो मातरं धयन् ।
रायस्पोषमस्मासु दीधरत् स्वाहा ॥

51. O married people, in this domestic life is delight, here is surety, here the accumulation of wealth and the performance of virtuous acts; enjoy yourselves here. Produce the child. Let it suck its mother. Give us riches and abundance with noble intentions!

५२. सत्रस्य ऋद्धिरस्यगन्म ज्योतिरमृता अभूम ।
दिवं पृथिव्या अध्याऽरुहामाविदाम देवान्त्स्वर्ज्योतिः ॥

52. O learned person thou contributest to the progress of our government. In thy company may we obtain the light of wisdom; and attain to final beatitude. May our rule extend from the earth to the sky. May we obtain spiritual enjoyment, knowledge and pleasure!

५३. युवं तमिन्द्रापर्वता पुरोयुधा यो नः पृतन्यादरतं तमिद्धतं वज्रेण तंतमिद्धतम् ।
दूरे चत्ताय च्छन्त्सद्गहनं यदिनक्षत् ।
अस्माकꣳ शत्रून्परि शूर विश्वतो दर्मा दर्षीष्ट विश्वतः ।
भूर्भुवः स्वः सुप्रजाः प्रजाभिः स्याम सुवीरा वीरैः सुपोषाः पोषैः ॥

53. O commander and soldiers, who march forward in a battle, kill the man with warlike instruments, who fain would war with us!
If the forces of the enemy approach our sturdy forces and try to increase their strength, kill them without fail, and drive them away, for your own happiness.
O Hero, the renderer of our foes, rend our foes in all possible ways, so that we may be rich in offspring, rich in brave soldiers, and rich in food to feed with, everywhere, on earth, in ether, and sky!

५४. परमेष्ठ्यभिधीतः प्रजापतिर्वाचि व्याहृतायामन्धो अच्छेतः ।
सविता सन्यां विश्वकर्मा दीक्षायां पूषा सोम क्रयण्याम् ॥

54. O married people; if ye truly realize God, the Lord of mankind, Who rests in the fullness of joy, as mentioned in the Vedas, revealed by Him: if ye understand the head of the State, who observes the laws of the land; if ye follow the physician, who effects cure through medicines, and take pure food; ye will ever remain happy!

५५. इन्द्रश्च मरुतश्च क्रयायोपोत्थितोऽसुरः पण्यमानो मित्रः क्रीतो विष्णुः शिपिविष्ट ऊरावासन्नो विष्णुर्नर्न्धिषः ॥

55. O learned persons understand, for success in your transactions the use of electricity, wind, and cloud. Know Ye the Dhananjay Vayu, which is praiseworthy, friendly, and pervades all objects. Know ye God, present in

---

[55]Dhananjaya: a kind of vital air nourishing the body.

our souls, ever near us for our protection, ever shining before us, and well-versed in His function!

५६. प्रोह्यमाणः सोम आगतो वरुण आसन्द्यामासन्नोऽग्निराग्नीध्र इन्द्रो हविर्द्धानिऽथर्वाणपाव-
ह्रियमाणः ॥

56. O married people in this world, just as ye honour and seat on a dais a learned person who visits your house, so should ye use electricity in well thought out sources of wealth, collection of waters, in fires to be burnt, in skilfully manufacturing all useful and serviceable articles!

५७. विश्वे देवा अꣳशुꣳ न्युप्तो विष्णुꣳराप्रीतपा आप्याय्यमानो यमः सूयमानो विष्णुः
सम्भ्रियमाणो वायुः पूयमानः शुक्रः पूतः ।
शुक्रः क्षीरश्रीर्मन्थी सक्तुश्री: ॥

57. O all learned people fully realise your conduct towards different objects of the universe, know ye the electricity that maintains all beautiful objects, the aged sun, the invisible matter brought into creation, the invigorating vital airs, pure semen and the noble, active suppressor of foes. Thus ye become the utilisers of all objects, and eaters of milk products!

५८. विश्वे देवाश्चमसेषूऽन्नीतोऽसुहर्मायोद्यतो रुद्रो हूयमानो वातोऽभ्यावृत्तो नृचक्षाः
प्रतिख्यातो भक्षो भक्ष्यमाणः पितरो नाराशꣳसाः ॥

58. Those who through Homa spread wide upto clouds the fragrant spices, have devoted their lives to noble deeds, are accepted as mighty souls, are the well known seers of men, and are known as powerful like a storm, are eaters of eatables, and should all be recognised as wise, learned preachers of humanity.

५९. सत्रः सिन्धरवभृथायोद्यतः समुद्रोऽभ्यवह्रियमाणः सलिलः प्रप्लुतो ययोरोजसा स्कभिता
रजाꣳसि वीर्येभिर्वीरतमा शविष्ठा या पत्येते अप्रतीता सहोभिर्विष्णू अगन्वरुणा पूर्वहूतौ ॥

59. Those, who for their bath manage to get pure water, construct canals, soar high in space, by their strength maintain the worlds, who in their prowess are most brave and powerful, whose power is not known to ordinary mortals, who are comprehensive in character and noble in nature, and whose praise is sung by the ancient sages, are received by the learned. They always remain happy.

६०. देवान्दिवमगन्यज्ञस्ततो मा द्रविणमष्टु मनुष्यानन्तरिक्षमगन्यज्ञस्ततो मा द्रविणमष्टु
पितृन् पृथिवीमगन्यज्ञस्ततो मा द्रविणमष्टु यं कं च लोकमगन्यज्ञस्ततो मे भद्रमभूत् ॥

60. The yajna grants us foodstuffs and spreads the light of knowledge,

---

[59] ययोः (yayo) refers to the priest and the worshipper according to Maharshi Dayananda and to God and यज्ञ yajna by some other commentators. In this verse is sung the praise of the priest (Hota) and worshipper (Yajman) who through their yajna purify and maintain the universe.

the learned perform it, may knowledge thence come to me. The yajna goes to men and clouds, the wise perform it; may riches come thence to me. The yajna goes to seasons and the Earth, the sages perform it, may come thence each season's comfort to me.

Whatever sphere the yajna (sacrifice) reaches, which the religious minded people perform, may happiness come thence to me.

६१. चतुस्त्रिꣳशत्तन्तवो ये वितत्निरे य इमं यज्ञꣳ स्वधया ददन्ते ।
तेषां छिन्नꣳ सम्वेतद्दधामि स्वाहा धर्मो अप्येतु देवान् ॥

61. Thirtyfour threads diffuse this yajna of the world. They sustain it with supply of food. I skilfully unify their different functions and duties. May this yajna be controlled by the learned.

६२. यज्ञस्य दोहो वितत: पुरुत्रा सो अष्टधा दिवमन्वाततान ।
स यज्ञ धुक्ष्व महि मे प्रजायाꣳ रायस्पोषं विश्वमायुरशीय स्वाहा ॥

62. The material of a yajna (sacrifice) goes far and wide in different objects. It extends to the heaven in eight directions. O sacrifice, pour on my offspring plenty of wealth and prosperity. May I through good conduct enjoy full age!

६३. आ पवस्व हिरण्यवदश्ववत्सोम वीरवत् ।
वाजं गोमन्तमा भर स्वाहा ॥

63. O married man, desirous of prosperity, with thy noble behaviour, become the master of gold, steeds and warriors. Perform the yajna with materials which strengthen the organs of the body, and purify the world.

---

[61]Thirty four threads that weave the fabric of this universe are eight vasus:—sun, moon, earth, water, fire, air, sky, lightning; eleven Rudras: Pran, Apan, Vyan, Udan, Sman, Nag, Kurma, Krikal, Devdutt, Dhananjaya, and Matrishwa, twelve Adityas:—the twelve months of the year, soul, God and matter.

I refers to God.

CHAPTER IX

१. देव सवित: प्रसुव यज्ञं प्रसुव यज्ञपतिं भगाय ।
दिव्यो गन्धर्व: केतपू: केतं न: पुनातु वाचस्पतिर्वाजं न: स्वदतु स्वाहा ॥

1. O virtuous and prosperous king, preach through vedas, the art of administration conducive to comfort and wealth. Direct duly the man at the helm of affairs!

May thou, the embodiment of noble qualities, the sustainer of earth, and purifier of our wisdom, the protector of knowledge through the spread of education, improve our intellect, and share our wealth as directed by the vedas.

२. ध्रुवसदं त्वा नृषदं मन:सदमुपयामगृहीतोऽसीन्द्राय त्वा जुष्टं गृह्णाम्येष ते योनिरिन्द्राय त्वा जुष्टतमम् ।

अप्सुषदं त्वा घृतसदं व्योमसदमुपयामगृहीतोऽसीन्द्राय त्वा जुष्टं गृह्णाम्येष ते योनिरिन्द्राय त्वा जुष्टतमम् । पृथिविसदं त्वान्तरिक्षसदं दिविसदं देवसदं नाकसदमुपयामगृहीतोऽसीन्द्राय त्वा जुष्टं गृह्णाम्येष ते योनिरिन्द्राय त्वा जुष्टतमम् ॥

2. O king elected by the learned, for carrying out the behest of God, I accept thee, well versed in knowledge, yoga practices, and full of humility. leader of leaders, expert in science, and full of affection, as my lord. This administration is thy mainstay. I accept thee, most beloved for attaining to prosperity!

Thou hast been elected by the people. I accept thee, that indulges in sea trade, is the master of strength-giving articles like ghee, fliest in space in an aeroplane, and is full of affection; as my lord. This kingdom is thy mainstay. I accept thee, most beloved for destroying foes.

Thou art full of plans, I accept thee, the traveller in all parts of the world, the flier in heavens, the bestower of justice, the devotee of duty and God, free from affliction; and the lover of humanity, as my lord. This kingdom is thy mainstay. I accept thee, most beloved for the attainment of happiness.

३. अपाꣳ रसमुद्वयसꣳ सूर्ये सन्तꣳ समाहितम् ।
अपाꣳ रसस्य यो रसस्तं वो गृह्णाम्युत्तममुपयामगृहीतोऽसीन्द्राय त्वा जुष्टं गृह्णाम्येष ते योनिरिन्द्राय त्वा जुष्टतमम् ॥

3. O king, I utilise the essence of waters, that infuse life, are gathered in the sun, and spread in all directions. I advise thee to preserve—'the essence of waters' essence for thy own good, Thou hast legally been elected. I accept thee, full of affection, as my lord, for the attainment of God!

²This verse mentions the various qualities of the person, who is elected as a king or head of the state by the people. The veda does not believe in autocrac yor totalitarianism It believes in democracy.

This kingdom is thy home. I accept thee most affectionate, for the attainment of happiness.

४. ग्रहा ऊर्जाहुतयो व्यन्तो विप्राय मतिम् ।
तेषां विशिप्रियाणां वोऽह्मिषमूर्जं ॐ समग्रभमुपयाम गृहीतोऽसीन्द्राय त्वा जुष्टं गृह्ळाम्येष ते योनिरिन्द्राय त्वा जुष्टतमम् ।
सम्पृचौ स्थ: सं मा भद्रेण पृङ्क्त्तं विपृचौ स्थो वि मा पाप्मना पृङ्क्तम् ॥

4. I grant wisdom to the learned, collect food for and give strength to you married people, charitably disposed, well-versed in vedic lore and engaged in various acts of religion. O learned person thou art equipped with the requisites of a ruler and married life. I accept thee full of happiness, for prosperity. This is thy home. I accept thee, most lovely, for destroying foes! United are ye twain, with bliss unite me apart from a wicked soul.

५. इन्द्रस्य वज्रोऽसि वाजसास्त्वयायं वाज ॐ सेत् ।
वाजस्य नु प्रसवे मातरं महीमदिति नाम वचसा करामहे ।
यस्यामिदं विश्वं भुवनमाविवेश तस्यां नो देव: सविता धर्म साविषत् ॥

5. O commander of the army thou art the thunderbolt of the king, who, expert in battles, wins the war, with thy assistance. May we speedily bring under us, according to vedic justice, the vast, undivided, honour-giving land; on which the whole mankind is settled. May God, the Illuminator of all, and Generator of the universe sustain us on it!

६. अप्स्वन्तरमृतमप्सु भेषजमपामुत प्रशस्तिष्वश्वा भवत वाजिन: ।
देवीरापो यो व ऊर्मि: प्रतूर्ति: ककुन्मान् वाजसास्तेनायं वाज ॐ सेत् ॥

6. In control of breath lies longevity, in waters lies the healing medicine. Having realised the praiseworthy qualities of breath and water, grow thee fleet and strong.
O noble-minded wife and broad-minded husband may the commander of the army, the winner of battles, win the campaign, with your strength, forceful like the waves of the ocean, and roaring like the fast sea!

७. वातो वा मनो वा गन्धर्वा: सप्तवि ॐ शति: ।
ते अग्रेऽश्वमयुञ्जँस्ते अस्मिन् जवमा दधु: ॥

7. The learned, who like the wind, mind and twenty seven articles, primarily harness swiftness in this world, may acquire alertness as well.

८. वातर ॐ हा भव वाजिन्युज्यमान इन्द्रस्येव दक्षिण: श्रियँ अधि ।
यज्जन्तु त्वा मरुतो विश्ववेदस आ ते त्वष्टा पत्सु जवं दधातु ॥

---

³Essence of waters' essence: Virya, semen. I may mean Purohita.
⁴I: King. Ye: husband and wife or subjects and officials.
⁶Thee: general of the army.
⁷Twenty seven articles: All encompassing air, Pran, Apan, Vyan, Udan, Sman, Nag, Kurma, Krikla, Devdutt, Dhananjya, Mind, five organs of action Karma Indriyas and five organs of perception (Gyan Indriyas) and five elements, earth, air, water, fire, and space.

8. O well equipped and qualified king, may the masters of all sciences harness thee to the work of administration and mechanical enterprises, may the expert in the science of velocity, put swiftness in thy feet! Be thou active like the wind.

Being ever wary, endowed with a religious bent of mind, like a powerful king, attain to greatness and glory, with splendid royal accomplishment.

९. जवो यस्ते वाजिन्निहितो गुहा य: श्येने परीत्तो अचरच्च वाते ।
तेन नो वाजिन् बलवान् बलेन वाजजिच्च भव समने च पार्यिष्णु: ।
वाजिनो वाजजितो वाजँ सरिष्यन्तो बृहस्पतेर्भागमवजिघ्रत ॥

9. O king, the swiftness laid in thee in secret, resembles the swiftness granted to a falcon, and the swiftness found in air. Be thou powerful for us, with that swiftness and army. Be thou the winner of battles, and our saviour-through war!

O nice, brave soldiers, serve your commander, acquire wisdom and food, win battles, and enjoy fragrant substances!

१०. देवस्याहँ सवितु: सवे सत्यसवसो बृहस्पतेरुत्तमं नाकँ रुहेयम् ।
देवस्याहँ सवितु: सवे सत्यसवस इन्द्रस्योत्तमं नाकँ रुहेयम् ।
देवस्याहँ सवितु: सवे सत्यप्रसवसो बृहस्पतेरुत्तमं नाकमरुहम् ।
देवस्याहँ सवितु: सवे सत्यप्रसवस इन्द्रस्योत्तमं नाकमरुहम् ॥

10. May I realise in this world, the nature of God free from pain and full of delight; Who is lustrous, and Generator of the universe. Whose cause and effect of the universe are true; Who nourishes all material objects, and is most high. May I rise, through the prosperity, and excellent gifts of the king, the creator of riches, the giver of comforts, and dispenser of justice.

May I rise through the highest pleasure I obtain from the knowledge imparted by my learned preceptor, the giver of imperishable knowledge, the embodiment of noble attributes and actions; and the encyclopaedia of learning.

May I rise through the victory-giving battle, and the persuasion of the commander, the subduer of wicked foes, the inciter to victory over opponents, the expert in the science of military warfare, the dispenser of justice and full of humility.

११. बृहस्पते वाजं जय बृहस्पतये वाचं वदत बृहस्पतिं वाजं जापयत ।
इन्द्र वाजं जयेन्द्राय वाचं वदतेन्द्रं वाजं जापयत ॥

11. O preacher, acquire knowledge. Let the learned speak to thee the ennobling language of the vedas. May they impart knowledge to the instructor!

O king win the battle. May the learned speak to thee the language of the duty of kingship, and bring victory to thee!

---

[10]I in the first part refers to the king, in the second part to a philanthropist, in the third to a student, the seeker after knowledge; and in the fourth to a warrior. Each in turn advises mankind to rise as he has done.

CHAPTER IX

१२. एषा व: सा सत्या संवागभूद्यया बृहस्पति वाजमजीजपताजीजपत बृहस्पति वाजं वनस्पतयो विमुच्यध्वम् ।
एषा व: सा सत्या संवागभूद्ययेन्द्रं वाजमजीजपताजीजपतेन्द्रं वाजं वनस्पतयो विमुच्यध्वम् ॥

12. O guardians of justice, advance thereby the knowledge of the vedas, and the learned who protect them. Bring victory to the king in the battle!

May ye be free in speech. O guardians of justice, bring thereby like the sun's beams victory to your commander in the battle. May ye grant to your king success in a wealth-producing pursuit. May this your utterance of statesmanship be true. May ye be free in speech!

१३. देवस्याहꣳ सवितु: सवे सत्यप्रसवसो बृहस्पतेर्वाजजितो वाजं जेषम् ।
वाजिनो वाजजितोऽध्वन स्कम्नुवन्तो योजना मिमाना: काष्ठां गच्छत ॥

13. May I, the general, stout in body and soul, win the battle with the help of God, in Whose universe reside the eternal causes, Who is the giver of all affluence, The Illuminator of all, Supreme in knowledge, and the Guardian of the Vedas. O active, learned persons, winners of battle, see the enemies from a distance and go towards different directions to check their onward march.

१४. एष स्य वाजी क्षिपणि तरण्यति ग्रीवायां बद्धो अपिकक्ष आसनि ।
क्रतुं दधिक्रा अनु सꣳ सनिष्यदत्पथामङ्कꣳस्यन्वापनीफणत् स्वाहा ॥

14. Just as this fast horse bound by the neck, and at the flanks and in the mouth, ever accelerating its speed, passes by the mile-stones, with full force and goes to the army; so does the commander of the army, with due orders, make it march on speedily.

१५. उत स्मास्य द्रवतस्तुरण्यत: पर्णं न वेरनुवाति प्रगधिन: ।
श्येनस्येव ध्रजतो अङ्कसं परि दधिक्राव्ण: सहोर्जा तरित्रत: स्वाहा ॥

15. O Government officials, he alone can conquer the foes, who marches speedily according to plan, on well constructed roads, with equipment and firm determination like the wings of a fast flying bird, the falcon that soars high desirous of prey, and the fleeting horse!

१६. शं नो भवन्तु वाजिनो हवेषु देवताता मितद्रव: स्वर्का: ।
जम्भयन्तोऽहिं वृकꣳ रक्षाꣳसि सनेम्यस्मद्युयवन्नमीवा: ॥

16. May the heroes expert in the science of warfare, marching uniformly, well respected and well fed, breaking the bodies of strong thieves and rascals, attain to everlasting happiness in battles, through the deeds of us the learned. May they banish for us all disease-like foes.

---
[12]Vanaspati, the guardian of justice is compared to the beams of the sun. Just as they impartially fall on all high and low, without distinction, so should the guardian of justice be impartial to all. वनस्मिति रश्मिनाम, निघंटु 1-5 van according to Nighantu means the beam to the sun.

१७. ते नो अर्वन्तो हवनश्रुतो हवं विश्वे शृण्वन्तु वाजिनो मितद्रव: ।
सहस्रसा मेधसाता सनिष्यवो महो ये धनꣳ समिथेषु जभ्रिरे ॥

17. The state officials, who are advanced in knowledge, listeners of religious books, full of wisdom, masters of their subjects, seekers after different branches of knowledge, lovers of their souls, leaders of social life, and acquirers of mighty wealth in battles, should all, listen to our learned discussions.

१८. वाजेवाजेऽवत वाजिनो नो धनेषु विप्रा अमृता ऋतज्ञा: ।
अस्य मध्व: पिबत मादयध्वं तृप्ता यात पथिभिर्देवयानै: ॥

18. O truthful, aged, steadfast and wise officials, protect us in each fray. Enjoy the reward of victory in the battle. Be joyful, be satisfied. Tread on paths, which sages are wont to tread!

१९. आ मा वाजस्य प्रसवो जगम्यादेमे द्यावापृथिवी विश्वरूपे ।
आ मा गन्तां पितरा मातरा चा मा सोमो अमृतत्वेन गम्यात् ।
वाजिनो वाजजितो वाजꣳ ससृवाꣳसो बृहस्पतेर्भागमबजिघ्रत निमृजाना: ॥

19. May I get in full, bounteous wealth of knowledge. May I get sovereignty over Heaven and Earth, in which reside all shining objects. May I get the knowledge of healing medicines. May I obtain learned father and mother.
Ye, mighty warriors, winners of battles, going to the battle-field, purified in heart, obey the orders of your general!

२०. आपये स्वाहा स्वापये स्वाहा ऽपिजाय स्वाहा क्रतवे स्वाहा वसवे स्वाहाऽहर्पतये स्वाहाऽहे मुग्धाय स्वाहा मुग्धाय वैनꣳ शिनाय स्वाहा विनꣳशिन आन्त्यायनाय स्वाहाऽन्त्याय भौवनाय स्वाहा भुवनस्य पतये स्वाहा ऽधिपतये स्वाहा ॥

20. For the attainment of full knowledge, noble deeds; for the attainment of happiness, religious life; for the attainment of definite object, activity, for the advancement of wisdom, the habit of reading and teaching, for retention of knowledge, truthful speech; for arithmetical measurement of day, the science of arithmetic; for checking the waste of time in infatuation, a word of wisdom, for the fool who revels in vice, a word of caution; for the degraded, wicked soul, advice to ward off evil deeds; for the strong person amongst the low and despicable, speech revealing the true nature of things; for the attainment of God, the Lord of the universe, the knowledge of yoga; for the king, the knowledge of all affairs, are essential.

२१. आयुर्यज्ञेन कल्पतां प्राणो यज्ञेन कल्पतां चक्षुर्यज्ञेन कल्पताꣳ श्रोत्रं यज्ञेन कल्पतां पृष्ठं यज्ञेन कल्पतां यज्ञो यज्ञेन कल्पताम् ।
प्रजापते: प्रजा अभूम स्वर्देवा अगन्मामृता अभूम ॥

21. May life be devoted to obeying the orders of God. May life-breath thrive through practice. May eye thrive by the study of natural objects. May ear thrive by listening to the vedas. May questioning improve through mutual

discussion. May worship of God thrive through celibacy. May we be the true sons of God. May the learned attain to final emancipation and thereby enjoy happiness.

२२. अस्मे वो अस्त्विन्द्रियमस्मे नृम्णमुत क्रतरस्मे वर्चाᳪसि सन्तु व: ।
नमो मात्रे पृथिव्यै नमो मात्रे पृथिव्या इयं ते राडचन्ताऽसि यमनो ध्रुवोऽसि धरण: ।
कृष्यै त्वा क्षेमाय त्वा रय्यै त्वा पोषाय त्वा ॥

22. I enjoin thee for agriculture, advancement, wealth, and prosperity. Thou art persevering, law-abiding, preserving and eminent. May food-grains be produced from this venerable Earth. May the worthy science of geology be studied, and water and food grains produced thereby from the Earth. May our physical force, wealth, wisdom, and knowledge be for your service.

२३. वाजस्येमं प्रसव: सुषुवेऽग्रे सोमᳪ राजानमोषधीष्वप्सु ।
ता अस्मभ्यं मधुमतीर्भवन्तु वयᳪ राष्ट्रे जागृयाम पुरोहिता: स्वाहा ॥

23. I, being First and Affluent, lend wisdom and prosperity to this king, the driver of all miseries and shining with knowledge, justice and humility.

May the medicines produced on the earth or grown in water, be highly efficacious for us. May we, the ministers, act tactfully for the betterment of the State, remaining alert, and always keeping the interests of the government foremost.

२४. वाजस्येमां प्रसव: शिश्रिये दिवमिमा च विश्वा भुवनानि सम्राट् ।
अदितसन्तं दापयति प्रजानन्त्स नो रयिᳪ सर्ववीरं नि यच्छतु स्वाहा ॥

24. I, the king, born in my state, afford shelter to all habitations, and enforce my policy.

May he, who truly knowing all his duties, realises taxes from those, unwilling to pay, receive from us riches, that bring us heroes.

२५. वाजस्य नु प्रसव आ बभूवेमा च विश्वा भुवनानि सर्वत: ।
सनेमि राजा परि याति विद्वान् प्रजां पुष्टिं वर्धयमानो अस्मे स्वाहा ॥

25. He is fit to be our King, who knows the course of conduct, as inculcated by the Vedas, who advances in knowledge, behaves properly, conduces to the prosperity of his old subjects, and all these provinces of the state, and tours throughout his territory.

२६. सोमᳪ राजानमवसेऽग्निमन्वारभामहे ।
आदित्यान्विष्णुᳪ सूर्यं ब्रह्माणं च बृहस्पतिᳪ स्वाहा ।

---

[21]Final emancipation: Mukti, salvation, deliverance, redemption.
[22]I: God. People should learn sacrifice, and place all their resources in the service of humanity. They should learn geology, cultivate land and grow more food.
[23]I: God.
[24]I: King. He: King. Us: Subjects.
He alone should be elected the King, who can protect the State, and realise taxes from the reluctant subjects.

26. Let us elect him, for our protection, after due deliberations, as king, who is amiable, and destroyer of foes like fire, who has received education from the learned, who has observed the vow of celibacy for forty eight years, who holds sway over administrative problems, is supreme among the learned, is master of all the four vedas, and protector of the sages.

२७. अर्यमणं बृहस्पतिमिन्द्रं दानाय चोदय ।
वाचं विष्णुꣳ सरस्वतीꣳ सवितारं च वाजिनꣳ स्वाहा ॥

27. O King, with a sound policy, for the spread of knowledge, urge, the lover of impartial justice, the teacher of all sciences, the master of riches and the vedas, the leader of men, the learned mistress, the lover of vedic lore and the brave warrior for noble deeds!

२८. अग्ने अच्छा वदेह न: प्रति न: सुमना भव ।
प्र नो यच्छ सहस्रजित्त्वꣳ हि धनदा असि स्वाहा ॥

28. O King, speak truthfully and kindly to us here, be graciously inclined to us. Winner of thousand warriors, grant us happiness, for thou art the giver of wealth!

२९. प्र नो यच्छत्वर्यमा प्र पूषा प्र बृहस्पति: ।
प्र वाग्देवी ददातु न: स्वाहा ॥

29. As the Lord of Justice gives us good instruction, as the nourisher gives us strength of body and soul, just as a learned man gives us knowledge, so let the mother, a sweet-tongued and nice instructor impart knowledge unto us.

३०. देवस्य त्वा सवितु: प्रसवेऽश्विनोर्बाहुभ्यां पूष्णो हस्ताभ्याम् ।
सरस्वत्यै वाचो यन्तुर्यन्त्रिये दधामि बृहस्पतेष्ट्वा साम्राज्येनाभि षिञ्चाम्यसौ ॥

30. O good-natured educated person, I, in this world created by the Effulgent God, appoint thee as King with the knowledge of the Vedas, with arms strong like the sun and moon, with hands swift like the wind. I anoint thee with supreme kingship in this state well organised by the learned!

३१. अग्निरेकाक्षरेण प्राणमुदजयत्तमुज्जेषमश्विनौ द्व्यक्षरेण द्विपदो मनुष्यानुदजयतां- तानुज्जेषं विष्णुस्त्र्यक्षरेण त्रीꣳल्लोकानुदजयत्तानुज्जेषꣳ सोमश्चतुरक्षरेण चतुष्पद: पशूनुदजयत्तानुज्जेषम् ॥

31. O King, just as thou, with the monosyllabic Om elevatest thy subjects, so may I elevate them. Just as the King and his men like the sun and moon,

---

[30] I refers to the priest who anoints the King.

[31] I: a high state official or any person of the state. Monosyllabic metre is Daivi Gayatri Chhand. Dissyllabic metre is Daivi Ushnik Chhand. Trisyllabic metre is Daivi Anushtup Chhand, Quadrisyllabic metre is Daivi Brihati Chhand. A king through the knowledge of vedic Mantras in these metres elevates and subdues the animate and inanimate objects.

CHAPTER IX

with dissyllabic metre, elevate bipeds, so may I elevate them. Just as the just King, with trisyllabic metre elevates the three worlds, so may I elevate them. Just as a King desirous for prosperity, with quadrisyllabic metre subdues the four-footed cattle, so may I subdue them!

३२. पूषा पञ्चाक्षरेण पञ्च दिश उदजयत्तां उज्जेषꣳ सविता षडक्षरेण षड्ऋतूनुदजय-तानुज्जेषम् ।
मरुतः सप्ताक्षरेण सप्त ग्राम्यान् पशूनदजयँस्तानुज्जेषं ।
बृहस्पतिरष्टाक्षरेण गायत्रीमुदजयत्तामुज्जेषम् ॥

32. O King, the nourisher of all, with penta-syllabic metre, thou hast won the five regions, may I also win them. Resplendent like the sun, thou, O' King, with six syllabic metre hast controlled the six seasons, may I also control them. O' King, fast like the sun, as thou with hepta syllabic metre rearest the seven domestic animals, so may I also rear them. O' learned King, as thou with octosyllabic metre followest the self-preserving policy, so may I also follow it!

३३. मित्रो नवाक्षरेण त्रिवृतꣳ स्तोममुदजयत्तमुज्जेषं ।
वरुणो दशाक्षरेण विराजमुदजयत्तामुज्जेषमिन्द्र एकादशाक्षरेण त्रिष्टुभमुदजयत्तामुज्जेषं ।
विश्वे देवा द्वादशाक्षरेण जगतीमुदजयँस्तामुज्जेषम् ॥

33. O King, the friend of all, just as thou knowest, with nine-syllabic metre, Him, deserving of praise with the aid of knowledge, action and meditation; Him may I know. O praiseworthy King, just as thou, with decasyllabic metre knowest Him mentioned in virat verses, so may I also know Him!

O giver of riches, just as thou with hendecasyllabic metre knowest Him mentioned in Trishtup verses, so may I also know Him. O ye all learned persons, just as you with, dodecasyllabic metre, know the teaching conveyed in Jagati metre, so may I also know it!

Three worlds: Earth, Atmosphere and Sun, or sun, lightning and fire, or high, mid, and low regions. According to Swami Dayananda's view they are birth, place and name.

[32]Pentasyllabic metre means Daivi Pankti Chhand. Five regions: North, South, East, West, and overhead direction.

Six-syllabic metre means Daivi Trishtup Chhand. Six seasons are Spring, Summer, Rains, Autumn, Winter, Dews.

Hepta-syllabic metre means Daivi Jagati Chhand. Seven domestic animals are cow, horse, buffalo, camel, goat, sheep and ass.

Octosyllabic metre means Yajushi Anushtup Chhand.

Gayatri according to Pt. Jaidev Vidyalankar, and Vedic Sansthan, Mathura mean earth, that protects and nourishes us all. Maharshi Swami Dayananda interprets it as self preserving policy.

[33]Nine-syllable metre means yajushi Brihati Chhand. Decasyllabic metre means yajushi Pankti. Hendecasyllabic metre means Asuri Pankti, Dodecasyllabic metre means Saamni Gayatri. The knowledge of the vedic verses in these metres leads one to the knowledge of God and worldly affairs.

३४. बसवस्त्रयोदशाक्षरेण त्रयोदशꣶ स्तोममुदजयँस्तमुज्जेषꣶ ।
रुद्राश्चतुर्दशाक्षरेण चतुर्दशꣶ स्तोममुदजयँस्तमुज्जेष-
मादित्या: पञ्चदशाक्षरेण पञ्चदशꣶ स्तोममुदजयँस्तमुज्जेषमदिति: षोडशाक्षरेण षोडशꣶ
स्तोममुदजयत्तमुज्जेषं ।
प्रजापति: सप्तदशाक्षरेण सप्तदशꣶ स्तोममुदजयत्तमुज्जेषम् ॥

34. Just as the Vasus, by thirteen syllabic metre, know the thirteenfold collection of laudable objects, so may I also know them. Just as the Rudras by fourteen-syllabic metre know the fourteenfold collection of laudable objects, so may I also know them. Just as the Adityas with fifteen Syllabic metre know the fifteenfold collection of laudable objects, so may I also know them. Just as the Aditi, with sixteen-syllabic metre knows the sixteenfold collection of laudable objects, so may I also know them. Just as Prajapati, with seventeen-syllabic metre, knows the seventeenfold collection of laudable objects, so may I also know them.

३५. एष ते निर्ऋ॑ते भागस्तं जुषस्व स्वाहा अग्निनेत्रेभ्यो देवेभ्य: पुर: सङ्रूच: स्वाहा यमनेत्रेभ्यो देवेभ्यो दक्षिणासङ्रूच: स्वाहा विश्वदेवनेत्रेभ्यो देवेभ्य: पश्चात्सङ्रूच: स्वाहा मित्रावरुणनेत्रेभ्यो वा महन्नेत्रेभ्यो वा देवेभ्य उत्तरासङ्रूच: स्वाहा सोमनेत्रेभ्यो देवेभ्य उपरिसङ्रूचो द्रुवस्वङ्रूच: स्वाहा ॥

³⁴Vasus are the Brahmcharis who have observed the vow of celibacy for 24 years. Thirteen-syllabic 'metre means Asuri Anushtup Chhand. Thirteenfold objects—Ten pranas, soul, Mahattatva (2nd of the 25 principles of the Sankhyas) and primordial matter.
Rudras: the Brahmcharis who have spent 44 years in celibacy and study.
Fourteen: syllabic metre means Saamni-Ushnik Chhand.
Fourteen-fold objects: Ten organs (5 Gyana and 5 Karma organs), mind, intellect, discernment and egotism.
Adityas: The Brahmcharis who have observed a vow of celibacy for 48 years, and studied all the four Vedas.
Fifteen: syllabic metre means Asuri Gayatri Chhand.
Fifteen-fold objects: Four Vedas, four-up-ved as (Ayurveda, Dhanurveda, Gandharva Veda, Artha Veda), Six Angas, Shiksha (the science which teaches the proper pronunciation of words), Kalpa (the science of rituals), Vyakarna (grammar), Nirukta (Etymology), Chhand (Prosody), Jyotish (Astronomy), and beauty in action.
Aditi :—the queen with immense wealth and glory.
Sixteen -syllabic metre means Samni Anushtup Chhand.
Sixteen-fold objects: (1) Pramana (Testimony) (2) Pramey (Theorem) (3) Sanshey (Doubts), (4) Prayojan (Application), (5) Drishtanta (Illustration), (6) Siddhanta (Principle), (7) Avayava (Syllogism), (8) Tarka (Logic), (9) Nirnaya (Decision), (10) Vada (Discussion), (11) Jalpa (Discourse), (12) Vitanda (Wrangling), (13) Hetvabhasa (Fallacy), (14) Chhala (Semblance), (15) Jaati (Futile answer), (16) Nigrhasthan (Flaw in an argument by which disputant is brought low). These sixteen objects are mentioned in Nayaya Darshan.
Prajapati: King who rears the subjects.
Seventeen-syllabic metre means Nichrid-Arshi Gayatri Chhand.
Seventeen-fold objects: Four Varnas (Brahman, Kshatriya; Vaish, Shudra), Four Ashramas (Brahmcharya, Grihastha, Banprastha, Sanyasa), Shravan (Hearing), Manan

CHAPTER IX

35. O King, the lover of truth, conduct thy rule with justice. Utter truthful words for the learned, whose policy shines like the fire. Behave in a religious spirit towards those lords of justice who work in the east. Be charitable to the learned, who are fast-witted like the wind and are put in charge of the southern part of the country. Use inspiring language towards the learned officials stationed in the west, who fully understand politics like all the wise. Behave respectfully like a state representative towards those just officials appointed in the north, who are regular in their duty like the in-going, and outcoming breath, and who give true lead to the subjects. Use the language of a sage towards those who brilliant like the moon, give happiness to all, and who acquire knowledge, cultivate humility, are religious-minded, and worship God!

३६. ये देवा अग्निनेत्राः पुरःसदस्तेभ्यः स्वाहा ये देवा यमनेत्रा दक्षिणासदस्तेभ्यः स्वाहा ये देवा विश्वदेवनेत्राः पश्चात्सदस्तेभ्यः स्वाहा ।
ये देवा मित्रावरुणनेत्रा वा मरुन्नेत्रा वोत्तरासदस्तेभ्यः स्वाहा ये देवाः सोमनेत्रा उपरिसदो दुवस्वन्तस्तेभ्यः स्वाहा ॥

36. O King, utter truthful words for the learned, who have mastered the science of electricity, and reside in the east. Behave in a religious spirit towards those yogis, who are well versed in the intricacies of the science of yoga, and reside in the south. Derive knowledge from the learned, who know the science of material objects, and reside in the west. Learn knowledge that benefits all, from those who grant happiness to all and reside in the north, preach Dharma to those, who are swift-witted like the mind. Learn medical science from t'ose who know the Ayur Veda, and the properties of medicinal herbs, are well placed in life and busy with their noble profession, and adore medical knowledge and religion!

३७. अग्ने सहस्व पृतना अभिमातीरपास्य ।
दुष्टरस्तरन्नरातीर्वर्चो धा यज्ञवाहसि ॥

37. O King, oppose the proud, happy powerful, and trained army, and drive our enemies away, subduing powerful foes. In this State advance knowledge, gain strength and practice justice.

३८. देवस्य त्वा सवितुः प्रसवेऽश्विनोर्बाहुभ्यां पूष्णो हस्ताभ्याम् ।
उपांशोर्वीर्येण जुहोमि हतँ रक्षः स्वाहा ।
रक्षसां त्वा बधायावधिष्म रक्षोऽबधिष्मामुमसौ हतः ॥

(Cogitation), Nidhidhyasan (Meditation), Desire for the non-obtained, Retention of the obtained, Development of the retained, proper use of the developed, Desire, and endeavour for salvation.

In the last four mantras 31 to 34, the duties of the king and the subjects are described, which they should realise, and derive happiness therefrom.

[36]Everybody should travel far and wide and add to his store of knowledge.

38. O King, rightly, I, with the glory of the just and prosperity-bringing commander of the army, with the strength of the nearby army, with the general's arms stout like the sun and moon, and with the skilful hands of a physician, accept thee for slaying the demons. Just as thou hast slain the demon so may we slay the demon. Just as we have slain that so may we slay all others!

३६. सविता त्वा सवाना᳕ सुवतामग्निगृ॒हपतीना᳕ सोमो वनस्पतीनाम् ।
बृहस्पतिर्वाचि इन्द्रो ज्यैष्ठचाय रुद्र: पशुभ्यो मित्र: सत्यो वरुणो धर्मपतीनाम् ।

39. O King, thou art the creator of supremacy, useful like fire for the domestic people, the lord of the trees, the friend, faithful companion, and religious leader of the lovers of religion, the master of the Vedas, aged among the aged, and the protector of the cattle. May the religious, truthful, learned people urge thee to serve thy people!

४०. इमं देवा असपत्न᳕ सुवध्वं महते क्षत्राय महते ज्यैष्ठचाय महते जानराज्यायेन्द्र-
स्येन्द्रियाय ।
इममुष्य पुत्रममुष्यै पुत्रमस्यै विश एष वोऽमी राजा सोमोऽस्माकं ब्रह्मणाना᳕ राजा ॥

40. O learned people, this lover of his subjects, is the King of you the Kshatriyas, and us the Brahmanas, and the people living afar. Him, the son of that father, and that mother, (for the protection of the people, for great supremacy), for sovereignty over the virtuous, and for obtaining huge wealth, do ye render free from foes!

---

[38]I: any person amongst the subjects.
[39]Just as Soma is the lord of medicines, so a King is the lord, the protector, the grower of trees.

CHAPTER X

१. अपो देवा मधुमतीरगृभ्णन्नूर्जस्वती राजस्वश्चितानाः ।
याभिर्मित्रावरुणावभ्यषिञ्चन्याभिरिन्द्रमनयन्नत्यरातीः ॥

1. O wise persons, the means through which ye control breath, create electric power, and conquer foes, should also be employed to acquire sweet, strength-infusing, refreshing, and sovereignty-bestowing waters!

२. वृष्ण ऊर्मिरसि राष्ट्रदा राष्ट्रं मे देहि स्वाहा ।
वृष्ण ऊर्मिरसि राष्ट्रदा राष्ट्रममुष्मै देहि ।
वृषसेनोऽसि राष्ट्रदा राष्ट्रं मे देहि स्वाहा ।
वृषसेनोऽसि राष्ट्रदा राष्ट्रममुष्मै देहि ॥

2. O people, ye are the givers of Kingship, that brings knowledge and showers happiness, bestow on me the kingdom, in a righteous manner. Ye are the knowers of government that showers happiness, and the givers of Kingship, bestow Kingdom on him, who can protect it. Ye are the definers of the duties of Kings, and masters of a strong army, bestow on me the Kingdom, in a beautiful speech. Ye are the givers of Kingship, and masters of a strong army, bestow the Kingdom on the deserving!

३. अर्थेत स्थ राष्ट्रदा राष्ट्रं मे दत्त स्वाहा अर्थेत स्थ राष्ट्रदा राष्ट्रममुष्मै दत्तौजस्वती स्थ राष्ट्रदा राष्ट्रं मे दत्त स्वाहौजस्वती स्थ राष्ट्रदा राष्ट्रममुष्मै दत्ताप: परिवाहिणी स्थ राष्ट्रदा राष्ट्रं मे दत्त स्वाहा अप: परिवाहिणी स्थ राष्ट्रदा राष्ट्रममुष्मै दत्तापां पतिरसि राष्ट्रदा राष्ट्रं मे देहि स्वाहा अपां पतिरसि राष्ट्रदा राष्ट्रममुष्मै देह्यपां गर्भोऽसि राष्ट्रदा राष्ट्रं मे देहि स्वाहा अपां गर्भोऽसि राष्ट्रदा राष्ट्रममुष्मै देहि ॥

3. O wealthy people, givers of Kingship, bestow on me the Kingdom in a righteous manner. Ye, the masters of knowledge, and givers of Kingship, bestow Kingdom on him who can protect it!

Ye royal women, imbued with knowledge, strength and supremacy, givers of Kingship, bestow kingdom on me in a righteous manner. Ye self-controlled ladies, the givers of Kingship, bestow kingdom on him, who deserves it!

Ye kind ladies, givers of kingship, bestow kingdom on me in a righteous manner!

Ye' kind ladies, givers of kingship, bestow kingdom on the self-controlled hero!

O ye protectors of the people, givers of kingship, bestow kingdom on me

---

[1] Water is sprinkled over the King at the time of the Coronation ceremony.
[2] It is the duty of the people to elect him as their ruler, who deserves the honour.
[3] This verse preaches the height of democracy. Men and women are equally and jointly entitled to elect a man as their King who fully deserves the honour.

in a righteous manner. Ye controllers of breath and givers of kingship, bestow kingdom on him, who protects his subjects!

O valiant King, guarded by the armies which give thee women-like protection, and are the givers of Kingship, help me a considerate successor in the election as a king!

O King, praised by the subjects, the electors of a ruler, help pass on the Kingship to the well-praised deserving person!

४. सूर्यंत्वचस स्थ राष्ट्रदा राष्ट्रं मे दत्त स्वाहा सूर्यंत्वचस स्थ राष्ट्रदा राष्ट्रममुष्मै दत्त सूर्यवर्चस स्थ राष्ट्रदा राष्ट्रं मे दत्त स्वाहा सूर्यवर्चस स्थ राष्ट्रदा राष्ट्रममुष्मै दत्त मान्दा स्थ राष्ट्रदा राष्ट्रं मे दत्त स्वाहा मान्दा स्थ राष्ट्रदा राष्ट्रममुष्मै दत्त ब्रजक्षित स्थ राष्ट्रदा राष्ट्रं मे दत्त स्वाहा ब्रजक्षित स्थ राष्ट्रदा राष्ट्रममुष्मै दत्त वाशा स्थ राष्ट्रदा राष्ट्रं मे दत्त स्वाहा वाशा स्थ राष्ट्रदा राष्ट्रममुष्मै दत्त शविष्ठा स्थ राष्ट्रदा राष्ट्रं मे दत्त स्वाहा शविष्ठा स्थ राष्ट्रदा राष्ट्रममुष्मै दत्त शक्वरी स्थ राष्ट्रदा राष्ट्रं मे दत्त स्वाहा शक्वरी स्थ राष्ट्रदा राष्ट्रममुष्मै दत्त जनभृत स्थ राष्ट्रदा राष्ट्रं मे दत्त स्वाहा जनभृत स्थ राष्ट्रदा राष्ट्रममुष्मै दत्त विश्वभृत स्थ राष्ट्रदा राष्ट्रं मे दत्त स्वाहा विश्वभृत स्थ राष्ट्रदा राष्ट्रममुष्मै दत्ताप: स्वराज स्थ राष्ट्रदा राष्ट्रममुष्मै दत्त ।

मधुमतीर्मधुमतीभि: पृच्यन्तां महि क्षत्रं क्षत्रियाय वन्वानां अनाधृष्टा: सीदत सहौजसो महि क्षत्रं क्षत्रियाय दधती: ॥

4. O people, protectors like the sun, with your spirit of true justice, ye are the givers of Kingship, bestow Kingdom on me!

Ye, protectors like the sun, ye, seekers after knowledge, are the givers of Kingship, bestow Kingdom on the deserving person. Ye people educationally brilliant like the sun, the givers of Kingship, bestow Kingdom on me in a befitting manner!

O people, ye are educationally brilliant like the sun and are the givers of Kingship, bestow Kingdom on the deserving person. Ye, bringers of joy, and givers of Kingship, bestow Kingdom on me in a befitting manner. Ye bringers of joy and givers of Kingship, bestow kingdom on him who is deserving!

Ye, builders of cow-sheds, and bestowers of kingship, bestow Kingdom on me in a befitting manner. Ye builders of cow-sheds and givers of Kingship, bestow Kingdom on him who is deserving, ye high-aimed people, and givers of Kingship, bestow Kingdom on me in a befitting manner. Ye high-aimed people, and givers of kingship, bestow Kingdom on him who is deserving. Most powerful are ye, and givers of kingship, bestow kingdom on me in a befitting manner!

Most powerful are ye, and givers of kingship, bestow kingdom on him who is deserving.

Endowed with might are ye and givers of kingship, bestow kingdom on me in a befitting manner.

⁴This excellent verse enjoins upon the people, possessing different sources of strength to exercise their vote carefully, fearlessly, cautiously and disinterestedly in electing the most deserving person as the head of the State. The Vedas favour democracy, and denounce autocracy.

CHAPTER X

Endowed with might are ye, and givers of Kingship, bestow kingdom on him who is deserving.

Man-nourishing are ye, and givers of Kingship, bestow Kingdom on me in a befitting manner. Man-nourishing are ye, and givers of Kingship, bestow kingdom on him who is deserving.

All-nourishing are ye, and givers of Kingship, bestow kingdom on me in a befitting manner. All-nourishing are ye, and givers of kingship. bestow kingdom on him, who is deserving. O people, full of knowledge and virtue, enjoying independence, ye are the givers of kingship, bestow kingdom on him who is most deserving. Let the sweet medicinal herbs, ripen in the spring and other seasons. O people procuring mighty power for the Kshatriya, rest in your place, inviolate and potent bestowing on the Kshatriya mighty power!

५. सोमस्य त्विषिरसि तवेव मे त्विषिर्भूयात् ।
अग्नये स्वाहा सोमाय स्वाहा सवित्रे स्वाहा सरस्वत्यै स्वाहा पूष्णे स्वाहा बृहस्पतये स्वाहेन्द्राय स्वाहा घोषाय स्वाहा श्लोकाय स्वाहाँशायं स्वाहा भगाय स्वाहा ऽर्यम्णे स्वाहा ॥

5. O king, thou art the light of greatness, may my light of knowledge grow like thine. Acquire truthful speech and knowledge coupled with practice for learning the science of electricity, and laborious nature of a doctor for learning medicine. Learn astronomy for acquiring the knowledge of sun. Learn grammar for understanding the vedas. Learn Yoga for the control of breath. Study the vedas for the knowledge of God. Acquire discrimination for the knowledge of soul. Acquire the art of eloquence for a good speech. Learn prosody for composing poems. Learn science for understanding the attributes of atoms. Learn to lead an active life for acquiring wealth. Learn politics for becoming a king!

६. पवित्रे स्थो वैष्णव्यौ सवितुर्वः प्रसव उत्पुनाम्यच्छिद्रेण पवित्रेण सूर्यस्य रश्मिभिः ।
अग्निभृष्टमसि वाचो बन्धुस्तपोजाः सोमस्य दात्रमसि स्वाहा राजस्वः ॥

6. O King, thou art the flawless, friend of the vedas. Thou, with the use of disease healing herbs, leadest the life of a Brahmchari. In this world created by God, ye, male and female students, engaged in study, lead a life of high morals. I purify ye, like the beams of the sun, with your unbroken pledge of celibacy. Ye are the producers of brave Kings in a nice way!

७. सधमादो द्युम्निनीराप एता अनाधृष्टा अपस्यो वसानाः ।
पस्त्यासु चक्रे वरुणः सधस्थमपाँ शिशुर्मातृतमास्वन्तः ॥

7. A good King should put in charge of educated and respectable nurses the children of women, well bred, ever happy, rich, famous, inviolate, calm

---

[5] In this verse different sciences a ruler should learn to become efficient have been enumerated.
[6] The King should arrange for the compulsory education of boys and girls in the State.
[7] The mother should not suckle the child for more than a few days, when an educated nurse should be put in its charge. The mother becomes weak by long suckling.

like water, well dressed and decorated with ornaments, expert in domestic affairs and advanced in Knowledge.

८. क्षत्रस्योल्वमसि क्षत्रस्य जरायवसि क्षत्रस्य योनिरसि क्षत्रस्य नाभिरसीन्द्रस्य वार्त्रघ्नमसि मित्रस्यासि वरुणस्यासि त्वयाऽयं वृत्रं बधेत् ।
द्रवाऽसि रुजाऽसि क्षुमाऽसि ।
पातैनं प्राञ्चं पातैनं प्रत्यञ्चं पातैनं तिर्य्यङ्चं दिग्भ्यः पात ॥

8. O King thou art the strength of the royal family, the giver of longevity to the warrior, the mainstay of princely power, and the administrator of your Kingdom. Thou art the destroyer of foes, as the sun is of clouds!

Thou art the friend of friends, the gentleman with gentlemen. Thou art the cleaver and tormentor of foes. Thou art the preacher of truth. With thee to aid may this hero slay like cloud the foe that dissembles justice. May the warrior protect the King in front, protect him rearwards; protect him sidewards; guard him from all quarters.

६. आविर्मर्या आवित्तो अग्निनर्गृहपतिराविन्त इन्द्रो वृद्धश्रवा आवित्तो मित्रावरुणौ धृतव्रता-वावित्तः पूषा विश्ववेदा आवित्ते द्यावापृथिवी विश्वशम्भुवावावित्तादितिरुरुशर्मा ॥

9. O men, know ye fully well, the learned householder, approach properly, the commander of the army who slays the foes, and has listened to the recitation of all the sacred religious books. Know fully well the friendly and noble persons, devoted to truth. Befriend fastly the doctor expert in the science of medicine. Understand thoroughly the uses of electricity and land, the givers of happiness for all. Get truly a learned mother, the giver of comforts.

१०. अवेष्टा दन्दशूकाः प्राचीमा रोह गायत्री त्वाऽवतु रथन्तरँ साम त्रिवृत्स्तोमो वसन्त ऋतुर्ब्रह्म द्रविणम् ॥

10. O King, conquer the opposing creatures who bite and torment others; and go forward to the East. May thou obtain Gayatri, the psalm of Rathantra, the triple praise-song, the spring season, God and the rich treasure of knowledge!

११. दक्षिणामा रोह त्रिष्टुप् त्वाऽवतु बृहत्साम पञ्चदश स्तोमो ग्रीष्म ऋतुः क्षत्रं द्रविणम् ॥

11. O King, conquer foes by advancing towards the south. May thou obtain, the knowledge conveyed in the Trishtup verse, the Brihat Sam, the fifteenfold praise-song, the summer season, the military force and riches!

---

[9] If men understand these personages, they will certainly be happy in life.

[10] Rathantra: One of the most important Samans, consisting of verses 22, 23 of Rigveda VII, 32 and Samveda II; 1. 1. II. Trivrit Stoma: a recitation in which first, the first, three verses of each triplet of Rigveda IX, 11 are sung together, then the second verses, and lastly the third.

Triple : that gives us the strength of mind, speech and body.

[11] Brihat: One of the most important Sama hymns. Samaveda, II. II. 1.12 taken from Rigveda VI. 46. 1. 2.

CHAPTER X

१२. प्रतीचीमा रोह जगती त्वाऽवतु वैरूप ॐ साम सप्तदश स्तोमो वर्षा ऋतुर्विड् द्रविणम् ॥

12. O King, advance towards the West. May thou obtain the knowledge conveyed in Jagati verse, the manifold knowledge of Sama Veda, the seventeenfold praise-song, the Rainy season, the store of wealth and the Vaishyas!

१३. उदीचीमा रोहानुष्टुप् त्वाऽवतु वैराज ॐ सामैकविꣳश स्तोमः शरदृतुः फलं द्रविणम् ॥

13. O King, advance towards the North. May thou obtain the knowledge conveyed in the Anushtup verse, the manifold knowledge of Sama Veda, the twentyonefold praise-song, the Autumn season, the rich treasurer, and Shudras (servants for service)!

१४. ऊर्ध्वामा रोह पङ्क्तिस्त्वऽवतु शाक्वररैवते सामनी त्रिणवत्रयस्त्रिꣳशौ स्तोमौ हेमन्त-शिशिरावृतू वर्चो द्रविणं प्रत्यस्तं नमुचेः शिरः ॥

14. O King, ascend the zenith. May thou obtain the Knowledge conveyed in the Pankti Shakvari and Rewati verses of the Sam Veda, the thirty-threefold praise-song, three divisions of time, both seasons, Winter and Dews. Arithmetic, the science of nine digits; thirtythree gods, the study through Brahmcharya and riches. Cast aside the head of a thief!

१५. सोमस्य त्विषिरसि तवेव मे त्विषिर्भूयात् ।
मृत्योः पाह्योजोऽसि सहोऽस्यमृतमसि ॥

15. O God! Thou art the brilliance of supremacy, may my knowledge shine like Thine. Save me from death. Thou art vigour and victory.

१६. हिरण्यरूपा उषसो विरोक उभाविन्द्रा उदिथः सूर्यश्च ।
आ रोहतं वरुण मित्र गर्तं ततश्चक्षाथामदितिं दितिं च
मित्रोऽसि वरुणोऽसि ॥

16. O Preacher! the friend of all and O commander! the destroyer of foes, ye both go to the house of a seeker after truth, and dilate upon the immortal and the mortal substances. Just as the sun and moon bring day and night, for the transaction of our various desirable dealings, so should ye both full of lustre and supremacy spread knowledge.

१७. सोमस्य त्वा द्युम्नेनाभि षिञ्चाम्यग्नेर्भ्राजसा सूर्यस्य वर्चसेन्द्रस्येन्द्रियेण ।
क्षत्राणां क्षत्रपतिरेध्यति दिद्यून् पाहि ॥

Fifteenfold: which contains mention of five Pranas i.e., Pran, Apan, Vyan, Udan, Sman. Five organs, i.e., ear, eye, nose, mouth and skin and five elements water, earth, fire, air and ether.

[15]Seventeen fold: Five Karma Indriyas (organs of action), Shabd (speech), Sparsh (touch), Rup (sight), Ras (taste), Gandh (smell), Five Bhutas (earth, water, air, fire and ether), Cause, and effect.

[16]फलम् has been translated as Shudras as well.
Twenty-one fold: Sixteen Kalas, Dharma, Arth, Kam, Moksha, and soul.

[17]Thirty-three fold:—8 vasus, 11 Rudras, 12 Adityas, Soul and God.

17. O King, I install thee with brilliance like the moon, lustre like the fire, splendour of knowledge like the sun, and the might of mind like the lightning. Be lord of princes. Guard constantly all acts conducive to knowledge and religion!

१८. इमं देवा असपत्नꣳ सुवध्वं महते क्षत्राय महते ज्यैष्ठ्याय महते जानराज्यायेन्द्रस्येन्द्रियाय ।
इममुष्य पुत्रममुष्यै पुत्रमस्यै विश एष वोऽमी राजा सोमोऽस्माकं ब्राह्मणानाꣳ राजा ॥

18. O learned generals, this is your King and of us Brahmanas, the devotees of God and of the Vedas. He is the well-qualified King of the subjects!

Produce such a foeless King, the son of such-a-man, and such a woman, for healthy teaching of his people, for adorable warrior-class, for mighty lordship, for mighty domination over princes, and for enhancing the wealth of the wealthy.

१९. प्र पर्वतस्य वृषभस्य पृष्ठान्नावश्चरन्ति स्वसिच इयानाः ।
ता आ ववृत्रन्नधरागुदक्ता अहिं बुध्न्यमनु रीयमाणाः ।
विष्णोर्विक्रमणमसि विष्णोविक्रान्तमसि विष्णोः क्रान्तमसि ॥

19. O royal skilled engineer, construct sea-boats, propelled on water by our experts, and aeroplanes, moving and flying up-ward, after the clouds that reside in the mid-region, that fly as the boats move on the sea, that fly high over and below the watery clouds. Be thou, thereby, prosperous in this world created by the Omnipresent God, and flier in both air, and lightning.

२०. प्रजापते न त्वदेतान्यन्यो विश्वा रूपाणि परि ता बभूव ।
यत्कामास्ते जुहुमस्तन्नो अस्तुवयममुष्य पितासावस्य पिता वयꣳ स्याम पतयो रयीणाꣳ स्वाहा ।
रुद्र यत्ते क्रिवि परं नाम तस्मिन्हुतमस्यमेष्टमसि स्वाहा ॥

20. O God, Thou only comprehendest all these created forms, and none besides Thee! Give us our heart's desire, when we invoke Thee. Just as Thou art the Lord of that invisible world, and this visible world, so, may we be righteous lords of rich possessions. O God! the Tormentor of the wicked, Thy remembrance relieves us of miseries. For that we worship Thee. We worship Thee at home in truthful words.

२१. इन्द्रस्य वज्रोऽसि मित्रावरुणयोस्त्वा प्रशास्त्रोः प्रशिषा युनज्मि ।
अव्यथायै त्वा स्वधायै त्वाऽरिष्टो अर्जुनो मरुतां प्रसवेन जयापाम मनसा समिन्द्रियेण ॥

21. O King, thou art invincible, admirably handsome, and a mighty bolt for the foes. I appoint thee for alleviating the miseries of humanity, for imparting instructions to all, for presiding over the Assembly and the army,

---
[17]I: Purohit.
See Manu, 9, 303, 311, for the qualities of Soma, Agni, Surya, and Indra in the King.
[19]Conveyances to be used on land, water and in air should be constructed by skilled engineers, which take us from one place to the other, from one country to the other. The use of these conveyances is essential for international intercourse.

and for government. I enjoin thee to guard thy state politically, with the advice of wise statesmen. May we be attached to thee with heart and soul. May thou be victorious!

२२. मा त इन्द्र ते वयं तुराषाडयुक्तासो अब्रह्मता विदसाम ।
तिष्ठा रथमधि यं वज्रहस्ता रश्मीन्देव यमसे स्वश्वान् ॥

22. O renowned King, equipped with arms, may we never behave unrighteously towards thee. May thou never shaken thy belief in the Vedas and God. May we never die in poverty. O conqueror of foes, ascend the chariot. Thou controllest the reins and noble horses!

२३. अग्नये गृहपतये स्वाहा सोमाय वनस्पतये स्वाहा मरुतामोजसे स्वाहेन्द्रस्येन्द्रिाय स्वाहा ।
पृथिवि मातर्मा मा हिँसीर्मो अहं त्वाम् ॥

23. We should behave righteously towards the religious-minded and learned householder, derive medical benefit from herbs and trees, inculcate the practice of yoga for the vigour of the priests, follow noble instructions for the improvement of physical organs controlled by the soul. O mother endowed with noble qualities like the Earth, don't injure me by wrong instructions. May I never injure thee!

२४. हँस: शुचिषद्सुरन्तरिक्षसद्धोता वेदिषदतिथिर्दुरोणसत् ।
नृषद्वरसदृतसद्व्योमसदञ्जा गोजा ऋतजा अद्रिजा ऋतं बृहत् ॥

24. Worship God alone, Who solidifies material objects, resides in the hearts of yogis, is Omnipresent, pervades the atmosphere, is the Giver of all gifts, pervades the earth, is Adorable, Ubiquitous, present in the hearts of godly persons, and in fine objects; dwells in space; is the Creator of waters, and Earth, Revealer of the Vedas, and Maker of clouds, mountains and trees. He is true in His nature and Mighty.

२५. इयदस्यायुरस्यायुर्मयि धेहि युङ्ङसि वर्चोऽसि वर्चो मयि धेह्योर्ँगंसूयर्ज मयि धेहि ।
इन्द्रस्य वां वीर्यकृतो बाहू अभ्युपाबहरामि ॥

25. O God, so great art Thou; life art thou, give me life. Thou yokest all in noble deeds; Thou art splendour, give me splendour. Strength art thou: give me strength. O King and subjects, I make the strength of your arms depend upon God, the Fountain of strength!

२६. स्योनासि सुषदासि क्षत्रस्य योनिरसि ।
स्योनामा सीद सुषदामा सीद क्षत्रस्य योनिमा सीद ॥

---

[21] I: Priest.
[22] Just as an expert driver sitting in the car controls the reins and horses, so should the King, at the helm of state affairs, manage them skilfully and efficiently.
[23] I:—Purohit.

26. O Queen, thou art happy, doer of virtuous deeds, and imparter of justice. So be eagerly engaged in delight-giving knowledge. Acquire carefully education that conduces to pleasure. Teach all the females the art of Kingship!

२७. नि षसाद धृतव्रतो वरुणः पस्त्यास्वा ।
साम्राज्याय सुक्रतुः ॥

27. O Queen, just as thy excellent husband, wedded to the vow of Brahmcharya, and master of nice wisdom, for universal sway, always sits in a court of law and administers justice, so shouldst thou!

२८. अभिभूरस्येतास्ते पञ्च दिशः कल्पन्तां ब्रह्माँस्त्वं ब्रह्माऽसि सविताऽसि सत्यप्रसवो वरुणोऽसि सत्यौजा इन्द्रोऽसि विशौजा रुद्रोऽसि सुशेवः ।
बहुकार श्रेयस्कर भूयस्करेन्द्रस्य वज्रोऽसि तेन मे रध्य ॥

28. O King, thou art the conqueror of foes, May these five regions be prosperous for thee. O King, the master of spiritual knowledge, thou art the maker of the state. Thou art the creator of prosperity through righteous dealings. Thou art affable in nature through real power. Thou art the giver of comforts, through the splendour of thy subjects. Thou makest the wicked and the enemy weep, and art full of happiness. Thou art the doer of many acts; contributor to the welfare of thy people. Thou endeavourest again and again. Thou art the grantor of prosperity. Therewith grant me strength to do my duty!

२९. अग्निः पृथुधर्मंणस्पतिर्जुषाणो अग्निः पृथुधर्मणस्पतिराज्यस्य वेतु स्वाहा ।
स्वाहाकृताः सूर्यस्य रश्मिभिर्यंतध्वꣳ सजातानां मध्यमेष्ठ्याय ॥

29. O King, just as spacious fire, dutiful and serviceable, residing in the midst of other allied objects, duly receives oblations of ghee, and gives happiness by diffusing them through the beams of the sun, so shouldst thou, the guardian of justice, large-hearted, and servant of the State, acquire sovereignty. So should the true workers exert!

३०. सवित्रा प्रसवित्रा सरस्वत्या वाचा त्वष्ट्रा रूपैः पूष्णा पशुभिरिन्द्रेणास्मे बृहस्पतिना ब्रह्मणा वरुणेनौजसाऽग्निना तेजसा सोमेन राज्ञा विष्णुना दशम्या देवतया प्रसूतः प्र सर्पामि ॥

30. I go forward urged onward by the impelling God, the truthful speech full of Vedic knowledge, the justice based on real facts, the Earth that rears

---

[26]In this verse, God preaches that there should be separate female magistrates to do justice to the females, and male-magistrates for the males, as in the presence of males, females, through shyness and fear, cannot speak out their mind and make a frank, oral or written statement. Males should teach the boys and females the girls. The vedas are against co-education.

[28]My-Purohit's.

CHAPTER X

different cattle, our supremacy, the mastery of vedic knowledge, the unperturbed tranquillity, the fiery strength to suppress the enemies, the pleasure-giving brilliance of the moon, and by the tenth, i.e., acting upon the qualities, actions, and nature of the Effulgent, Omnipresent God.

३१. अश्विभ्यां पच्यस्व सरस्वत्यै पच्यस्वेन्द्राय सुत्राम्णे पच्यस्व ।
वायुः पूतः पवित्रेण प्रत्यङ्क्सोमो अतिसुतः ।
इन्द्रस्य युज्यः सखा ॥

31. O King and people try to be good teachers and preachers like the sun and moon, try hard to obtain the knowledge of the Vedas, exert your utmost, for supremacy that affords protection. By leading a religious life, being pure like the air, endowed with noble qualities, full of knowledge, be friend unto God, by practising yoga!

३२. कुविदङ्ग यवमन्तो यवं चिद्यथा दान्त्यनुपूर्वं वियूय ।
इहैहैषां कृणुहि भोजनानि ये बर्हिषो नम उक्तिं यजन्ति ।
उपयामगृहीतोऽस्यश्विभ्यां त्वा सरस्वत्यै त्वेन्द्राय त्वा सुत्राम्णे ॥

32. O learned King, full of supremacy, thou, the observer of the vow of celibacy, art accepted by us, for the betterment of the learned teachers, for acquisition of the knowledge of the Vedas, for power and protection. Just as agriculturists whose fields are full of barley, reap the ripe corn, and remove the chaff in order, so bring food in a decent way to the aged, who deserve respect and homage!

३३. युवँ सुराममश्विना नमुचावासुरे सचा ।
विपिपाना शभस्पती इन्द्रं कर्मस्ववातम् ॥

33. O Speaker of the Assembly and Commander of the Army, ye, the united protectors of the State, and doers of altruistic deeds, protect from evil deeds and carnal pleasures, the rich cultivator, nicely busy with agricultural performances!

३४. पुत्रमिव पितरावश्विनोभेन्द्रावथः काव्यैर्दंसनाभिः ।
यत्सुरामं व्यपिबः शचीभिः सरस्वती त्वा मघवन्नभिष्णक् ॥

34. O wealthy and adorable King, with the force of wisdom, enjoy the gladdening rule of thine; may a learned and devoted wife serve thee. O' Speaker of the Assembly and Commander of the Army, protect the State, following the usages framed by the learned, as father and mother protect their child!

---

[30] In this verse ten qualities, a King should possess have been enumerated.
And the tenth: Nine qualities have been mentioned before, this tenth quality, a King should possess is the inner urge by God.

CHAPTER XI

१. युञ्जानः प्रथमं मनस्तत्त्वाय सविता धियः ।
श्रग्नेर्ज्योतिर्निचाय्य पृथिव्या अध्याऽभरत् ॥

1. An aspirant after superhuman power for the acquisition of spiritual knowledge, should first of all harness his mind and intellect with yoga. Having fully realised the high light of Omniscient God, he should show it to others on this earth.

२. युक्तेन मनसा वयं देवस्य सवितुः सवे ।
स्वर्गाय शक्त्या ॥

2. We, the yogis, with full concentration of mind, according to our resources, in this world created by the Supreme Lord, should strive to acquire His Light, for our happiness.

३. युक्त्वाय सविता देवान्त्स्वर्यतो धिया दिवम् ।
बृहज्ज्योतिः करिष्यतः सविता प्र सुवाति तान् ॥

3. The master of the knowledge of yoga, having concentrated his mind on God, should with his intellect cultivate noble qualities, which spread the light of knowledge, and add to happiness. God guides them who advance scientific knowledge.

४. युञ्जते मन उत युञ्जते धियो विप्रा विप्रस्य बृहतो विपश्चितः ।
वि होत्रा दधे वयुनाविदेक इन्महीदेवस्य सवितुः परिष्टुतिः ॥

4. The learned, who give and take knowledge, unite their mind and intellect riveted upon God, Who is Mighty and the fountain of knowledge. He alone, the Knower of all acts, worlds and sciences, declares law. Mighty is the praise of God, Who is the Creator of the universe and Giver of knowledge.

५. युजे वां ब्रह्म पूर्व्यं नमोभिर्वि श्लोक एतु पथ्येव सूरे¹ ।
शृण्वन्तु विश्वे अमृतस्य पुत्रा आ ये धामानि दिव्यानि तस्थुः ॥

5. O seekers after yoga, I wedded to truth, unite my soul with God, realised by past sages through prayer and meditation!
May that God be realised by ye both through diverse efforts, just as a learned person finds the true path and sticks to it. All noble souls should listen to yoga vidya, so that they may acquire salvation and reach regions full of joys.

६. यस्य प्रयाणमन्वन्य इद्ययुर्देवा देवस्य महिमानमोजसा ।
यः पार्थिवानि विममे स एतशो रजाꣳसि देवः सविता महित्वना ॥

¹ I : Purohit.
Ye both:—Who preach and practise yoga.

6. O yogis, the learned souls, should follow through contemplation, God, the Embodiment of happiness, and the Giver of peace. The Omnipresent, Effulgent Lord, the Creator of the universe, brings into existence the material worlds through His glory and power. He alone deserves worship!

७. देव सवितः प्र सुव यज्ञ' प्र सुव यज्ञपतिं भगाय ।
दिव्यो गन्धर्वः केतपूः केतं नः पुनातु वाचस्पतिर्वाचं नः स्वदतु ॥

7. O God, the Bestower of knowledge, and Father of all accomplishments, create for our advancement the pleasant usages, and their protectors. O Sustainer of the Earth, Master of fine qualities, acts and nature, and Purifier through knowledge, purify our thought and will. O Guardian of the Vedas, by their revelation unto us sweeten our speech!

८. इमं नो देव सवितर्यज्ञं प्र नय देवाव्यꣳ सखिविदꣳ सत्राजितं धनजितꣳ स्वर्जितम् ।
ऋचा स्तोमꣳ समर्धय गायत्रेण रथन्तरं बृहद्गायत्रवर्त्तनि स्वाहा ॥

8. O God, the Fulfiller of our noble desires, our Impeller through Omnipresence, direct rightly our yajna, the protector of the learned, the bringer of friends, the promoter of truth, the giver of wealth, the developer of happiness, performed with Rig-vedic hymns. Speed praise-song with the sacred verse. Speed the journey we make in good planes!

९. देवस्य त्वा सवितुः प्रसवेऽश्विनोर्बाहुभ्यां पूष्णो हस्ताभ्याम् ।
आ ददे गायत्रेण छन्दसाऽङ्गिरस्वत्पृथिव्याः सधस्थादग्निं पुरीष्यमङ्गिरस्वदा भर त्रैष्टुभेन छन्दसाऽङ्गिरस्वत् ॥

9. O Vedic speech, in this world created by the Omniscient Lord, I with the forces of sun and moon and the pran and apan forces of the air, with the teachings of verses in Gayatri metre, accept thee dear as breath!
O vedic speech, bestow on me, from this altar knowledge, the benefactor of humanity. Grant me the strength of knowledge dear as breath, through verses in Trishtup metre!

१०. अश्मिरसि नार्यसि त्वया वयमग्निꣳ शकेम खनितुꣳ सधस्थ आ ।
जागतेन छन्दसाऽङ्गिरस्वत् ॥

10. O vedic speech, thou art the bestower of knowledge, beneficial for the people like woman. Through thee, in this place of knowledge, may we be able to explore learning. With a life of celibacy for 48 years, may we improve our learning!

११. हस्त आधाय सविता बिभ्रदग्निꣳ हिरण्ययीम् ।
अग्नेर्ज्योतिर्निचाय्य पृथिव्या अध्याऽभरदानुष्टुभेन छन्दसाऽङ्गिरस्वत् ॥

11. The skilled artisan, following the instructions given in the Anushtap

---

[11]Swami Dayananda gives its purport as such :—People should know that electricity exists in all substances just as it does in iron and stones. Having its full knowledge, and using it well they should construct fiery instruments and aeroplanes.

१२. प्रतूर्त्तं वाजिन्ना द्रव वरिष्ठामनु संवतम् ।
दिवि ते जन्म परममन्तरिक्षे तव नाभिः पृथिव्यामधि योनिरित् ॥

12. O learned person, with the skill of art, thou hast attained to fame under the sun, thou art connected with air's mid-realm through electricity, thy asylum is on earth. Being the master of aeroplanes, go ahead with nice well-balanced speed!

१३. युञ्जाथाꣳ रासभं युवमस्मिन् यामे वृषण्वसू ।
अग्निं भरन्तमस्मयुम् ॥

13. O artisan and his master, ye both, the bestowers of happiness like the sun and air, harness electricity in this aeroplane, possessing the speed of fire and water, seating and taking us afar!

१४. योगे-योगे तवस्तरं वाजे-वाजे हवामहे ।
सखाय इन्द्रमूतये ॥

14. O friends, in every deed and battle, we call for succour, our King, the mightiest of all!

१५. प्र तूर्वन्नेह्यवक्रामन्नशस्ती रुद्रस्य गाणपत्यं मयोभूरेहि ।
उर्वन्तरिक्षं वीहि स्वस्तिगव्यूतिरभयानि कृण्वन् पूष्णा सयुजा सह ॥

15. O King, thou whose paths are pleasant, with thy powerful and devoted army, come, destroying the forces of thy wicked foes. Come, overtaking the territories of the enemies. Spreading gladness all around, accept the chieftainship of thy commander of the army, who makes the enemies weep. Granting fearlessness to all thy subjects, speed through the wide air!

१६. पृथिव्याः सधस्थादग्निं पुरीष्यमङ्गिरस्वदा भरग्निं पुरीष्यमङ्गिरस्वदच्छेमोऽग्निं पुरीष्यमङ्गिरस्वद्‌धरिष्याम: ॥

16. O learned person, just as we skilfully evolve from a part of the earth, electricity, dear as breath, and the giver of comfort, and just as we procure atmospheric electricity, dear as breath, and the giver of comfort, so shouldst thou skillfully prepare electricity which like the sun conduces to our comforts!

१७. अन्वग्निरुषसामग्रमख्यदन्वहानि प्रथमो जातवेदाः ।
अनु सूर्यस्य पुरुत्रा च रश्मीननु द्यावापृथिवी आ ततन्थ ॥

17. The First and Foremost God illuminates the sun before twilight. He also illuminates the days, and multiple beams of the sun. He alone establishes the Heaven and Earth.

CHAPTER XI

१८. आगत्य वाज्यध्वान्ॐ सर्वा मृधो वि धूनुते ।
अग्निॐ सधस्थे महिते चक्षुषा नि चिकीषते ॥

18. O learned King, just as a swift horse, having started on his way, causes terror in all battles, and just as a householder wants to see with his eyes, fire arranged in a beautiful place, so shouldst thou shake all battles and spread knowledge to each house!

१९. आक्रम्य वाजिन् पृथिवीमग्निमिच्छ रुचा त्वम् ।
भूम्या वृत्वाय नो ब्रूहि यतः खनेम तं वयम् ॥

19. O learned King, according to thy desire, trample upon the foes, hanker after sovereignty and knowledge, and having accepted us as thy subjects on the earth, instruct us in geology and electricity; so that we may use that knowledge!

२०. द्यौस्ते पृष्ठं पृथिवी सधस्थमात्माऽन्तरिक्षॐ समुद्रो योनिः ।
विख्याय चक्षुषा त्वमभि तिष्ठ पृतन्यतः ॥

20. O learned King, thy humility and dealings are resplendent like the sun, thy seat is firm like the Earth, thy soul is indestructible, like the space, thy goal is vast like the ocean. Having measured thy strength carefully attack the enemy with thy army!

२१. उत्क्राम महते सौभगायास्मादास्थानाद् द्रविणोदा वाजिन् ।
वयॐ स्याम सुमतौ पृथिव्या अग्निं खनन्त उपस्थे अस्याः ॥

21. O prosperous, learned person, just as we, the givers of wealth, from the surrounding of each dwelling place of ours, exploring the science of fire, acquire wisdom for worldly prosperity, so shouldst thou elevate thy self!

२२. उदक्रमीद् द्रविणोदा वाज्यर्वाक् सुलोकॐ सुकृतं पृथिव्याम् ।
ततः खनेम सुप्रतीकमग्निॐ स्वो रुहाणा अधि नाकमुत्तमम् ॥

22. O learned geologist, wealth-giver, just as a strong horse jumps up, so should'st thou attain to greatness in this world; acquire absolute, beautiful happiness free from pain, derivable from a saintly life. May we, in the enjoyment of happiness, explore the pervading electricity full of brilliance!

२३. आत्वा जिघर्मि मनसा घृतेन प्रतिक्षियन्तं भुवनानि विश्वा ।
पृथुं तिरश्चा वयसा बृहन्तं व्यचिष्ठमन्नॐ रभसं दृशानम् ॥

23. O seeker after knowledge, just as I with learning and ghee, clearly manifest the properties of air, that pervades all substances, that moves

---

[21]The verse can also be translated as such. 'O' learned persons, ye are the givers of wealth. God forward from the present position for great prosperity. Digging, according to your instructions from the bosom of the earth, the lustrous metals like gold, let us be devoted to the good of humanity."

[23]I: God.

transversely, is vast in vitality, highly powerful with the oblations of corn, vast in velocity, and visible, so I make thee also understand the properties of air!

२४. आ विश्वत: प्रत्यङ्ञ्चं जिघर्म्यरक्षसा मनसा तज्जुषेत ।
मर्यंश्री स्पृहयद्वर्णो ऽग्निर्नाभिमृशे तन्वा जर्भुराण: ॥

24. O man, just as heat and air pervading the body are useful to their sustainer, who fastly moves the organs of the body, like one attempting to fulfil his desire; So I, for the grandeur of man, manifest, with immaculate reason, the properties of the heat that sets in motion the air inside the body; so shouldst thou enjoy that heat!

२५. परि वाजपति: कविरग्निर्हव्यान्यक्रमीत् ।
दधद्रत्नानि दाशुषे ॥

25. O learned person, know thou, the handsome, charitably-disposed renowned person, giving in charity gold to the learned person who acquires from all sides substances fit for charity, like the householders who preserve foodstuffs!

२६. परि त्वाऽग्ने पुरं वयं विप्रᳰ सहस्य धीमहि ।
धृष्द्वर्णं दिवे-दिवे हन्तारं भङ्गुरावताम् ॥

26. O learned person, aspirant after power, we unanimously select thee, as our commander, the day by day destroyer of the citadel of our treacherous foes, possessing iron determination, good looking features, and vast knowledge!

२७. त्वमग्ने द्युभिस्त्वमाशुशुक्षणिस्त्वमद्भ्यस्त्वमश्मनस्परि ।
त्वं वनेभ्यस्त्वमोषधीभ्यस्त्वं नृणां नृपते जायसे शुचि: ॥

27. Thou, Sovereign Lord of men, just King, resplendent like fire, brilliant like the sun, speedy destroyer of the wicked, with air and waters, with clouds and stones, with forests and beams, with medicinal herbs, art adorned in every way, being pure amongst the subjects.

२८. देवस्य त्वा सवितु: प्रसवेऽश्विनोर्बाहुभ्यां पूष्णो हस्ताभ्याम् ।
पृथिव्या: सधस्थादग्निं पुरीष्यमङ्गिरस्वत्खनामि ।
ज्योतिष्मन्तं त्वाऽग्ने सुप्रतीकमजस्रेण भानुना दीद्यतम् ।
शिवं प्रजाभ्योऽहिᳰसन्तं पृथिव्या: सधस्थादग्निं पुरीष्यमङ्गिरस्वत्खनाम: ॥

28. O geologist and artisan, just as I, in this world created by the Effulgent Lord, like the powers of attraction and retention of the atmosphere and

---

²⁴I : God.
²⁶A man possessing the virtues mentioned in the verse should be selected as a commander of the army.
²⁷The King should make full use of the air, waters, clouds, stones, forests, beams and medicinal herbs for the good of his subjects.

CHAPTER XI

earth, and like the force and swiftness of air, following in your wake, explore from a part of the earth, electricity, giver of full comfort, luminous, resplendent with imperishable lustre, gracious like air; and just as, with your assistance, we, explore from a part of the atmosphere, electricity, pervading like refined air, doing no harm, excellent amongst all nourishing substances, and administering to the prosperity of the people, so should all do!

२९. अपां पृष्ठमसि योनिरग्ने: समुद्रमभित: पिन्वमानम् ।
वर्धमानो महाँ२ आ च पुष्करे दिवो मात्रया वरिम्णा प्रथस्व ॥

29. O learned person, thou knowest the qualities of integration and disintegration of the All pervading electricity, thou art worthy of respect. Mayest thou progress with the aid of knowledge and scientific skill, having known the all round raining clouds, the support of water, the ocean and the material substances embedded in it, from which the sun, residing in the atmosphere, takes up with its beams; and adds amply to thy comforts!

३०. शर्म च स्थो वर्म च स्थोऽच्छिद्रे बहुले उभे ।
व्यचस्वती सं वसाथां भूतमग्निं पुरीष्यम् ॥

30. O wife and husband, ye have entered the domestic life with all its responsibilities, like the two faultless objects which are full of comforts, fit for service in many ways. There are in your house deeds of virtue and worldly gain, which are the props of your domestic life.
Dwell peacefully in that house, making full use of the nourishing and protecting electricity.

३१. सं वसाथाॐ स्वविदा समीची उरसा त्मना ।
अग्निमन्तर्भरिष्यन्ती ज्योतिष्मन्तमजस्रमित् ॥

31. O wife and husband, ye full well knowers of objects, protectors of all, enjoyers of happiness, make use with your thinking faculty, of ceaseless, ever flowing brilliant, and all pervading electricity.

३२. पुरीष्योऽसि विश्वभरा अथर्वा त्वा प्रथमो निरमन्थदग्ने ।
त्वाम् पुष्करादध्यथर्वा निरमन्थत ।
मूर्ध्नो विश्वस्य वाघत: ॥

---

[28]Powers of attraction and retention found in the atmosphere have figuratively been described in the verse as its arms, and the force and swiftness of the air as its hands. Electricity is to be explored from the earth and atmosphere.
I: a scientist. We: Workers.
[30]The purport of this verse as given by Swami Dayananda is, that we should construct houses full of doors, comfortable in all seasons, affording all round protection, and installed with electricity.
[31]He who knows the use and science of electricity never leads a life of poverty.

32. O learned person, well versed in religious lore, thou art the caretaker of cattle. The harmless, and advanced well read person, the nourisher of all, accepts thee, having derived electricity from the sky, high above the world.

३३. तमु त्वा दध्यङ्ङ्ङ्ऋषिः पुत्र ईधे अथर्वणः ।
वृत्रहणं पुरन्दरम् ॥

33. O King, may the noble pupil of the harmless scholar, having mastered the comforts-giving objects like electricity, possessing the knowledge of the vedas, and master of all sciences, make thee, the killer of foes, and breaker of their forts, shine.

३४. तमु त्वा पाथ्यो वृषा समीधे दस्युहन्तमम् ।
धनञ्जयँ रणे-रणे ॥

34. O warrior, thou art well equipped with food-stuffs and water, and imbued with valour. May the army of heroes, with the teaching of the art of government illuminate thee, the destroyer of the wicked and winner of wealth in every battle-field.

३५. सीद होतः स्व उ लोके चिकित्वान्त्सादया यज्ञँ सुकृतस्य योनौ ।
देवावीर्देवान्हविषा यजास्यग्ने बृहद्यजमाने वयो धाः ॥

35. O learned person, fond of charity, full of knowledge, reside in pleasant happiness. On the basis of virtue, establish good relations between the King and the subjects. Taught by the sages, thou shouldst justly respect noble qualities. Give long life to the king and his people.

३६. नि होता होतृषदने विदानस्त्वेषो दीदिवाँ२ असदत्सुदक्षः ।
अदब्धव्रतप्रमतिर्वसिष्ठः सहस्रम्भरः शुचिजिह्वो अग्निः ॥

36. He acquires happiness, who follows the charitably disposed learned persons, is an aspirant after religious practices, resplendent with noble traits, a seeker after knowledge, pure-tongued, passing mighty, wise through religious austerities, foremost amongst the celibates, a possessor of thousands of virtues, a grasper of noble characteristics, and pure like fire.

३७. सँ सीदस्व महाँ२ असि शोचस्व देववीतमः ।
वि धूममग्ने अरुषं मियेध्य सृज प्रशस्त दर्शतम् ॥

37. O learned person, praiseworthy, chastiser of the wicked, deeply loved by the sages, and sinless, acquire beautiful and attractive complexion. Be pure. Thou art full of noble qualities. Assume the role of a teacher!

३८. अपा देवीरुप सृज मधुमतीरयक्ष्माय प्रजाभ्यः ।
तासामास्थानादुज्जिहतामोषधयः सुपिप्पला ॥

---

[37] A teacher should possess the qualities mentioned in the verse.

CHAPTER XI

38. O skilled physician, arrange for the supply of pure and sweet waters, with their help, let medicinal plants with goodly berries spring for the cure of consumption-like diseases of the people!

३९. सं ते वायुर्मातरिश्वा दधातूत्तानाया हृदयं यद्विकस्तम् ।
यो देवानां चरसि प्राणथेन कस्मै देव वषडस्तु तुभ्यम् ॥

39. O wife, the embodiment of fine qualities, may the air blowing in the mid-region, purified through yajna, strengthen thy well-trained heart!
O learned husband, giver of comforts, thou hast got a heart disciplined by the wise through the pleasant exercises of breath, may I bring thee, the source of happiness, reverence, glory, strength and well-being!

४०. सुजातो ज्योतिषा सह शर्म वरूथमासदत्स्वः ।
वासो अग्ने विश्वरूपँ सं व्ययस्व विभावसो ॥

40. O householder, full of riches, blazing like fire, well-renowned for knowledge, reside in a comfortable nice house, and robe thyself in many-hued attire!

४१. उदु तिष्ठ स्वध्वरावा नो देव्या धिया ।
दृशे च भासा बृहता सुशुक्वनिराग्ने याहि सुशस्तिभिः ॥

41. O householder, lord of good deeds, arise. With Godlike thought protect us well. Shining like fire, sharer of all good things, verily splendid to behold like the resplendent sun; study all sciences with thy praiseworthy qualities!

४२. ऊर्ध्व ऊ षु ण ऊतये तिष्ठा देवो न सविता ।
ऊर्ध्वो वाजस्य सनिता यदञ्जिभिर्वाघद्भिर्विह्वयामहे ॥

42. O learned teacher, arise erect, for our protection, like the brilliant sun high up in the sky. May thou, like shining beams, follow the pursuit of knowledge, with disciplined intelligent pupils trained in the art of grappling with knowledge. We specially invoke thee!

४३. स जातो गर्भो असि रोदस्योरग्ने चारुर्विभृत ओषधीषु ।
चित्रः शिशुः परि तमाँस्यक्तून्प्र मातृभ्यो अधि कनिक्रदद्गाः ॥

43. O learned person, just as the sun, well-known on the Earth and the Sky, beautiful, infuser of strength in medicinal plants, wonderful, moving all around, subdues the glooms of nights, so should the child obtain knowledge!

४४. स्थिरो भव वीडवङ्ग आशुर्भव वाज्यर्वन् ।
पृथुर्भव सुपदस्त्वमग्नेः पुरीषवाहणः ॥

44. O intelligent son, steady be thou to acquire knowledge, learn statesmanship, be stout in body, be active, learn the use of fiery instruments, be diffuser of happiness, and teacher of moral duty of protecting the weak!

⁴²We: the pupils.
⁴⁴The father instructs the son as to the qualities he should possess.

४५. शिवो भव प्रजाभ्यो मानुषीभ्यस्त्वमङ्गिरः ।
मा द्यावापृथिवी अभि शोचीर्मान्तरिक्षं मा वनस्पतीन् ॥

45. O beloved son, be propitious to creatures of the human race. Weep not for the objects between the heaven and earth, in air's mid region, and for trees.

४६. प्रेतु वाजी कनिक्रदन्नानदद्रासभः पत्वा ।
भरन्नग्निं पुरीष्यं मा पाद्यायुषः पुरा ।
वृषाग्निं वृषणं भरन्नपां गर्भᳪ समुद्रियम् ।
अग्न आ याहि वीतये ॥

46. O noble son, like the fast moving, neighing, running, strong horse, die not ere thy time. Utilising electricity for thy safety, waste not thy energy. Just as the powerful, adorable sun takes away waters from the sea, and causes rain, so shouldst thou come hither for bestowing happiness!

४७. ऋतᳪ सत्यमृतᳪ सत्यमग्निं पुरीष्यमङ्गिरस्वद्व्रराम: ।
ओषधयः प्रति मोदध्वमग्निमेतᳪ शिवमायन्तमभ्यत्र यूयमा ।
व्यस्यन् विश्वा अनिरा अमीवा निषीदन्नो अप दुर्मतिं जहि ॥

47. O good children, just as we realise, like air, the true, indestructible, steady, excellent, protection-affording electricity, so should ye remain happy, after mastering this auspicious electricity. The medicinal food like barley, which ye obtain, is secured by us also!

O physician, remove from us in various ways the unimpartible pain of diseases, and being well versed in medical science, banish all our evil thoughts!

४८. ओषधयः प्रति गृभ्णीत पुष्पवतीः सुपिप्पलाः ।
अयं वो गर्भ ऋत्वियः प्रत्नᳪ सधस्थमाऽसदत् ॥

48. O women, use medicinal plants laden with bloom and goodly fruit, so that your conception experienced at the time of menstruation may stay in the womb in its proper place. Use the medicines prepared from nice flowery herbs full of fruits!

४९. वि पाजसा पृथुना शोशुचानो बाधस्व द्विषो रक्षसो अमीवाः । सुशर्मणो बृहतः शर्मणि स्यामग्नेरहᳪ सुहवस्य प्रणीतौ ॥

49. O husband, resplendent with thy wide-extending strength, chastise the voluptuous and degraded women, painful to mankind like fell diseases. May I remain in your comfortable house, as the wife of one, highly graceful, pure in dealings, and lustrous like fire!

---

⁴⁵"One should not weep over the wordly objects, but should try to protect and utilise them.
⁴⁷"We : parents.
⁴⁸"For the preservation of their conception, women should use medicines which help in its proper growth.

CHAPTER XI

५०. आपो हि ष्ठा मयोभुवस्ता न ऊर्जे दधातन ।
महे रणाय चक्षसे ॥

50. O wives, be pure and sweet like waters, and full of happiness. Stick to us steadfastly, for energy, valour, and highly memorable battle-fields!

५१. यो वः शिवतमो रसस्तस्य भाजयतेह नः ।
उशतीरिव मातरः ॥

51. O wives, we have got to perform a highly pleasant, joyful duty in this domestic life. Just as mothers in their longing love feed the child, so should ye perform it in a spirit of love and devotion!

५२. तस्मा अरं गमाम वो यस्य क्षयाय जिन्वथ ।
आपो जनयथा च नः ॥

52. O wives, calm like waters, be contented in our house, and rear good sons. May we nobly attain to ye!

५३. मित्रः सँ सृज्य पृथिवीं भूमिं च ज्योतिषा सह ।
सुजातं जातवेदसमयक्ष्माय त्वा सँ सृजामि प्रजाभ्यः ॥

53. O husband, friend unto all, for the health of the people, with the aid of knowledge, justice and instruction, having determined the earth and space, thou givest me pleasure: I bring fame unto thee, master of the vedas, and enjoying good reputation!

५४. रुद्राः सँ सृज्य पृथिवीं बृहज्ज्योतिः समिधिरे ।
तेषां भानुरजस्र इच्छुको वेवेषु रोचते ॥

54. O husband and wife, just as airs, making the sun shine, set the earth aglow with lofty light: and as the brilliant sun, born of airs, sheds constant light on material objects, so shoudst ye enlighten the people, with knowledge and justice and bring happiness unto them!

५५. सँसृष्टां वसुभी रुद्रैर्धीरैः कर्मण्यां मृदम् ।
हस्ताभ्यां मृद्वीं कृत्वा सिनीवाली कृणोतु ताम् ॥

55. O husband, just as a potter with the dexterity of his hand and skill, utilizes the clay, so render soft-hearted the celibate girl, well trained by the vasus, the Rudras, and the self-controlled instructors. Take her as thy wife, who through love makes the girls strong!

५६. सिनीवाली सुकपर्दा सुकुरीरा स्वौपशा ।
सा तुभ्यमदिते महोखां दधातु हस्तयोः ॥

---

[50]Husband and wife should always remain together and be never separated, even on the battle-field. This is the grand vedic ideal of their constant companionship.

[55]Vasus: Learned persons who observe celibacy for 24 years.

Rudras: Persons who observe celibacy for 44 years.

Girls strong: Improves the girls physically, intellectually and morally.

56. O venerable, ever-happy wife, utilise the services of a maid servant, who, full of love, with lovely looks, nobieminded, cooker of nice meals, places the cooking-pan in thy hands!

५७. उखां कृणोतु शक्त्या बाहुभ्यामदितिर्धिया ।
माता पुत्रं यथोपस्थे साऽग्निं विभर्त्तु गर्भे श्रा । मखस्य शिरोऽसि ॥

57. O householder, thou art the head of domestic yajna. Prepare medicines with thy cooking skill, thy arms, and thy intellect, May thy wife bear semen in her womb, as a mother bears her son in her lap!

५८. वसवस्त्वा कृणवन्तु गायत्रेण छन्दसाऽङ्गिरस्वद्ध्रुवासि पृथिव्यसि धारया मयि प्रजाँ-रायस्पोषं गौपत्यँ सुवीर्यँ सजातान्यजमानाय रुद्रास्त्वा कृणवन्तु त्रैष्टुभेन छन्दसाऽङ्गि-रस्वद-ध्रुवाऽस्यन्तरिक्षमसि धारया मयि प्रजाँ रायस्पोषं गौपत्यँ सुवीर्यँ सजाता-न्यजमानायादित्यास्त्वा कृणवन्तु जागतेन छन्दसाऽङ्गिरस्वद्ध्रुवासि द्यौरसि धारया मयि प्रजाँ रायस्पोषं गौपत्यँ सुवीर्यँ सजातान्यजमानाय विश्वे त्वा देवा वैश्वानरा: कृणवन्त्वानुष्टुभेन छन्दसाऽङ्गिरस्वद्ध्रुवासि दिशोऽसि धारया मयि प्रजाँ रायस्पोषं-गौपत्यँ सुवीर्यँ सजातान्यजमानाय ॥

58. O learned celibate young woman, thou art steady like air, and giver of happiness, may the learned Vasu Brahmcharis, with the teachings of Gayatri verses, as given in the Vedas, make thee my wife. O celibate young man, thou art steady like vital air, and full of forbearance like the earth, may the learned Vasu Brahmcharis, with the teachings of Gayatri verses as given in the Vedas, make thee my husband. Establish in me, thy wife, good progeny, abundant wealth, mastery of speech and land, and excellent valour. May we both hand-over the children born alike, to a learned teacher for acquiring knowledge. O learned celibate young woman, thou art stead-fast like the sky, and highly lovely, may the learned Rudra Brahmcharis, with the teachings of Trishtup verses as given in the vedas, make thee my wife. O celibate young man, thou art steadfast like the sky, and full of love may Rudra Brahmcharis, with the teachings of Trishtup verses, as given in the Vedas, make thee my husband. May thou establish in me, virtuous children, abundant wealth, art of teaching, and excellent valour. May we both, hand over the children born of the same womb, to a learned teacher, the master of the Vedas, for learning the vedic lore from him.

O learned celibate young woman, thou art steady like the sky, and brilliant like the sun. May the learned Aditya Brahmcharis, with the teachings of

[56]Trained and intelligent maid-servants should be employed by householders to cook meals.

[57]Medicines should be used for the preservation of conception.

[58]A Vasu Brahmchari is one who observes the vow of celibacy of 24 years. A Rudra Brahmchari remains celibate for 44 years, and an Aditya Brahmchari for 48 years. These learned persons unite the young man and woman in wedlock, reciting the vedic verses dilating upon the respective duties and responsibilities of domestic life.

Born alike means born of the same womb, without distinction.

Jagati verses as given in the vedas, make thee my wife. O celibate young man, thou art steadfast like the sky and brilliant like the sun. May the learned Aditya Brahmcharis, with the teachings of Jagati verses as given in the Vedas, make thee my husband. Establish in me good progeny, abundant wealth, full mastery of knowledge, and excellent valour. May we both hand over the children giving them instructions from their infancy, to a learned teacher, for receiving education. O beautiful and glorious wife, thou art steadfast like the vital air, and famous in all directions. May all the sages and preachers, with the teachings of Anushtup verses as given in the Vedas, entrust thee to my care. O husband, thou art steadfast like the vital air, and famous in all directions, may all the sages and teachers place thee in my charge. Establish in me, good progeny, abundant wealth, wisdom of speech, and excellent valour. May we both hand over our children for receiving education, to a learned teacher who preaches truth!

५९. अदित्यै रास्नास्यदितिष्टे बिलं गृभ्णातु ।
कृत्वाय सा महीमुखां मृन्मयीं योनिमग्नये ।
पुत्रेभ्य: प्रायच्छददिति: श्रपयानिति ॥

59. O learned teachress, thou art the bestower of education. Let the son and daughter, observing celibacy, receive education from thee. Thou, like a mother, handest over the big earthen cooking-pan to thy pupils, to be placed near the fire, so that being trained in the art of cooking, they cook nicely their meals!

६०. वसवस्त्वा धूपयन्तु गायत्रेण छन्दसाऽङ्गिरस्वद्रुद्रास्त्वा धूपयन्तु त्रैष्टुभेन छन्दसाऽङ्गिरस्वदादित्यास्त्वा धूपयन्तु जागतेन छन्दसाऽङ्गिरस्वद्विश्वे ।
त्वा देवा वैश्वानरा धूपयन्त्वानुष्टुभेन छन्दसाऽङ्गिरस्वदिन्द्रस्त्वा धूपयतु वरुणस्त्वा धूपयतु विष्णुस्त्वा धूपयतु ।

60. O male or female student, may the Vasu Brahmcharis, with the Gayatri verses as given in the vedas coach thee dear as life. May the Rudra Brahmcharis with the Trishtup verses as given in the vedas, coach thee, a seeker after knowledge. May the Aditya Brahmcharis, with the Jagati verses as given in the vedas coach thee, pure like air. May all the noble teachers and religious preachers, with the Anushtup verses as given in the vedas, coach thee, lustrous like electricity. May the King coach thee in statesmanship. May the Lord of justice coach thee in the art of administering justice. May the yogi coach thee in yogic practices!

६१. अदितिष्ट्वा देवी विश्वदेव्यावती पृथिव्या: सधस्थे अङ्गिरस्वत् खनत्ववट देवानां त्वा पत्नीर्देवीर्विश्वदेव्यावती: पृथिव्या: सधस्थे अङ्गिरस्वद्दधतुखे ।
घिपणास्त्वा देवीर्विश्वदेव्यावती: पृथिव्या: सधस्थे अङ्गिरस्वदभीन्धतामुखे वरूत्रीष्ट्वा

---

[59] A teachress should give instruction to her pupils in the art of cooking also, besides teaching them other branches of knowledge.

देवीर्विश्वदेव्यावती: पृथिव्या: सधस्थे अङ्ङिरस्वच्छुपयन्तूखेग्नास्त्वा देवीर्विश्वदेव्यावती: पृथिव्या: सधस्थे अङ्ङिरस्वत्पचन्तुखे जनयस्त्वाच्छिन्नपत्रा देवीर्विश्वदेव्यावती: पृथिव्या: सधस्थे अङ्ङिरस्वत्पचन्तूखे ॥

61. O child free from sin and blame, may the lady advanced in knowledge amongst the learned, expert in teaching, well read, in any part of the earth, educate thee, brilliant like fire!

O educated young girl, may the wife of a learned person, most advanced in knowledge amongst the learned, well read, in any part of the earth, educate thee, dear as life!

O girl, seeker after knowledge, may the lady advanced in knowledge amongst the learned, wise, sweet-tongued and well read, in any part of the earth, enlighten thee, strong as vital air!

O girl, receiving education, may a learned, noble, beautiful lady, in any part of the earth make thee glorious like the sun!

O girl students, may a lady advanced in knowledge amongst the learned, full of pure knowledge, and well versed in the vedas, in any part of the earth, make thee forceful like electricity!

O girl desirous of knowledge, may a learned lady, attired in beautiful clothes, and air-minded, well-known for her virtues, the bestower of fine moral qualities, in a good place of the earth, make thee sweet, like the juice of medicinal herbs!

६२. मित्रस्य चर्षणीधृतोऽवो देवस्य सानसि ।
द्युम्नं चित्रश्रवस्तमम् ॥

62. O woman, protect the valuable ancestral property of thy glorious husband, who loves thee, is the guardian of the people, and master of various nice foodstuffs!

६३. देवस्त्वा सवितोद्वपतु सुपाणि: स्वङ्गुरि: सुबाहुरुत शक्त्या ।
अव्यथमाना पृथिव्यामाशा दिश आ पृण ॥

63. O woman, let thy majestic husband, with lovely arms, with lovely hands, with lovely fingers, by the power he hath, make thee, residing on the earth, pregnant. Thou shouldst serve thy husband without fear, and fill all directions with thy desire and fame!

६४. उत्थाय बृहती भवोदु तिष्ठ ध्रुवा त्वम् ।
मित्रैतां त उखां परि ददाभ्यभित्या एषा मा भेदि ॥

---

[61]Just as earth is dug, well is constructed and water drawnout, so the teacher draws out the latent faculties of the head and heart of the pupil. The word खनतु which means digging, has figuratively been used for developing the mental and intellectual faculties of the child.

The student girl is advised in this verse, to lead a life of celibacy, and acquire knowledge from different ladies mentioned therein.

[62]Wife should inherit the property of her husband, and keep it in-tact.

64. O educated girl, be highly active, and firm in noble resolves. Get ready, and shedding idleness, marry this husband. O friend, I hand over this girl to thee, to remain without fear. Never separate her from thyself!

६५. वसवस्त्वाऽऽच्छन्दन्तु गायत्रेण छन्दसाऽङ्गिरस्वद्रुद्रास्त्वाऽऽच्छन्दन्तु त्रैष्टुभेन छन्दसाऽङ्गिरस्व-दादित्यास्त्वाऽऽच्छन्दन्तु जागतेन छन्दसाऽङ्गिरस्वद्विश्वे त्वा देवा वैश्वानरा आच्छन्दन्त्वानु-ष्टुभेन छन्दसाऽङ्गिरस्वत् ॥

65. O man or woman, may the Vasu Brahmcharis, illuminate thee like fire, with Gayatri verses. May the Rudra Brahmcharis, strengthen thee like vital breath with Trishtup verses. May the Aditya Brahmcharis make thee pure and lustrous, with Jagati verses. May all the sages and preachers of truth, make thee pure like medicinal herbs, with Anushtup verses!

६६. आकूतिमग्निं प्रयुजῶ स्वाहा मनो मेधामग्निं प्रयुजῶ स्वाहा चित्तं विज्ञातमग्निं प्रयुजῶ स्वाहा वाचो विधृतिमग्निं प्रयुजῶ स्वाहा । प्रजापतये मनवे स्वाहाग्नये वैश्वानराय स्वाहा ॥

66. Realise, through the practice of truth, the thoughtful soul, fit to understand the true essence of things and their use.
Realise through yoga, mind, wisdom, and soul their impeller, know fully the fire like soul, the impeller of thought and knowledge.
Realise well speech and steady abstraction of the mind, and their urger, the yogic force.
Revere the wise ruler, the Protector of the people.
Eulogise the Self Effulgent Lord, the Friend of all.

६७. विश्वो देवस्य नेतुर्मर्तो वुरीत सख्यम् । विश्वो राय इषुध्यति द्युम्नं वृणीत पुष्यसे स्वाहा ॥

67. Let all mortals seek the friendship of God, the Maker of the universe. Let all use arms for glory and wealth, and possess truthful speech, fame and food. Just as thou prosperest thereby, let all of us prosper.

६८. मा सु भित्था मा सु रिषोऽम्ब धृष्णु वीरयस्व सु । अग्निश्चेद् करिष्यथ: ॥

68. O mother, wean us not from education, harm us not. Accomplish with determination the task undertaken. May thou and thy son thus, resolute like fire, finish this task worth doing!

[64] I : Priest.
[65] Gayatri verses: which preach high sciences.
Trishtup verses: which dilate upon action, meditation and knowledge.
Jagati verses: which reveal the nature of material objects.
Anushtup verses: which remove our miseries.
[67] Thou: a learned person.

६९. दृ॒ꣳह॑स्व देवि पृथिवि स्वस्तय॒ आसु॒री मा॒या स्व॒धया॑ कृ॒तासि॑ ।
जु॒ष्टं दे॒वेभ्य॑ इ॒दम॑स्तु ह॒व्यम॑रिष्टा॒ त्वमु॒दिहि॑ य॒ज्ञे अ॒स्मिन् ॥

69. O wife, equipped with knowledge, and possessing learning vast like the earth, thou hast corrected the low mentality of self-interested persons, with food and water, for their good. Make me thy husband prosper. Being non-violent, attain to fame in this domestic life. May this oblation be accepted by the learned!

७०. द्रु॒व॒न्नः स॑र्पिरासुतिः प्र॒त्नो होता॒ वरे॑ण्यः ।
सह॑सस्पु॒त्रो अद्भु॑तः ॥

70. O husband, fed on fruits of trees, and clarified butter, ever worthy of respect, giver and taker, the son of the strong, wonderful in qualities, deeds and temperament, be famous in this domestic life for enjoying happiness!

७१. पर॒स्या अधि॑ संव॒तो॑ऽव॒राꣳ अ॒भ्या त॑र ।
य॒त्राह॒मस्मि॒ ताꣳ अव॑ ॥

71. O well qualified girl, reject those who are equal or inferior to thee in strength and learning. I want to marry thee!
Protect the good persons of the family, which I belong to.

७२. पर॒स्याः पा॑रा॒वतो॑ रोहिद॒श्व इ॒हा ग॑हि ।
पु॒रीष्यः॑ पुरुप्रि॒योऽग्ने॒ त्वं तरा॒ मृधः॑ ॥

72. O learned and dignified husband, lord of conveyances propelled by fire, excellent in affording protection, loved by many, come hitherward from the farthest distance, for marrying this beautiful renowned and well-behaved girl, and overcome our foes along with her!

७३. यद॑ग्ने॒ कानि॒ कानि॑ चि॒दा ते॒ दारू॑णि द॒ध्मसि॑ ।
सर्वं॒ तद॑स्तु ते घृ॒तं तज्जु॑षस्व यविष्ठ्य ॥

73. O most youthful young man or woman, may we put in the earthen pot all eatables belonging to thee. All that belongs to us, is thine. Eat the ghee that belongs to us. All that belongs to thee is ours. May we use the ghee that belongs to thee!

७४. यदा॒त्युप॑जि॒ह्विका य॒द्वम्रो॒ अति॒सर्प॑ति ।
सर्वं॒ तद॑स्तु ते घृ॒तं तज्जु॑षस्व यविष्ठ्य ॥

---

[70] Giver and taker: The husband gives sound advice to the wife, and takes good counsel from her.

[72] The veda condemns the near and advocates the distant marriages. Swami Dayananda, in his immortal book the *Satyarth Prakash* mentions in details the drawbacks of near, and advantages of distant marriages. Our: Parents.

[73] We, us: The near relatives of the boy or girl.

74. O most youthful husband, whatever thou eatest, or whatever thy wife, free from greed, with control over her palate, eatest and the breath that comes sharply out of her mouth, that all is thine. Eat the ghee that is thine!

७५. ब्रह्नरहरप्रयावं भरन्तोऽश्वायेव तिष्ठते घासमस्मै ।
रायस्पोषेण समिषा मदन्तोऽग्ने मा ते प्रतिवेशा रिषाम ॥

75. Just as we, with unceasing care bring fodder day after day to a stabled courser, so may we, amassing all the enjoyable objects of life, pleased with food and growth of riches, leading a religious life, never injure this learned householder, fit for domestic life, free from injustice!

७६. नाभा पृथिव्याः समिधाने अग्नौ रायस्पोषाय बृहते हवामहे ।
इरम्मदं बृहदुक्थं यजत्रं जेतारमग्निं पृतनासु सासहिम् ॥

76. Just as we put oblations in the fire enkindled on earth's navel, so we for ample increase of our riches, hail the commander of the army, most calm in the midst of armies, relisher of meals, much applauded, warrior, fast like electricity, and conqueror.

७७. याः सेना अभीत्वरीराव्याधिनीरुगणा उत ।
ये स्तेना ये च तस्करास्तांस्ते अग्नेऽपि दधाम्यास्ये ॥

77. Whatever hosts there are, fiercely assailant, charging all round with weapons, drawn up in order with arms. Whatever thieves there are, whatever robbers, all these I put under the care of the King for deserving chastisement.

७८. दंष्ट्राभ्यां मलिम्लूञ्जम्भ्यैस्तस्करारँ2 उत ।
हनुभ्यां3 स्तेनान् भगवस्तांस्त्वं खाद सुखादितान् ॥

78. O King, devour the burglars, with both tusks, destroy the robbers, with thy teeth. With both thy jaws, eat up the thieves and cheats!

७९. ये जनेषु मलिम्लव स्तेनासस्तस्करा वने ।
ये कक्षेष्वघायवस्तांस्ते दधामि जम्भयोः ॥

79. The burglars living among men, the thieves and robbers in the wood, criminals lurking in their lairs, these do I lay between thy jaws.

---

[74]There should be no distinction between the belongings of the husband and wife. What belongs to the husband is the property of the wife, and vice versa.

[75]We: relatives and neighbours.
Householder: Wife.

[77]Just as everything put in the mouth of the fire is burnt, so boisterous enemies, thieves and robbers are placed under the King for due punishment.

[78]The language is figurative. The tusks, teeth and jaws of the King are his policy, punishments, discipline and diverse means of suppressing the evil-minded people.

[79]I: Commander of the army.
Thy: the King. Just as grass is laid in the jaws of an animal to be chewn, so wicked persons are placed at the disposal of the King for punishment.

८०. यो अस्मभ्यमरातीयाद्यश्च नो द्वेषते जन: ।
निन्दाद्यो अस्मान्धिप्साच्च सर्वं तं मस्मसा कुरु ॥

80. Turn thou to ashes, him, who would seek to injure us, the man who looks on us with hate, and the man who slanders and deceives us.

८१. स꣡ शितं मे ब्रह्म स꣡ शितं वीर्यं बलम् ।
स꣡ शितं क्षत्रं जिष्णु यस्याहमस्मि पुरोहित: ॥

81. Praiseworthy be my and his knowledge of the vedas.
Praiseworthy be his manly strength and force. Praiseworthy be his victorious power and dynasty of whom I am the household priest.

८२. उदेषां बाहु अतिरमुद्वर्चो अथो बलम् ।
क्षिणोमि ब्रह्मणामित्रानुन्नयामि स्वाँर अहम् ॥

82. May I, with the strength of vedic knowledge and aid of God excel the wicked persons, in strength, and might. I ruin the foes and lift my friends to a high position.

८३. अन्नपतेऽन्नस्य नो देह्यनमीवस्य शुष्मिण: ।
प्र-प्र दातारं तारिष ऊर्जं नो धेहि द्विपदे चतुष्पदे ॥

83. O Lord of Food, vouchsafe us a share of food that invigorates us, and brings on sickness. Onward, still onward lead the giver. Grant us maintenance both for quadrupeds and bipeds.

[80]Thou: King.
[81]My: the purohit or priest.
His: the householder, i.e., Yajman.
[82]I: Household priest.
[83]Lord of food: Priest or yajman (Sacrificer).

CHAPTER XII

१. दृशानो रुक्म उर्व्या व्यद्यौद् दुर्मर्षमायु: श्रिये रुचान: ।
अग्निरमृतो अ्रभवद्वयोभिर्यदेनं द्यौरजनयत्सुरेता: ॥

1. Just as the shining beaming sun, exhibits the diverse material objects on this vast solid earth, so does a man, desirous of wealth, extremely lovely, full of vitality, enjoy undaunted life, free from the injury of foes, in his long life, and beget this learned offspring.

२. नक्तोषासा समनसा विरूपे धापयेते शिशुमेकँसमीची ।
द्यावाक्षामा रुक्मो अ्रन्तर्वि भाति देवा अ्रग्निं धारयन्द्रविणोदा: ॥

2. Night and Dawn, different in hue, accordant, meeting together, suckle like two mothers one same infant the sun, which, pleasant in sight, shines between the heaven and earth. The powerful divine forces support him.

३. विश्वा रूपाणि प्रति मुञ्चते कवि: प्रासावीद्भद्रं द्विपदे चतुष्पदे ।
वि नाकमख्यत्सविता वरेण्योऽनु प्रयाणमुषसो वि राजति ॥

3. God is adorable, Omniscient, Maker of the universe, Worthy of worship at dawn, Shaper of all material objects, Bringer of good for the quadrupeds and bipeds, and Remover of their troubles.

४. सुपर्णोऽसि गरुत्मान्स्त्रिवृत्ते शिरो गायत्रं चक्षुर्बृहद्रथन्तरे पक्षौ । स्तोम आत्मा छन्दाँ-स्यङ्गानि यजूँषि नाम ।
साम ते तनूर्वामदेव्यं यज्ञायज्ञियं पुच्छं धिष्ण्या: शफा: ।
सुपर्णोऽसि गरुत्मान्दिवं गच्छ स्व: पत ॥

4. O learned person thou hast action, contemplation and learning for thy head. Gayatri is thy eye. Brihat and Rathantra are thy wings. Rigveda is thy soul. Metres are thy limbs. The hymns of the yajurveda are thy name. The vamdevya saman is thy body. The deeds worth doing and shunning are thy tail. The yajnas are thy hooves. Thou art high souled, and master of noble qualities. Acquire knowledge and attain to happiness!

³Him: the sun.
Just as mother and nurse suckle the child, so do day and night protect and support the sun.
⁴Head: Whereby a learned person removes all miseries.
Gayatri: The knowledge given in the Gayatri verses.
Brihat and Rathantra: The well known songs of the Samveda.
Name: The source of glory and fame.
Vamdevya: The portion of the Samveda, named so, as it is revealed by Vam, the one worshipful God.
Tail: The source of support.
Hooves: Just as hooves are the supporters of an animal, so the yajnas are the props of a learned person.

५. विष्णो: क्रमोऽसि सपत्नहा गायत्रं छन्द आ रोह पृथिवीमनु वि क्रमस्व
विष्णो: क्रमोऽस्यभिमातिहा त्रैष्टुभं छन्द आ रोहान्तरिक्षमनु वि क्रमस्व ।
विष्णो: क्रमोऽस्यरातीयतो हन्ता जागतं छन्द आ रोह दिवमनु वि क्रमस्व
विष्णो: क्रमोऽसि शत्रूयतो हन्ताऽऽनुष्टुभं छन्द आ रोह दिशोऽनु वि क्रमस्व ॥

5. O learned person, purified by the instruction of God, thou art the rival-slayer. Follow the teachings of Gayatri verses; and utilise all earthly objects for thy benefit. Thou knowest the law of cause and effect, and art the destroyer of the proud. Know the significance of verses in Trishtup metre; and control the mid-air!

Thou knowest the pervading electricity, art the chastiser of the opponents of the spread of learning. Master the knowledge derived from the verses in Jagati metre, and utilise the heat of the sun.

Thou knowest the pervading air, and art the foeman-slayer, understand the instructions given in verses revealed in Anushtup metre, and master all directions.

६. अक्रन्ददग्नि स्तनयन्निव द्यौ: क्षामा रेरिह्द्वीरुध: समञ्जन् ।
सद्यो जज्ञानो वि हीमिद्धो अख्यदा रोदसी भानुना भात्यन्त: ॥

6. O people, just as a ruler attains to fame in a day, and thundering like the lightning meets with the foes; just as the earth fills the trees with fruits, so he rewards soon, for the happiness of his subjects, their good and bad deeds. Just as the sun, blazing and manifesting visibly all the material objects, adorns the Earth and Heaven, and fills the universe with lustre, so a person possessed of noble qualities, be elected as a ruler!

७. अग्नेऽअभ्यावर्तिन्नभि मा नि वर्तस्वायुषा वर्चसा प्रजया धनेन ।
सन्या मेधया रय्या पोषेण ॥

7. Return to me, thou ever-returning learned person, with life, literary lustre, progeny, and treasure, with wisdom that explains all departments of knowledge, with intellect and abundance.

८. अग्ने अङ्गिर: शतं ते मन्त्वावृत: सहस्रं न उपावृत: ।
अधा पोषस्य पोषेण पुनर्नो नष्टमा कृधि पुनर्नो रयिमा कृधि ॥

8. O scientist filled with the delight of knowledge; may thy visits be a hundred, and thy returns a thousand. With the increase of strength-giving wealth, give us anew the knowledge unknown before, give us again wealth!

९. पुनरूर्जा नि वर्तस्व पुनरग्न इषाऽऽयुषा ।
पुनर्न: पाह्य‌ँहस: ॥

⁵Trishtup verses: They deal with the spiritual and physical enjoyments and those derived from the forces of nature. Jagati verses give us the knowledge of the science of universe. Anushtup verses give us the desired happiness.

⁷A learned person visits the house of a householder now and then, and grants him through his instructions the objects mentioned in the verse.

9. O learned teacher, save us again and again from vices. Protect us again and again. Grant us again and again noble resolves, nourishing diet, and valorous deeds!

१०. सह रय्या नि वर्तस्वाग्ने पिन्वस्व धारया ।
विश्वप्स्न्या विश्वतस्परि ॥

10. O learned person, shun evil deeds, and enjoy happiness, with wealth, and speech, the imparter of all enjoyable objects and the retainer of all knowledge!

११. आ त्वाऽहार्षमन्तरभूर्ध्रुवस्तिष्ठाविचाचलि: ।
विशस्त्वा सर्वा वाञ्छन्तु मा त्वद्राष्ट्रमधिभ्रशत् ॥

11. O King, enter the Assembly, I declare thee as the ruler. Stand steadfast and immovable. Let all thy subjects long for thee. Let not thy Kingship fall away!

१२. उदुत्तमं वरुण पाशमस्मदवाधमं वि मध्यमं श्रथाय ।
अथा वयमादित्य व्रते तवानागसो अदितये स्याम ॥

12. O ruler, the controller of foes and dispenser of justice, controller of thy kingdom like the eternal sun, release us from the up-most bond, let down the lowest and remove the midmost. So may we, for thy kingship, be sinless in the observance of thy true and just laws!

१३. अग्ने बृहन्नुषसामूर्ध्वो अस्थान्निर्जगन्वान् तमसो ज्योतिषा ऽऽ अगात् ।
अग्निर्भानुना रुशता स्वङ्ग आ जातो विश्वा सद्मान्यप्रा: ॥

13. O king, just as the brilliant sun rising early, resides beautifully in the sky before the dawns, removes darkness with its light and lustre, reaches the universe, and fills with splendour all material objects, so shouldst thou live amongst thy subjects!

१४. हँस: शुचिषद्वसुरन्तरिक्षसद्धोता वेदिषदतिथिर्दुरोणसत् ।
नृषद्वरसदृतसद् व्योमसदजा गोजा ऋतजा अद्रिजा ऋतं बृहत् ॥

14. God is the Destroyer of evil deeds, the Embodiment of purity, the Supporter of the virtuous, Steadfast in the laws of religion, the Imbiber of Truth, Omnipresent, Adorable, Present in the minds of the people and sages, Wedded to Truth, Ubiquitous, Creator of vital breaths, animals, and the Vedas, the Bringer of clouds, True and Mighty.

---
[11]I: Purohit, who anoints the King.
[12]The bonds fastened in the upper, middle and lower parts of the body can be released by the order of the King.
[14]The verse is the same as 10-24 but with a different interpretation and thus free from the charge of repetition.

१५. सीद् त्वं मातुरस्या उपस्थे विश्वान्यग्ने वयुनानि विद्वान् ।
मैनां तपसा मार्चिषाऽभि शोचीरन्तरस्याꣳ शुक्रज्योतिर्वि भाहि ॥

15. O aspirant after knowledge, shine thou in the presence of thy mother. Filled with the lustre of pure character and knowledge, sit in the lap of this thy mother, thy support like earth. Learn from her all holy ordinances. Never think of putting her to grief with distress and violence!

१६. अन्तरग्ने रुचा त्वमुखाया: सदने स्वे ।
तस्यास्त्वꣳ हरसा तपञ्जातवेद: शिवो भव ॥

16. O majestic King, master of the Vedas, tormenting the foes, seated in thy study room, live in the midst of thy subjects, with love. Be gracious, suppressing the enemies with the glowing strength of thy subjects!

१७. शिवो भूत्वा मह्यमग्ने अथो सीद शिवस्त्वम् ।
शिवा: कृत्वा दिश: सर्वा: स्वं योनिमिहासद: ॥

17. O King, the destroyer of foes, being propitious unto us thy subjects, be gracious in this world. Filling thy subjects living in all directions with grace, sit on thy seat of government, and be calm in thy task of administration!

१८. दिवस्परि प्रथमं जज्ञे अग्निरस्मद् द्वितीयं परि जातवेद: ।
तृतीयमप्सु नृमणा अजस्रमिन्धान एनं जरते स्वाधी: ॥

18. O King thou art firstly born like the sun in heaven; thou art secondly full of knowledge from amongst us. Thou art thirdly, most thoughtful among men, with control over senses!
Just as a learned person constantly applauds and stimulates thee, so shouldst thou praise thy subjects.

१९. विद्मा ते अग्ने त्रेधा त्रयाणि विद्मा ते धाम विभृता पुरुत्रा ।
विद्मा ते नाम परमं गुहा यद्विद्मा तमुत्सं यत आजगन्थ ॥

19. O learned person, may we know thy three duties in three stages. May we know thy name, parentage and birth place, worthy of acceptance. May we know what peculiar name supreme thou hast hidden in intellect. In order to approach thee well, may we know thee as our assuager like the well !

२०. समुद्रे त्वा नृमणा अप्स्वन्तर्नृचक्षा ईधे दिवो अग्न ऊधन् ।
तृतीये त्वा रजसि तस्थिवाꣳ समपामुपस्थे महिषा अवर्धन् ॥

[16] A king makes all plans for attacking the enemies, in a calm silent contemplative mood seated in his study room.

[18] The threefold qualities of a King are mentioned in this verse. (1) he should be full of lustre and brilliance like the sun, (2) full of knowledge (3) a deep thinker and self controlled. The verse may also refer to Ashramas in which people should acquire knowledge, twealth, practise penance and spread vedic light.

[19] Three duties: Knowledge, Action and Contemplation.
Three Stations: Brahmcharya, Grihastha and Vanprastha Ashramas.

20. O learned person, I, the Lover of leaders, illuminate thee, like lightning in the sky. I, the Judge of the worth of men, spread thy fame over seas. The high-souled literary persons, like the sun in the third high region, elevate thee in the midst of the subjects!

२१. अक्रन्ददग्नि स्तनयन्निव द्यौ: क्षामा रेरिह्द्धीरुध समञ्जन् ।
सद्यो जज्ञानो वि हीमिद्धो अरूयदा रोदसी भानुना भात्यन्त: ॥

21. The sun, like the roaring lightning, helping the growth of medicinal herbs, speedily sets in motion the material objects, strikes against the earth with its beams, rising in full glory, kindles on all sides the Heaven and Earth with its rays; and shines with full lustre in the universe.

२२. श्रीणामुदारो धरुणो रयीणां मनीषाणां प्रार्पण: सोमगोपा: ।
वसु: सूनु: सहसो अप्सु राजा वि भात्यग्र उषसामिधान: ॥

22. Elect him as a ruler who is lustrous like the sun in fore-front of the dawns, the giver of wealth, the master of riches, the bestower of wisdom, the protector of prosperity, the observer of the vow of celibacy, the son of a strong father, and the controller of his senses.

२३. विश्वस्य केतुर्भुवनस्य गर्भ आ रोदसी अपृणाज्जायमान: । वीडुं चिद्द्रिमभिनत् परायञ्जना यदग्निमयजन्त पञ्च ॥

23. Elect him as a ruler, who is the protector of the whole world, springs to life in its midst; fills the Earth and Heaven opposing the foes, cuts to pieces the powerful enemy, just as the sun cuts asunder the dense cloud, is full of knowledge, and respected by five classes of persons.

२४. उशिक्पावको अरति: सुमेधा मर्तेष्वग्निरमृतो नि धायि ।
इयर्ति धूममरुषं भरिभ्रदुच्छुक्रेण शोचिषा द्यामिनक्षन् ॥

24. God has established among mortals, knowledge, which is acceptable, purifier, knowable, wise and immortal. The same knowledge, with its active brilliance, pervading the universe, and sustaining the world, dispels darkness devoid of light.

२५. दृशानो रुक्म उर्व्या व्यद्यौद्दुर्मर्षमायु: श्रिये रुचान: ।
अग्निरमृतो अभवद्वयोभिर्यदेनं द्यौरजनयत्सुरेता: ॥

25. Know God, Who manifests the universe, is fascinating, full of grace, the Giver of life free from calamities, displays Himself in imperishable, lustrous earth, is All-pervading, Self-illuminating, full of manifold vitalities, and Creator of this world.

[20]I: God.
[25]Panch jana: Brahman, Kshatriya, Vaish, Shudra, and Nishad. It may also mean, the four Ritvijas, Hota, Adhwaryu, Udgata, Brahma, and the yajman, sacrificer. It may also mean; five pranas, as a ruler is expected to have control over his breaths.

२६. यस्ते अद्य कृणवन्द्भद्रशोचेऽपूपं देव घृतवन्तमग्ने ।
प्र तं नय प्रतरं वस्यो अच्छाभि सुम्नं देवभक्तं यविष्ठ ॥

26. O lovely, young learned person, the bestower of enjoyments, always select him as thy cook, who can prepare highly delicious, palatable meals, mixed with butter, fit to be taken by the wise!

२७. आ तं भज सौश्रवसेष्वग्न उवथ उवथ आ भज शस्यमाने ।
प्रिय: सूर्ये प्रियो अग्ना भवात्युज्जातेन भिनददुज्जनित्वै: ॥

27. O learned person, appoint him as thy cook, who has worked with the rich, who feels pleased with praise and acts upon the instructions given, is dear to respectable persons, and knows the use of fire, lives peacefully with your sons and grandsons, and tears asunder the foes!

२८. त्वामग्ने यजमाना अनु द्यून् विश्वा वसु दधिरे वार्याणि ।
त्वया सह द्रविणमिच्छमाना व्रजं गोमन्तमुशिजो वि वव्रु: ॥

28. O learned person, the wise householders, under thy shelter, daily acquire with thy assistance, all sorts of riches worthy of acceptance. Desirous of wealth they resort to thee, as an agriculturist resorts to the stable filled with cattle, or wishes for clouds filled with rain!

२९. अस्ताव्यग्निर्नरां सुशेवो वैश्वानर ऋषिभि: सोमगोपा: ।
अद्वेषे द्यावापृथिवी हुवेम देवा धत्त रयिमस्मे सुवीरम् ॥

29. O learned sages, ye have applauded God, the Comforter of the people, and the Support of all. Give us wealth and heroic children; whereby we, guardians of supremacy, free from hatred, attain to the sovereignty of the earth and political sagacity!

३०. समिधाऽग्निं दुवस्यत घृतैर्बोधयतातिथिम् ।
आस्मिन् हव्या जुहोतन ॥

30. O householders, just as fire is kindled with fuel, so serve the learned preacher with well-cooked food. Welcome thy preacher guest with ghee, just as fire is aroused with it in oblations. Give in charity, in this world, all things worth giving!

३१. उदु त्वा विश्वे देवा अग्ने भरन्तु चित्तिभि: ।
स नो भव शिवस्त्वꣳ सुप्रतीको विभावसु: ॥

31. O learned person, may all the sages nourish thee with their knowledge. Thou, rich in light of learning, and endowed with noble qualities, preach unto us elevating thoughts!

३२. प्रेद्धने ज्योतिष्मान् याहि शिवेभिरर्चिभिष्ट्वम् ।
बृहद्भिर्भानुभिर्भासन्मा हिꣳसीस्तन्वा प्रजा: ॥

32. O King, the preacher of knowledge, just as the sun, resplendent with its auspicious flames of fire, and shining with mighty beams of light, works in the universe, so attain to happiness, and destroy not the bodies of the subjects deserving protection!

३३. अक्रन्ददग्नि स्तनयन्निव द्यौ: क्षामा रेरिह्द्वीरुध: समञ्जन् ।
सद्यो जज्ञानो वि हीमिद्धो अरूयदा रोदसी भानुना भात्यन्त: ॥

33. He alone is fit to rule, who spreads knowledge, and administers justice, kills the foes, roars like the lightning, protects the forest trees, wages battles on the earth, is expert in statesmanship, and endowed with noble qualities, speedily preaches religion, keeps with his power under control, the Sun and Earth, and spreads around his lustre.

३४. प्र-प्रायमग्निर्भरतस्य शृण्वे वि यत्सूर्यो न रोचते बृहद्भा: ।
अभि य: पूरुं पृतनासु तस्थौ दीदाय देव्यो अतिथि: शिवो न: ॥

34. He should be put at the head of the army, who, full of brilliance, shines like the sun with lofty splendour, stands with the officers in our battles; is loved by the learned, constantly on tour, full of bliss, the advocate of learning and religion, and known as the protector of the State.

३५. आपो देवी: प्रति गृभ्णीत भस्मैतत्स्योने कृणुध्वꣳ सुरभा उ लोके ।
तस्मै नमन्तां जनय: सुपत्नीमतिव पुत्रं विभृताप्स्वेनत् ॥

35. O learned persons, take in wedlock the girls, who like the pure water are full of vast intellect and learning, good looking and well-behaved, full of glory, please their husbands in their beautiful homes; and make them happy and contented. Just as the beautiful and well educated wives bow unto ye so should you bow unto them. The husband and wife should love this child like life, as a mother does her son!

३६. अप्स्वग्ने सधिष्टव सौषधीरनु रुध्यसे ।
गर्भे सञ्जायसे पुन: ॥

36. O learned and tolerant soul, after roaming in waters and plants, thou enterest the womb, and art born again and again!

३७. गर्भोऽस्योषधीनां गर्भो वनस्पतीनाम् ।
गर्भो विश्वस्य भूतस्याग्ने गर्भो अपामसि ॥

37. O soul thou art born in plants, thou art born in trees, thou art born in all created animate objects, thou art born in waters!

[32]Destroy not the body of any person. Don't give capital punishment. Hanging on the gallows is thus prohibited in the Vedas.
[33]This verse is the same as revealed in 12.6 and 12.21. The interpretation of each is different from the other.
[36]The soul after leaving the body at the time of death roams in air, waters and plants, before it enters the womb for rebirth. The doctrine of the transmigration of soul is propounded in this verse.
[37]After leaving the body, soul is reborn. By nature it is eternal, immortal and unborn, but takes birth to reap the fruit of its actions. It is eternal with God and matter.

३८. प्रसद्य भस्मना योनिमपश्च पृथिवीमग्ने ।
सꣳसृज्य मातृभिष्ट्वं ज्योतिष्मान् पुनरा ऽसदः ॥

38. O soul, blazing like the sun, after cremation, having reached the fire and the earth for rebirth, and residing in the belly of thy mother, thou art born again!

३९. पुनरासद्य सदनमपश्च पृथिवीमग्ने ।
शेषे मातुर्यथोपस्थेऽन्तरस्याꣳ शिवतमः ॥

39. O soul, having reached the womb, again and again, thou auspiciously liest in thy mother, as a child sleeps in her mother's lap!

४०. पुनरूर्जा नि वर्तस्व पुनरग्न इषाऽऽयुषा ।
पुननः पाह्यꣳहसः ॥

40. O noble parents, advance us with food and life, protect us again and again from sinful conduct. O son, remain aloof from vices, with thy force of character, and keep us away from evil intentions!

४१. सह रय्या नि वर्तस्वाग्ने पिन्वस्व धारयो ।
विश्वप्स्न्या विश्वतस्परि ॥

41. O learned person, travel constantly in the world, with wealth and seasoned speech, the sources of enjoyment, and serve the people!

४२. बोधा मे अस्य वचसो यविष्ठ मꣳहिष्ठस्य प्रभृतस्य स्वधावः ।
पीयति त्वो अनु त्वो गृणाति वन्दारुष्टे तन्वं वन्दे अग्ने ॥

42. O most youthful, and resourceful pupil, understand the significance of the eloquent speech of mine, thy protector and sustainer. One will hate thee and another sing thy praises; but never renounce the truth. I, an adorer of thine bow at thy feet!

४३. स बोधि सूरिर्मघवा वसुपते वसुदावन् ।
युयोध्यस्मद् द्वेषाꣳसि विश्वकर्मणे स्वाहा ॥

43. O preacher, the guardian of wealth, giver of riches to the beserving, full of commendable knowledge and wisdom, thou knowest the truth. For the

---

[38] The soul, after cremation, before it enters the womb, roams in waters, earth, fire, and material objects, the cause of creation.
[40] The verse is the same as 12.9, but with a different interpretation.
[41] The verse is the same as 12.10, but with a different interpretation.
[42] I:pupil. Mine the preceptor,
In the first part the teacher instructs the pupil; and in the second, the pupil expresses his gratitude towards his teacher.
[43] A preacher is the guardian of the wealth of knowledge. He imparts this wealth to others. A preacher is expected to be a man of knowledge and truthful speech. His duty is to save humanity from evil thoughts.

performance of all noble needs, and preaching the truth, keep far away from us all evil designs!

४४. पुनस्त्वाऽऽदित्या रुद्रा वसव: समिन्धतां पुनर्ब्रह्माणो वसुनीथ यज्ञै: ।
घृतेन त्वं तन्वं वर्धयस्व सत्या: सन्तु यजमानस्य कामा: ॥

44. O imparter of vedic knowledge and wealth, in the company of the learned, may thou improve thy body with butter. After the completion of study, let the Adityas, Rudras, Vasus and Brahmas, make thee renowned. Let the sacrificer's wishes be fulfilled!

४५. अपेत वीत वि च सर्पतातो येऽत्र स्थ पुराणा ये च नूतना: ।
अदाद्यमोऽवसानं पृथिव्या अक्रन्निमं पितरो लोकमस्मै ॥

45. O learned persons, may all the aged and young scholars living at present in the world acting as teachers and preachers impart spiritual knowledge to this disciple filled with noble resolves. May thy teacher grant thee a dignified position. Shun unrighteousness, and follow Dharma, and stick to it particularly!

४६. संज्ञानमसि कामधरणं मयि ते कामधरणं भूयात् ।
अग्नेर्भस्मास्यग्ने: पुरीषमसि चित्त स्थ परिचित ऊर्ध्वचित: श्रयध्वम् ।

46. O learned teacher, thou art the embodiment of knowledge. May I obtain thy strength for the accomplishment of wishes. Thou removest my evils as the fire reduces the fuel to ashes. Thou art full of strength like the lightning. Give me that strength. O' pupils, ye are the achievers of knowledge, ye are the observers of the real spirit of religion, hence always follow religion!

४७. अयꣳ सो अग्निर्यस्मिन्त्सोममिन्द्र: सुतं दधे जठरे वावशान: ।
सहस्रियं वाजमत्यं न सप्तिꣳ ससवान्त्सन्त्स्तूयसे जातवेद: ॥

47. O highly cultured person, thou art worthy of praise, being charitable in nature. Lightning and sun, ripen the juices of plants, for thee. I take in my belly the juice thus ripened. I full of intense desire receive my wife, as my companion. Along with thee, I preserve the foodstuffs, like a fast horse!

४८. अग्ने यत्ते दिवि वर्च: पृथिव्यां यदोषधीष्वप्स्वा यजत्र ।
येनान्तरिक्षमुर्वाततन्थ त्वेष: स भानुरर्णवो **नृचक्षा:** ॥

⁴⁴Adityas: Brahmcharis who lead a life of celibacy for 48 years, and acquire knowledge.
Rudras: Those who remain celibate up to 36 years, and study the vedas.
Vasus: Who remain celibate and study the vedas for 24 years.
Brahmas: Who have mastered all the four vedas.
⁴⁶This verse is a dialogue between the teacher and pupils.
⁴⁷I: A householder.
As a fast horse preserves the rider and speedily takes him to his destination, so I preserve the foodstuffs for proper use.

48. O social learned person, the splendour of thy knowledge is found in the soul, in the earth, in plants, and in waters. Wherewith thou hast overspread mid air's vast region. The light of the sun, that gives sight to man, is the bringer of rain.

४९. अग्ने दिवो अर्णमच्छा जिगास्यच्छा देवाँ॒२ ऊचिषे धिष्ण्या ये ।
या रोचने परस्तात् सूर्यस्य याश्चावस्तादुपतिष्ठन्त आप: ॥

49. O learned person, with the light of thy knowledge, thou duly singest the praise of waters beyond the light of sun, and those that are beneath it here. Thou well preachest knowledge to the students who are expert in the art of speaking!

५०. पुरीष्यासो अग्नय: प्रावणेभि: सजोषस: ।
जुषन्तां यज्ञमद्रुहोऽनमीवा इषो मही: ॥

50. All learned persons, endowed with various sorts of knowledge, free from disease and malice, friendly towards all, shrewd in actions should spread education and entertain high aims.

५१. इडामग्ने पुरुदर्२सँ सनि गो: शश्वत्तमँ हवमानाय साध ।
स्यान्न: सूनुस्तनयो विजावाग्ने सा ते सुमतिर्भूत्वस्मे ॥

51. O preceptor, vouchsafe thy wisdom unto us. May the son born to us, be the begetter of different sorts of supremacy. Teach him while receiving education, praiseworthy eloquence, eternal knowledge of the Vedas, and the Rigveda, the granter of success in all our actions.!

५२. अयं ते योनिर्ऋत्वियो यतो जातो अरोचथा: ।
तं जानन्नग्न आ रोहाथा नो वर्धया रयिम् ॥

52. O fire-like pure soul this is thine ordered birth, the giver of happiness and remover of misery, whence sprung to life, thou shinest forth. Knowing this do noble deeds, and cause our riches increase!

५३. चिदसि तया देवतयाऽङ्गिरस्वद् ध्रुवा सीद ।
परिचिदसि तया देवतयाऽङ्गिरस्वद् ध्रुवा सीद ॥

53. O girl, thou art the imparter of knowledge; with vedic lore remain steady like breaths. O celibate girl, thou art the master of different sciences, with thy religious life, remain steady like God!

५४. लोकं पृण छिद्रं पृणाथो सीद ध्रुवा त्वम् ।
इन्द्राग्नी त्वा बृहस्पतिरस्मिन् योनावसीषदन् ॥

"Our: Parents.
The Ritugami parents produce a noble child, who adds to the wealth and fame of the parents.

54. O girl, thy father, mother, and teachress who know the vedas, impart thee knowledge for the emancipation of thy soul. Preserve that knowledge with iron determination. Henceforth fill up all thy weaknesses, and please the people with thy knowledge!

५५. ता अस्य सूददोहसः सोमꣳ श्रीणन्ति पृश्नयः ।
जन्मन्देवानां विशस्त्रिष्वा रोचने दिवः ॥

55. The wives of learned persons, with beautiful bodies and tender limbs, having good cooks and servants to milch the cows, being reborn with knowledge, cook well prepared diet, in this beautiful domestic life. They observing the laws of Brahmcharya, give happiness to their husbands in past, present and future, in all pleasant domestic tasks and give birth to good offspring.

५६. इन्द्रं विश्वा अवीवृधन्त्समुद्रव्यचसं गिरः ।
रथीतमꣳ रथीनां वाजानाꣳ सत्पतिं पतिम् ॥

56. O men and women, just as all vedic sacred speech, deep like the sea, protector of the vedas and noble souls, master of supremacy, magnifies on battlefields, the best amongst the warriors, and adds to his glory, so shouldst ye magnify all!

५७. समितꣳ सं कल्पेथाꣳ संप्रियौ रोचिष्णू सुमनस्यमानौ ।
इषमूर्जमभि संवसानौ ॥

57. O husband and wife, be dear to each other, shun sensuality, be one-minded, dress nicely. Attain together to your goal, and use your vigour for a common cause!

५८. सं वां मनाꣳसि सं व्रता समु चित्तान्याकरम् ।
अग्ने पुरीष्याधिपा भव त्वं न इषमूर्जं यजमानाय धेहि ॥

58. Together have I brought your minds, your vows, and your thoughts. O teacher, our protector, be thou our guardian; give food, physical and spiritual strength to the sacrificer.

५९. अग्ने त्वं पुरीष्यो रयिमान् पुष्टिमाꣳर् असि ।
शिवाः कृत्वा दिशः सर्वाः स्वं योनिमिहाऽसदः ॥

59. O learned preacher, in this world, thou art the follower of one principle, wealthy, physically and spiritually strong. Having made all the people blest, stick to thy duty of preaching; thou giver of happiness, and the dispeller of miseries!

⁵⁸I: Acharya, preceptor.
Your: Husband and wife.
⁵⁹One principle: vedic truth.
An updeshak should be a true follower of vedic principles, above want, physically and spiritually strong. He should never forsake his duty of preaching the truth.

६०. भवतं न: समनसौ सचेतसावरेपसौ ।
मा यज्ञ ॐ हिꣳसिष्टं मा यज्ञपतिं जातवेदसौ शिवौ भवतमद्य न: ॥

60. Be ye one-minded unto us, both of one thought, free from fault, Harm not the Dharma worth-attaining. Harm not him who preaches religion. Be ever gracious unto us, ye knowers of all knowledge.

६१. मातेव पुत्रं पृथिवी पुरीष्यमग्निꣳ स्वे योनावभारुखा ।
तां विश्वेदेवैॠतुभि: संविदान: प्रजापतिर्विश्वकर्मा वि मुञ्चतु ॥

61. The learned woman, calm like the earth, preserves in her womb, like a mother, the healthy and beautiful son.
May the Omniscient God, the source of all noble actions, relieve the child from pain, in all seasons, with His divine powers.

६२. अ्रसुन्वन्तमयजमानमिच्छ स्तेनस्येत्यामन्विहि तस्करस्य ।
अ्न्यमस्मदिच्छ सा त इत्या नमो देवि निॠ्ते तुभ्यमस्तु ॥

62. O learned woman, calm like the earth, seek some one else besides our relatives of thievish and plundering nature. Don't wish for an irreligious or uncharitable husband. Whatever course of action thou choosest, may that succeed. To thee be homage!

६३. नम: सु ते निॠते तिग्मतेजोऽयसमयं वि चृता बन्धमेतम् ।
यमेन त्वं यम्या संविदानोत्तमे नाके अधि रोहयैनम् ॥

63. O woman, the embodiment of true conduct, thine are the foodstuffs, and substances brilliant like gold; cut asunder ignorance, the source of bondage. In unanimity with yama and yami, uplift thy husband to the sublimest vault of happiness!

६४. यस्यास्ते घोर आसञ्जुहोम्येषां बन्धानामवसर्जनाय ।
यां त्वा जनो भूमिरिति प्रमन्दते निॠति त्वाऽहं परिवेद विश्वत: ॥

64. O woman, awe-inspiring to the wicked, I put in thy mouth palatable food for the removal of thy physical ailments. People please thee invoking thee as Bhoomi. May I know thee in every way as the producer of good progeny, as earth produces foodstuffs!

⁶⁰Ye: Husband and wife.
Us: Teacher and preacher.
⁶¹Just as the earth preserves electricity and fire in its womb, so should the mother preserve the child.
⁶³Yama: the male administrator of justice.
Yami: the female administrator of justice.
In unanimity means in consonance with, according to the wishes of the king and queen.
⁶⁴Bhoomi: A woman is compared to earth, Just as earth produces nice fruits, flowers and grains, so does a woman give birth to noble children.

६५. यं ते देवी निऋँ'तिराबबन्ध पाशं ग्रीवास्वविचृत्यम् ।
तं ते वि ष्याम्यायुषो न मध्यादथैतं पितुमद्धि प्रसूत: ।
नमो भूत्यै येदं चकार ॥

65. O husband, calm like the earth, I fasten on thy neck, the unbreakable binding noose of pure married life. The same do I fasten unto me for thee. I enter this life for longevity. Let none of us disobey the law of domestic life. Eat thou young man this food, which I eat!

O wife, the embodiment of virtue, follow strictly the duties of married life. I give thee foodstuffs for thy prosperity!

६६. निवेशन: सङ्गमनो वसूनां विश्वा रूपाऽभि चष्टे शचीभि: ।
देव इव सविता सत्यधर्मेन्द्रो न तस्थौ समरे पथीनाम् ॥

66. He alone is fit to lead a married life, who, like God, the Creator of the universe, and master of eternal laws, keeps constant company with his wife and behaves properly, who, like the sun, opposes the warriors on the battle-fields.

६७. सीरा युञ्जन्ति कवयो युगा वि तन्वते पृथक् ।
धीरा देवेषु सुम्नया ॥

67. The intelligent ply the ploughs. The wise for the comfort of the learned, carry the yokes in different directions.

६८. युनक्त सीरा वि युगा तनुध्वं कृते योनौ वपतेह बीजम् ।
गिरा च श्रुष्टि: सभरा असन्नो नेदीय इत्सृण्य: पक्वमेयात् ॥

68. O people, use various implements for cultivating the earth. Employ ploughs and yokes. Sow seed in a well prepared field. With the knowledge of the science of agriculture and full consideration, be quick to sustain and nourish yourselves. May we get the corn fully grown and ripened in the near fields!

⁶⁵The married couple should lead together a life of purity, and mutual love; being free from sensuality.

Unbreakable: The vedic marriage is indissoluble and irrevocable, being a sacrament and not a contract.

⁶⁶Just as the sun wages fight with the clouds, to make them rain, so should a true Grihasthi wage war with the enemies in a battle and subdue them. He should be brave like a warrior, and not timid. Just as God, with His constant law creates the universe, and protects all men, so should the husband always remain in the company of his wife for her protection and behave properly towards her.

⁶⁷Agriculture is considered to be highly essential for the good of humanity. The learned should follow this profession, and grow more food by scientific methods of cultivation, say the use of fertilizers and tractors.

This verse can be applied for yoga as well, and interpreted like this. The yogis concentrate on different organs through samadhi. Through Sushumna, they control their breaths in different ways.

६९. शुनं सु फाला वि कृपन्तु भूमिं शुनं कीनाशा अभि यन्तु वाहै: ।
शुनासीरा हविषा तोशमाना सुपिप्पला ओषधी: कर्तनास्मै ॥

69. Happily let the ploughshares turn up the plough land, happily go the hard-working ploughers with the oxen. O air and sun, nourishing the earth with water, cause ye our plants bear abundant fruit!

७०. घृतेन सीता मधुना समज्यतां विश्वेर्देवैरनुमता मरुद्भि: ।
ऊर्जस्वती पयसा पिन्वमानास्मान्सीते पयसाऽभ्या ववृत्स्व ॥

70. Approved by all the learned persons, strengthened and sprinkled with water and milk, the furrow be balmed with butter and honey. The furrow will give us ghee so we should water it again and again.

७१. लाङ्गलं पवीरवत्सुशेवं सोमपित्सरु ।
तदुद्वपति गामविं प्रफर्व्यं च पीवरीं प्रस्थावद्रथवाहनम् ।

71. O farmers, the keen-sheared plough, the bringer of bliss, the protector of foodstuffs, moves away. It is the giver of fast, comfortable conveyances. With it dig the solid earth for protection's sake!

७२. कामं कामदुघे ध्रुक्ष्व मित्राय वरुणाय च ।
इन्द्रायाश्विभ्यां पूष्णे प्रजाभ्य ओषधीभ्य: ॥

72. O cook, the preparer of palatable meals, please with thy vegetarian preparations, thy friends, the learned, the guests, the officials, and the Pranas and Apanas, the protecting parents, and the children!

७३. वि मुच्यध्वमघन्या देवयाना अगन्म तमसस्पारमस्य ।
ज्योतिरापाम ॥

73. O persons, just as ye become free from ailments by getting good food from inviolable cows, the source of prosperity, so should we. Just as ye attain to the end of night at dawn, so should we. Just as ye receive the light of this sun, so should we!

७४. सजूर्ऋद्वो अयवोभि: सजूरुषा अरुणीभि: ।
सजोपसाविश्विना दं सोभि: सजु: सूर एतशेन सजूर्वैश्वानर इडया घृतेन स्वाहा ॥

74. We all should live together amicably, as the year lives with its parts, the dawn with its ruddy beams, the husband and wife with their wonderful achievements, the sun together with his dappled courser, the air, the earth with water, and the lightning with its exact thunder.

[70] The orthodox commentators interpret Sita as the wife of Shri Ram Chandra. There is no history in the vedas. This is a wrong interpretation. Sita is the furrow traced in a field when it is ploughed. The furrow should be fed with milk, honey and water so that it may grow sweet, fresh, good and pleasant corn.

[71] Plough is the instrument of agriculture, which gives us prosperity and wealth wherewith we can buy comfortable conveyances like motor cars and aeroplanes.

७५. या ओषधी: पूर्वा जाता देवेभ्यस्त्रियुगं पुरा ।
मने नु बभ्रूणामहँ शतं धामानि सप्त च ॥

75. May I know the herbs that were born three years ago in the earth, that pervade all the 107 vital parts of the body of the patients.

७६. शतं वो अम्ब धामानि सहस्रमुत वो रुह: ।
अधा शतक्रत्वो यूयमिमं मे अगदं कृत ॥

76. O physicians imbued with manifold wisdom and deeds, protect my body from disease, with medicines having hundred, and thousand growths. Cure your bodies as well. Know the innumerable vital parts of your body. O mother thou shouldst also do like this!

७७. ओषधी: प्रति मोदध्वं पुष्पवती: प्रसूवरी: ।
अश्वा इव सजित्वरीर्वीरुध: पारयिष्णव: ॥

77. O people derive happiness by the use of herbs full of blossoms and fruits, conquerors of diseases like horses, and assuagers of physical discomforts!

७८. ओषधीरिति मातरस्तद्वो देवीरुप ब्रुवे । सनेयमश्वं गां वास आत्मानं तव पूरुष ॥

78. O learned mother comforting like the herbs, may I speak unto thee in proximity, wholesome words. O active, virtuous son, may I, your mother, enjoy your horse, cow, land, home, clothes and soul-force!

७९. अश्वत्थे वो निषदनं पर्णे वो वसतिष्कृता ।
गोभाज इत्किलासथ यत्सनवथ पूरुषम् ॥

79. O souls, this unstable body like the decaying herbs is your home. God has given ye abode in this ephemeral world like water on the lotus-leaf. Enjoy this earth, nourish the body with food and medicine, and attain to happiness!

८०. यत्रौषधी: समग्मत राजान: समिताविव ।
विप्र: स उच्यते भिषग्रक्षोहामीवचातन: ॥

80. O men go to places where there are herbs, just as kings go to the battle-fields!

[75]I: A physician.
Three years old: The herbs that grow to full maturity in three years; and are fully ripened.
One hundred and seven vital parts of this body as given in the text mean the several vital parts in which the herbs pervade.
[77]Just as swift horses help us in conquering foes, so do the medicinal herbs conquer our diseases and physical discomforts.
[80]Him: Physician.
Them: herbs.

The sagacious physician, the slayer of fiendish ailments and chaser of diseases, tells ye the qualities of the herbs. Take service from him and them both.

८१. अश्वावतीꣳ सोमावतीमूर्जयन्तीमुदोजसम् ।
आविन्त्सि सर्वा श्रोषधीरस्मा अरिष्टतातये ॥

81. May I know for the health of this patient, all medicines, efficacious in nature, full of juice, rich in nourishments, and possessing strength-giving power. May they all give me ease.

८२. उच्छुष्मा श्रोषधीनां गावो गोष्ठादिवेरते ।
धनꣳ सनिष्यन्तीनामात्मानं तव पूरुष ॥

82. O man, just as strong cows go forth from their stalls and feed their calves, so do the healing virtues of the wealth-giving medicinal herbs, used properly, strengthen thy body and soul!

८३. इष्कृतिर्नाम वो माताऽथो यूयꣳ स्थ निष्कृती: ।
सीरा: पतत्रिणी स्थन यदामयति निष्कृथ ॥

83. O men, know the medicine that brings ye relief like the mother. Like flowing streams pay back the debt of gratitude. Keep afar whatever brings disease!

८४. अति विश्वा: परिष्ठा स्तेन इव व्रजमक्रमु: ।
श्रोषधी: प्राच्च्यवुर्यत्किं च तन्वो रप: ॥

84. Lust as a thief steals into the cattle-fold, by breaking through the wall, so do all well-known healing plants, come out of the earth tearing it asunder, and drive out from the body whatever malady there is.

८५. यदिमा वाजयन्नहमोषधीर्हस्त आदधे ।
आत्मा यक्ष्मस्य नश्यति पुरा जीवगृभो यथा ॥

85. When I, obtaining them beforehand, hold these medicinal herbs within my hand, the root of life-killing disease like tuberculosis disappears.

८६. यस्यौषधी: प्रसर्पथाङ्गमङ्गं परुष्परु: ।
ततो यक्ष्मं वि बाधध्व उग्रो मध्यमशीरिव ॥

---

[81]I: Physician.

[83]Any medicine or a physician that brings disease should be shunned.
Just as a flowing stream, into which the people throw their filth does them good by watering their fields, so should you do good unto them in return, who are kind or unkind to you.

[85]People should prepare medicines with their dexterous hands, and use them for eradicating fell diseases.
I: Physician.

86. O medicines, when ye creep in a patient part by part, joint by joint, ye destroy his pulmonary disease, as a strong man destroys the delicate bodily parts of the foe!

८७. साकं यक्ष्म प्र पत चाषेण किकिदीविना ।
साकं वातस्य ध्राज्या साकं नश्य निहाकया ॥

87. O physician, try to extirpate tuberculosis through well-regulated nourishing diet, through control of breath (Pranayam) and through medicines which fully relieve the patient of its pain!

८८. ग्रन्या वो अन्यामवत्वन्यान्यस्या उपावत ।
ता: सर्वा: संविदाना इदं मे प्रावता वच: ॥

88. O women discussing together the merits of the qualities of medicines, follow these words of mine, that all medicines help each other. Just as one helps the other, so should your teachress protect you!

८९. या: फलिनीर्या अफला अपुष्पा याश्च पुष्पिणी: ।
बृहस्पतिप्रसूतास्ता नो मुञ्चन्त्व॑ऺहस: ॥

89. Let fruitful and fruitless herbs, those that blossom and the blossomless, created by God, relieve us from disease.

९०. मुञ्चन्तु मा शपथ्यादथो वरुण्यादुत ।
अथो यमस्य पड्वीशात्सर्वस्मादेवकिल्विषात् ॥

90. O learned persons, just as medicines relieve me from sickness, so should ye, relieve me from the curse's evil, the offence committed towards the virtuous, violation of the orders of the ruler, and the entire sin against the sages!

९१. अवपतन्तीरवदन्निदव ओषधयस्परि ।
यं जीवमश्नवामहै न स रिष्याति पूरुष: ॥

91. The learned talk about the medicines, that like the rays emanating from the sun, come from an experienced physician. No disease shall attack the man, whom, while he liveth, these pervade.

९२. या ओषधि: सोमराज्ञीर्बह्वी: शतविचक्षणा: ।
तासामसि त्वमुत्तमारं कामाय श॑ऺ हृदे ॥

92. O woman, thou knowest fully all the herbs, whose King is Soma, and which possess innumerable healing properties. Thou art most advanced in their knowledge, prompt for the fulfilment of wishes, and sweet to the heart!

९३. या ओषधी: सोमराज्ञीर्विष्ठिता: पृथिवीमनु ।
बृहस्पतिप्रसूता अस्यै संदत्त वीर्यम् ॥

---
⁸⁸Mine : Physician's.
⁹⁰Curse : The wishing of evil for others.
⁹¹These : medicines.

93. O married man, God has created the various herbs, whose king is Soma, that overspread the earth. With their aid, grant semen for this woman, and spread the knowledge of these medicines unto all!

६४. याश्चेदमुपशृण्वन्ति याश्च दूरं परागताः ।
सर्वाः संगत्य वीरुधोऽस्यै संदत्त वीर्यम् ॥

94. O learned persons, collect all medicinal herbs, which are known to ye, and which ye hear of, which are near at hand, or are found at a distance. Advance the strength of the body with their use, and impart their knowledge to this girl!

६५. मा वो रिषत् खनिता यस्मै चाहं खनामि वः ।
द्विपाच्चतुष्पादस्माकꣳ सर्वमस्त्वनातुरम् ॥

95. May not the herb I dig for some purpose, harm you, while being dug. May our and your bipeds and quadrupeds be free from disease by its use.

६६. ओषधयः समवदन्त सोमेन सह राज्ञा ।
यस्मै कृणोति ब्राह्मणस्तꣳ राजन् पारयामसि ॥

96. O physicians, discuss together the healing properties of the herbs, with Soma as their head. O King we save from death the man whose cure a learned physician knowing the vedas and up-vedas undertakes!

६७. नाशयित्री बलासस्यार्शस उपचितामसि ।
अथो शतस्य यक्ष्माणां पाकारोरसि नाशनी ॥

97. O physicians, know ye the medicines that cure catarrh, piles, tumours, consumption in diverse forms, fistula, diseases of the mouth, and those that cause excruciating pain in vital parts of the body!

६८. त्वां गन्धर्वा अखनँस्त्वामिन्द्रस्त्वां बृहस्पतिः ।
त्वामोषधे सोमो राजा विद्वान् यक्ष्मादमुच्यत ॥

98. O people, use the medicine that cures the patient suffering from phthisis. It should be dug by a man expert in the art of smelling, by an exalted person, by a knower of the vedas, by a well qualified person, by a learned man and by a famous king!

६९. सहस्व मे अराती: सहस्व पृतनायतः ।
सहस्व सर्व पाप्मानꣳ सहमानास्योषधे ॥

⁹³The use of medicines during the conception days is essential for the preservation and growth of the foetus. At the time of conception also the use of medicines is necessary.

⁹⁶We: Physicians.

Upvedas: Arth Veda, Dhanur Veda, Ayur Veda, Gandharva Veda.

⁹⁸A novice, inexperienced person ignorant of the nature and qualities of herbs should not dig them, so that they may not be destroyed. Expert and intelligent persons alone, having some knowledge of the medicinal herbs, should dig them so that they may not be destroyed and uprooted.

CHAPTER XII

99. O medically trained wife, just as medicine is the source of strength for me, removes my ailments and gives me power, so should'st thou conquer my enemies, subdue the men who challenge me. Conquer thou every kind of disease!

१००. दीर्घायुस्त ओषधे खनिता यस्मै च त्वा खनाम्यहम् ।
अथो त्वं दीर्घायुर्भूत्वा शतवल्शा विरोहतात् ॥

100. O man, thou knowest the merits and demerits of the herbs. Whatever herb I dig, for whatever purpose or for whom I dig, mayest thou be long-lived, with its use; and having attained to long age, be happy and famous by using the herb with a hundred shoots!

१०१. त्वमुत्तमास्योषधे तव वृक्षा उपस्तयः ।
उपस्तिरस्तु सोऽस्माकं यो अस्माँ२ अभिदासति ॥

101. O physician, be thou our companion, who givest heartfelt delight, Grant us happiness through the most excellent herb, whose retainers are the trees!

१०२. मा मा हिꣳसीज्जनिता यः पृथिव्या यो वा दिवꣳ सत्यधर्मा व्यानट् ।
यश्चापश्चन्द्राः प्रथमो जजान कस्मै देवाय हविषा विधेम ॥

102. God, whose laws are immutable, creates the Earth. He pervades the sun, fire, waters and air. He, being Primordial, creates the lustrous moon. Let us worship with devotion, Him, Who is the Embodiment of happiness. May He not harm me.

१०३. अभ्या वर्तस्व पृथिवि यज्ञेन पयसा सह ।
वपां ते अग्निरिषितो अरोहत् ॥

103. O man, utilise fully this earth, worthy of contact and full of water. Its impelled, internal heat makes thy seed grow!

१०४. अग्ने यत्ते शुक्रं यच्चन्द्रं यत्पूतं यच्च यज्ञियम् ।
तद्देवेभ्यो भरामसि ॥

104. O learned person, whatever swiftness, purity, brightness and fitness for sacrifice, there is in fire, may we acquire them all for thee and for being virtuous!

१०५. इषमूर्जमहमित आदमृतस्य योनि महिषस्य धाराम् ।
आ मा गोष विशत्वा तनुषु जहामि सेदिमनिराममीवाम् ॥

105. May I get from this heat of the earth, corn and all strengthening foods. May I get the vedic speech, the repository of the true knowledge of the Mighty God, and the source of truth.
May I banish diseases, that cause excruciating pains, disallow the taking of meals, as are the source of trouble to my organs of sense and body.

१०६. अग्ने तव श्रवो वयो महि भ्राजन्ते अर्चयो विभावसो ।
बृहद्भानो शवसा वाजमुक्थ्यं दधासि दाशुषे कवे ॥

106. O learned person, possessing the light of knowledge blazing like fire, brilliancy of diverse forms, and height of wisdom; thou art the giver of laudable knowledge to a worthy disciple. Thereby shine forth, thy lustre, life-strength, and knowledge worthy of adoration and hearing!

१०७. पावकवर्चाः शुक्रवर्चा अनूनवर्चा उदियर्षि भानना ।
पुत्रो मातरा विचरन्नुपावसि पृणक्षि रोदसी उभे ॥

107. O man, just as a son, passing through Brahmcharya Ashram (student life) acquires knowledge and with the light of his learning, imparts justice like the lustre of the sun, carries on his studies uninterruptedly, just as the sky and earth are allied together, so shouldst thou receive education, manage the affairs of the State, and serve thy father and mother!

१०८. ऊर्जो नपाज्जातवेदः सुशस्तिभिर्मन्दस्व धीतिभिर्हितः ।
त्वे इषः सन्दधुर्भूरिवर्पसश्चित्रोतयो वामजाताः ॥

108. O son, imbued with wisdom and wealth, to thee, the learned teachress and the mother nobly born, doing wondrous deeds for thy protection, and master of admirable qualities, give food to eat. Rejoice thyself, always occupied with thy own praiseworthy hands in serving others, and never swerving from the path of rectitude.

१०९. इरज्यन्नग्ने प्रथयस्व जन्तुभिरस्मे रायो अमर्त्यं ।
स दर्शतस्य वपुषो वि राजसि पृणक्षि सानसिं क्रतुम् ॥

109. O man, active like fire, possessing unusual strength unlike mortals, gaining power, possessing beautiful appearance, and preserving ancient wisdom, thou acquirest splendour thereby. Increase our wealth with the co-operation of other persons!

११०. इष्कर्तारमध्वरस्य प्रचेतसं क्षयन्तं राधसो महः ।
राति वामस्य सुभगां महीमिषं दधासि सानसिं रयिम् ॥

110. O learned person, thou art the performer of prosperous sacrifice (yajna), exceedingly wise, laudable, giver of huge riches, nice dweller, protector of foodstuffs and earth, and preserver of immemorial vedic wealth, hence thou art fit for veneration!

१११. ऋतावानं महिषं विश्वदर्शतमग्निं सुम्नाय दधिरे पुरो जनाः ।
श्रुत्कर्णं सप्रथस्तमं त्वा गिरा दैव्यं मानुषा युगा ॥

111. O man, just as learned persons accept with praise songs for their happiness, the auspicious amongst the wise, the well-read, the expounder of all sciences, the master of vast learning, the embodiment of truth, and the

leader of scholars, so shouldst thou do. They revere the past generations of men. Thus do I instruct thee!

११२. आ प्यायस्व समेतु ते विश्वतः सोम वृष्ण्यम् ।
भवा वाजस्य सङ्गथे ॥

112. O king, may thy power spread in all directions. May thou advance. May thou, the master of knowledge and the science of fighting, succeed in all battles!

११३. सं ते पयाꣳसि समु यन्तु वाजाः सं वृष्ण्यान्यभिमातिषाहः ।
आप्यायमानो अमृताय सोम दिवि श्रवाꣳस्युत्तमानि धिष्व ॥

113. O man of peaceful nature may juicy nutriments be procured by thee, may thou learn military science for subduing the arrogant foes. May thou amass strength. May thou, thus progress, win immortality, following the noble teachings of God!

११४. आ प्यायस्व मदिन्तम सोम विश्वेभिरꣳशुभिः ।
भवा नः सप्रथस्तमः सखा वृधे ॥

114. O most gladdening, prosperous fellow, make progress through different means, like the sun with its beams. Strive for our prosperity, O friend of vast happiness!

११५. आ ते वत्सो मनो यमत्परमाच्चित्सधस्थात् ।
अग्ने त्वाङ्कामया गिरा ॥

115. O learned person, just as a calf is fastened with its mother, the cow, so thou, desirous for spiritual advancement, concentrate thy mind with vedic speech obtained from God, the Support of all !

११६. तुभ्यं ता अङ्गिरस्तम विश्वाः सुक्षितयः पृथक् ।
अग्ने कामाय येमिरे ॥

116. O King, the foremost realiser of the essence of problems, all loyal subjects turn to thee for the fulfilment of their wishes. Always protect them!

११७. अग्निः प्रियेषु धामसु कामो भूतस्य भव्यस्य ।
सम्राडेको वि राजति ॥

117. He alone is fit to rule, who, full of brilliance, like the One Self-sufficient Lord, is worthy of homage, self-resplendent, and shines forth in God's attributes in the past and future.

---

[111]I: God.
[113]Juicy nutriments; Milk and water.

CHAPTER XIII

१. मयि गृह्लाम्यग्रे अग्निꣳ रायस्पोषाय सुप्रजास्त्वाय सुवीर्याय ।
मामु देवताः सचन्ताम् ॥

1. I realise within me God first of all, for increase of my knowledge, good offspring and manly strength. So may noble virtues wait upon me.

२. अपां पृष्ठमसि योनिरग्नेः समुद्रमभितः पिन्वमानम् ।
वर्धमानो महाꣳ२ आ च पुष्करे दिवो मात्रया वरिम्णा प्रथस्व ॥

2. O God, Thou art the Support of waters, the Cause of fire, the Enveloper of ocean as it swells and surges, the Loftiest of all, Worthy of adoration by humanity, and full of Majesty in space. Shine forth for us with Omnipresence and Omniscience.

३. ब्रह्म जज्ञानं प्रथमं पुरस्ताद्वि सीमतः सुरुचो वेन आवः ।
स बुध्न्या उपमा अस्य विष्ठाः सतश्च योनिमसतश्च वि वः ॥

3. That God alone is Adorable, Who, in the beginning of the universe, created everything, is wide in expansion. Highest of all, Effulgent, and Worthy of worship. The sun, moon and other worlds in the atmosphere, stationed in their orbits, testify to His knowledge. He pervades them all through His Omnipresence and comprehends the visible and the invisible in space.

४. हिरण्यगर्भः समवर्तताग्रे भूतस्य जातः पतिरेक आसीत् ।
स दाधार पृथिवीं द्यामुतेमां कस्मै देवाय हविषा विधेम ॥

4. God is the Creator of the universe, its one Lord, the Sustainer of luminous objects like the sun. He was present before the creation of the world. He sustains the earth, the sun and this world. Let us worship with full devotion of our soul, Him, the Embodiment of happiness.

५. द्रप्सश्चस्कन्द पृथिवीमनु द्यामिमं च योनिमनु यश्च पूर्वः ।
समानं योनिमनु सञ्चरन्तं द्रप्सं जुहोम्यनु सप्त होत्रा ॥

5. Seven forces realise Him. He engulfs this earth, the sun and the sky. In His fullness, He favourably possesses happiness and energy. Moving in Him, I willingly perceive complete pleasure.

६. नमोऽस्तु सर्पेभ्यो ये के च पृथिवीमनु ।
ये अन्तरिक्षे ये दिवि तेभ्यः सर्पेभ्यो नमः ॥

---
³This verse is the same as 11—29, but with a quite different interpretation.
⁵Seven: soul, mind and five Pranas. Soul realises God, with the aid of the mind and five pranas.

CHAPTER XIII

6. May the denizens of all planets of the universe obtain food. May all the living creatures residing in the atmosphere, the sun and roaming on the earth obtain food.

७. या इषवो यातुधानानां ये वा वनस्पतीँ१रन् ।
ये वावटेषु शेरते तेभ्यः सर्पेभ्यो नमः ॥

7. Suppress through arms the movements of dacoits and plunderers who live in forests; and lie hidden in unknown paths.

८. ये वामी रोचने दिवो ये वा सूर्यस्य रश्मिषु ।
येषामप्सु सदस्कृतं तेभ्यः सर्पेभ्यो नमः ॥

8. Subdue with arms, all these evil-minded persons, who generally remain hidden, and now and then appear in the day time, or walk freely in the light of the sun, or dwell in waters.

९. कृणुष्व पाजः प्रसितिं न पृथ्वीं याहि राजेवामवाँ२ इभेन ।
तृष्वीमनु प्रसितिं द्रूणानोऽस्ताऽसि विध्य रक्षसस्तपिष्ठैः ॥

9. O Commander of the army, increase thy vigour, master the earth well-ordered like a net. Thou art the extirpator of foes, attack them like a king equipped with ministers and military paraphernalia. Strengthening thy hold with most deadly weapons, facing and killing the fiends, subdue them soon!

१०. तव भ्रमास आशुया पतन्त्यनु स्पृश धृषता शोशुचानः ।
तपूँष्यग्ने जुह्वा पतङ्गानसन्दितो वि सृज विष्वगुल्काः ॥

10. O Commander the specimen of morality, keep thy fast moving brave soldiers, well disciplined in the army. Like the swift movements of lightning, let them fall falcon-like on the enemies. With uninterrupted force, let fire-arms, brilliant like the flames of fire fed with ghee, rain over the foes; and train well thy horses!

११. प्रति स्पशो वि सृज तूर्णितमो भवा पायुर्विशो अस्या अदब्धः ।
यो नो दूरे अधशँ२सो यो अन्त्यग्ने मा किष्टे व्यथिरा दधर्षीत् ॥

11. O destroyer of foes like fire, put shackles on and speedily punish the troublesome evil-minded enemy of yours and ours, may he be far or near, so that he may not harm us. May thou be the harmless guardian of the people of thine!

१२. उदग्ने तिष्ठ प्रत्या तनुष्व न्यमित्राँ२ ओषतात्तिग्महेते ।
यो नो अरातिँ समिधान चक्रे नीचा तं धक्ष्यतसं न शुष्कम् ॥

---

⁶God supplies food to all creatures living on the earth, in space and in the sun. This means there are living creatures in the Sun, Mercury, Mars, Uranus, and Neptune etc., whom God supplies sustenance. सर्प does not mean serpent here, as Griffith interprets it, but moving, living creatures, as interpreted by Swami Dayananda.

12. O king, make progress in thy duty of administration, extend happiness to the virtuous. O terrible chastiser, burn down the irreligious foes. O splendid person, humiliate and consume utterly like dried up stubble, him, who encourages our foe!

१३. ऊर्ध्वो भव प्रति विध्याध्यस्मदाविष्कृणुष्व दैव्यान्यग्ने ।
अव स्थिरा तनुहि यातुजूनां जामिमजामिं प्र मृणीहि शत्रून् ।
अग्नेष्ट्वा तेजसा सादयामि ॥

13. O King, rise high, punish the wicked foes righteously, manifest the objects prepared by our steady scholars, enhance pleasures. Destroy the kitchens and other places of plundering of the vigorous enemies. Kill the foes, I settle thee with fire's ardour!

१४. अग्निर्मूर्धा दिवः ककुत्पतिः पृथिव्या अयम् ।
अपाꣳ रेताꣳसि जिन्वति ।
इन्द्रस्य त्वौजसा सादयामि ॥

14. O king, just as this sun, in the midst of luminous sky, as the head of earth, foremost of all, the protector of all, satisfies men with the strength of waters, so shouldst thou be. I appoint thee for kingship, with the strength of the sun!

१५. भुवो यज्ञस्य रजसश्च नेता यत्रा नियुद्भिः सचसे शिवाभिः ।
दिवि मूर्धानं दधिषे स्वर्षां जिह्वामग्ने चक्षुषे हव्यवाहम् ॥

15. O learned person, know, that country flourishes, in which, there are men like thee active as air, leaders of supremacy, and heads of justice; where there are men to carry on the administration of the land with good statesmanship; where the country is preserved by efficient officials; and where the wisdom-inspiring and pleasure-giving speech is used!

१६. ध्रुवासि धरुणाऽऽस्तृता विश्वकर्मणा ।
मा त्वा समुद्र उद्वधीन्मा सुपर्णोऽव्यथमाना पृथिवीं दृꣳह ॥

16. O queen, living in the company of thy religious-minded husband, and adorned with dress, ornaments and good qualities, acquiring knowledge and practising religion, remain steadfast. Being free from distress, advance the country under thy rule. Let no lascivious person torment thee, let not thy husband with beautiful body, harm thee!

१७. प्रजामतिष्ट्वा सादयत्वपां पृष्ठे समुद्रस्येमन् ।
व्यचस्वतीं प्रथस्वतीं प्रथस्व पृथिव्यसि ॥

---
[13]I: Purohit or general.
[14]I: The priest.
[16]Samudra has been compared to lust. Just as ocean is endless so is lust, vide Pt. Jaidev vidyalankar's interpretation.

17. O learned queen, the King establishes thee, full of knowledge, reverence, and wide fame, on the seat of justice, like a canoe at a suitable place on the waters of the ocean. Thou art comforting like the Earth. Be famous in doing justice unto females, as thy husband does unto men!

१८. भूरसि भूमिरस्यदितिरसि विश्वधाया विश्वस्य भुवनस्य धर्त्री ।
पृथिवीं यच्छ पृथिवीं दृ̐ह पृथिवीं मा हि̐सीः ॥

18. O Queen, thou art patient like the earth, hence control the earth. Thou, the organiser of household affairs, and the conductor of full administration, art firm like the earth, hence steady the earth. Thou art unagitated like the glorious sky, hence do the earth no injury!

१९. विश्वस्मै प्राणायापानाय व्यानायोदानाय प्रतिष्ठायै चरित्राय ।
अग्निष्ट्वाऽभि पातु मह्या स्वस्त्या छ्दिषा शन्तमेन तया देवतयाङ्गिरस्वद् ध्रुवा सीद ॥

19. O woman, may thy learned husband, protect thee, with pleasure-giving deeds and beautiful peaceful acts, for full longevity, removal of misery, acquisition of various noble performances, vigour, veneration, and religious duties. May thou attain to fame, living permanently with thy husband, as cause and effect are inseparable!

२०. काण्डात्काण्डात्प्ररोहन्ती परुषः-परुषस्परि ।
एवा नो दूर्वे प्र तनु सहस्रेण शतेन च ॥

20. O woman, just as the grass increases widely from all sides, with hundreds and thousands of joints and knots, so lengthen out our line of descendants with sons and grandsons!

२१. या शतेन प्रतनोषि सहस्रेण विरोहसि ।
तस्यास्ते देवीष्टके विधेम हविषा वयम् ॥

21. O beautiful, well-built woman, just as hundreds and thousands of bricks build and magnify a house, so dost thou increase our family with hundreds of sons and grandsons, and profusely enrich it with thousands of articles. We serve thee with nice presents!

२२. यास्ते अग्ने सूर्ये रुचो दिवमातन्वन्ति रश्मिभिः ।
ताभिर्नो अद्य सर्वाभी रुचे जनाय नस्कृधि ॥

22. O brilliant learned teachress, gladden us with all thy tastes, just as lights in the sun, with their beams, spread brilliance all around. With all those tastes make us always friendly towards the lovely famous person!

२३. या वो देवः सूर्ये रुचो गोष्वश्वेषु या रुचः ।
इन्द्राग्नी ताभिः सर्वाभी रुचं नो धत्त बृहस्पते ॥

---

[12]Lovely famous person may mean the husband of the teachress.
Tastes: Likings, hobbies.

23. O learned persons, whatever love ye have got for the sun, the cows and horses, with all that inculcate love in us, just as the teacher and preacher incite our love for learning. O unbiassed learned examiner, examine us!

२४. विराड्ज्योतिरधारयत्स्वराड्ज्योतिरधारयत् ।
प्रजापतिष्ट्वा सादयतु पृष्ठे पृथिव्या ज्योतिष्मतीम् । विश्वस्मै प्राणायापानाय व्यानाय विश्वं ज्योतिर्यच्छ । अग्निष्टेऽधिपतिस्तया देवतयाऽङ्गिरस्वद् ध्रुवा सीद ॥

24. The woman, who, filled with the light of different sorts of knowledge, spreads learning, and the morally advanced person, who shines like lightning, may both these husband and wife attain to happiness.

Live permanently like soul, with thy husband, who is learned and godly in nature. O woman, thy husband, the guardian of his progeny, establishes thee, endowed with learning on this earth, in a place of responsibility, for the acquisition of happiness, removal of suffering, and the practice of yoga for preaching noble qualities, actions and attributes. Imbibe thou full knowledge!

२५. मधुश्च माधवश्च वासन्तिकावृतू अग्नेरन्तः श्लेषोऽसि कल्पेतां द्यावापृथिवी कल्पन्तामाप ओषधयः कल्पन्तामग्नयः पृथङ् मम ज्येष्ठचाय सव्रताः ।
ये अग्नयः समनसोऽन्तरा द्यावापृथिवी इमे । वासन्तिकावृतू अभिकल्पमाना इन्द्रमिव देवा अभिसंविशन्तु तया देवतयाऽङ्गिरस्वद् ध्रुवे सीदतम् ॥

25. Let the Chetra and Baisakh months, parts of spring, born of heat, mutually inter-related, contribute to my prosperity. Let these months be the source of happiness to all. In those months let sun and earth, and water be pleasure-giving. Let medicinal herbs grow in them, and heat be useful to us. O learned persons, wedded to truth, keeping before ye in spring time, the fervent seekers after knowledge, attain to prosperity. Just as the sun and earth, through the dispensation of God, steadfastly work together like breath, so should you wife and husband live constantly together.

२६. अषाढासि सहमाना सहस्वारातीः सहस्व पृतनायतः ।
सहस्रवीर्याऽसि सा मा जिन्व ॥

26. O wife, thou art unconquerable by foes. Being patient, tolerate me thy husband. Possessing a thousand manly powers, anxious to oppose an army, overpower the foes, Just as I keep thee satisfied so shouldst thou keep me pleased!

२७. मधु वाता ऋतायते मधु क्षरन्ति सिन्धवः ।
माध्वीनं: सन्त्वोषधीः ॥

27. In spring the zephyrs blow coolly like water, the rivers and oceans flow calmly, and medicinal herbs are filled with sweet juice.

---
[24]Students address their teachers.
[25]Chetra is March-April, Vaishakha is April-May. The heat of these months is useful to us in ripening the wheat crop.

२८. मधु नक्तमुतोषसो मधुमत्पार्थिवᳬ रज: ।
मधु द्यौरस्तु न: पिता ॥

28. In spring the nights are sweet, the days are sweet, the terrestrial atmosphere is sweet, and light, our protector, is sweet unto us.

२९. मधुमान्नो वनस्पतिर्मधुमाᳬ अस्तु सूर्य: ।
माध्वीर्गावो भवन्तु न: ॥

29. In spring, let trees give us sweet fruits, sun physical strength and cows sweet milk.

३०. अपां गम्भन्त्सीद मा त्वा सूर्योऽभि ताप्सीन्मात्रिन्बैश्वानर: ।
अच्छिन्नपत्रा: प्रजा अनुवीक्षस्वानु त्वा दिव्या वृष्टि: सचताम् ॥

30. O man, in spring, seat thyself in the deepness of waters, lest sun, lest heat burning in all men, should afflict thee. Let well-built subjects be under thy control. Let highly useful rain pour. Think deeply and favourably over these points!

३१. त्रीन्त्समुद्रान्त्समसृपत् स्वर्गानिपां पतिर्वृषभ इष्टकानाम् ।
पुरीषं वसान: सुकृतस्य लोके तत्र गच्छ यत्र पूर्वे परेता: ॥

31. O learned person, as sun, the protector of our vital organs, the cause of rain, the sustainer of pleasant water, attains to all pleasure-giving regions, the mainstay of achieving our desires on earth, space and sky, in past, present and future, so shouldst thou. Tread thou the path of virtue, as did thy ancestors!

३२. मही द्यौ: पृथिवी च न इमं यज्ञं मिमिक्षताम् ।
पिपृतां नो भरीमभि: ॥

32. O mother and father just as the Mighty Sun and Earth nourish the world, so shouldst ye desire for the completion of our noble task of getting education and rear us full with nourishments!

३३. विष्णो: कर्माणि पश्यत यतो व्रतानि पस्पशे ।
इन्द्रस्य युज्य: सखा ॥

33, God is the Adorable, Inseparable Companion of the soul; which realises through His grace the actions and laws of the Omnipresent God. O man, ye should also observe them!

३४. ध्रुवासि धरुणेतो जज्ञे प्रथममेभ्यो योनिभ्यो अधि जातवेदा: ।
स गायत्र्या त्रिष्टुभाऽनुष्टुभा च देवेभ्यो हव्यं वहतु प्रजानन् ॥

[30]गाव : may also mean rays of the sun and lands. They also give us pleasure.
[32]This verse is the same as 8-32, but with a different meaning.
[33]The verse is the same, as 6-4.
Actions: creation, sustenance and annihilation of the universe.
Laws: Righteousness and performance of noble deeds.

34. O woman, thou art firm, and the master of noble qualities. A learned person is first born of thee, and afterwards is born of virtuous, talented gurus. Thy husband, equipped with the knowledge conveyed by the Gayatri, Trishtup, and Anushtup vedic verses; improving his talent thereby, derives learning worthy of exchange!

३५. इषे राये रमस्व सहसे द्युम्न ऊर्जे अ्रपत्याय ।
सम्राडसि स्वराडसि सारस्वतौ त्वोत्सौ प्रावताम् ॥

35. O man thou art self-effulgent through knowledge. O woman thou art graceful through learning and virtuous conduct. Strive together for knowledge, riches, strength, fame, food, heroism and offspring. I enjoin ye, to protect your bodies and foodstuffs, being sweet like the water of a well, and observing the teachings of the vedas!

३६. अग्ने युक्ष्वा हि ये तवाश्वासो देव साधव: ।
अरं वहन्ति मन्यवे ॥

36. O learned, powerful person, verily harness thou thy steeds, which are well disciplined and trained, and carry the conveyance with full force in thy attacks on the foe with righteous indignation!

३७. युक्ष्वा हि देवहूतमाँ२ अश्वाँ२ अग्ने रथीरिव ।
नि होता पूर्व्य: सद: ॥

37. O learned person, trained by ancient scholars, and charitable in nature; yoke like a charioteer thy steeds, well disciplined by the experts. Seat thyself on the seat of justice!

३८. सम्यक् स्रवन्ति सरितो न धेना अन्तर्हृदा मनसा पूयमाना: ।
घृतस्य धारा अभि चाकशीमि हिरण्ययो वेतसो मध्ये अग्ने: ॥

38. Just as rivers flow, so do speeches, purified in the inmost recesses of the heart and mind, come out of the mouth of a learned person. I, full of brilliance, acquire those speeches, coming like the fast-moving showers of rain from the midst of lightning.

३६. ऋचे त्वा रुचे त्वा भासे त्वा ज्योतिषे त्वा ।
अभूदिदं विश्वस्य भुवनस्य वाजिनमग्नेवैश्वानरस्य च ॥

39. O learned person, thou hast acquired the knowledge of all objects of the universe, and the wisdom of lightning-like brilliant persons, being lovely of all human beings, We resort to thee for praise, for love for the acquisition of spiritual knowledge, and for the light of justice!

४०. अग्निज्र्योतिषा ज्योतिष्मान् रुक्मो वर्चसा वर्चस्वान् ।
सहस्रदा असि सहस्राय त्वा ॥

"A man takes his physical birth from his mother, and spiritual birth from his guru the teacher, hence he is called Dwijanma (twice born).
Worthy of exchange: Knowledge is a commodity which is received, and imparted.

40. O learned person, thou art luminous like fire, with the light of thy knowledge. Thou art the giver of knowledge with thy splendour. Like gold thou art the giver of innumerable comforts. We pay homage to thee for acquiring vast knowledge!

४१. आदित्यं गर्भं पयसा समङ्ग्धि सहस्रस्य प्रतिमां विश्वरूपम् ।
परि बृङ्ग्धि हरसा माऽभि मँ ॐ स्था: शतायुषं कृणुहि चीयमान: ॥

41. O learned person, just as lightning supports with water, the sun, that measures innumerable objects, and exhibits the whole universe, and is worthy of praise, so shouldst thou purify the inmost recesses of thy heart. With thy glowing strength keep afar all diseases. Making due progress, make your son live for a hundred years. Always shun pride!

४२. वातस्य जूतिं वरुणस्य नाभिमश्वं जज्ञानँ ॐ सरिरस्य मध्ये ।
शिशुं नदीनाँ ॐ हरिमद्रिबुध्नमग्ने मा हिँ ॐ सी: परमे व्योमन् ॥ ४२

42. O learned person, in the vast space, harm not the wind's impetuous rush, the bond of ocean-wide water, and the cloud the tawny child of rivers!

४३. अजस्रमिन्दुमरुषं भरण्युमग्निमीडे पूर्वचित्तिं नमोभि: ।
स पर्वभिऋतुष: कल्पमानो गां मा हिँ ॐ सीरदिति विराजम् ॥

43. O learned person, just as I constantly search for electricity, newly produced, full of accomplishments, creator of foodstuffs, pure like water, powerful like the horse, knowable by the highly learned, and using it skilfully in each season, do not harm the indivisible beautiful earth, so thou shouldst not harm electricity and this earth!

४४. वरूत्रीं त्वष्टुर्वरुणस्य नाभिमविं जज्ञानाँ ॐ रजस: परस्मात् ।
महीँ ॐ साहस्रीमसुरस्य मायामग्ने मा हिँ ॐ सी: परमे व्योमन् ॥

44. O learned person, residing in the supreme Lord, vast like the space, harm not the vast Earth, attracted by the sun, the repository of water, created by the Pre-eminent God, the Giver of countless fruits, and the Cause of our protection, nor harm the lightning, the precursor of the clouds!

४५. यो अग्निरग्नेरध्यजायत शोकात्पृथिव्या उत वा दिवस्परि ।
येन प्रजा विश्वकर्मा जजान तमग्ने हेड: परि ते वृणक्तु ॥

45. O learned person, may thy displeasure spare the fire that has its being from the heat of the Earth, or from the lightning of the sun, whereby the Omnific Lord engenders creatures!

---

⁴²Learned persons through the performance of yajnas should get timely rain, and thereby prolong their life.

⁴³In the text all commentators use पूर्वचित्तिम् but Maharshi Dayananda uses the word पूर्वचितिम् ।

⁴⁵This verse can be translated thus as well:—
O learned person, don't show disrespect to God. Who is more learned than a yogi, more illuminating than the luminous sun and beautiful earth, who creates all creatures.

४६. चित्रं देवानामुदगादनीकं चक्षर्मित्रस्य वरुणस्याग्ने: ।
आप्रा द्यावापृथिवी अन्तरिक्षᳪ सूर्यं आत्मा जगतस्तस्थुषश्च ॥

46. God is Wonderful and Powerful amongst all material objects. He is the Manifestor of Pran, Udan, and fire. He pervades the air, earth and heaven. He is the Creator and Sustainer of all that moveth and moveth not.

४७. इमं मा हिᳪसीद्विपादं पशुᳪसहस्राक्षो मेधाय चीयमान: ।
मयुं पशुं मेधमग्ने जषस्व तेन चिन्वानस्तन्वो नि षीद ।
मयुं ते शुगृच्छतु यं द्विष्मस्तं ते शुगृच्छतु ।

47. O King, born as man, and wide-awake, possessing thousand-fold vision, progressing for the attainment of happiness, don't destroy the bipeds and quadrupeds, and useful denizens of the forest; but protect them. Increase thy wealth with those cattle, and possess a strong body. The injurious beast of the forest should be put to grief by thee. Let thy enemy, whom we dislike, be put to grief!

४८. इमं मा हिᳪसीरेकशफं पशुं कनिक्रदं वाजिनं वाजिनेषु ।
गौरमारण्यमनु ते दिशामि तेन चिन्वानस्तन्वो नि षीद ।
गौरं ते शुगृच्छतु यं द्विष्मस्तं ते शुगृच्छतु ॥

48. O King, don't destroy this one-hoofed beautiful horse, soon agitated and writhing with pain in battlefields. I point out to thee the forest rhinoceros. With his protection add to thy prosperity and physical strength. Let the wild and uncontrolled rhinoceros be put to grief by thee. Let thy enemy, whom we detest, be put to grief!

४९. इमᳪ साहस्रᳪ शतधारमुत्सं व्यच्यमानᳪ सरिरस्य मध्ये ।
घृतं दुहानामदिति जनायाग्ने मा हिᳪसी: परमे व्योमन् ।
गवयमारण्यमनु ते दिशामि तेन चिन्वानस्तन्वो नि षीद ।
गवयं ते शुगृच्छतु यं द्विष्मस्तं ते शुगृच्छतु ॥

49. O sagacious King, in this world, don't harm this bull, the giver of thousands of comforts, the source of immense milk, and worthy of protection. Harm not in God's creation, the cow, the giver of milk for mankind, and innocent in nature. I point out to thee the forest cow. With her destruction add to thy prosperity and physical strength in the midst of vast space and under God's guidance. Let the wild forests cow be put to grief by thee. Let thy foe, whom we dislike, be put to grief!

५०. इममूर्णायुं वरुणस्य नाभि त्वचं पशूनां द्विपदां चतुष्पदाम् ।
त्वष्टु: प्रजानां प्रथमं जनित्रमग्ने मा हिᳪसी: परमे व्योमन् ।

⁴⁶I: God.
A king should protect the useful, and tame beasts of the forest, and subdue the wild and ferocious ones.
One hoofed: Having one hoof in each foot.

CHAPTER XIII

उष्ट्रमारण्यमनु ते दिशामि तेन चिन्वानस्तवो नि षीद ।
उष्ट्रं ते शुगृच्छतु यं द्विष्मस्तं ते शुगृच्छतु ॥

50. O learned King, don't kill the two-footed men and birds, and four-footed cattle, the source of comforts. Don't kill the sheep that covers our bodies with blankets, and is foremost worthy of protection amongst God's creatures. I point out to thee the forest camel. With his protection add to thy prosperity and physical strength. Let the wild, uncontrollable camel be put to grief by thee. Let thy foe, whom we dislike be put to grief!

५१. अजो ह्यग्नेरजनिष्ट शोकात्सो अपश्यज्जनितारमग्रे ।
तेन देवा देवतामग्रमायँस्तेन रोहमायन्नुप मेध्यास: ।
शरभमारण्यमनु ते दिशामि तेन चिन्वानस्तन्वो नि षीद ।
शरभं ते शुगृच्छतु यं द्विष्मस्तं ते शुगृच्छतु ॥

51. The unborn soul is educated through the power of God. He then sees God, existing before the creation of the universe, and the Generator of all. The learned, through that soul, attain to pre-eminent godly life; and the virtuous to an exalted position. I point out to thee, O king, the forest porcupine. Utilising her add to thy prosperity and physical strength. Let the untamed porcupine be put to grief by thee. Let thy foe, whom we dislike be put to grief by thee.

५२. त्वं यविष्ठ दाशुषो नॄँ: पाहि शृणुधी गिर: ।
रक्षा तोकमुत त्मना ॥

52. O most youthful leader, protect the pleasure-giving persons, hear their songs. With thy soul, protect their offspring!

५३. अग्नं त्वेमन्त्सादयाम्यपां त्वोदन्त्सादयाम्यपां त्वा भसन्त्सादयाम्यपां त्वा ज्योतिषि सादयाम्यपां त्वाऽयने सादयाम्यर्णवे त्वा सदने सादयामि समुद्रे त्वा सदने सादयामि ।
सरिरे त्वा सदने सादयाम्यपां त्वा क्षये सादयाम्यपां त्वा सधिषि सादयाम्यपां त्वा सदने सादयाम्यपां त्वा सधस्थे सादयाम्यपां त्वा योनौ सादयाम्यपां त्वा पुरीषे सादयाम्यपां त्वा पाथसि सादयामि गायत्रेण त्वा छन्दसा सादयामि त्रैष्टुभेन त्वा छन्दसा सादयामि जागतेन त्वा छन्दसा सादयाम्यानुष्टुभेन त्वा छन्दसा सादयामि पाङ्क्तेन त्वा छन्दसा सादयामि ॥

53. O man, I give thee the knowledge of the moving air for the medicinal herbs fielled with the wetness of water, clouds, brilliant electricity, open space, control of breath, fleeting mind, acquirable speech, a well-furnished house, ear that hears various sounds, the sky and mid region full of water,

---

[50]I: God.
Even the wild forest beasts like camel, cow, rhinoceros should be tamed, protected and utilised, but the ferocious and uncontrollable destroyed.

[51]Aj means the eternal soul and goat. The goat should not be killed. The porcupine which is uncontrollable should be destroyed, but not the one that can be tamed.
I: God.

ocean full of water, sandy tracts of water, foodstuffs that grow through water. I preach unto thee the significance of vedic texts couched in Gayatri, Trishtup, Jagati, Anushtup, and Pankti metres!

५४. अयं पुरो भुवस्तस्य प्राणो भौवायनो वन्सत: प्राणायनो गायत्री वासन्ती गायत्र्यं गायत्रं
गायत्रादुपाꣽशुरुपाꣽशोस्त्रिववृत् त्रिवृतो रथन्तरं वसिष्ठ ऋषि: ।
प्रजापतिगृहीतया त्वया प्राणं गृह्णामि प्रजाभ्य: ॥

54. O wife, this fire is primordial. It is the cause of Prana (breath), the source of life. Spring is the result of Prana. Spring is the cause of Gayatri, whereby we sing the praise of God. From the Gayatri comes the Gayatri metre. From the Gayatri comes the prayer. From the prayer come action, contemplation, and knowledge (Karma, Upasana and Jnana)!

As the fruit of these three comes the pleasure of liberation (Moksha). A learned person is the cause of producing intense pleasure like Prana. Thou accept me as thy husband, the protector of progeny. I gain strength to create offspring from thee.

५५. अयं दक्षिणा विश्वकर्मा तस्य मनो वैश्वकर्मणं ग्रीष्मो मानसस्त्रिष्टूब्ग्रैष्मी त्रिष्टुभ:
स्वारꣽ स्वारादन्तर्यामो अन्तर्यामात्पञ्चदश: पञ्चदशाद् बृहद् भरद्वाज ऋषि: प्रजापति-
गृहीतया त्वया मनो गृह्णामि प्रजाभ्य: ॥

55. O wife, in the south resides this air, the source of all acts. From that air the doer of all deeds, comes the mind. From the heat of the mind comes the summer. The eulogiser of summer is the Trishtup metre. From the warmth of Trishtup comes the intense glow. From the intense glow comes the mid-day. From mid-day comes the day of the full moon. From that comes the ear, the organ of receiving and strengthening knowledge. Just as a king, with his knowledge, administers justice to his subjects, so do I, with thee, cultivate a contemplative mind for the people!

५३. अयं पश्चाद्विश्वव्यचास्तस्य चक्षुर्वैश्वव्यचसं वर्षाश्चाक्षुष्यो जगती वार्षीं जगत्या
ऋक्सममृक्समाच्छुक्र:
शुक्रात्सप्तदश: सप्तदशाद्ध्रुवरूपं जमदग्निऋꣳषि: प्रजापतिगृहीतया त्वया चक्षुर्गृह्णामि
प्रजाभ्य: ॥

56. O wife, this sun rising in the East goes to the West, illuminating the universe. The lustrous rays of the sun are its eyes. The eye enjoys the rainy season. The Jagati verse is the expositor of the rainy season. From Jagati is

---

⁵³I: Teacher or God.
The teacher teaches his pupil different sciences, to equip him fully with knowledge.
⁵⁴In spring Gayatri verses are generally recited.
Vasishtha Rishi: Prana.
Moksha: Emancipation, salvation.
⁵⁵The subtle connection between the things mentioned has not been understood by me. Bhardwaj Rishi means ear and is not the name of a Rishi.

derived the knowledge of vedic verses. From that knowledge comes prosperity. From prosperity we get the knowledge of seventeenfold powerful soul. From that knowledge comes the knowledge of different phases and objects of the world. The eye makes us receive light.

Just as a husband, the guardian of offspring attains to discerning knowledge with his educated wife, so do I with thee gain power from the world.

५७. इदमुत्तरात् स्वस्तस्य श्रोत्रꣳ सौवꣳ शरच्छ्रौत्र्यनुष्टुप् शारद्यनुष्टुभ ऐडेमैदान्मन्थी मन्थिन एकविꣳश एकविꣳशाद्वैराजं विश्वामित्र ऋषि: प्रजापतिगृहीतया त्वया श्रोत्रं गृह्णामि प्रजाभ्य: ॥

57. O wife, this North direction is the giver of comforts. Ear is the source of its pleasantness. The ear is related to autumn. The significant Anushtup verse is the expositor of autumn. From Anushtup is derived the verse that explains speech. From that verse is derived the means of churning the objects. From that means is derived the principle of perfecting twenty one sciences. From that principle, we derive the ear, the cause of friendship with all, the receiver of the significance of words, the manifestor of various objects, and listener to the singing of Sama Veda. I, thy husband, the guardian of the offspring, along with thee, use the ear for the good of the people!

५८. इयमुपरि मतिस्तस्यै वाङ्माल्या हेमन्तो वाच्य: पङ्क्तितहैमन्ती पङ्क्त्यै निधनवन्निधनवत् आग्रयण आग्रयणात् त्रिणवत्रयस्त्रिꣳशौ त्रिणवत्रयस्त्रिꣳशाभ्याꣳ शाक्वररैवते विश्वकर्मं ऋषि: प्रजापतिगृहीतया त्वया वाचं गृह्णामि प्रजाभ्यो लोकं ता इन्द्रम् ॥

58. O learned wife, the highest of all things is intellect. From intellect is born speech. Winter is the offspring of speech. The Pankti verse is the expositor of winter. From Pankti springs Nidhanvat a part of Sama Veda, that comments on the mystery of Death. From that springs knowledge, the source of acquisition. From that knowledge are derived the twelve and thirty three songs of the Sama Veda. With those songs, knowing strength and the objects that contribute to wealth, the doer of noble deeds and the master of vedic lore, behaves rightly. I, thy husband, the guardian of offspring, with thee, acquire speech full of knowledge and sound instructions.

---

[56]Jamadagni Rishi means eye, and is not the name of any person, vide Shatapatha 8-1-2-3. The verse is not fully understood by me. Seventeen fold powerful means possessing various powers. Vide Shatapatha 8-1-2-4.

[57]Vishwamitra Rishi means the ear. This verse is not well understood by me.

[58]Vishvakarma Rishi means speech, vide Shatapath 8-1-2-9.

CHAPTER XIV

१. ध्रुवक्षितिर्ध्रुवयोनिर्ध्रुवाऽसि ध्रुवं योनिमा सीद साधुया ।
उरुयस्य केतुं प्रथमं जुषाणाऽश्विनाऽध्वर्यू सादयतामिह त्वा ॥

1. O woman, thou belongest to a firm nation. Thou hast got a permanent house. Thou art resolute. Enter in a religious spirit the stable domestic life (Grihastha Ashrama). Use the vast knowledge of the art of cooking. May the learned teachers and preachers, themselves admirers of pure domestic life, settle thee in it!

२. कुलायिनी घृतवती पुरन्धि: स्योने सीद सदने पृथिव्या: ।
अभि त्वा रुद्रा वसवो गृणन्त्विमा ब्रह्म पीपिहि सौभगायाऽश्विनाऽध्वर्यू सादयतामिह त्वा ॥

2. O woman, thou belongest to a noble family. Thou hast plenty of water. Thou art full of pleasures, and givest them to others. Settle in thy house on this earth. The Rudras and vasus instruct thee. Imbibe these vedic instructions for thy auspiciousness. May the learned teachers and preachers, themselves admirers of pure domestic life, settle thee in it!

३. स्वैर्दक्षैर्दक्षपितेह सीद देवानाꣳसुम्ने बृहते रणाय ।
पितेवैधि सूनव आ सुशेवा स्वावेशा तन्वा सं विशस्वाऽश्विनाऽध्वर्यू सादयतामिह त्वा ॥

3. O woman, just as the master of forces and employees, with their aid, standing in the midst of learned persons, advances for battle and pleasure, so shouldst thou advance in this world. Just as a father looks to the comforts of his son, so shouldst thou. With pleasure adorning thy body with clothes and ornaments enter bodily the domestic life with thy husband. May the teachers and preachers, themselves admirers of pure domestic life, settle thee in it!

४. पृथिव्या: पुरीषमस्यप्सो नाम तां त्वा विश्वे अभि गृणन्तु देवा: ।
स्तोमपृष्ठा घृतवतीह सीद प्रजावदस्मे द्रविणा ऽऽ यजस्वाऽश्विनाऽध्वर्यू सादयतामिह त्वा ॥

4. O woman, thou art aspirant after vedic eulogies. Thou art the protectrix of the earth, handsome and well-named; full of butter and other good edibles. May all the learned persons revere thee. Stay in this domestic life. Give us wealth that produces good children. May the learned teachers and preachers, themselves admirers of pure domestic life, settle thee in it!

५. अदित्यास्त्वा पृष्ठे सादयाम्यन्तरिक्षस्य धर्त्रीं विष्टम्भनीं दिशामधिपत्नीं भुवनानाम् ।
ऊर्मिर्द्रप्सोऽअपामसि विश्वकर्मा त ऋषिरश्विनाऽध्वर्यू सादयतामिह त्वा ॥

---

[1]Ashwina may also mean father and mother, who settle their daughter is domestic life, just as learned teachers and preachers settle her.

5. O wife, I, thy learned husband, engaged in the performance of noble deeds, establish thee on the surface of the earth, as mistress of the house, thee, the recipient of deathless mental knowledge, the mainstay of all directions, the guardian of the house, the place of bearing children. I establish thee on the earth like the rays of sun, as mistress of the house. Thou art pleasant like the wave of waters. May the learned teachers and preachers, the performers of sacrifice for self-protection, establish thee in this domestic life.

६. शुक्रश्च शुचिश्च ग्रैष्मावृतू अग्नेरन्त: इलेषोऽसि कल्पेतां द्यावापृथिवी कल्पन्तामाप ओषधय: कल्पन्तामग्नय: पृथङ्मम ज्येष्ठचाय सव्रता: ।
ये अग्नय: समनसोऽन्तरा द्यावापृथिवी इमे । ग्रैष्मावृतू अभिकल्पमाना इन्द्रमिव देवा अभिसंविशन्तु तया देवतयाङ्गिरस्वद् ध्रुवे सीदतम् ॥

6. May-June (Jayeshth), and June-July (Asarh) constitute the summer. This season due to intense heat, removes cough. May Heaven and Earth, may waters, medicinal plants, and fires, obeying the exact laws of nature, separately contribute to my prosperity in this season.

May fires, similar in nature, that exist between the heaven and earth, make the summer strong, just as spiritual forces strengthen the soul. O husband and wife, receiving life from God, remain steady like Heaven and Earth.

७. सजूऋँतुभि: सजूर्विधाभि: सजूर्देवैं: सजूर्देवैर्वयोनाधैरग्नये त्वा वैश्वानरायाश्विनाऽध्वर्यूं सादयतामिह त्वा
सजूऋँतुभि: सजूर्वंसुभि: सजूर्देवैर्वयोनाधैरग्नये त्वा वैश्वानरायाश्विनाऽध्वर्यूं सादयतामिह त्वा सजूऋँतुभि: सजूर्विधाभि: सजू रुद्रै: सजूर्देवैर्वयोनाधैरग्नये त्वा वैश्वानरायाश्विनाऽध्वर्यूं सादयतामिह त्वा सजऋँतुभि: सजूर्विधाभि: सजूरादित्यै: सजूर्देवैर्वयोनाधैरग्नये त्वा वैश्वानरायाश्विनाऽध्वर्यूं सादयतामिह त्वा सजूऋँतुभि: सजूर्विधाभि: सजूर्विश्वैर्देवै: सजूर्देवैर्वयोनाधैरग्नये त्वा वैश्वानरायाश्विनाऽध्वर्यूं सादयतामिह त्वा ॥

7. O man or woman, the learned teachers and preachers, thy guardians, establish thee in this world, for the acquisition of all objects, and mastering the science of fire, and we too establish thee!

Associate thyself with seasons, love waters, cultivate virtuous traits, try to prolong life and recite the Gayatri Mantra, hold dear thy breaths, the source of happiness.

O active man or woman, the learned teachers and preachers, thy guardians, establish thee in this domestic life, for the attainment of God, the Leader of the universe, and we too establish thee. Associate thyself with seasons, love waters, be friendly towards Vasus, live in the company of highly learned persons, the imparters of knowledge!

*Compare 13-25, where the praise of spring has been sung.
In this verse the praise of summer is sung.

O celibate man or woman, seeker after knowledge, the learned teachers and preachers, thy guardians, establish thee in this Brahmcharya Ashram (student life) for the study of religious books, the source of happiness for all; and we too establish thee!

Associate thyself with seasons, hold dear thy Pranas (vital breaths) which retain all objects, love the Rudras; befriend the learned, who arrange for the study of the vedas.

O learned man or woman, the learned teachers and preachers, thy guardians, establish thee in this world, for spreading knowledge and happiness unto all, and we too establish thee. Lead thy life according to seasons, love all noble deeds, regulate thy diet and sport according to twelve months of the year. Be friendly towards the highly learned persons, who arrange for the preaching of full knowledge!

O man or woman, the preacher of true ideas, the learned teachers and preachers, the guardians of vedic lore, establish thee in this world, for the diffusion of knowledge useful to humanity, and we too establish thee!

Regulate thy life according to seasons, perform pleasure-giving acts, love all the preachers of truth, and cultivate friendly relations, with the discriminators between truth and falsehood for the good of others, and for the dispensers of pleasant life.

८. प्राणं मे पाह्यपानं मे पाहि व्यानं मे पाहि चक्षुर्म उर्व्या वि भाहि श्रोत्रं मे श्लोकय ।
अप: पिन्वौषधीर्जिन्व द्विपादव चतुष्पात् पाहि दिवो वृष्टिमेरय ॥

8. O husband, guard thou my prana guard my apana guard my vyana through different nice devices. Illumine my eye. Fill my ear with religious sermons. Strengthen my vital breaths. Get medicinal plants. Protect bipeds. Protect quadrupeds. Manage well the household affairs, as sun, with its brilliance pours the rain!

९. मूर्धा वय: प्रजापतिश्छन्द: क्षत्रं वयो मयन्दं छन्दो विष्टम्भो वयोऽधिपतिश्छन्दो विश्वकर्मा वय: परमेष्ठी छन्दो वस्तो वयो विवलं छन्दो वृष्णिर्वयो विशाल छन्द: पुरुषो त्रयस्तन्द्र छन्दो व्याघ्रो व्योऽनाधृष्टं छन्द: सिꣳहो वयश्छदिश्छन्द: पष्ठवाड्वयो बृहती छन्द उक्षा वय: ककुप् छन्द ऋषभो वय: सनोबृहती छन्द: ॥

9. The Brahman is foremost in the society, like head in the body. His force lies in the protection of humanity through knowledge, religion and austerity. The Kshatriya is a class amongst men. His power lies in affording

---

⁷Vasus: Fire, Earth, air, space, sun, moon, sky, stars.
Rudras: Pran, Apan, Vyan, Udan, Saman, Nag, Kurma, Krikal, Dev Dutt, Dhananjaya, and soul. The first ten are the names of breaths.
Adityas: the twelve months of the year.
We: Learned persons or parents.
⁸Pran: the air that goes upward from the navel.
Apan: the air that goes downward from the navel, and is emitted through the anus.
Vyan: the air that is diffused in different joints of the body.

happiness to humanity through justice, humility and strength. The Vaishya is another class, who amasses foodstuffs. His strength lies in becoming the lord of riches. The artisan, Shudra is another class of men, whose strength lies in doing hard work.

The king, the doer of all good acts, is lovable, lord of all subjects and independent. It is the duty of man at the helm of affairs, to muster different forces for the protection of his body. It is the duty of the strong man, who is competent to give happiness to others, to attain to supremacy, and grant power to others.

It is the duty of an affluent person to nourish his family. It is the duty of a man heroic like a tiger, to be invincible by an enemy. He, who is powerful to subdue foes, powerful like the lion, should afford protection to his people, like the roof of the house.

He, who like the camel can take upon his shoulders this responsibility of managing the affairs of the State, should like the earth take upon himself the burden of all enterprises.

It is the duty of a man, strong like an ox, to protect his subjects and treat all straightly and justly.

It is the duty of a person well-known for his intellect and honour, to undertake projects that lie before him.

१०. अनड्वान्वय: पङ्क्तिशछन्दो धेनुर्वयो जगती छन्दस्त्र्यविर्वयस्त्रिष्टुप् छन्दो दित्यवाड्वयो विराट् छन्द: पञ्चाविर्वयो गायत्री छन्दस्त्रिवत्सो वय उष्णिक् छन्दस्तुर्यवाड्वयोऽनुष्टुप् छन्दो लोकं ता इन्द्रम् ॥

10. Like the bull that conveys the cart, the physically developed person should ripen his semen and undertake duties of a house-holder. The souls that like the milch-cow nourish others, are fit to rear the world.

The master of the three vedas should praise God through action, contemplation and knowledge.

The person brilliant like the sun, should through eminence and knowledge illumine himself and others. He who controls his five organs, can control his five breaths. He, who is engrossed in action, contemplation and knowledge, is fit to eradicate his sins.

He who knows all the four vedas, constantly prays to God.

११. इन्द्राग्नी अव्यथमानामिष्टकां दृ ँहतं युवम् ।
पृष्ठेन द्यावापृथिवी अन्तरिक्षं च वि बाधसे ॥

11. O husband and wife, behaving like lightning and earth, with mature intellect, make your domestic life cemented like a brick. Just as the sun and earth with their might restrict the atmosphere, so should ye bind your foes and remove miseries. O man just as thou removest the affliction of thy wife, so shouldst she remove thine!

[10]The last two sentences can be interpreted as a Banprasthi in the third Ashram, or Sanyasi in the fourth Ashram.
Three Vedas: Mean the Vedas that dilate upon Gyan, Karma and Upasana.

१२. विश्वकर्मा त्वा सादयत्वन्तरिक्षस्य पृष्ठे व्यचस्वतीं प्रथस्वतीमन्तरिक्षं यच्छान्तरिक्षं
दृꣳहान्तरिक्षं मा हिꣳसीः ।
विश्वस्मै प्राणायापानाय व्यानायोदानाय प्रतिष्ठायै चरित्राय । वायुष्ट्वाभि पातु मह्या
स्वस्त्या छदिषा शन्तमेन तया देवतयाङ्गिरस्वद् ध्रुवा सीद ॥

12. O woman, may thy husband well-versed in doing various noble deeds, fix in his heart thee, full of reverence, praiseworthy knowledge, and vast store of learning. Thou shouldst offer water to all, for the safety of their Pran, Vyan, Udan, and Saman, for their prosperity and preservation of character. Increase the store of laudable, pure water. Don't destroy the sweet and disease-uprooting water. May thy husband, loving thee like life, keep thee safe with great well-being, his splendour and pleasant knowledge. Live constantly with thy godly husband like the soul!

१३. राज्ञ्यसि प्राची दिग्विराडसि दक्षिणा दिक् सम्राडसि प्रतीची दिक् स्वराडस्युदीची
दिगधिपत्न्यसि बृहती दिक् ॥

13. O woman, thou art brilliant like the East, modest like the South, calm and lustrous like the West, self-effulgent like the North. Like the vast upper and lower directions, thou hast been made the mistress of the house. Please thou thy husband and other relatives!

१४. विश्वकर्मा त्वा सादयत्वन्तरिक्षस्य पृष्ठे ज्योतिष्मतीम् ।
विश्वस्मै प्राणायापानाय व्यानाय विश्वं ज्योतिर्यच्छ ।
वायुष्टेऽधिपतिस्तया देवतयाङ्गिरस्वद् ध्रुवा सीद ॥

14. O woman, may thy husband, the doer of various noble deeds, establish like sun-light on water, in his heart, thee, full of knowledge. Grant full light to all the members of the family for strengthening their Pran, Apan, Vyan. Thy husband dear like vital breath, is thy Lord. Live constantly with thy godly husband like the sun!

१५. नभश्च नभस्यश्च वार्षिकावृतू अग्नेरन्तः श्लेषोऽसि कल्पेतां द्यावापृथिवी कल्पन्तामाप
ओषधयः कल्पन्तामग्नयः पृथङ्मम ज्येष्ठाय सव्रताः ।
ये अग्नयः समनसोऽन्तरा द्यावापृथिवी इमे । वार्षिकावृतू अभिकल्पमाना इन्द्रमिव देवा
अभिसंविशन्तु तया देवतयाङ्गिरस्वद् ध्रुवे सीदतम् ॥

15. Shravan (July-August) and Bhadrapada (August-September) constitute the rainy season, and they contribute to my prosperity. In them there is the touch of heat and cold.
Just as the Sky and Earth thrive in these months, so shouldst ye, husband and wife, prosper with your enjoyment.

[12] Pran, Vyan, Udan, Saman are different vital airs or breaths in the body.
[15] Just as breath is never separated from the body, so should husband and wife be not separated from each other.
My: Preceptor.

Just as waters, plants and fires separately thrive in the rainy season, so should noble persons, with unanimity of purpose, and sameness of knowledge, prosper.

Just as the Sky and Earth thrive in the rainy season, so should learned persons utilizing the rainy season for their comfort, come in contact with it like lightning. O husband and wife, live together in this season firmly and affectionately like breath!

१६. इषश्चोर्जश्च शारदावृतू अग्नेरन्तः श्लेषोऽसि कल्पेतां द्यावापृथिवी कल्पन्तामाप ओष-
धयः कल्पन्तामग्नयः पृथङ्मम ज्येष्ठाय सव्रताः । ये अग्नयः समनसोऽन्तरा द्यावापृथिवी
इमे । शारदावृतू अभिकल्पमाना इन्द्रमिव देवा अभिसंविशन्तु तया देवतयाऽङ्गिरस्वद् ध्रुवे
सीदतम् ॥

16. O men, Aswin (September-October) and Kartik (October-November) constitute the Autumn season. Both these months contribute to my enjoyable comforts. In them there is the touch of heat and cold. Let them make the Sky and Earth thrive. Let waters and plants grow by their means. Let the fires of our body that regulate all actions function separately. Let the learned people enter these two months gloriously, desiring for happiness. O husband and wife live together firmly like space, in this good season!

१७. आयुर्मे पाहि प्राणं मे पाह्यपानं मे पाहि व्यानं मे पाहि चक्षुर्मे पाहि श्रोत्रं मे पाहि
वाचं मे पिन्व मनो मे जिन्वात्मानं मे पाहि ज्योतिर्मे यच्छ ॥

17. Preserve my life, Preserve my Pran. Guard my Apan. Guard my Vyan. Preserve my eyes. Preserve my ears. Strengthen my speech with good instructions. Satisfy my mind. Preserve my soul. Vouchsafe me light of knowledge.

१८. मा छन्दः प्रमा छन्दः प्रतिमा छन्दो अस्रीवयश्छन्दः पङ्क्तिश्छन्दः उष्णिक् छन्दो बृहती
छन्दो अनुष्टुप् छन्दो विराट् छन्दो गायत्री छन्दस्त्रिष्टुप् छन्दो जगती छन्दः ॥

18. Wisdom gives pleasure. Intellect grants strength. Discernment gives freedom. Food gives physical force. Yoga with five components gives light. Affection gives fame. Matter affords shelter. Intense attachment to pleasure creates sexual enjoyment. The manifestation of different sciences gives knowledge. The worshipper of God knows Him. Dependence on physical, mental, and spiritual enjoyments gives happiness. The force that rules the universe is the source of strength and pleasure. People should take advantage of these and add to their store of happiness.

१९. पृथिवी छन्दो ऽन्तरिक्षं छन्दो द्यौश्छन्दः समाश्छन्दो नक्षत्राणि छन्दो वाक् छन्दो मनश्छन्दः
कृषिश्छन्दो हिरण्यं छन्दो गौश्छन्दो अजाश्छन्दो अश्वश्छन्दः ॥

19. Earth is full of freedom. Heaven is extremely pleasant. Light is knowledge. Years enhance our wisdom. The stars are free in their movements.

---

[17]The husband addresses this verse to his wife, or vice versa.

Let speech be truthful and mind free from fraud. Husbandry leads to produce. Gold gives comforts. Cow is the source of happiness. Goat gives us pleasure. Horses are free in motion.

२०. अग्निर्देवता वातो देवता सूर्यो देवता चन्द्रमा देवता वसवो देवता रुद्रा ऽदित्या देवता मरुतो देवता विश्वे देवा देवता बृहस्पतिर्देवतेन्द्रो देवता वरुणो देवता ॥

20. Fire, wind, sun, moon, vasus, Rudras, Adityas, learned men of contemplative mood, all good objects, God the protector of the universe and the vedas, well earned riches, and water are devatas, *i.e.*, highly useful things. Men and women should take advantage of these devatas.

२१. मूर्धासि राड् ध्रुवाऽसि धरुणा धर्त्र्यसि धरणी ।
आयुषे त्वा वर्चसे त्मा कृष्यै त्वा क्षेमाय त्वा ॥

21. O woman, thou art excellent like the sun, thou art pure and firm like the lustrous sun that moves in its orbit. Thou art the rearer of progeny like the nourishing earth. I accept thee for longevity, for food, for agriculture, for peace and happiness!

२२. यन्त्री राड् यन्त्र्यसि यमनी ध्रुवाऽसि धरित्री ।
इषे त्वोर्जे त्वा रय्यै त्वा पोषाय त्वा लोकं ता इन्द्रम् ॥

22. O wife, thou art stable like a machine, full of brilliance, for bearing like the earth, firm like the sky, full of determination, and embodiment of virtue. I accept thee for the fulfilment of desires, for the attainment of valour, riches and prosperity!

२३. आशुस्त्रिवृड्भ्रान्तः पञ्चदशो व्योमा सप्तदशो धरुण एकविꣳशः प्रतूतिरष्टादशस्तपो नवदशो ऽभीवर्तः सविꣳशो वर्चो द्वाविꣳशः सम्भरणस्त्रयोविꣳशो योनिश्चतुर्विꣳशो गर्भाः पञ्चविꣳश ओजस्त्रिणवः ऋतुरेकत्रिꣳशः प्रतिष्ठा त्रयस्त्रिꣳशो ब्रह्मणस्य विष्टपं चतुस्त्रिꣳशो नाकः पट्त्रिꣳशो विवर्तोऽष्टाचत्वारिꣳशो धर्त्र चतुष्टोमः ॥

²³Seventeen-fold: Twelve months and five seasons.
Twenty-one-fold: Twelve months, five seasons three worlds and itself.
Eighteen-fold: Twelve months, five seasons and itself.
Nineteen-fold: Twelve months, six seasons and itself.
Twenty-two-fold: Twelve months, seven seasons, day and night, and itself.
Twenty-three-fold: Consisting of thirteen months (one intercalary), seven seasons, day and night and itself.
Twenty-four-fold: Twenty-four half months.
Twenty-five-fold: 24 half months and itself.
Twenty-seven-fold: 24 half months, day and night and itself.
Thirty-one-fold: 24 half months, six seasons and itself.
Thirty-three-fold: 24 half months, 6 seasons, day and night and itself.
Thirty-four-fold: 24 half months, 7 seasons, day and night and itself.
Thirty-six-fold: 24 half months and 12 months.
Forty-eight-fold: 26 half months, 13 months seven seasons, day and night.

CHAPTER XIV

23. The year contains heat, cold and moderate heat, cold. The moon waxes and wanes for fifteen days. The year, like the vast atmosphere is seventeenfold. The year, the support of all substances is twentyonefold.
The fast fleeting year is eighteenfold.
The year giving warmth to all like the sun, is nineteenfold.
The year that confronts men is twentyfold.
The powerful year is twentytwofold.
The year, the nourisher of all is twentythree-fold.
The year, the resort of all beings is twentyfour-fold.
The year that keeps human beings under its control is twentyfive-fold.
The vigorous year is twentyseven-fold.
The year, the field for work is thirtyone-fold.
The year, the cause of the residence of all, is thirty-three-fold.
The year, pervaded by the Almighty Father, is thirty-four-fold.
The year, the giver of happiness is thirtysix-fold.
The year, in which we move in various ways, is forty eight-fold.
The year, is the retainer of all objects, and the support of praises in the four directions.
O men know this to be the year!

२४. अग्नेर्भागोऽसि दीक्षाया आधिपत्यं ब्रह्म स्पृतं त्रिवृत्स्तोम
इन्द्रस्य भागोऽसि विष्णोराधिपत्यं क्षत्रꣳ स्पृतं पञ्चदश स्तोमो
नृचक्षसां भागोऽसि धातुराधिपत्यं जनित्रꣳ स्पृतꣳ सप्तदश स्तोमो
मित्रस्य भागोऽसि वरुणस्याधिपत्यं दिवो वृष्टिर्वति स्पृतं एकविꣳश स्तोम: ॥

24. O learned person, thou art like the year. Practising celibacy, attain to the sovereignty of a Brahmin family. Being pure in body, word and mind, and worthy of praise, thou art the embodiment of supremacy; attain to the sovereignty of a royal Kshatriya family, loved by the All-pervading God. Being fifteen-fold praiser, thou art like the part of objects described by the people; attain to the desired birth and right of a sustainer. Laudable in seventeen ways, thou art the part of Pran; attain to the sovereignty of waters. Served by air, thou art like the twenty-one-fold praiser, draw rain from the sun through Homa (sacrificial fire)!

२५. वसूनां भागोऽसि रुद्राणामाधिपत्यं चतुष्पात् स्पृतं चतुर्विꣳश स्तोम
आदित्यानां भागोऽसि मरुतामाधिपत्यं गर्भा स्पृता: पञ्चविꣳश स्तोमो
अदित्यै भागोऽसि पूष्ण आधिपत्यमोज स्पृतं त्रिणव स्तोमो
देवस्य सवितुर्भागोऽसि बृहस्पतेराधिपत्यꣳ **समीचीर्दिश** स्पृताश्चतुष्टोम स्तोम: ॥

---
[24]The word Panchdash in the verse may mean vigour, lustre or vitality, vid$_e$ तां० 11-6-11.
The word panchdash may also mean the fifteen days in which the moon waxes and wanes.
The word Saptdash in the text may also mean food-grain vide तां० 2-7-7.
The word Ekvinsha in the text may mean, respect, honour vide तां० 16-13-4. The verse is not fully understood by me. Sustainer means preserver of the people.

25. O learned person, thou art served by the Vasu Brahmcharis, Control thou the ten Pranas and the soul. Twentyfour-fold praiser, thou art honoured by the Aditya-Brahmcharis; rear the cattle like cows; and be the master of men. Deserving praise in twenty-five ways, thou art like a part of light!

Acquiring the serviceable power of the earth, attain to sovereignty. Deserving praise in twenty seven ways, thou art the creation of pleasant God, acquire the strength granted thee by God, the Protector of the vedas. Thou, the worshipper with vedic verses, filled with knowledge and noble qualities, shouldst know all the directions, fit for affection, deserving to be fully mastered, and knowable by good people.

२६. यवानां भागोऽस्ययवानामाधिपत्यं प्रजा स्पृताश्चतुश्चत्वारिꣳश स्तोम
ऋभूणां भागोऽसि विश्वेषां देवानामाधिपत्यं भूतꣳ स्पृतं त्रयस्त्रिꣳश स्तोम: ॥

26. O man, thou usest the mixed substances, as is done in autumn. Having sovereignty over objects with different natures, with affection, thou shouldst nourish the people worthy of sustenance. Thou art worthy of praise in forty-four ways, and fit to be revered by the wise. Having acquired the power exercised by all the learned persons in the past, and being worthy of praise in thirty-three ways; thou deservest respect from us!

२७. सहश्च सहस्यश्च हैमन्तिकावृतू अग्नेरन्त: श्लेषोऽसि कल्पेतां द्यावापृथिवी कल्पन्तामाप
ओषधय: कल्पन्तामग्नय: पृथङ्ममम ज्येष्ठघाय सव्रता: ।
ये अग्नय: समनसोऽन्तरा द्यावापृथिवी इमे । हैमन्तिकावृतू अभिकल्पमाना इन्द्रमिव देवा
अभिसंविशन्तु तया देवतयाङ्गिरस्वद् ध्रुवे सीदतम् ॥

27. For my aged elders, the mid November to mid January months constitute the winter season. These two months are the life and soul of winter. In this season there is a slight touch of heat. In that season let Sky and Earth be competent to do their duty; let waters, medicinal plants, and bright fires be separately vigorous.

Men of contemplative mood, regulated in life, unanimous in purpose should make the strong Earth and Sky perform their duty. Let the learned keeping in view these two glorious months, enter them. Let the good people full of affection for God attain to happiness by regulating their diet and recreation.

२८. एकयास्तुवत प्रजा अधीयन्त प्रजापतिरधिपतिरासीत्
तिसृभिरस्तुवत ब्रह्मासृज्यत ब्रह्मणस्पतिरधिपतिरासीत्
पञ्चभिरस्तुवत भूतान्यसृज्यन्त भूतानां पतिरधिपतिरासीत्
सप्तभिरस्तुवत सप्त ऋषयोऽसृज्यन्त धाताऽधिपतिरासीत् ॥

---

[25]The word chaturvinsha in the text may also mean beauty, dignity, and power, vide तां॰ 15-10-6.

The word Trinava, i.e., 27 may also mean strength, power vide तां॰ 10-1-15.

[26]The word Trayastrinsha may mean body, vide तां॰ 19-10-10. Forty-four and thirty three ways of praise are not clear to me.

28. O men, God is the Creator and Protector of all. Praise Him with your speech. He has educated humanity through the vedas. God is the Guardian of the vedas and the Lord of all. He has revealed the vedas full of knowledge. Praise Him with the movement of three Pran, Udan and Vyan breaths. He has created all the worlds. He is their Protector, and Protector of the protectors. Praise Him with the help of Saman breath, perception, intellect, self consciousness and mind. He has created the seven Rishis. He is the Sustainer and Lord of all. Praise Him with the help of Nag, Kurma, Krikal, Deva Dutta, Dhananjaya (breaths), desire and effort!

२९. नवभिरस्तुवत पितरोऽसृज्यन्तादितिरधिपत्न्यासी-
देकादशभिरस्तुवत ऋतवोऽसृज्यन्तार्तवा अधिपतय आसँ
स्त्रयोदशभिरस्तुवत मासा असृज्यन्त संवत्सरोऽधिपतिरासीत्
पञ्चदशभिरस्तुवत क्षत्रमसृज्यतेन्द्रोऽधिपतिरासीत्
सप्तदशभिरस्तुवत ग्राम्या: पशवोऽसृज्यन्त बृहस्पतिरधिपतिरासीत् ॥

29. O men, God has created wise persons. The mother-like nourishing Earth is our lord. Praise God with nine breaths. He has created the seasons. The attributes of those seasons respectively reign supreme in them. Praise God with ten pranas and soul. He has created the twelve months. The year is the master of time. Praise God with thirteen objects. He has created the Kshatriyas. The sun lords over us through his intense glory. Praise God with fifteen objects. He has created the village cattle, and the vaisha-, who are our supporters. Praise God through seventeen objects!

३०. नवदशभिरस्तुवत शूद्रार्यावसृज्येतामहोरात्रे अधिपत्नी आस्ता-
मेकविँशत्यास्तुवतैकशफा: पशवोऽसृज्यन्त वरुणोऽधिपतिरासीत्
त्रयोविँशत्यास्तुवत क्षुद्रा: पशवोऽसृज्यन्त पूषाऽधिपतिरासीत्
पञ्चविँशत्यास्तुवतारण्या: पशवोऽसृज्यन्त वायुरधिपतिरासीत्
सप्तविँशत्यास्तुवत द्यावापृथिवी व्यैतां वसवो रुद्रा आदित्या अनुव्यायँस्त एवाधिपतय
आसन् ॥

---

[28]Three Breaths: Out-breath, upward breath, diffusive breath.
  Seven Rishis: Two eyes, two ears, two nostrils and mouth. According to Swami Dayananda Seven Rishis are five principal breaths, Intellect and Ego.
[29]Nine: Seven vital airs of the head, and two below.
  Eleven: Ten vital airs and the soul.
  Thirteen: Ten vital airs, two feet and the soul.
  Fifteen: The fifteen tithis lunar days as interpreted by Swami Dayananda; or ten fingers, two arms, two legs, and the part above the navel vide Shatapatha 8-4-3-11.
  Seventeen: Ten toes, two knees, two legs, two feet, and the part below the navel.
[30]Nineteen: Ten pranas, five great elements, mind, intellect, perception and egotism; or ten fingers and nine pranas vide Shatapatha 8-4-3-12.
  Twenty-one: Ten fingers, ten toes, and soul, vide Shatapatha 8-4-3-13.
  Twenty-three: Ten fingers, ten toes, two feet and soul. Shatapatha 8-4-3-14.

30. O men, God has created the day and night for work, and the Shudra and Arya. Praise Him through nineteen objects. He has created water, which is dear like life. He has created one-hoofed animals. Praise Him through twenty-one objects. He has created this strong Earth, the cause of our protection, and that of small animals. Praise Him through twenty-three objects. He has created the forest animals, and the air that rears us. Praise Him through twenty five objects!

He has created the Heaven and Earth, the Vasus, the Rudras, and the Adityas. Those forces of nature and learned persons are our protectors. Praise Him through twenty-seven objects.

३१. नवविꣳशत्याऽस्तुवत वनस्पतयोऽसृज्यन्त सोमोऽधिपतिरासी-
देकत्रिꣳशताऽस्तुवत प्रजा अ़सृज्यन्त यवाश्चायवाश्चाधिपतय आसꣳ-
स्त्रयस्त्रिꣳशताऽस्तुवत भूतान्यशाम्यन् प्रजापति: परमेष्ठ्यधिपतिरासील्लोकꣳ ता इन्द्रम् ॥

31. O men, God has created the trees, Soma is their head. Praise Him with twenty-nine objects. He has created the important plants, the forests, the dust-rays, the different parts of the matter with their attributes of Satva, Rajas and Tamas. Atoms are their over-lord. Praise Him with thirty one objects. Through His grace all big forces of Nature attain to calmness, God, the Sustainer of men, the Pervader of the universe, is over-lord, Praise Him through thirty-three objects!

Twente-five: Ten fingers, ten toes, two arms, two legs and soul. Shatapatha 8-4-3-15.

Twenty-seven: Ten fingers, ten toes, two arms, two legs, two feet and soul. Shatapatha 8-4-3-16.

Vasus, Rudras and Adityas have already been explained, they are respectively 8, 11 and 12. They may also mean the Vasus, Rudra and Aditya Brahmcharis who observe a vow of celibacy for 24, 36 and 48 years.

[31]Twenty-nine: Ten fingers, ten toes, and nine vital airs. Shatapatha 8-4-3-17.

Thirty-one: Ten fingers, ten toes, ten vital airs and soul, Shatapatha 8-4-3-18.

Thirty-three: Ten fingers, ten toes, ten vital airs, two feet and soul. Shatapatha 8-4-3-19.

Swami Dayananda interprets these figures of 29, 31, and 33 as the forces of nature, and the qualities of trees, medicines, and other created objects.

CHAPTER XV

१. अग्ने जातान् प्र णुदा नः सपत्नान् प्रत्यजातान् नुद जातवेदः ।
अधि नो ब्रूहि सुमना अहेडँस्तव स्याम शर्म त्रिवरूथ उद्भौ ॥

1. O King, drive away our known enemies. O powerful king, put our unknown foes aright. Graciously-minded, showing no disrespect, give us good instructions; wherewith we may live happily in a thrice-guarded house, well-provided by thee with all necessary things!

२. सहसा जातान् प्र णुदा नः सपत्नान् प्रत्यजाताञ्जातवेदो नुदस्व ।
अधि नो ब्रूहि सुमनस्यमानो वयँ स्याम प्र णुदा नः सपत्नान् ॥

2. O learned King, drive away with might our known foes. Keep off those who oppose us secretly. Benevolent in thought and spirit, teach us the art of victory. May we be thy supporters. Drive away our foes!

३. षोडशी स्तोम ओजो द्रविणं चतुश्चत्वारिँश स्तोमो वर्चो द्रविणम् ।
अग्नेः पुरीषमस्यप्सो नाम तां त्वा विश्वे अभि गृणन्तु देवाः ।
स्तोमपृष्ठा घृतवतीह सीद प्रजावदस्मे द्रविणा यजस्व ॥

3. She, the master of sixteen arts, worthy of praise, grants strength and wealth, laudable celibacy of forty-four years, learning and power. She has acquired the completion of sacrificial fire. She is free from covetousness for the wealth of others. All learned people should praise her. Enriched with songs of praise and butter, stay thou in this domestic life, and give us wealth with store of children.

४. एवश्छन्दो वरिवश्छन्दः शम्भूश्छन्दः परिभूश्छन्द आच्छच्छन्दो मनश्छन्दो व्यचश्छन्दः
सिन्धुश्छन्दः समुद्रश्छन्दः सरिरं छन्दः ककुप्छन्दस्त्रिककुप्छन्दं काव्यं छन्दो अङ्कुपं
छन्दो अक्षरपङ्क्तिश्छन्दः पदपङ्क्तिश्छन्दो विष्टारपङ्क्तिश्छन्दः क्षुरो भ्रजश्छन्दः ॥

4. Knowledge gives pleasure. The practice of truth gives ease. Experience of comfort gives delight. Action brings light of truth. Avoidance of sins gives life. The mental conceptions and aversions give light.
The cultivation of noble traits gives peace of mind.
The free movement like a river gives independence.
The depth of mind, like the ocean, solves all problems.
The sweetness of speech like water gives calmness.

---

[1] Thrice guarded: A house in which one finds spiritual, physical happiness, and protection against the forces of nature, i.e., Adhi-Atmika, Adhi-Bhautika and Adhi-Daivik pleasures.

[3] She means womankind.

[4] Three kinds: They are mentioned in verse 1.

Our fame wide like directions adds to our greatness.
The deed that is the bringer of three kinds of comforts gives us delight.
The works of far-sighted poets give knowledge.
Meandering water brings usefulness.
Life after death give solace.
This world is a place of happiness.
All directions are the source of delight.
Sun gives us knowledge.
Light of knowledge brings happiness.

५. आच्छच्छन्दः प्रच्छच्छन्दः संयच्छन्दो वियच्छन्दो बृहच्छन्दो रथन्तरञ्छन्दो निकायश्छन्दो विवधश्छन्दो गिरश्छन्दो भ्रजश्छन्दः सँस्तुप् छन्दो ऽनुष्टुप् छन्द एवश्छन्दो वरिवश्छन्दो वयश्छन्दो वयस्कृच्छन्दो विष्पर्धाश्छन्दो विशालं छन्दश्छदिश्छन्दो दूरोहणं छन्दस्तन्द्रं छन्दो श्रङ्काङ्कं छन्दः ॥

5. The action that removes sins, gives light.
The action that with exertion removes evil propensity, lends determination.
Concentration of mind gives strength.
Perseverance leads to various efforts.
Increase in prosperity leads to independence.
Emancipator from this world is worthy of adoration.
Air is useful.
Space in which reside different objects is full of light.
Food worth enjoying is acceptable.
Brilliant fire is acceptable.
Speech gives enjoyment.
The mental attitude, that after hearing, makes us understand the religious books serves as our mentor.
Acquisition is the result of exertion.
Service of the learned is worthy of resort.
Life is synonymous with independence.
Means for prolonging life are exercisable.
Emulation is laudable.
Enterprise is praiseworthy.
Removal of obstacles is the bringer of happiness.
Conquest of affliction demands strength.
Independence is splendour.
Arithmetic is a useful science.

६. रश्मिना सत्याय सत्यं जिन्व प्रेतिना धर्मणा धर्म जिन्वान्वित्या दिवा दिवं जिन्व सन्धिनाऽन्तरिक्षेणान्तरिक्षं जिन्व प्रतिधिना पृथिव्या पृथिवीं जिन्व विष्टम्भेन वृष्ट्या वृष्टिं जिन्व प्रवयाऽह्नाऽह्र्जिन्वानुया रात्र्या रात्रीं जिन्वोषिजा वसुभ्यो वसूञ्जिन्वं प्रकेतेना-दित्येभ्य आदित्याञ्जिन्वं ॥

6. O learned person with lustre, perform virtuous deed for happiness and control over material objects. Know religion, with the observance of enlightened noble justice!

CHAPTER XV

For investigation, get the light of truth, with the light of religion.
Know mid-air as uniting the Earth with Heaven.
Know Earth through geology.
Know rain through the science of rain that nourishes the body.
Know day with the beautiful science of light.
Know night by the science of night that follows light.
Know the eight Vasus through their desirable science.
Know the Adityas (twelve months) intelligently with their science.

७. तन्तुना रायस्पोषेण रायस्पोषं जिन्व सꣳ सर्पेण श्रुताय श्रुतं जिन्वैडेनौषधीभिरोष-
धीजिन्वोत्तमेन तनूभिस्तनूर्जिन्व वयोधसाधीतेनाधीतं जिन्वाभिजिता तेजसा तेजो जिन्व ॥

7. O man gain the strength of wealth, through the extended application of wealth!
Learn to listen to religious lore, for acquiring it properly.
Acquire medicines through the sciences of medicine, and agriculture.
Attain to physical strength, through pure bodies, well regulated according to religious instructions.
Acquire knowledge through study, that gives life.
Learn perseverance for conquering the opposing foes, with a firm hand.

८. प्रतिपदसि प्रतिपदे त्वा ऽनुपदस्यनुपदे त्वा सम्पदसि सम्पदे त्वा तेजोऽसि तेजसे त्वा ॥

8. O wife, thou art an embodiment of wealth, for wealth do I accept thee. Thou art obedient, obtainable after the completion of studies. I accept thee!
Thou art riches, for riches do I accept thee Thou art brilliance, for brilliance do I accept thee.

९. त्रिवृदसि त्रिवृते त्वा प्रवृदसि प्रवृते त्वा विवृदसि विवृते त्वा सवृदसि सवृते त्वा ऽऽक्रमो-
ऽस्याक्रमाय त्वा संक्रमोऽसि संक्रमाय त्वोत्क्रमोऽस्युत्क्रमाय त्वोत्क्रान्तिरस्युत्क्रान्त्यै त्वा अधि-
पतिनोर्जोर्जं जिन्व ॥

9. O husband, thou knowest the primordial matter with three qualities. For knowing that matter, do I accept thee!
Thou knowest this world, the effect of matter. For knowing this world do I accept thee. Thou art the manifold benefactor of the world. I accept thee for doing good to humanity. Thou knowest all objects similar in nature. For knowing them do I accept thee.
Thou possessest the knowledge of atmosphere, for knowing the atmosphere, do I accept thee. Thou accurately knowest all the objects. For knowing them do I accept thee.
Thou knowest the movements of clouds on high. For knowing them do I accept thee. O wife, thou knowest the science wherewith we cross the accessible and inaccessible regions. For knowing the art of flying, do I accept thee. Living with thy husband, with thy energy attain to strength!

⁶Eight Vasus, the forces of nature have already been explained.
⁹Three qualities: The matter has got three qualities of Satva, Rajas, Tamas.

१०. राज्यसि प्राची दिग्वसवस्ते देवा अधिपतयोऽग्निर्हेतीनां प्रतिधर्ता त्रिवृत् त्वा स्तोम: पृथिव्याꣳश्रयत्वाज्यमुक्थमव्यथायै स्तभ्नातु रथन्तरꣳ साम प्रतिष्ठित्या अन्तरिक्ष ऋषयस्त्वा प्रथमजा देवेषु दिवो मात्रया वरिम्णा प्रथन्तु विधर्ता चायमधिपतिश्च ते त्वा सर्वे संविदाना नाकस्य पृष्ठे स्वर्गे लोके यजमानं च सादयन्तु ॥

10. O Woman, thou art queen brilliant like the East. Eight Vasus are thy protectors. Thou possessest the fire that resides in arms and weapons, that pervades the sun, lightning and Earth, and is full of praise. Get butter on the Earth for enjoyment. For thy prosperity, possess the military force of aeroplanes. May the aged vedic seers, with great power, and brilliance of knowledge, fill thee with good qualities and wisdom. This husband of thine is thy protector in diverse ways. May all the learned persons, unanimously settle thee and thy husband in a happy place on this comfortable Earth!

११. विराडसि दक्षिणा दिग्रुद्रास्ते देवा अधिपतय इन्द्रो हेतीनां प्रतिधर्ता पञ्चदशस्त्वा स्तोम: पृथिव्याꣳ श्रयतु प्र उगमुक्थमव्यथायै स्तभ्नातु बृहत्साम प्रतिष्ठित्या अन्तरिक्ष ऋषयस्त्वा प्रथमजा देवेषु दिवो मात्रया वरिम्णा प्रथन्तु विधर्ता चायमधिपतिश्च ते त्वा सर्वे संविदाना नाकस्य पृष्ठे स्वर्गे लोके यजमानं च सादयन्तु ॥

11. O woman thou art like the bright South. Eleven Rudras (airs) are thy protectors. Thy husband, the wielder of arms and weapons, the knower of the meanings of vedic verses in fifteen ways, and the sun serve thee on earth. He, being fearless of man, preaches unto thee firmly the narrable and instructible words!

For stability he recites the significant verses of the Sama Veda, The aged, learned persons, the significant plenteous airs in beautiful objects in the atmosphere, and the particles of blazing fire make thee renowned. The sustainer and nourisher of the Earth through attraction, the sun, the foremost amongst the brilliant objects, strengthens thee. May all the learned persons, unanimously establish thee and thy husband in a happy place in the space, where there is plenty of water.

१२. सम्राडसि प्रतीची दिगादित्यास्ते देवा अधिपतयो वरुणो हेतीनां प्रतिधर्ता सप्तदशस्त्वा स्तोम: पृथिव्याꣳ श्रयतु मरुत्वतीयमुक्थमव्यथायै स्तभ्नातु वैरूपꣳ साम प्रतिष्ठित्या अन्तरिक्ष ऋषयस्त्वा प्रथमजा देवेषु दिवो मात्रया वरिम्णा प्रथन्तु विधर्ता चायमधि-पतिश्च ते त्वा सर्वे संविदाना नाकस्य पृष्ठे स्वर्गे लोके यजमानं च सादयन्तु ॥

12. O woman, thou art brilliant like the West. The learned persons are thy overlords. Thy husband, possessing seventeen vital parts of the body,

---

[10] Vasus: The eight forces of nature mentioned before.

[11] Fifteen: Five organs of knowledge (Gyan Indriya) and five of action (Karma Indriyas) and five airs, Pran, Apan, Vyan, Udan and Saman.

[12] Seventeen: Pt. Jaidev, Vidyalankar, in his commentary describes seventeen to be 17 parts of the body. i.e., 10 fingers, two arms, two legs, head, belly and soul.

Seventeen may also mean food vide तां० 2-7-7.

worthy of praise, the subduer of foes, master of fiery spirits, may serve thee on earth!

May he, unfaltering in nature, full of instructions from many learned persons, and vedic lore, full of various teachings of great men, learn the Sama Veda for greatness.

There are in the atmosphere many lustrous objects, created from the limitless material cause, and serviceable moving airs spread in all parts. The learned should instruct thee so. The master of riches, the king, keeps the people contented, so should all learned persons unanimously establish thee and thy husband in a happy abode, in a part of the earth, free from affliction.

१३. स्वराडस्युदीची दिङ्मरुतस्ते देवा अधिपतयः सोमो हेतीनां प्रतिधर्तंकविँ॑शस्त्वा स्तोमः पृथिव्याँ॑ श्रयतु निष्केवल्यमुक्थमव्यथायै स्तभ्नातु वैराजँ॑ साम प्रतिष्ठत्या अन्तरिक्ष ऋषयस्त्वा प्रथमजा देवेषु दिवो मात्रया वरिम्णा प्रथन्तु विधर्ता चायमधि-पतिश्च ते त्वा सर्वे संविदाना नाकस्य पृष्ठं स्वर्गे लोके यजमानं च सादयन्तु ॥

13. O woman, Just as North is self luminous, so is thy husband. The beautiful airs are the presiding forces of the North!

May the husband worthy of praise like the moon that preserves rays in twenty one ways, live with thee on this earth.

Being free from the sway of passions, may he, for thee, learn that part of the veda which deals with the unity of God. For stability, may he study that portion of the Sama Veda, that deals with the universal aspect of God. In thy body there are many chief strong vital airs, in the organs, coupled with perception. He is the sustainer and lord of those airs.

May all the learned persons, with one mind make thee renowned, and establish thee and thy husband in a happy place on a comfortable part of the earth.

१४. अधिपत्न्यसि बृहती दिग्विश्वे ते देवा अधिपतयो बृहस्पतिहेतीनां प्रतिधर्ता त्रिणवत्रय-स्त्रिँ॑शौ त्वा स्तोमौ पृथिव्याँ॑ श्रयतां वैश्वदेवा निमारुते उक्थे अव्यथायै स्तभ्नीताँ॑ शाक्वररैवते सामनी प्रतिष्ठत्या अन्तरिक्ष ऋषयस्त्वा प्रथमजा देवेषु दिवो मात्रया वरिम्णा प्रथन्तु विधर्ता चायमधिपतिश्च ते त्वा सर्वे संविदाना नाकस्य पृष्ठे स्वर्गे लोके यजमानं च सादयन्तु ॥

14. O woman, thou art the lady paramount like the lofty region. All the shining bodies like the sun, are thy protectors. May thy husband, like the

---

¹³Twenty-one: The real significance of this number is not clear. In Tandya Brahman Granth it is written प्रतिष्ठेकविंश: । 16-3-4. According to this Brahman, Twentyone means greatness, superiority.

¹⁴The word त्रिनवत्रयस्त्रिंशौ meaning twenty-seven and thirty-three has not been understood. No commentator has thrown light on it. Tandya Brahman Granth describes twenty-seven to mean strength and thirty-three to mean rain, vide तां॰ 10-1-15, 16-10-10.

sun, the guardian of the world, and the sustainer of big planets, adore thee. For freedom from pain on this earth, through twenty-seven and thirty-three means of praise, let all the learned persons, knowing the sciences of fire and air, resort to two parts of the veda. For progress let them have knowledge of the two parts of the Sama Veda, with verses in Shakvari and Raivati metres!

Just as in the atmosphere, the first-born minute and bulky airs like Dhananjaya etc. residing in divine objects, make thee renowned, so should people make them known. This sun, the lord, and sustainer of all in diverse ways, and the learned persons with one mind establish thee and thy husband in a happy house on a comfortable part of the earth.

१५. अयं पुरो हरिकेश: सुर्यरश्मिस्तस्य रथगृत्सश्च रथौजाश्च सेनानीग्रामण्यौ ।
पुञ्जिकस्थला च ऋतुस्थला चाप्सरसौ
दङ्क्षणव: पशवो हेति: पौरुषेयो वध: प्रहेतिस्तेभ्यो नमो अस्तु ते नोऽवन्तु ते नो मृडयन्तु ते यं द्विष्मो यश्च नो द्वेष्टि तमेषां जम्भे दधम: ॥

15. In the East there are golden-tressed sunbeams. There are other beams also, which work like a wise driver and horses of a conveyance, and like the head of an army and a village chieftain.

Their chief direction and sub-direction, both are called Apsaras that move in the Pranas. Let injurious animals like lions and others that eat flesh and grass be destroyed. Let murderous crowds of men that destroy others like a powerful weapon, be killed. Let virtuous rulers protect us from those animals, and make us comfortable. In the jaws of these animals we place the ferocious man whom we hate and who hates us.

१६. अयं दक्षिणा विश्वकर्मा तस्य रथस्वनश्च रथेचित्रश्च सेनानीग्रामण्यौ ।
मेनका च सहजन्या चाप्सरसौ यातुधाना हेती रक्षाꣳसि प्रहेतिस्तेभ्यो नमो अस्तु ते नोऽवन्तु ते नो मृडयन्तु ते यं द्विष्मो यश्च नो द्वेष्टि तमेषां जम्भे दधम: ॥

16. O men, this vishvakarma breeze blows in the south. These two kinds of air, that give sound like the sound of a chariot, and are the doers of wonderous acts like a chariot, are like the head of an army and the chieftain of a village, which help meditation, and are born together, are called Apsaras which live in the atmosphere. Those who tease the people should be destroyed. Those who commit unrighteous deeds should be subdued through arms. Use weapons against those who torment mankind. Let just rulers protect us and make us comfortable. In the lion-like jaws of these airs we place the depraved man whom we hate and who hates us!

[15]Just as the driver and horses work in unison, and the military and civil powers work together, so do the different airs.
Apsaras: Two airs that course through our veins.
Their: sunbeams.
[16]Apsaras: Two kinds of air which blow in the atmosphere.
Vishvakarma: Air with which all actions are performed.

१७. अयं पश्चाद्विश्वव्यचास्तस्य रथप्रोतश्चासमरथश्च सेनानीग्रामण्यौ ।
प्रम्लोचन्ती चानुम्लोचन्ती चाप्सरसौ
व्याघ्रा हेति: सर्पा: प्रहेतिस्तेभ्यो नमो अस्तु ते नोऽवन्तु ते नो मृडयन्तु ते यं द्विष्मो यश्च नो द्वेष्टि तमेषां जम्भे दध्म: ॥

17. O men, there is all pervading lightning in the West. Like the head of the army and the village chieftain, are its Rathprota, and Asamaratha. Both these Apsaras, active beams in the atmosphere, dry all the medicinal plants, and shed lustre.

Those who like tigers and serpents torture mankind, should be subdued through arms. Let the rulers protect us from these animals and make us comfortable. In the jaws of these animals we place the degraded man whom we hate and who hates us.

१८. अयमुत्तरात्संयद्वसुस्तस्य तार्क्ष्यश्चारिष्टनेमिश्च सेनानीग्रामण्यौ ।
विश्वाची च घृताची चाप्सरसावापो हेतिर्वात: प्रहेतिस्तेभ्यो नमो अस्तु ते नोऽवन्तु ते नो मृडयन्तु ते यं द्विष्मो यश्च नो द्वेष्टि तमेषां जम्भे दध्म: ॥

18. In the North, the autumn is associated with the yajna. Its Aswin and Kartik are like the head of the army and the village chieftain. The fire that pervades the universe and the fire that receives ghee (butter) are its Apsaras, i.e., the motion of the Pranas. In this season water is in abundance, and air highly pleasant. Those who enjoy this air properly deserve honour. May they protect us and make us comfortable. In the jaws of destructive power of water and air, we place the man whom we hate and who hates us.

१६. अयमुपर्यर्वाग्वसुस्तस्य सेनजिच्च सुषेणश्च सेनानीग्रामण्यौ ।
उर्वशी च पूर्वचित्तिश्चाप्सरसाववस्फूर्जन् हेतिर्विद्युत्प्रहेतिस्तेभ्यो नमो अस्तु ते नोऽवन्तु ते नो मृडयन्तु ते यं द्विष्मो यश्च नो द्वेष्टि तमेषां जम्भे दध्म: ॥

19. This one direction above, is the source of wealth after rains. Its army conqueror and well-armed lords are both Margshirsh and Paush months of winter, like the head of an army and the village chieftain. The internal fire that is the cause of eating much, and intellect the recipient of eternal knowledge are two forces that reside in the Pranas. Thundering is its weapon and lightning its missile weapon. We offer food to persons who are our guardians like them. May they protect us and make us comfortable. We place in the jaws of thunder and lightning the man whom we hate and who hates us!

---

[17] Rathaprota: Beautiful, lustrous air.
Asamaratha: Peerless air.
Both the haters deserve punishment.
According to Jaidev Vidyalankar, Rathaprota and Asamaratha are two military Commanders. Rathaprota is he who fights always sitting in the chariot. Asamaratha is he whose chariot is unparalleled.
[19] Hate means dislike. Hate in the sense of enmity, with a view to do harm or injury is prohibited by the vedas, which preach love for all. Both the haters deserve punishment.

२०. अग्निर्मूर्धा दिव: ककुत्पति: पृथिव्या अयम् ।
अपाँ रेताँसि जिन्वति ॥

20. This Agni, resides between the Earth and Heaven, like head in the shape of the Sun. Being the protector of all directions, it satisfies the forces of our breaths.

२१. अयमग्नि: सहस्त्रिणो वाजस्य शतिनस्पति: ।
मूर्धा कवी रयीणाम् ॥

21. This fire in winter, present in thousands of nice objects, and possessing hundreds of characteristics, is the lord of foodgrains and riches, and beautiful like the head.

२२. त्वामग्ने पुष्करादध्यथर्वा निरमन्थत ।
मूर्ध्नो विश्वस्य वाघत: ॥

22. O learned person, I instruct thee that a harmless, wise scholar, dispels ignorance with instructive speech, creates fire from the atmosphere, by churning, and is mighty like the head!

२३. भुवो यज्ञस्य रजसश्च नेता यत्रा नियुद्भि: सचसे शिवाभि: ।
दिवि मूर्धानं दधिषे स्वर्षां जिह्वामग्ने चकृषे हव्यवाहम् ॥

23. O learned person, this visible fire, with its properties of alliance and division, full of blissful flames, helps in the performance of yajna, and worldly deeds. It imbibes in its lustrous nature the lofty sun!
It stimulates the pleasant speech, worthy of acceptance and giver of enjoyments.
Like fire, the learned person, full of noble qualities should preach all sciences.

२४. प्रबोध्यग्नि: समिधा जनानां प्रति धेनुमिवायतीमुषासम् ।
यह्वा इव प्र वयामुज्जिहाना: प्र भानव: सिस्त्रते नाकमच्छ ।

24. With fuel the fire is kindled. Just as calf is pleased seeing the cow coming, so are people delighted by seeing the Dawn. Just as highly religious people fairly well resort to permanent devices of happiness, so do the rays wholly attain to heaven.

२५. अवोचाम कवये मेध्याय वचो वन्दारु वृषभाय वृष्णे ।
गविष्ठिरो नमसा स्तोममग्नौ दिवीव रुक्ममुरुव्यञ्चमश्रेत् ॥

25. Let us use respectful language for a person, who is pure, intelligent, wise, strong, and virtuous. Let him who expounds the vedic lore, humbly divulge the praises of the Effulgent God, as the sun seated in its rays, sheds in heaven the lustre that spreads to various places.

²¹I: Acharya.
²²see Yajur 13-15.

२६. अयमिह प्रथमो धायि धातृभिर्होता यजिष्ठो अध्वरेष्वीड्यः ।
यमप्नवानो भृगवो विरुरुचुर्वनेषु चित्रं विभ्वं विशे-विशे ॥

26. In this world, this visible fire, serviceable in works of protection, worthy of investigation, the paramount accomplisher of sacrifice (yajna), the recipient of ghee, and ubiquitous, is acknowledged by the learned. The beautiful persons, adequately advanced in knowledge expound for all people this fire pervading the beams wondrously.

२७. जनस्य गोपा अजनिष्ट जागृविरग्निः सुदक्षः सुविताय नव्यसे ।
घृतप्रतीको बृहता दिविस्पृशा द्युमद्वि भाति भरतेभ्यः शुचिः ॥

27. Fire, the guardian of the created world, ever active, full of strength, developing with ghee and pure, is born for fresh prosperity. Illumined by the suns, it glitters with the intense touch of light.

२८. त्वामग्ने अङ्गिरसो गुहा हितमन्वविन्दञ्छिश्रियाणं वने-वने ।
स जायसे मथ्यमानः सहो महत्त्वामाहुः सहसस्पुत्रमङ्गिरः ॥

28. O learned person, dear like life, thou shinest with knowledge, like fire with attrition!
Fire, highly serviceable, residing in the inmost recesses of our heart, present in all rays and objects, is called the son of highly strong and powerful air. The learned master it. I preach unto thee its significance.

२९. सखायः सं वः सम्यञ्चमिषं स्तोमं चाग्नये ।
वर्षिष्ठाय क्षितीनामूर्जो नप्त्रे सहस्वते ॥

29. O men, just as the learned, your associates, offer seemly oblations and praises to fire, supreme, and highly powerful, behaving as your grandson, so should you proceed with it!

३०. सं समिद्युवसे वृषन्नग्ने विश्वान्यर्य आ ।
इडस्पदे समिध्यसे स नो वसून्या भर ॥

30. O mighty, enlightened vaishya, having adequate trade relations with others, and worthy of adoration, thou lookest graceful, seated in a desirable position of vantage; bring us all riches!

३१. त्वां चित्रश्रवस्तम हवन्ते विक्षु जन्तवः ।
शोचिष्केशं पुरुप्रियाग्ने हव्याय वोढवे ॥

[27]Suns: There are various suns in the solar system. The one we see is for the planet Earth, but there are other planets also.
[29]Grandson: Just as a grandson is helpful and serviceable to the parents, so is fire useful and serviceable to the learned.
[30]Vaishya: A trader, businessman, merchant, representing the third division of men, the first two being Brahmana and Kshatriya.

31. O noble learned person, loved of many people invoke thee, powerful like the scorching rays of the sun acquiring necessary nice foodstuffs for the subjects!

३२. एना वो अग्निं नमसोर्जो नपातमा हुवे ।
प्रियं चेतिष्ठमरतिᳪ स्वध्वरं विश्वस्य दूतममृतम् ।

32. O men, just as I acknowledge for ye, through desirable foodgrains, Agni, steadfast in nature, lovely, giver of life, devoid of consciousness, united with harmless usages, eternal in nature, world's messenger, and your enterprises, so should ye do for me!

३३. विश्वस्य दूतममृतं विश्वस्य दूतममृतम् ।
स योजते अरुषा विश्वभोजसा स दुद्रवत्स्वाहुत: ॥

33. I acknowledge the immortal sun, the warmer of the universe. I acknowledge the immortal fire present in water, the scorcher of all objects of the world.

The protector of the universe, this beautiful fire is present in all things. It acts as a uniting force. Well-comprehended, it courses through the body. The learned should realise it.

३४. स दुद्रवत्स्वाहुत: स दुद्रवत्स्वाहुत: ।
सुब्रह्मा यज्ञ: सुशमी वसूनां देवᳪ राधो जनानाम् ॥

34. Agni moves like an invited friend. It goes like an invited scholar. Use properly the fire, that is the desired treasure of persons and material objects, like the master of the four vedas, companionable and calm in nature.

३५. अग्ने वाजस्य गोमत ईशान: सहसो यहो ।
अस्मे धेहि जातवेदो महि श्रव: ॥

35. O son of a strong man, possessing knowledge of the objects created, dignified and well-read, thou like fire, with land and laudable cow, art the master of foodgrains. Vouchsafe great wealth unto us!

३६. स इधानो वसुष्कविरग्निरीडेन्यो गिरा ।
रेवदस्मभ्यं पुर्वणीक दीदिहि ॥

---

[32] World's messenger: Agni moves in the whole world, and puts life in it.
Foodgrains: Agni through yajna brings rain, which produces foodgrain. Agni is thus the source of ripening the harvest.
Eternal in nature: It is eternal in its cause the Matter, not in itself.
Agni: Fire, Electricity.
I: Acharya.
[33] There are two kinds of fire: the rough and the subtle.
The repetition of the words in the first line of the verse denotes the double nature of fire.
[34] Just as a scholar of the vedas, who is calm and affable is liked by all, so fire is liked by all persons. Just as an invited friend and an invited learned person go hastily so does fire move quickly.

36. O ruler equipped with a good army, worthy of praise with words, provider of dwelling to his subjects, affluent, brilliant, and resembling fire, grant us laudable riches!

३७. क्षपो राजन्नुत तमनाऽग्ने वस्तोरुतोषस: ।
स तिग्मजम्भ रक्षसो दह प्रति ॥

37. O resplendent learned person, with powerful limbs, just as the sharp fire creates the night, day, morning and evening, so shouldst thou spread good instruction. Like fire burn the wicked with the force of thy soul!

३८. भद्रो नो अग्निराहुतो भद्रा राति: सुभग भद्रो अध्वर: ।
भद्रा उत प्रशस्तय: ॥

38. O man of power and supremacy, just as lovely Agni through oblations brings us bliss, just as gift brings bliss, just as harmless dealing brings bliss, just as our praises bring us bliss, so shouldst thou be blissful unto us!

३९. भद्रा उत प्रशस्तयो भद्रं मन: कृणुष्व वृत्रतूर्ये ।
येना समत्सु सासह: ॥

39. O man of power and supremacy behave in a manner, wherewith we may get in battles, optimistic mind, praiseworthy followers, and calm, determined soldiers!

४०. येना समत्सु सासहोऽव स्थिरा तनुहि भूरि शर्धताम् ।
वनेमा ते अभिष्टिभि: ॥

40. O man of power and supremacy, with thy strength, grant us daring courage in battles, add to the resources of our resolute army, exerting to its utmost for victory. Acting in obedience to thy desires, let us utilise the resources of the army!

४१. अग्निं तं मन्ये यो वसुरस्तं यं यन्ति धेनव: ।
अस्तमर्वन्त आशवोऽस्तं नित्यासो वाजिन इषं स्तोतृभ्य आ भर ॥

41. O learned person, I value the omnipresent fire, led by which the king go to their home. The fleet-foot, steady and active steeds seek the indestructible fire, as their home. I bring food to the learned who sing thy glory. So shouldst thou realise that fire!

४२. सो अग्निर्यो वसुगृर्णे सं यमायन्ति धेनव: ।
समर्वन्तो रघुद्रुव: संसुजातास: सूरय इषं स्तोतृभ्य आ भर ॥

42. O learned person, I laud fire, that provides shelter; whom the speeches attain to. Just as the praiseworthy scholars walk slowly, and the learned, famous for their knowledge, thoroughly imbibe learning for the pupils who

---

38-40Man of power may mean the head of the army.
41In the evening, in the light of the sun the kine go home.

sing their praise, and just as the teacher explains the merits of God and other objects, so shouldst thou acquire the knowledge of all these things.

४३. उभे सुश्चन्द्र सर्पिषो दर्वी श्रीणीष आसनि ।
उतो न उत्पुपूर्या उक्थेषु शवसस्पत इषँ स्तोतृभ्य आ भर ॥

44. O beautiful, pleasurable teacher, just as two ladles of ghee cook food, so fill in the mouth both the practices of reading and teaching. O lord of strength, teach us the vedic lore, and give food to us and the learned!

४४. अग्ने तमद्याश्वं न स्तोमैः क्रतुं न भद्रँ हृदिस्पृशम् ।
ऋध्यामा त ओहैः ॥

44. O teacher, we derive today from thee like a disciplined horse, the pleasant knowledge of the vedas. May we always make progress, having received the knowledge which touches our soul, and is blissful like intellect!

४५. अधा ह्यग्ने क्रतोर्भद्रस्य दक्षस्य साधोः ।
रथीर्ऋतस्य बृहतो बभूथ ॥

45. O learned person, just as thou art in the possession of conveyances for journey, having the intellectual wisdom of a truthful person, following the noble path of virtue, filled with pleasurable, physical and spiritual strength, so shouldst we blissfully and certainly be!

४६. एभिर्नो अर्कैर्भवा नो अर्वाङ् स्वर्ण ज्योतिः ।
अग्ने विश्वेभिः सुमना अनीकैः ॥

46. O learned person, be thou well-disposed towards us, like a king with his armies. With these worshipful learned persons be thou for us the expositor of knowledge; and the uplifter of the down-trodden, granting us pleasure!

४७. अग्निँ होतारं मन्ये दास्वन्तं वसुँ सूनुँ सहसो जातवेदसं विप्रं न जातवेदसम् ।
य ऊर्ध्वया स्वध्वरो देवो देवाच्या कृपा ।
घृतस्य विभ्राष्टिमनु वष्टि शोचिषाऽऽजुह्वानस्य सर्पिषः ॥

47. He, who with his superior knowledge, deserves harmlessness, is fit to be honoured by the learned, is powerful in deeds, is imbued with noble qualities, and displays diverse kinds of lustre, with extreme loveliness, by performing Havan, using ghee and water, him do I honour. He is the giver of happiness, the knower of all created objects, charitably disposed like the son of a great man, giver of gifts, foremost amongst the wise, and a trustworthy, highly learned person, brilliant like fire.

[43]The word उभय in the text may also mean knowledge and action.
[44]Just as a well fed disciplined horse takes us fast to our destination, so a student properly looked after and well taught soon becomes learned.
[46]These: mentioned in the previous verses.
[47]A leader should possess these qualities.

CHAPTER XV

४८. अग्ने त्वं नो अन्तम उत त्राता शिवो भवा वरूथ्यः।
वसुरग्निर्वसुश्रवा अच्छा नक्षि द्युमत्तमꣳ रयिं दाः।
तं त्वा शोचिष्ठ दीदिवः सुम्नाय नूनमीमहे सखिभ्यः॥

48. O learned person, be thou nearest friend, our protector, most prosperous, and blissful unto us, like fire that gives us riches, food-grains, and wealth. O learned person, actuated by noble aspirations, just as we pray unto thee with our friends for happiness, so may all pray. Just as I goodly meet thee full of desirable intentions, so shouldst thou meet us!

४९. येन ऋषयस्तपसा सत्रमायन्निन्धाना अग्निꣳ स्वराभरन्तः।
तस्मिन्नहं नि दधे नाके अग्निं यमाहुर्मनव स्तीर्णबर्हिषम्॥

49. With whatever penance, the sages, well-read in vedic lore, securing illuminating pleasure, and full of true knowledge, explore fire; with similar devotion, for the acquisition of happiness, do I grasp the fire, described by the thoughtful learned persons as pervader of the atmosphere.

५०. तं पत्नीभिरनु गच्छेम देवाः पुत्रैर्भ्रातृभिरुत वा हिरण्यैः।
नाकं गृभ्णानाः सुकृतस्य लोके तृतीये पृष्ठे अधि रोचने दिवः॥

50. O learned persons, just as ye, mastering that fire, engaged in the performance of virtuous vedic deeds, residing in a beautiful, knowable, pleasant place, built scientifically, attain to happiness with your wives, sons, brothers, other relatives, and with gold, so may we also be happy in all these respects!

५१. आ वाचो मध्यमरुह्द्रुꣳ रण्वुरयमग्निः सत्पतिश्चेकितानः।
पृष्ठे पृथिव्या निहितो दविद्युतदधस्पदं कृणुतां ये पृतन्यवः॥

51. O learned person, full of knowledge, protector of the virtuous, having understood the essence of vedic speech, cast under foot those who would fight against him, who is well read, firmly established on the earth, benefits all with his advice, and sticks to religion!

५२. अयमग्निर्वीरतमो वयोधाः सहस्रियो द्योततामप्रयुच्छन्।
विभ्राजमानः सरिरस्य मध्य उप प्र याहि दिव्यानि धाम॥

52. May this commander of the army, most manly, supporter of the lives of all, powerful like thousand soldiers, shining with knowledge and justice like sun in the midst of heaven, free from carelessness, shine, and attain to nice birth, deeds and position.

५३. सम्प्रच्यवध्वमुप सम्प्रयाताग्ने पथो देवयानान् कृणुध्वम्।
पुनः कृण्वाना पितरा युवानाऽन्वाताꣳसीत् त्वयि तन्तुमेतम्॥

---

[48] see Yajur 3-25, 26. Interpretation given there is different from that given here.
Fire: Electricity.

53. O people, learn well all sciences, follow the path of the virtuous, be religious-minded. O learned grandfather, in thy lifetime, let thy sons, leading a life of Brahmcharya, in the bloom of their youth, marry according to their own selection, and produce afterwards children, according to the rules of eugenics!

५४. उद् बुध्यस्वाग्ने प्रति जागृहि त्वमिष्टापूर्तेे सꣳसृजेथामयं च ।
अस्मिन् सधस्थे अध्युत्तरस्मिन् विश्वे देवा यजमानश्च सीदत ॥

54. O highly learned man or woman acquire knowledge thoroughly, avoid ignorance, and be full of learning. Thou wife and this husband both, in this present place and in future, should acquire desired happiness, honour the learned, pray to God, keep good company, give true knowledge as a free gift, possess full strength, cultivate Brahmcharya, acquire the glory of knowledge, attain to puberty, and try for the attainment of final beatitude through helpful means!

Let all the learned and the sacrificers be seated in this place.

५५. येन वहसि सहस्रं येनाग्ने सर्ववेदसम् ।
तेनेमं यज्ञं नो नय स्वर्देवेषु गन्तवे ॥

55. O learned man or woman, just as thou, for the happiness of the wise, with a resolute vow, solvest the thousand problems of domestic life, and with knowledge observest the injunction of the vedas, so help us in discharging our domestic duties!

५६. अयं ते योनिऋ्त्विियो यतो जातो अरोचथा ।
तं जानन्नग्न आ रोहाथा नो वर्धया रयिम् ॥

56. O learned man or woman, this is thy house comfortable in all seasons. Stick fast to religion keeping in mind the education received, whereby thou hast attained to name and fame. Cause then our riches to increase!

५७. तपश्च तपस्यश्च शैशिरावृतू अग्नेरन्तः श्लेषोऽसि कल्पेतां द्यावापृथिवी कल्पन्तामाप ओषधयः कल्पन्तामग्नयः पृथङ्मम ज्यैष्ठ्याय सव्रताः ।
ये अग्नयः समनसोऽन्तरा द्यावापृथिवी इमे । शैशिरावृतू अभिकल्पमाना इन्द्रमिव देवा अभिसंविशन्तु तया देवतयाङ्गिरस्वद्ध्रुवे सीदतम् ॥

57. O God, for my prosperity, the Magh (January-February) and Phagan (February-March) these two months constituting the dewy-winter, add to my pleasure. Thou pervadest them and fire! In those months let sky and earth, and water be pleasure-giving. Let medicinal plants grow in them. Let lightning-fires, following the same laws, be separately useful to us. These lightning-

---

⁵³Rules of conception are given in the *Sanskar Vidhi* by Swami Dayananda, while dealing with Garbhadhan Sanskar.

⁵⁴In this present place: domestic life, Grihastha Ashrama.
In this place: In Yajnashala for performing the yajna.
Puberty: full youth.

fires residing in between the Sky and Earth, unanimously the cause of Dewy-winter, create the Magh and Phagan months. The learned should use these mighty fires. Just as the Sky and Earth, through the dispensation of God work together like breath, so should you wife and husband live constantly together.

५८. परमेष्ठी त्वा सादयतु दिवस्पृष्ठे ज्योतिष्मतीम् ।
विश्वस्मै प्राणायापानाय व्यानाय विश्वं ज्योतिर्यच्छ ।
सूर्यस्तेऽधिपतिस्तया देवतयाऽङ्गिरस्वद् ध्रुवा सीद ॥

58. O woman, may God seat thee, full of admirable knowledge, on the back of learning, for strengthening the Pran, Apan and Vyan breaths of all thy family members. Diffuse the full light of knowledge to all women!
Remain tenaciously firm like the sun, with thy husband, endowed with noble traits, and lustrous like the sun.

५९. लोकं पृण छिद्रं पृणाथो सीद ध्रुवा त्वम् ।
इन्द्राग्नी त्वा बृहस्पतिरस्मिन्योनावसीषदन् ॥

59. O woman, make this life and the next comfortable. Remove thy weaknesses; and stay at home with firmness of purpose. May the glorious, learned teachers establish thee in this domestic life!

६०. ता अस्य सूददोहसः सोमᳪ श्रीणन्ति पृश्नयः ।
जन्मन्देवानां विशस्त्रिष्वा रोचने दिवः ॥

60. The subjects endowed with knowledge and good training, enquiring about the birth of the learned, equipped with cooks and servants expert in the performance of their duties, devoted to vedic action, worship, and knowledge, living in the presence of the Effulgent God, provide everywhere, for their ruler edible foods mixed with the juices of medicinal herbs.

६१. इन्द्रं विश्वा अवीवृधन्त्समुद्रव्यचसं गिरः ।
रथीतमᳪ रथीनां वाजानाᳪ सत्पतिं पतिम् ॥

61. May all sacred songs coupled with knowledge and learning, magnify the king, full of wealth, protector of the doings of the learned, and master of the people, most valiant among the valorous, extensive in fame like the sky.

६२. प्रोथदश्वो न यवसेऽविष्यन्यदा महः संवरणाद्व्यचस्थात् ।
आदस्य वातो अनुवाति शोचिरध स्म ते व्रजनं कृष्णमस्ति ।

62. O King, just as thou makest the horse strong with fodder, so shouldst thou make thy subjects strong, so that they may be well established, shielded and protected by thee. When thou marchest forth with thy attractive splendour; thy followers march in thy wake!

---

59 60.61see Yajur 12-54-55-56 with different meanings.

६३. आयोष्ट्वा सदने सादयाम्यवतश्छायाया ँ समुद्रस्य हृदये ।
रश्मीवतीं भास्वतीमा या द्यां भास्यापृथिवीमोर्वन्तरिक्षम् ॥

63. O woman, thou illuminest the Sky, the Earth, and airs broad realm between them. Thou art full of grace, and the light of pure knowledge, I set thee in the house of thy husband, who will live long, I place thee under his care, thy protector. I set thee in heart, deep like the ocean.

६४. परमेष्ठी त्वा सादयतु दिवस्पृष्ठे व्यचस्वतीं प्रथस्वतीं दिवं यच्छ दिवं दृ ँ ह दिवं मा हि ँ सी: ।
विश्वस्मै प्राणायापानाय व्यानायोदानाय प्रतिष्ठायै चरित्राय ।
सूर्यस्त्वाभि पातु महया स्वस्त्या छर्दिषा शन्तमेन तया देवतयाङ्गिरस्वद् ध्रुवे सीदतम् ॥

64. O woman, God places thee, worthy of praise and well-read, in charge of the house, for the full enjoyment of life, for the eradication of misery, for the acquisition of knowledge, for amassing strength, for eliciting universal respect, and for the improvement of character!

Spread thou the light of justice, strengthen the lustre of learning. Violate not the truths of religion.

God guards thee on all sides, bestowing due respect and extreme delight; and distinguishing truth from untruth.

May thou and thy husband live constantly together, holding God dear as life.

६५. सहस्रस्य प्रमासि सहस्रस्य प्रतिमासि सहस्रस्योन्मासि साहस्रोऽसि सहस्राय त्वा ॥

65. O learned man or woman, thou knowest the world full of countless objects; thou measurest the intrinsic worth of countless precious objects, thou servest as balance for judging the nature of countless material objects. Thou art the master of innumerable sciences. God sets thee in life for numberless achievements!

**See Yajur 14-12, 14-14, 15-58 with different meanings.

CHAPTER XVI

१. नमस्ते रुद्र मन्यव उतो त इषवे नम. ।
बाहुभ्यामुत ते नमः ॥

1. O King, the chastiser of the wicked, may thy indignant soldiers get arms. May thou, the destroyer of foes, get food. May the enemies be attacked with weapons by thy arms!

२. या ते रुद्र शिवा तनूरघोराऽपापकाशिनी ।
तया नस्तन्वा शन्तमया गिरिशन्ताभि चाकशीहि ॥

2. O learned person, the comforter of people with thy noble teachings, the administrator of fear for the miscreants and happiness for the good, educate us again and again, with thy system of teaching, which is highly delightful, conducive to progress, expository of true principles, and free from violence!

३. यामिषुं गिरिशन्त हस्ते विभर्ष्यस्तवे ।
शिवां गिरित्र तां कुरु मा हिꣳसीः पुरुषं जगत् ॥

3. O commander of the army, the giver of comforts like a cloud, whatever shaft thou takest in hand to shoot, make that auspicious. O protector of the preachers of knowledge, destroy not this world full of enterprising men!

४. शिवेन वचसा त्वा गिरिशाच्छा वदामसि ।
यथा नः सर्वमिज्जगदयक्ष्मꣳ सुमना असत् ।

4. O physician, dweller on the mountains, and analyser of waters, we praise thee with propitious speech. Full of happiness, let all our living beings be free from tuberculosis and well satisfied!

५. अध्यवोचदधिवक्ता प्रथमो दैव्यो भिषक् ।
अहीꣳश्च सर्वाञ्जम्भयन्त्सर्वाश्च यातुधान्योऽधराची: परा सुव ॥

5. O physician, the dispeller of ailments, chief amongst the learned, the teacher of the first class science of medicine, the remover of diseases by diagnosing them, the sure banisher of diseases deadly like serpents, with efficacious medicines, preach unto us the laws of health, cast away all drugs that aggravate the disease, and lower our vitality!

६. असौ यस्ताम्रो अरुण उत बभ्रुः सुमङ्गलः ।
ये चैनꣳ रुद्रा अभितो दिक्षु श्रिताः सहस्रशोऽवैषाꣳ हेड ईमहे ॥

---

[1] A physician has often to visit mountains in search after medicinal herbs, hence he is spoken of as a dweller on the mountains. He has to test and analyse waters, and find out their efficacy. The word गिरिश may also mean God, whose characteristics are mentioned in the vedas, or whose true nature can be known from the vedas or figuratively, who dwells in the vedas.

6. O people, your king is most auspicious, with limbs strong like copper, brilliant like fire, slightly red and brown. Thousands of brave soldiers remain under his shelter in all directions. With these soldiers at our back, we never entertain any evil designs!

७. असौ योऽवसर्पति नीलग्रीवो विलोहित: ।
उतैनं गोपा अदृश्रन्नदृश्रन्नुदहार्य: स दृष्टो मृडयाति न: ॥

7. The commander of the army, with a necklace of precious gems round the neck full of good qualities, actions and disposition, goes against the vicious. The faithful servants and the girls who carry water behold him May he when seen be kind to us.

८. नमोऽस्तु नीलग्रीवाय सहस्राक्षाय मीढुषे ।
अथो ये अस्य सत्वानोऽहं तेभ्योऽकरं नम: ॥

8. The commander-in-chief, with a clear throat and voice, who watches the actions of thousands of soldiers, and is full of valour, receives food from me. I offer food to the well-behaved and brave soldiers as well, who work under him.

९. प्रमुञ्च धन्वनस्त्वमुभयोरात्न्योर्ज्याम् ।
याश्च ते हस्त इषव: परा ता भगवो वप ॥

9. O powerful commander of the army, loosen both the extremities of the bow, put the arrows in thy hand, in the bowstring, throw them on the enemy, and ward off the arrows the enemy throws on thee!

१०. विज्यं धनु: कपर्दिनो विशल्यो बाणवाँ२ उत ।
अनेशन्नस्य या इषव आभुरस्य निषङ्गधि: ॥

10. O masters of the science of archery, let not the bow of this commander with coiled and braided hair, be ever unstrung, let him never be devoid of arrows, and warlike instruments, let not the treasure of arrows and weapons of this commander who always keeps himself well-armed, be ever empty. May he possess many arrows. Equip him anew with arrows whenever they are destroyed!

११. या ते हेतिर्मीढुष्टम हस्ते वभूव ते धनु: ।
तयाऽस्मान्विश्वतस्त्वमयक्ष्मया परि भुज ॥

11. O virile commander, protect us well on all sides with thy army, the remover of the pain of defeat, with thy weapon, and the bow in thy hand!

१२. परि ते धन्वनो हेतिरस्मान्वृणक्तु विश्वत: ।
अथो य इषुधिस्तवारे अस्मन्नि धेहि तम् ॥

---

⁸¹I and me: The minister in charge of food.

12. O commander of the army, protect us in all directions from the attack of thy bow. Lay thou the quiver that thou hast in place away from us!

१३. अवतत्य धनुष्ट्वं सहस्राक्ष शतेषुधे ।
निशीर्य शल्यानां मुखा शिवो नः सुमना भव ॥

13. O commander of the army, the seer of countless scenes on the battle-field filled with the lustre for innumerable weapons and missiles, extend thy bow; sharpen the front edges of thy arms, kill thy foes, and be kind and gracious unto us!

१४. नमस्त आयुधायानाततताय धृष्णवे ।
उभाभ्यामुत ते नमो बाहुभ्यां तव धन्वने ॥

14. O King, skilled in fighting, keeper of thy designs in secret, full of eloquence, may thou get foodstuff. I offer food for thee to eat. I offer food to thy warriors acting as thy arms with their strength and valour!

१५. मा नो महान्तमुत मा नो अर्भकं मा न उक्षन्तमुत मा न उक्षितम् ।
मा नो बधीः पितरं मोत मातरं मा नः प्रियास्तन्वो रुद्र रीरिषः ॥

15. O commander of the army, kill not our revered elders, nor our children. Harm not our full grown youths, harm not our progeny in embryo. Slay not our rearing father, slay not our loving mother. Harm not the dear bodies of our women!

१६. मा नस्तोके तनये मा न आयुषि मा नो गोषु मा नो अश्वेषु रीरिषः ।
मा नो वीरान् रुद्र भामिनो वधीर्हविष्मन्तः सदमित् त्वा हवामहे ॥

16. O commander of the army, harm not our newly born child, nor him over five years in age. Make no attack on our life, our cows, sheep and goats and harm not our horses, elephants and camels. Kill not our heroes full of wrath. We with oblations ever call on thee, firm in justice!

१७. नमो हिरण्यबाहवे सेनान्ये दिशां च पतये नमो नमो वृक्षेभ्यो हरिकेशेभ्यः पशूनां पतये नमो नमः
शष्पिञ्जराय त्विषीमते पथीनां पतये नमो नमो हरिकेशायोपवीतिने पुष्टानां पतये नमः ॥

17. O commander of the army, may thou with strong sparkling arms, and leader of hosts, get arms. May thou lord of the regions get food. Take thou in hand the axe to cut the mango trees exposed to the rays of the sun. Homage to thee, the protector of cattle like cows. Homage to thee, free from the bondage of passions, full of the light of justice. Homage to thee, the guardian of the way-farers. Food to thee, the golden-haired wearer of the yajnopavit (sacrificial cord). Homage to thee the protector of the healthy!

---

[14] I means the spokesman of the subjects.

१८. नमो बभ्लुशाय व्याधिने ऽन्नानां पतये नमो नमो भवस्य हेत्यै जगतां पतये नमो नमो रुद्रायाततायिने क्षेत्राणां पतये नमो नमः सूतायाहन्त्यै वनानां पतये नमः ॥

18. Let the state-officials give food to the patient who lives in their midst. Let them pay homage to the growers of corn. Let them grant grain for the progress of the world. Let them offer homage to the lord of human beings. Let them give food to the tormentor of the foes, and the fighter from all directions against vast armed foes. Let them give food to the brave warrior, and the queen who injures none. Let them give food to the Lord of forest.

१६. नमो रोहिताय स्थपतये वृक्षाणां पतये नमो नमो भुवन्तये वारिवस्कृतायौषधीनां पतये नमो नमो मन्त्रिणे वाणिजाय कक्षाणां पतये नमो नम उच्चैर्घोषायाक्रन्दयते पत्तीनां पतये नमः ॥

19. Let the officials and the people give food to the commander of the army, the enhancer of delights. Let them give food to the lord of trees. Let them give food to servants of good character. Let them give food to the physician, the guardian of medicinal herbs. Let them pay homage to the thoughtful minister, and the expert in trade. Let them give food to the protector of the householders. Homage to the shouting lord of justice who makes the wicked weep. Homage to the guardian of different parts of the army.

२०. नमः कृत्स्नायतया धावते सत्वनां पतये नमो नमः सहमानाय निव्याधिन आव्याधिनीनां पतये नमो नमो निषङ्गिणे ककुभाय स्तेनानां पतये नमो नमो निचेरवे परिचरायारण्यानां पतये नमः ॥

20. Food for the person who is active for obtaining full conquest. Homage to the protector of the substances secured. Food for the powerful and chastiser of the foes. Homage to the general who subdues the armies of the enemies with his own army. Food for the master of arrow, sword, gun and cannon. Homage to the self-contented, enterprising person who serves religion, knowledge, mother, master and friends. Arms for him who keeps the thieves under control. Food for the forest-guard.

२१. नमो वञ्चते परिवञ्चते स्तायूनां पतये नमो नमो निषङ्गिण इषुधिमते तस्कराणां पतये नमो नमः सृकायिभ्यो जिघांसद्भ्यो मुष्णतां पतये नमो नमोऽसिमद्भ्यो नक्तंचरद्भ्यो विकृन्तानां पतये नमः ॥

21. Thunderbolt to the cheat, to the arch-deceiver; and the lord of stealers. Food to the sword-bearer for the protection of the State. Thunderbolt to the lord of robbers; to the bolt-armed homicides. Homage to the chastiser of the pilferers. Thunderbolt to the roamers at night with arms. Homage to the killer of pickpockets.

---

[18] सूत means the brave son of a Kshatriya from a Brahman woman. Griffith translates भव as Bhava, whereas Rishi Dayananda translates it as the world.

२२. नम उष्णीषिणे गिरिचराय कुलुञ्चानां पतये नमो नम इषुमद्भ्यो धन्वायिभ्यश्च वो नमो नम आतन्वानेभ्य: प्रतिदधानेभ्यश्च वो नमो नम आयच्छद्भ्यो ऽस्यद्भ्यश्च वो नम: ॥

22. Homage to the turban-wearing villager, the haunter of mountains, the suppressor of the evil-minded dacoits. Food to you who bear arrows and to you who carry bows. Homage to you who add to our happiness, and take up arms against foes. Food to you who dissuade the wicked from evil deeds, and homage to you who use arms against them.

२३. नमो विसृजद्भ्यो विध्यद्भ्यश्च वो नमो नम: स्वपद्भ्यो जाग्रद्भ्यश्च वो नमो नम: शयानेभ्य आसीनेभ्यश्च वो नमो नमस्तिष्ठद्भ्यो धावद्भ्यश्च वो नम: ॥ १

23. Food to you who use arms against the enemies, and you who kill them. Punishment to you who sleep on the battle-field, and food to you who keep awake. Food to you who lie, and to you who sit. Food to you who stand and to you who run.

२४. नम: सभाभ्य: सभापतिभ्यश्च वो नमो नमोऽश्वेभ्यो ऽश्वपतिभ्यश्च वो नमो नम आव्याधिनीभ्यो विविध्यन्तीभ्यश्च वो नमो नम उगणाभ्यस्तृंहतीभ्यश्च वो नम: ॥

24. Homage to you ladies endowed with the display of justice, and to you Kings, lords of Assemblies. Food to horses and to you masters of horses. Food to our armies that kill the armies of the foes. Homage to you ladies, who kill the heroes of the enemies. Homage to you ladies, masters of the science of logic, and the ladies who kill foes in the battle.

२५. नमो गणेभ्यो गणपतिभ्यश्च वो नमो नमो व्रातेभ्यो व्रातपतिभ्यश्च वो नमो नमो गृत्सेभ्यो गृत्सपतिभ्यश्च वो नमो नमो विरूपेभ्यो विश्वरूपेभ्यश्च वो नम: ।:

25. Food to the servants, and to you their masters. Homage to the people and to you their guardians. Homage to the learned who expatiate on the qualities of objects, and to you the protectors of the wise. Homage to those who assume various garbs, and to you who wear all forms.

३६. नम: सेनाभ्य: सेनानिभ्यश्च वो नमो नमो रथिभ्यो ऽरथेभ्यश्च वो नमो नम: क्षतृभ्य: संग्रहीतृभ्यश्च वो नमो नमो महद्भ्यो ऽर्भकेभ्यश्च वो नम: ॥

26. Homage to armies, and food to you the leaders of armies. Homage to you car-borne, and homage to you the pedestrians. Food to you born through intermarriage. Homage to you who collect materials for war. Food to the aged and the learned. Homage to you the students.

---

[14]This verse ordains women also to fight at times of emergency. A separate army of women may be trained, if needed.

[15]Buffoons, who through mimickry imitate different forms, deserve respect for their tact and intelligence.

२७. नमस्तक्षभ्यो रथकारेभ्यश्च वो नमो नमः कुलालेभ्यः कर्मारिभ्यश्च वो नमो नमो निषादेभ्यः पुञ्जिष्ठेभ्यश्च वो नमो नमः श्वनिभ्यो मृगयुभ्यश्च वो नमः ॥

27. Food to the carpenters. Homage to you the manufacturers of aeroplanes. Food to the potters. Homage to you the manufacturers of arms. Food to the denizens of forest who subdue wild creatures. Homage to the masters of different languages. Food to the trainers of dogs. Homage to you the lovers of deer.

२८. नमः श्वभ्यः श्वपतिभ्यश्च वो नमो नमो भवाय च रुद्राय च नमः शर्वाय च पशुपतये च नमो नीलग्रीवाय च शितिकण्ठाय च ।

28. Food to the dogs, and to you the rearers of dogs. Homage to him well-known for noble characteristics. Homage to him who makes the wicked weep. Food to those who kill the depraved, and to those who rear the cattle. Homage to him with a beautiful neck, and to him with a black throat.

२९. नमः कपर्दिने च व्युप्तकेशाय च नमः सहस्राक्षाय च शतधन्वने च नमो गिरिशयाय च शिपिविष्टाय च नमो मीढुष्टमाय चेषुमते च ॥

29. Food to the celibate with braided hair. Homage to the shavenhaired recluse. Homage to the scholar who keeps an eye on thousand subjects, and to the Kshatriya who teaches manifold sciences of armoury. Homage to the Banprasthi who lives in mountains, to the Vaisha who protects the cattle, and to the Shudra. Homage to the gardener, and to the well-armed soldier.

३०. नमो ह्रस्वाय च वामनाय च नमो बृहते च वर्षीयसे च नमो वृद्धाय च सवृधे च नमो-ऽग्र्याय च प्रथमाय च ।

30. Food to the child and the learned. Homage to the strong and those advanced in knowledge. Homage to the aged, and the eminent amongst the associates. Homage to the foremost in doing noble deeds and to the well-known.

३१. नम आशवे चाजिराय च नमः शीघ्र्याय च शीभ्याय च नम ऊर्म्याय चावस्वन्याय च नमो नादेयाय च द्वीप्याय च ॥

31. Food to the horse swift like air, and to the horse that throws down a novice rider. Food to the hasty and to the rapid mover. Food to the zealous and to the silent workers. Food to him who dwells in rivers and on islands.

३२. नमो ज्येष्ठाय च कनिष्ठाय च नमः पूर्वजाय चापरजाय च नमो मध्यमाय चापगल्भाय च नमो जघन्याय च बुध्न्याय च ॥

[27]Carpenters and blacksmiths who manufacture arms should be well paid and respected.
[29]Celibate: Brahmchari.
Recluse: Sanyasi.

32. Namaste (Homage) to the aged and to the children. Homage to the first born and to the last born. Homage to the relatives and to the simple-minded. Homage to the Shudra and to the charitably disposed.

३३. नमः सोम्याय च प्रतिसर्याय च नमो याम्याय च क्षेम्याय च नमः श्लोक्याय चा-
वसान्याय च नम उर्वर्याय च खल्याय च ॥

33. Food to the prosperous and the virtuous. Food to the lovers of justice, and to the protectors. Homage to the scholars of the Vedas, and to the expert in finishing projects. Homage to the great, and to the skilled in making collection of provisions.

३४. नमो वन्याय च कक्ष्याय च नमः श्रवाय च प्रतिश्रवाय च नम आशुषेणाय चाशुरथाय
च नमः शूराय चावभेदिने च ॥

34. Food to those who live in wood, bushes and caves. Homage to the teacher and the taught, and to him who fulfils his vow. Food to him with swift conveyances. Homage to the hero, and to him who rends asunder the foes.

३५. नमो बिल्मिने च कवचिने च नमो वर्मिणे च वरूथिने च नमः श्रुताय च श्रुतसेनाय
च नमो दुन्दुभ्याय चाहनन्याय च ॥

35. Homage to him who wears a helmet, and to him who wears a cuirass. Food to him who wears mail and defensive armour, and to him who possesses a nice house. Homage to the renowned and to him whose army is renowned. Homage to the skilled drummer, and to the efficient player on military musical instruments that encourage the soldiers.

३६. नमो धृष्णवे च प्रमृशाय च नमो निषङ्गिणे चेषुधिमते च नमस्तीक्ष्णेषवे चायुधिने च
नमः स्वायुधाय च सुधन्वने च ॥

36. Food to the bold, the prudent and the mild. Homage to him who carries sword and quiver. Homage to him who hath sharp weapons, and is equipped with brave warriors. Food to him who possesses good weapons and good bows.

३७. नमः स्रुत्याय च पथ्याय च नमः काट्याय च नीप्याय च नमः कुल्याय च सरस्याय
च नमो नादेयाय च वैशन्ताय च ॥

37. Food to him who dwells in rivulets, to him who keeps the paths clean. Homage to him expert in constructing wells, and water-falls. Homage to him who knows how to construct canals and tanks. Homage to him who lives on

---

[32] This verse preaches that the elder should greet the younger with Namaste and vice-versa. Brahmans, Kshatriyas, Vaishas and Shudras should greet each other with Namaste. No sense of superiority or inferiority should prevail amongst the great and small, high and low.

[34] Food means wages, pay, remuneration.

[37] People should utilise the water of the streams, canals, wells and tanks to grow fruits, food and trees.

the banks of streams and food for compassion to the animalcules residing in small ponds.

३८. नमः कूप्याय चावटच्याय च नमो वीध्रयाय चातप्याय च नमो मेघ्याय च विद्युत्याय च नमो वर्ष्याय चावर्ष्याय च ॥

38. Food to the creatures who dwell in wells, pits and forests. Food to him who lives in diverse lights, to him who works in heat, and manages his fields. Homage to him who knows the science of clouds, and to him who knows the science, of electricity. Homage to him who lives in a rainy place, and to him who lives in an arid place.

३९. नमो वात्याय च रेष्म्याय च नमो वास्तव्याय च वास्तुपाय च नमः सोमाय च रुद्राय च नमस्ताम्राय चारुणाय च ॥

39. Food to him who knows the science of air, and to him who is the chief killer. Homage to the expert in the construction of houses, and to their protector. Food to the wealthy, and to him who makes the wicked weep. Homage to him who abhors sin and to him who practices virtue.

४०. नमः शङ्ग्वे च पशुपतये च नम उग्राय च भीमाय च नमोऽग्रेवधाय च दूरेवधाय च नमो हन्त्रे च हनीयसे च नमो वृक्षेभ्यो हरिकेशेभ्यो नमस्ताराय ॥

40. Food to the giver of meal, and to the protector of cows. Homage to the fierce and to the awe-inspiring. Food to him who slays the enemy in front, and to him who slays him at a distance. Food to the slayer of the wicked and to the extirpator of the evil-minded. Homage to the killer of foes, and the green-tressed soldiers. Food to the deliverer from misery.

४१. नमः शम्भवाय च मयोभवाय च नमः शङ्कराय च मयस्कराय च नमः शिवाय च शिवतराय च ॥

41. Homage to God, the Source of happiness, and the Source of delight. Homage to God, the Bestower of happiness and the Bestower of delight. Homage to the Auspicious, homage to the most Auspicious God.

४२. नमः पायाय चावार्याय च नमः प्रतरणाय चोत्तरणाय च नमस्तीर्थ्याय च कूल्याय च नमः शष्प्याय च फेन्याय च ॥

42. Homage to him who is beyond misery, and to him who is struggling for release. Homage to him who crosses over and to him who crosses back. Food to the teachers of the vedas, and speakers of truth, and to the dwellers on the banks of seas and rivers. Food to him who knows the science of grass, and to him who knows the science of foam.

४३. नमः सिकत्याय च प्रवाह्याय च नमः किँ शिलाय च क्षयणाय च नमः कपर्दिने च पुलस्तये च नम इरिण्याय च प्रपथ्याय च ॥

---

38 In diverse lights means who lives not in dark but well ventilated places.
41 This is the last Mantra of the Vedic Sandhya.

43. Food to the expert in extracting gold from sand, and to the expert in driving oxen. Food to him who knows the use of stones, and to him who constructs houses for dwelling. Food to him who wears braided hair, and to him who knows the use of instruments for lifting heavy objects. Homage to him who utilises properly the barren land, and to him who is skilled in treading the noble paths of virtue.

४४. नमो व्रज्याय च गोष्ठ्याय च नमस्तल्प्याय च गेह्याय च नमो हृदय्याय च निवेष्याय च नम: काट्याय च गह्वरेष्ठाच च ॥

44. Food to the expert in deeds, and to the manager of cow-pens. Food to the efficient couch-maker, and to him who lives peacefully in his house. Homage to him who is skilled in mental deliberations, and to him who is proficient in diving deep into intricate topics. Food to him who explores the mysteries of nature, and to him who dwells in inaccessible mountain caves.

४५. नम: शुष्क्याय च हरित्याय च नम: पांस्य्याय च रजस्याय च नमो लोप्याय चोलप्याय च नम ऊर्व्याय च सूर्व्याय च ॥

45. Homage to him who deals in dry fruits, and to him who deals in green vegetables. Respects to him who lives in a sandy place, and to him who lives in distant places. Homage to him who is expert in the knowledge of invisible things, and to him who is expert in the knowledge of visible things. Homage to him who is skilled in murdering, and to him who gives condign punishment.

४६. नम: पर्ण्याय च पर्णशद्याय च नम उद्गुरमाणाय चाभिघ्नते च नम आखिदते च प्रखिदते च नम इषुकृद्भ्यो धनुष्कृद्भ्यश्च वो नमो नमो व: किरिकेभ्यो देवानां हृदयेभ्यो नमो विचिन्वत्केभ्यो नमो विक्षिणत्केभ्यो नम आनिर्हतेभ्य: ॥

46. Food to him who shows gratitude in return, and to him who shears leaves. Food to the enterprising and to him who kills the wicked foes in front. Homage to the poor and the pauper. Food to the arrow-makers, and homage to you the bow-makers. Food to the learned dear like soul, and to you the dischargers of arrows. Homage to the embodiments of virtues, to the destroyers of enemies and to the vanquished.

४७. द्रापे अन्धसस्पते दरिद्र नीललोहित ।
आसां प्रजानामेषां पशूनां मा भेर्मा रोड्मो च न: किंचनाममत् ॥

47. O King, our saviour from degradation, lord of wealth, driver of foes to the abyss of poverty, robed in blue and red dress, terrify not these people and cattle, nor make them diseased. Let not us or any one else be sick!

४८. इमा रुद्राय तवसे कर्पदिने क्षयद्वीराय प्र भरामहे मती: ।
यथा शमसद् द्विपदे चतुष्पदे विश्वं पुष्टं ग्रामे अस्मिन्ननातुरम् ॥

⁴⁵Skilled in murdering, refers to a commander who kills the soldiers of the opposing army on the battlefield.

⁴⁶An enemy, being defeated deserves protection, honour and respect, and not annihilation.

48. O King, we honour these wise persons, advisers of the commander of the army, who makes the sinful weep, is accompanied by heroes who destroy the wicked, leads a life of celibacy; and is powerful, so that in this universe all human beings and cattle of the world be happy, free from misery and disease!

४६. या ते रुद्र शिवा तनू: शिवा विश्वाहा भेषजी ।
शिवा रुतस्य भेषजी तया नो मृड जीवसे ॥

49. O royal physician, thy auspicious, vast and fascinating skill, is like medicine the killer of disease. It gives comfort to the patient and removes his affliction. Make us enjoy this life with pleasure for all days!

५०. परि नो रुद्रस्य हेतिर्वृणक्तु परि त्वेषस्य दुर्मतिरघायो: ।
अव स्थिरा मघवद्भ्यस्तनुष्व मीढ्वस्तोकाय तनयाय मृड ॥

50. O King, giver of pleasure unto us, keep us away from the weapons of the valiant, save us from the evil-mindedness of the indignant sinners. Extend unto our babes and youths, the stable intellect derived from the rich, and make us all delightful with it!

५१. मीढुष्टम शिवतम शिवो न: सुमना भव ।
परमे वृक्ष आयुधं निधाय कृत्तिं वसान आ चर पिनाकं बिभ्रदा गहि ॥

51. O most bounteous, most auspicious King, be auspicious, well inclined to us. Take up thy weapons, put on the deer-skin cloak, wear the armour, thy protector, and come for our safety. Attack the strong army of the enemy worthy to be torn asunder.

५२. विकिरिद्र विलोहित नमस्ते अस्तु भगव: ।
यास्ते सहस्रꣳ हेतयोऽन्यमस्मन्नि वपन्तु ता: ॥

52. O King, sound sleeper like a powerful swine, bent on inaugurating various projects, holy Lord, to thee be homage. May all the thousand darts of thine strike dead against the foe different from us!

५३. सहस्राणि सहस्रशो बाह्वोस्तव हेतय: ।
तासामीशानो भगव: पराचीना मुखा कृधि ॥

53. O auspicious commander of the army, thou hast got thousands of weapons in thy possession. Thou art their Lord. Turn back with them the faces of thousands of our foes!

५४. असंख्याता सहस्राणि ये रुद्रा अधि भूम्याम् ।
तेषाꣳ सहस्रयोजनेऽव धन्वानि तन्मसि ॥

---

[52]विलोहित may mean free from sin according to Mahidhar's interpretation. Swami Dayananda translates it as, 'bent on inaugurating various projects'.

54. Innumerable, thousands are the creatures on the face of the earth. In their connection we should send weapons to places a thousand leagues away.

५५. अस्मिन् महत्यर्णवे ऽन्तरिक्षे भवा अधि ।
तेषाꣳ सहस्रयोजनेऽव धन्वानि तन्मसि ॥

55. In this mighty, subtle, watery space above us there are creatures and airs. We should make use of them; and transport weapons to places a thousand leagues away.

५६. नीलग्रीवाः शितिकण्ठा दिवꣳ रुद्रा उपश्रिताः ।
तेषाꣳ सहस्रयोजनेऽव धन्वानि तन्मसि ॥

56. Creatures are dwelling in the sky, whose necks are blue, whose throats are white. We should make use of them, and send weapons to places a thousand leagues away.

५७. नीलग्रीवाः शितिकण्ठाः शर्वा अधः क्षमाचराः ।
तेषाꣳ सहस्रयोजनेऽव धन्वानि तन्मसि ॥

57. The injurious creatures, whose necks are blue and whose throats are white, live down below on the earth. Let us use weapons for their extermination in places a thousand leagues away.

५८. ये वृक्षेषु शष्पिञ्जरा नीलग्रीवा विलोहिताः ।
तेषाꣳ सहस्रयोजनेऽव धन्वानि तन्मसि ॥

58. There are injurious serpents, living in the dens of trees, awful in appearance, full of poison, with blue necks and different in colours. We should use our arms for their extinction in places a thousand leagues afar.

५९. ये भूतानामधिपतयो विशिखासः कपर्दिनः ।
तेषाꣳ सहस्रयोजनेऽव धन्वानि तन्मसि ॥

59. The Sanyasis with no hair-tufts, and the Brahmcharis with braided hair, are the lords of the animate and inanimate world. For their safety, we roam in distant places a thousand leagues afar, and use the weapons of knowledge for the removal of the evil of ignorance.

६०. ये पथां पथिरक्षय ऐलबृदा आयुर्युधः ।
तेषाꣳ सहस्रयोजनेऽव धन्वानि तन्मसि ॥

60. For them, who are the protectors of paths and pedestrians, the producers of corn on the earth, who fight with full force, against their enemies, we transport our weapons to places a thousand leagues afar.

⁵⁶⁻⁵⁷It may mean, they are unreliable. They show different phases of character. They behave in one way from the front and in another from behind. They are double faced, sweet tongued before the authorities, and evil intentioned in the back.

६१. ये तीर्थानि प्रचरन्ति सृकाहस्ता निषङ्गिणः ।
तेषाᳪ सहस्रयोजनेऽव धन्वानि तन्मसि ॥

61. For them, who with arrows in their hand, and armed with sword, preach the study of the vedas and the use of ships, we send our weapons to places a thousand leagues afar.

६२. येऽन्नेषु विविध्यन्ति पात्रेषु पिबतो जनान् ।
तेषाᳪ सहस्रयोजनेऽव धन्वानि तन्मसि ॥

62. The degraded persons, who harm the men taking food and drink from their cups, deserve to be uprooted by the use of our arms, though they be a thousand leagues afar.

६३. य एतावन्तश्च भूयाᳪ सश्च दिशो रुद्रा वितस्थिरे ।
तेषाᳪ सहस्रयोजनेऽव धन्वानि तन्मसि ॥

63. We use the forces of nature against the creatures, mentioned above and still more, lodged in different directions, though they be a thousand leagues afar.

६४. नमोऽस्तु रुद्रेभ्यो ये दिवि येषां वर्षमिषवः ।
तेभ्यो दश प्राचीर्दश दक्षिणा दश प्रतीचीर्दशोदीचीर्दशोर्ध्वः ।
तेभ्यो नमो अस्तु ते नोऽवन्तु ते नो मृड्यन्तु ते यं द्विष्मो यश्च नो द्वेष्टि तमेषां जम्भे दध्मः ॥

64. Homage to the heroes, who work selflessly like vital breaths, who like sun's light are shining in humility and knowledge, who are powerful like the rain. To them ten eastward, southward ten, ten to the west, ten to the north, ten to the region uppermost. To them we offer food. May they guard and delight us. Within their jaws we lay the man who dislikes us and whom we dislike.

६५. नमोऽस्तु रुद्रेभ्यो येऽन्तरिक्षे येषां वात इषवः ।
तेभ्यो दश प्राचीर्दश दक्षिणा दश प्रतीचीर्दशोदीचीर्दशोर्ध्वः ।
तेभ्यो नमो अस्तु ते नोऽवन्तु ते नो मृड्यन्तु ते यं द्विष्मो यश्च नो द्वेष्टि तमेषां जम्भे दध्मः ॥

65. Homage to the heroes, who sitting in planes fly in the airs, who work selflessly like vital breaths, who are powerful like the wind. To them ten

---

[61]There are two channels or expedients तीर्थ for man. The first is the vow of celibacy, study of the vedas, service of the preceptor, contemplation of God, and truthfulness, which make us overcome the miseries of life. The second is the use of ships and boats that carry us from one corner of the river to the other and make us cross it.

[64]Ten: In each direction they enjoy the delights and comforts of ten directions; or the ten fingers of both the hands be raised in supplication to God, for their prosperity. Just as a mouse in the mouth of a cat is put to inconvenience so we put the hater and the hated in the hands of heroes punishment.

eastward, southward ten, ten to the west, ten to the north, ten to the region uppermost. To them we offer food. May they guard and delight us. Within their jaws we lay the man who dislikes us and whom we dislike.

६६. नमोऽस्तु रुद्रेभ्यो ये पृथिव्यां येषामन्नमिषव: ।
तेभ्यो दश प्राचीर्दश दक्षिणा दश प्रतीचीर्दशोदीचीर्दशोर्ध्वा: ।
तेभ्यो नमो अस्तु ते नोऽवन्तु ते नो मृडयन्तु ते य द्विष्मो यश्च नो द्वेष्टि तमेषां जम्भे दध्म: ॥

66. Homage to the heroes who sitting in conveyances travel on the earth, who work selflessly like the vital breaths, whose arms are foodstuffs. To them ten eastward, southward ten, ten to the west, ten to the north, ten to the region uppermost. To them we offer food. May they guard and delight us. Within their jaws we lay the man who dislikes us and whom we dislike.

CHAPTER XVII

१. श्रश्मभ्रूर्जं पर्वते शिश्रियाणामड्डच श्रोषधीभ्यो वनस्पतिभ्यो अधि सम्भृतं पय: ।
तां न इषमूर्जं वत्त मरुत: सपरराणा श्रश्मेंस्ते क्षन्मयि त ऊर्यं द्विष्मस्तं ते शुगृच्छतु ॥

1. O fully charitably disposed persons, ever active like the wind, grant us food and strength contained in lightning and clouds, formidable in appearance mountain-like!
Grant us food, strength and juice gathered from the plants, trees and waters. O man may I possess thy cloudwise strength and thy appetite. Let thy pain reach the man we dislike.

२. इमा मे श्रग्न इष्टका धेनव: सन्त्वेका च दश च दश च शतं च शतं च सहस्रं च सहस्रं चायुतं चायुतं च नियुतं च नियुतं च प्रयुतं चार्बुदं च न्यर्बुदं च समुद्रश्च मध्यं चान्तश्च पराधंश्चेता मे श्रग्न इष्टका धेनव: सन्त्वमुत्रामुष्मिँल्लोके ॥

2. O learned person, may the materials of my yajna, like milch kine, be the givers of happiness to me!
They may be one, and ten, and ten tens, a hundred, and ten hundred, a thousand and ten thousand and a hundred thousand, a lac and ten lacs, a million, and ten millions, a crore, ten crores, hundred crores, thousand crores, its ten times Maha Padma, its ten times Shankh, its ten times Samudra, its ten times Madhya, its ten times Prardh. May these bricks of my altar be a source of happiness to me, like milch-kine in this world and the next world.

३. ऋतव स्थ ऋतावृध ऋतुष्ठा स्थ ऋतावृध: ।
घृतश्चुतो मधुश्चुतो विराजो नाम कामदुधा श्रक्षीयमाणा: ॥

3. O women, ye are pleasant like the spring season, full of truth like canals with water, enjoyers of seasons like spring, advancers of truth, givers of butter, givers of sweet juices, worthy of protection, full of various noble qualities, fulfillers of our desires like kine, make us happy!

४. समुद्रस्य त्वाऽवकयाग्ने परि व्ययामसि ।
पावको श्रस्मभ्यँ शिवो भव ॥

4. O ruler, just as we conversant with the knowledge of self-protection in space, approach thee from all sides, be thou our purifier and auspicious unto us!

---

[1] Husband and wife should share the weal and woe of each other.

[2] Millions and billions of bricks are used in the construction of a big house or a grand altar. The house and the altar (वेदी) strongly built are a source of comfort and happiness like the milch-kine. Daily performance of Havan is necessary to elevate our soul in this world and the world to come. God has in this verse preached the science of Arithmetical digits, which can be multiplied ad-infinitum.

CHAPTER XVII

५. हिमस्य त्वा जरायुणाऽग्ने परि व्ययामसि ।
पावको अस्मभ्यꣳ शिवो भव ॥

5. O ruler, we rally round thee for safety, just as fire or cloth removes cold. Be thou our purifier, and auspicious unto us!

६. उप ज्मन्नुप वेतसेऽव तर नदीष्वा ।
अग्ने पित्तमपामसि मण्डूकि ताभिरा गहि सेमं नो यज्ञं पावकवर्णꣳ शिवं कृधि ।

6. O noble and well-decorated woman, live on this earth in the midst of riches, enhancing thy resources. Just as fire is the emblem of the essence of life, so shouldst thou approach us with sweetness and vigour. Make our resplendent domestic life successful!

७. अपामिदं न्ययनꣳ समुद्रस्य निवेशनम् ।
अन्याँस्ते अस्मत्तपन्तु हेतयः पावको अस्मभ्यꣳ शिवो भव ॥

7. O learned person, this space in full is the decided home of waters and creatures. Lead the life of a domestic person with certainty like the ocean of vapours in space. Doing virtuous deeds, be propitious unto us. Let thy shafts trouble others different from us!

८. अग्ने पावक रोचिषा मन्द्रया देव जिह्वया ।
आ देवान् वक्षि यक्षि च ॥

8. O excellent diffuser and preacher of knowledge, the gratifier of the hearts of men, with thy pleasant and truthful tongue; and thy light of knowledge, preach unto the learned, and associate with them!

९. स नः पावक दीदिवोऽग्ने देवाँ२ इहा वह ।
उप यज्ञꣳ हविश्च नः ॥

9. O learned person; pure, foe-destroyer, distinguisher of truth from untruth; just as fire carries afar our fragrant oblations, so dost thou in this world bring hither for us domestic life and learned persons!

१०. पावकया यश्चितयन्त्या। कृपा क्षामन् रुरुच उषसो न भानुना ।
तूर्वन् न यामन्नेतशस्य नू रण आ यो घृणे न ततृषाणो अजरः ॥

10. The Commander of the army, who with purifying conscious force shines upon the earth like dawns with sun's light, who kills speedily like strong horses, the foes that come in the way; who in the heat of battle tolerate thirst, whom old age does not touch, is fit for rule.

११. नमस्ते हरसे शोचिषे नमस्ते अस्त्वर्चिषे ।
अन्याँस्ते अस्मत्तपन्तु हेतयः पावको अस्मभ्यꣳ शिवो भव ॥

11. O ruler, our obeisance to thee, the remover of afflictions. Our obeisance to thee pure and worthy of respect. May thy armed forces trouble others than

us. Be thou our purifier, and propitious unto us!

१२. नृषदे वेड्प्सुषदे वेड् बर्हिषदे वेड् वनसदे वेट् स्वर्विदे वेट् ॥

12. O King, the leader of men, occupy the seat of justice. Administer justice unto sailors in ships. Thou art the chief for improving thy subjects. Be thou a dweller in the solitude of forests, and a lover of justice. Be thou the enjoyer of pleasure, full of perseverance!

१३. ये देवा देवानां यज्ञियां यज्ञियानाᳪ संवत्सरीणमुप भागमासते ।
अहुतादो हविषो यज्ञे अस्मिन्त्स्वयं पिबन्तु मधुनो घृतस्य ॥

13. The hermits (Sanyasis) learned of the learned, who take their meals without performing Havan, lead a life of sacrifice, and contemplation amongst the performers of usual sacrifice (yajna), and worship the Adorable God, after a year's penance, take themselves the honey and butter of oblations in this yajna.

१४. ये देवा देवेष्वधि देवत्वमायन् ये ब्रह्मणः पुर एतारो अस्य ।
येभ्यो न ऋते पवते धाम किञ्चन न ते दिवो न पृथिव्या अधि स्नुषु ॥

14. The learned yogis who amongst the learned attain to Godhead, who first of all acquire communion with God, without Whose aid no place of happiness is sanctified, dwell neither on heaven's heights nor on the face of the earth.

१५. प्राणदा अपानदा व्यानदा वर्चदा वरिवोदाः ।
अन्यास्ते अस्मत्तपन्तु हेतयः पावको अस्मभ्यᳪ शिवो भव ॥

15. O King, thy powers are the givers of life and strength unto us, the givers of resources for the removal of affliction, the givers of knowledge, the helpers for studying all sciences, the preachers of true religion and service of the learned. May thy weapons trouble others than us. Be thou our purifier and propitious unto us!

१६. अग्निस्तिग्मेन शोचिषा यासद्विश्वं न्यत्रिणम् ।
अग्निर्नो वनते रयिम् ॥

16. O learned person, just as fire with its sharpened blaze, gives us all eatables, and just as electricity adds to our wealth, so shouldst thou be helpful for us!

[13] A sanyasi kindles the inner and not the outer fire. It is not necessary for him to perform havan.

[14] The yogis attain to salvation, i.e., final beatitude (Moksha). and being absorbed in God, their souls roam throughout the universe.

[16] Just as fire burns grass dry or wet, so we should burn all our vices and imbibe virtues. Just as electricity pervades all objects, so should we learn all sciences and dispel ignorance.

१७. य इमा विश्वा भुवनानि जुह्वृषिर्होता न्यसीदत् पिता नः ।
स आशिषा द्रविणमिच्छमानः प्रथमच्छदवराँ२ आ विवेश ॥

17. The Omniscient God, the Creator and Dissolver of all objects, our Father, pervading all these regions, is ever-present. He sustains the universe. With His blessing, He grants us riches; and pervades the subtle primordial vast matter, and the world created therefrom.

१८. किꣳ स्विदासीदधिष्ठानमारम्भणं कतमत्स्वित्कथाऽऽसीत् ।
यतो भूमिं जनयन् विश्वकर्मा वि द्यामौर्णोन्महिना विश्वचक्षाः ॥

18. What is the support of this universe? What is the material cause of the world in the beginning? What was its nature? Whence God, the Doer of myriad deeds, the Seer of all, producing the earth and the heavens, covers them with His mighty power.

१९. विश्वतश्चक्षुरुत विश्वतोमुखो विश्वतोबाहुरुत विश्वतस्पात् ।
सं बाहुभ्यां धमति सं पतत्रैर्द्यावाभूमी जनयन् देव एकः ॥

19. God keeps an eye on the whole world, preaches morality to humanity, is full of immense strength, is present everywhere. The Incomparable One Effulgent Lord, with mobile atoms, producing the Earth and Heaven, with His mighty force puts the universe in motion.

२०. किꣳ स्विद्वनं क उ स वृक्ष आस यतो द्यावापृथिवी निष्टतक्षुः ।
मनीषिणो मनसा पृच्छतेदु तद्यदध्यतिष्ठद्भुवनानि धारयन् ॥

20. Let the Yogis with mind under control, intelligently question the learned. What was the adorable cause, what the transitory resultant universe? Who created separately the heaven and Earth and how? Know God the Creator of the universe, Who sustaining all regions where human beings dwell, reigns supreme over them.

२१. या ते धामानि परमाणि याऽवमा या मध्यमा विश्वकर्मन्नुतेमा ।
शिक्षा सखिभ्यो हविषि स्वधावः स्वयं यजस्व तन्वं वृधानः ॥

21. O God, the Lord of foodgrains, and Doer of noble deeds, whatever high, low, and medium sized places there are in Thy universe. Thou Thyself providest them with food. Developing our body, give us Thy devoted friends, good instructions!

---

¹⁷God was present in matter the cause of the universe, and is present in all heavenly bodies, created therefrom.
²⁰Adorable cause is matter, from which results this universe, which is ephemeral and is dissolved into atoms by God.
The process of creating the universe from indestructible matter by God, and dissolving it again into atoms is eternal.

२२. विश्वकर्मन् हविषा वावृधानः स्वयं यजस्व पृथिवीमुत द्याम् ।
मुह्यन्त्वन्ये अभितः सपत्ना इहास्माकं मघवा सूरिरस्तु ॥

22. O noble King, just as God, the Embodiment of virtues, through His grandeur, connects the earth and the sun, so shouldst thou associate with all. Let the venerable rich learned person throw all our foes into confusion.

२३. वाचस्पतिं विश्वकर्माणमूतये मनोजुवं वाजे अद्या हुवेम ।
स नो विश्वानि हवनानि जोषद्विश्वशम्भूरवसे साधुकर्मा ॥

23. Let us invoke for our protection in battle, the high souled individual, who is the preserver of the vedas, swift like mind, and expert in all deeds. May he, the giver of comfort to all, the doer of virtuous deeds, for our safety, approve of our invocations.

२४. विश्वकर्मन् हविषा वर्धनेन त्रातारमिन्द्रमकृणोरवध्यम् ।
तस्मै विशः समनमन्त पूर्वीरयमुग्रो विहव्यो यथासत् ॥

24. O King, the lover of noble actions, the head of all Assemblies, select him as thy minister for advice in state affairs, who is highly serviceable, dignified, unworthy of harm, protector, and wealthy. Let the good subjects bow unto him; so that this minister be quick to hurt, and fit to be respected in various ways!

२५. चक्षुषः पिता मनसा हि धीरो घृतमेने अजनन्नम्नमाने ।
यदेदन्ता अददृह्न्त पूर्व आदिद् द्यावापृथिवी अप्रथेताम् ॥

25. Ye people, when you elect as your ruler the man, who is the guardian of the lovers of justice; has a patient mind peaceful through austerity, grants us dainties, and makes the officials and the subjects respect each other, and live together like the ancient far extended Heaven and Earth, and make progress working unitedly like feet the lowest portion of the body, then alone is the government stabilised!

२६. विश्वकर्मा विमना आद्विहाया धाता विधाता परमोत सन्दृक् ।
तेषामिष्टानि समिषा मदन्ति यत्रा सप्त ऋषीन् पर एकमाहुः ॥

26. God is the Creator of the whole universe, full of knowledge, Ubiquitous, Sustainer, Maker, Seer, and Foremost of all. He is known as the Incomparable One. In Him the souls controlling the seven rishis live in enjoyment according to their desire. He fulfils their lofty ambitions.

---

[22] Heaven and earth are connected through mutual attraction.
[23] The high-souled individual means the ruler. He should possess the qualities mentioned in this verse. see 8.45.
[24] see 8.46.
[26] Seven Rishis: Five breaths, Pran, Apan, Vyan, Udan, Saman, Dhananjaya and soul. Their: Souls.
Seven Rishis may also mean two eyes, two ears, two nostrils and mouth.

२७. यो नः पिता जनिता यो विधाता धामानि वेद भुवनानि विश्वा ।
यो देवानां नामधा एक एव तं सम्प्रश्नं भुवना यन्त्यन्या ॥

27. God is the Father, Who made us. Who rewards our acts, and creates the universe. Who knoweth all worlds and all things existing. He is the name-giver of all the forces of nature. He is One. Him do all created beings seek for information.

२८. त आ्ऽयजन्त द्रविणं समस्मा ऋषयः पूर्वे जरितारो न भूना ।
असूर्ते सूर्ते रजसि निषत्ते ये भूतानि समकृण्वन्निमानि ॥

28. Highly learned persons, the nourishers of all, the knowers of the significance of the vedas, like a praiser, thoroughly educate these living beings, in invisible and visibly settled worlds, and amass wealth for carrying out the commands of God.

२६. परो दिवा पर एना पृथिव्या परो देवेभिरसुर्यं यदस्ति ।
कं स्विद् गर्भं प्रथमं दध्र आपो यत्र देवाः समपश्यन्त पूर्वे ॥

29. God is higher than this Earth and Heaven, higher than learned living beings, and beyond the divisions of time. Through His persuasion souls enter the numerous assumable bodies. Him do the devotees of knowledge see with a spiritual eye.

३०. तमिद्गर्भं प्रथमं दध्र आपो यत्र देवाः समगच्छन्त विश्वे ।
अजस्य नाभावध्येकमर्पितं यस्मिन् विश्वानि भुवनानि तस्थुः ॥

30. Know Him to be God, in Whom souls sustain the vast eternal matter, the source of creation; to Whom all yogis attain. Who acts as Lord over eternal soul and matter. Who is Self Existent. In Whom abide all things existing.

३१. न तं विदाथ य इमा जजानान्यद्युष्माकमन्तरं बभूव ।
नीहारेण प्रावृता जल्प्या चासुतृप उक्थशासश्चरन्ति ॥

31. O people, ye do not know God, Who has produced these creatures, Who is away from the irreligious and separate from soul and matter, and being present in all is still distant; as ye are sunk in the darkness of ignorance; occupied with the discussion of partial truth and untruth, engaged in the enjoyment of carnal pleasures, and abandoning the practice of yoga, are busy with controversy over the meanings of words!

३२. विश्वकर्मा ह्यजनिष्ट देव आदिद्गन्धर्वो अभवद् द्वितीयः ।
तृतीयः पिता जनितौषधीनामपां गर्भं व्यदधात् पुरुत्रा ॥

27For information: to learn who is the supreme God.
28Vedic teachings are meant for the inhabitants of earth and other invisible planets where dwell men.
31Distant: Though near, God is distant from those engrossed in ignorance and lack of knowledge.

32. Firstly was created the air, in which are performed all good deeds; secondly was created the sun, which sustains the earth; thirdly was created the cloud, that fosters plants, waters and souls, and helps the retention of life in material objects, is the guardian of many, and begetter of rain.

३३. आशुः शिशानो वृषभो न भीमो घनाघनः क्षोभणश्चर्षणीनाम् ।
संक्रन्दनोऽनिमिष एकवीरः शतꣳ सेना अजयत् साकमिन्द्रः ॥

33. He is an ideal commander of the army, who is swift, keeps his arms sharpened, fearless like a strong bull, a zealous killer of foes, strikes terror in men; makes the enemies weep bitterly, works day and night, a sole hero, rends asunder the opponents, and subdues with us a hundred armies.

३४. संक्रन्दनेनानिमिषेण जिष्णुना युत्कारेण दुश्च्यवनेन धृष्णुना ।
तदिन्द्रेण जयत तत्सहध्वं युधो नर इषुहस्तेन वृष्णा ॥

34. Ye warriors, win the opposing forces, and bear the brunt of their speed with the commander, who makes the enemies weep, is ever exerting, is fond of victory, arranges his soldiers in different divisions, puts the enemies to inconvenience, is steady, energetic, and strong, with arms in hand!

३५. स इषुहस्तैः स निषङ्गिभिर्वशी सꣳस्रष्टा स युध इन्द्रो गणेन ।
सꣳ सृष्टजित्सोमपा बाहुशर्ध्युप्रधन्वा प्रतिहिताभिरस्ता ॥

35. The Commander of the army, with arms in hand, with welltrained and armed soldiers, keeper in stock of arms and weapons, the master of passions, the conqueror of foes, the maintainer of peace in the country, strong in arms, with sharp shafts fond of fight, discharges his weapons, kills his enemies, and with his disciplined army achieves victory over the opposing forces.

३६. बृहस्पते परि दीया रथेन रक्षोहाऽमित्राꣳर् अपबाधमानः ।
प्रभञ्जन्त्सेनाः प्रमृणो युधा जयन्नस्माकमेध्यविता रथानाम् ॥

36. O protector of the religious minded, the aged and the forces, the slayer of demons, the remover of our foes, their killer, the breaker-up of the enemy's forces, their destroyer in the battle with military accoutrements, be thou protector of our conveyances that are used on the earth, the sea, and in the air!

३७. बलविज्ञाय स्थविरः प्रवीरः सहस्वान् वाजी सहमान उग्रः ।
अभिवीरो अभिसत्वा सहोजा जैत्रमिन्द्र रथमा तिष्ठ गोवित् ॥

37. O Commander of the army, well-equipped with military warfare, thou knowest how to strengthen thy army, art an experienced statesmen, a foremost fighter, mighty, the master of the science of war, the endurer of plea-

---

[37]Conveyance: refers to the conveyance used on land, on water and in the air. Cars, ships and aeroplanes are covered by this word.

sure and pain, the fierce slayer of the wicked, the possessor of nice warriors, and martial intelligent employees, famous for strength, conquering land, surrounded by victorious heroes, mount thy conquering conveyance!

३८. गोत्रभिदं गोविदं वज्रबाहुं जयन्तमज्म प्रमृणन्तमोजसा ।
इम‌ सजाता अनु वीरयध्वमिन्द्र‌ सखायो अनु स‌ रभध्वम् ॥

38. O friendly countrymen, encourage the commander of the army, and begin the battle with him, who with his physical, mental and military strength, cleaves the enemies' families, usurps their land, is armed with weapons, slays the foes, subdues the enemy in the battle, and conquers him!

३६. अभि गोत्राणि सहसा गाहमानोऽदयो वीरः शतमन्युरिन्द्रः ।
दुरच्यवनः पृतनाषाड्युध्योऽस्माक‌ सेना अवतु प्र युत्सु ॥

39. May the commander of the army, who, with surpassing vigour pierces in the battles the families of the enemies, is pitiless, wild with anger, unconquerable by foes, conqueror of the enemy's forces, unequalled in fight, and victor, protect our armies.

४०. इन्द्र आसां नेता बृहस्पतिर्दक्षिणा यज्ञः पुर एतु सोमः ।
देवसेनानामभिभञ्जतीनां जयन्तीनां मरुतो यन्त्वग्रम् ॥

40. In battle, the commander, the leader of these armies of the learned, the conqueror and demolisher of the enemies should march behind. The organiser of the army should march in front. The leader of big bands should march on the right. The encourager of the army should march on the left. The warriors swift like air should march ahead.

४१. इन्द्रस्य वृष्णो वरुणस्य राज्ञ आदित्यानां मरुता‌ शर्ध उग्रम् ।
महामनसां भुवनच्यवानां घोषो देवानां जयतामुदस्थात् ॥

41. Musical instruments, to infuse valour and energy should be played upon before the commencement of the battle, by the learned soldiers of the powerful commander, and mighty king, who possess decent homes, lofty ideas, are able to conquer the enemies, have led a life of celibacy for forty eight years, are highly learned and strong, full of terrible power.

४२. उद्धर्षय मघवन्नायुधान्युत्सत्वनां मामकानां मना‌ सि ।
उद्वृत्रहन् वाजिनां वाजिनान्युद्रथानां जयतां यन्तु घोषाः ॥

42. O adorable commander, the slayer of foes, like the sun of clouds, make the weapons of our soldiers flourish, excite the spirits of our warring heroes, increase the speed of our horses, and let the din of conquering cars go upward!

39Pitiless: A commander is full of pity for the virtuous, but is devoid of pity for the foes.

४३. अस्माकमिन्द्र: समृतेषु ध्वजेष्वस्माकं या इषवस्ता जयन्तु ।
अस्माकं वीरा उत्तरे भवन्त्वस्मार्२ उ देवा अवता हवेषु ॥

43. O learned persons desirous of victory, may the commander and our forces, under different flags, the emblems of justice and truth, win in the battle. May our brave men enjoy after war. May ye protect us everywhere at the time of war!

४४. अमीषां चित्तं प्रतिलोभयन्ती गृहाणाङ्गान्यप्वे परेहि ।
अभि प्रेहि निर्दह हृत्सु शोकैरन्धेनामित्रास्तमसा सचन्ताम् ॥

44. O queen, the slayer of foes, organise the bands of thy army, that bewilders the hearts of the forces of the enemy, remain aloof from sin, convey thy aim to thy soldiers, burn down the foes, whereby they may abide in utter darkness with hearts full of griefs!

४५. अवसृष्टा परा पत शरव्ये ब्रह्मसं शिते ।
गच्छामित्रान् प्र पद्यस्व माऽमीषां कं चनोच्छिष: ॥

45. O wife of the commander-in-chief, expert in the art of archery, trained by a learned person knowing the vedas, on persuasion, go afar, encounter the foes, achieve victory by slaying them. Let not even one of those distant foes escape!

४६. प्रेता जयता नर इन्द्रो व: शर्म यच्छतु ।
उग्रा व: सन्तु बाहवोऽनाधृष्या यथाऽसथ ॥

46. Advance, O heroes, win the day. May the commander of the army provide ye with shelter, food and clothes. Exceeding mighty be your arms, that none may threaten or injure you!

४७ असौ या सेना मरुत: परेषामभ्येति न ओजसा स्पर्धमाना ।
तां गूहत तमसाऽपव्रतेन यथाऽमी अन्यो अन्यं न जानन् ॥

47. O learned persons, the army of our enemies, that comes against us in a jealous mood, with its might, meet ye and enwrap it harshly in the darkness of the smoke arising out of the use of cannons so that they may not recognise one another!

४८. यत्र बाणा: सम्पतन्ति कुमारा विशिखा इव ।
तत्र इन्द्रो बृहस्पतिरदिति: शर्म यच्छतु विश्वाहा शर्म यच्छतु ॥

---

[45]अप्वे According to Sayana, a female deity who presides over sin; according to Mahidhar, sickness or fear. According to Swami Dayananda, it means the queen who leads the army of women and kills the foes. This verse advocates the formation of the army of women.

[47]Darkness: the use of fiery weapons produces smoke, that envelops the enemy's forces, and being blinded one soldier cannot recognise the other. It may also refer to the use of gases which darken the eyes of the soldiers.

48. There where the flights of arrows fall like boys whose locks are unshorn, may the Commander, the protector of the big army grant us shelter, may the entire Assembly adorned with members, grant us a happy home through all our days.

४८. मर्माणि ते वर्मणा छादयामि सोमस्त्वा राजाऽमृतेनानुवस्ताम् ।
उरोर्वरीयो वरुणस्ते कृणोतु जयन्तं त्वानु देवा मदन्तु ॥

49. O valiant warrior, thy vital parts I cover with armour. May this calm, considerate king protect thee with efficacious medicine. May the exalted King give thee what is more than ample. May the learned encourage thee in thy triumph over the wicked!

५०. उदेनमुत्तरां नयाग्ने घृतेनाहुत ।
रायस्पोषेण सꣳ सृज प्रजया च बहुं कृधि ॥

50. O Commander of the army, well satisfied with ghee, lead this conquering hero to a high position; vouchsafe him growth of riches and multiply his progeny!

५१. इन्द्रेमं प्रतरां नय सजातानामसद्वशी ।
समेनं वर्चसा सृज देवानां भागदा असत् ॥

51. O Commander, lead to eminence, this hero amongst the learned of the same age. May he have control over his passions. Vouchsafe him lustre of knowledge, so that he may give each his share!

५२. यस्य कुर्मो गृहे हविस्तमग्ने वर्धया त्वम् ।
तस्मै देवा अधि ब्रुवन्नयं च ब्रह्मणस्पतिः ॥

52. O learned family priest prosper the King in whose house we perform Homa (offer oblation). May the learned teach him, and may the master of the vedas teach them!

५३. उद्‌ उ त्वा विश्वे देवा अग्ने भरन्तु चित्तिभिः ।
स नो भव शिवस्त्वꣳ सुप्रतीको विभावसुः ॥

53. O learned King, may all the intellectuals bear and lift thee upward.

---

⁴⁸Like boys: The arrows fall where they list, as boys before the Mundan Sanskar, (tonsure ceremony) play about vigorously wherever they like.
Professor Roth separates Visikha from Kumara, and translates 'where the arrows fly, young and old'; that is feathered and unfeathered. Swami Dayananda translates arrows to mean weapons and arms.

⁴⁹The armour or coat of mail, protects the shoulders, back, chest, and lower parts of the body.

⁵¹His share: The wealth obtained through defeating the enemy should not be usurped by the King, but distributed amongst the warring soldiers.

⁵²The priests teach the King, and the King the Knower of the Vedas teaches them. Knowledge is thus preserved and expanded through deliberations.

⁵³The text has occurred in 12-31, with a different interpretation.

May thou endowed with convincing knowledge, shining with the light of mastery of various subjects, be propitious unto us!

५४. पञ्च दिशो देवीर्यज्ञमवन्तु देवीरपामति दुर्मति बाधमाना: ।
रायस्पोषे यज्ञपतिमाभजन्ती रायस्पोषे अधि यज्ञो अस्थात् ॥

54. Casting aside dense ignorance and evil genius, these educated wives of the learned, engaged in different duties like the five regions, for the growth of riches, serving their husbands should yearn for domestic life, whereby this domestic life be made firm in the aquisition of wealth.

५५. समिद्धे अग्नावधि मामहान उक्थपत्र ईड्यो गृभीत: ।
तप्तं धर्म परिगृह्यायजन्तोजाँ यद्यज्ञमयजन्त देवा: ॥

55. Just as the learned, in enkindled fire, perform Agnihotra yajna, so should a highly revered person, the singer of vedic hymns, adorable, lovable sacrificer perform the well lighted yajna, accepting it with vigour.

५६. देव्याय धर्त्रे जोष्ट्रे देवश्री: श्रीमना: शतपया: ।
परिगृह्य देवा यज्ञमायन् देवा देवेभ्यो अध्वर्यन्तो अस्थु: ॥

56. Just as learned persons, desirous of performing yajna, engage themselves in the performance of Agni Hotra yajna for the happiness of the learned, and just as for the loving, benign, and virtuous priest, the wealth of knowledge, and a sacrificer (Yajman) intent on acquiring riches, and lord of a hundred drinkable objects like milk and its ilk, are there, so should ye the imparters of knowledge, having acquired learning perform the Agni Hotra yajna.

५७. वीतꣳ हवि: शमितꣳ शमिता यजध्यै तुरीयो यज्ञो यत्र हव्यमेति ।
ततो वाका आशिषो नो जुषन्ताम् ॥

57. The householder, who with a tranquil mind, puts into the fire, for performing the yajna, the oblation which moves above and removes foul smell, performs the fourth yajna. May prayers and the fulfilment of our desires bless us in the yajna where we get material fit for Homa.

५८. सूर्यरश्मिहरिकेश: पुरस्तात्सविता ज्योतिरुदयाँ अजस्त्रम् ।
तस्य पूषा प्रसवे याति विद्वान्त्सम्पश्यन्विश्वा भुवनानि गोपा: ॥

58. Sun gives us light from the beginning of creation. Its rays are green. In the created world it incessantly gives us strength. A learned person per-

---

⁵⁶Priest means Hota.
⁵⁷Fourth yajna: Excellent yajna. In Shatapatha Brahmana 9-2-3-11 the Turiya (fourth) yajna is described as one in which the Adhwaryu sings verses from the Yajur Veda, and then Hota recites hymns from the Rig Veda, and then Brahma recites the Apratirath or irresistible Sukta (R.V. 10-103). Professor Eggeling remarks that these verses (33-44) are enigmatical, but his view is incorrect, as the verses are clear.

ceiving fully realises its science. With its light, the Earth, planets and stars, the protectors of the world, manifest all regions.

५९. विमान एष दिवो मध्य आस्त आपप्रिवान् रोदसी अन्तरिक्षम् ।
स विश्वाचीरभि चष्टे घृताचीरन्तरा पूर्वमपरं च केतुम् ॥

59. This sun, in the midst of heaven, like an aroplane, sits, filling the earth, sky and air's mid region, with its light. It spreads its beams that illumine the world and give us water. It sheds its lustre on the day, the night and the intervening period.

६०. उक्षा समुद्रो अरुण: सुपर्ण: पूर्वस्य योनि पितुरा विवेश ।
मध्ये दिवो निहित: पृश्निरश्मा वि चक्रमे रजसस्पात्यन्तौ ॥

60. God has set the sun in the midst of heaven. It attracts rain-water and pours it down, is red, protects us thoroughly, possesses diverse coloured rays, rotates, keeps under check the clouds and different worlds, and guards them. It pervades lightning, the efficient cause of light.

६१. इन्द्रं विश्वा अवीवृधन्त्समुद्रव्यचसं गिर: ।
रथीतमः रथीनां वाजानाः सत्पतिं पतिम् ॥

61. All vedic songs glorify God, expansive like the space, the most delightful of all pleasant objects, the Lord of the wise, the Guardian of eternal matter and souls.

६२. देवहूयज्ञं आ च वक्षत्सुम्नहूयज्ञं आ च वक्षत् ।
यक्षदग्निर्देवो देवाँर् आ च वक्षत् ॥

62. God is the Invoker of the learned, Adorable, our Instructor in truth and Relinquisher from untruth, the Bestower of pleasures, Worshipful, the giver of comfort and remover of discomforts. May the Effulgent God grant and procure us noble qualities.

६३. वाजस्य मा प्रसव उद्ग्राभेणोदग्रभीत् ।
अधा सपत्नानिन्द्रो मे निग्राभेणाधरांर् अक: ॥

63. Just as God, the Sustainer, the Producer of Knowledge, through devices of elevation lifts me up, so elect him as General of the army who with his subjugating power keeps my foemen down.

६४. उद्ग्राभं च निग्राभं च ब्रह्म देवा अवीवृधन् ।
अधा सपत्नानिन्द्राग्नी मे विष्वञ्चीनान्व्यस्यताम् ॥

64. May the learned increase wealth through strenuous exertion and renunciation; and may the military and civil heads of the State, drive away my opposing foes.

---

[59]Like an aeroplane : Just as aeroplanes fly high in the sky and look wonderful, so does the sun appear beautiful and wonderous when it shines in the sky.
The night : Moon receives light from the sun, and illumines the night.

६५. क्रमध्वमग्निना नाकमुख्यꣳ हस्तेषु बिभ्रतः ।
दिवस्पृष्ठꣳ स्वर्गंत्वा मिश्रा देवेभिराध्वम् ॥

65. Ye heroes, with spiritual force in your hand, attain to happiness through the science of electricity. Having procured the desired happiness resulting from justice and humility, live in the company of the learned!

६६. प्राचीमनु प्रदिशं प्रेहि विद्वानग्नेरग्ने पुरो अग्निर्भवेह ।
विश्वा आशा दीद्यानो वि भाह्य जं नो धेहि द्विपदे चतुष्पदे ॥

66. O King, go forward to the eastern region. In thy state, with the use of fiery weapons, be a skilled leader full of passion like fire. Illumining all the quarters, shine with splendour; supply food to our quadrupeds and bipeds!

६७. पृथिव्या अहमुदन्तरिक्षमारुहमन्तरिक्षाद्दिवमारुहम् ।
दिवो नाकस्य पृष्ठात् स्वर्ज्योतिरगामहम् ॥

67. Through yoga, from physical force I rise higher to mental force; from mental force I rise higher to spiritual force; from spiritual force I rise higher to God, the Blissful Light.

६८. स्वर्यन्तो नापेक्षन्त आ द्यांꣳ रोहन्ति रोदसी ।
यज्ञं ये विश्वतोधारꣳ सुविद्वाꣳसो वितेनिरे ॥

68. The learned yogis, who attain to God, the Sustainer of the universe, on their march to salvation, pay no attention to worldly pleasures, but rise to salvation, that frees them from birth and death.

६९. अग्ने प्रेहि प्रथमो देवयतां चक्षुर्देवानामुत मर्त्यानाम् ।
इयक्षमाणा भृगुभिः सजोषाः स्वर्यन्तु यजमानाः स्वस्ति ॥

69. Foremost of those who exert, O learned person, come forward, thou art the eye of the literate and the illiterate!

The sacrificers, fain to worship, friendly to all, accordant with the highly learned persons, attain to ordinary and extreme happiness.

७०. नक्तोषासा समनसा विरूपे धापयेते शिशुमेकꣳ समीची ।
द्यावाक्षामा रुक्मो अन्तर्वि भाति देवा अग्निं धारयन् द्रविणोदाः ॥

70. Just as the nurse and mother with different characteristics, but with one mind, working in harmony suckle the same child, so do the night and dawn, with different hues nourish the world. Just as the brilliant sun shines between the Heaven and Earth, so do the imparters of knowledge imbibe the glow of knowledge.

---

[65] Ukha : Spiritual force.
[67] Antrikshaloka is described in the Shatapatha Brahmana as mind, vide Shatapatha 14/4/3/11. The verse may also mean, a yogi through yogic practices, can rise from the earth to the space, from the space to the sun, from the sun rise to the height of happiness.
[69] Eye: who keeps a watch over their doings, and shows them the right path.
[70] See 12-2. The text is the same, but meanings are different.

CHAPTER XVII

७१. अग्ने सहस्राक्ष शतमूर्धञ्छतं ते प्राणाः सहस्रं व्यानाः ।
तव ँ साहस्रस्य राय ईशिषे तस्मै ते विधेम वाजाय स्वाहा ॥

71. O yogi, thou hast the knowledge of innumerable usages, immense power of meditation, hundreds of accomplishments of life, and thousands of modes of activity. Thou art the Lord of thousandfold possessions. To thee full of knowledge may we offer our obeisance in truthful words!

७२. सुपर्णोऽसि गरुत्मान् पृष्ठे पृथिव्याः सीद ।
भासाऽन्तरिक्षमा पृण ज्योतिषा दिवमुत्तभान तेजसा दिश उद्दृ ँ ह ॥

72. O learned yogi, with thy light, thou art endowed with excellent noble qualities, yoked with high soul-power. Just as the sun shines in the midst of heaven, so do thou be seated on earth. Grant happiness to the people like air. As the sun fills air's mid-region with its glow, so shouldst thou strengthen sovereignty with thy statesmanship. Just as fire with its intense heat fills the quarters, so shouldst thou elevate the people!

७३. आजुह्वानः सुप्रतीकः पुरस्तादग्ने स्वं योनिमा सीद साधुया ।
अस्मिन्त्सधस्थे अध्युत्तरस्मिन्विश्वे देवा यजमानश्च सीदत ॥

73. Thou, whose soul is enlightened with yoga, who invitest respect from those who contact thee, the master of good traits, the teacher of the science of yoga, through thy virtuous deeds, seat thyself firmly in God thy nearest home. Ye all yogis, with laudable acts, stick fast to truth after discussion!

७४. ता ँ सवितुर्वरेण्यस्य चित्रामाऽहं वृणे सुमतिं विश्वजन्याम् ।
यामस्य कण्वो अदुहत्प्रपीना ँ सहस्रधारां पयसा महीं गाम् ॥

74. Just as a wise person, knows the exalted vedic speech of God, the Adorable, the Giver of the glory of yoga, and enhances his knowledge with that speech, that is wondrous, explains the creation of the universe, is full of knowledge, explains each topic lucidly and gives us wisdom and food, so do I rightly accept it.

७५. विधेम ते परमे जन्मन्नग्ने विधेम स्तोमैरवरे सधस्थे ।
यस्माद्योनेरुदारिथा यजे तं प्र त्वे हवी ँ षि जुहुरे समिद्धे ॥

75. O Yogi, we adore thee with praise-songs for thy past life, and for thy present life, in which we live with thee. May we worship God through whose shelter thou hast risen. Just as the performers of Homa, put oblations in the well kindled fire, so do we remove our moral weaknesses through the fire of yoga!

७६. प्रेद्धो अग्ने दीदिहि पुरो नोऽजस्रया सूर्म्या यविष्ठ ।
त्वा ँ शश्वन्त उप यन्ति वाजाः ॥

[74] It refers to vedic speech.

76. O most youthful yogi, first enkindled with dignity, with continuous supremacy, long for us. Constantly unto thee come the learned.

७७. अग्ने तमद्याश्वं न स्तोमैः क्रतुं न भद्रꣳ हृदिस्पृशम् ।
ऋध्यामा त ओहैः ॥

77. O learned person, just as a horse is fed with fodder, and intellect sharpened with prayers, so art thou beneficent and pleasing to our heart; may we approach thee with praises, and advance under thy protections.

७८. चित्तिं जुहोमि मनसा घृतेन यथा देवा इहागमन्वीतिहोत्रा ऋतावृधः ।
पत्ये विश्वस्य भूमनो जहोमि विश्वकर्मणे विश्वाहाऽदाभ्यꣳ हविः ॥

78. Just as an oblation is put with butter, into the fire, filled with fuel, so with a contemplative mind do I acquire discernment so that the learned, who strengthen truth, and are devoted to knowledge, may come here. To God, Lord of the Earth, and Master of all deeds, I offer up day after day the inviolable sacrifice of knowledge.

७९. सप्त ते अग्ने समिधः सप्त जिह्वाः सप्त ऋषयः सप्त धाम प्रियाणि ।
सप्त होत्राः सप्तधा त्वा यजन्ति सप्त योनीरा पृणस्व घृतेन स्वाहा ॥

79. O Sage, seven breaths are thy fuel, seven flames are thy flames of knowledge, seven organs of perception are thy sources of wisdom. Thou hast seven beloved mansions. Seven priests in sevenfold manner pay thee worship. With knowledge and fine speech fill full these seven sources of learning!

८०. शुक्रज्योतिश्च चित्रज्योतिश्च सत्यज्योतिश्च ज्योतिष्माँश्च ।
शुक्रश्च ऋतपाश्चात्यꣳहाः ॥

80. God is Purely Bright. Wonderfully Bright, Eternally Bright, All Luminous, Bright, Truth's Protector, and free from Sin.

८१. ईदृङ् चान्यादृङ् च सदृङ् च प्रतिसदृङ् च ।
मितश्च सम्मितश्च समराः ॥

[76]Most youthful : most advanced in knowledge.
[77]See 15-44. The text is the same, but interpretation different. Protections means qualities of protection.
[79]प्राणो वै समिधः श० 9-2-3-44.
Seven breaths : Pran, Apan, Saman, Vyan, Udan, Devdutt, Dhananjaya.
Seven flames : Kali, Karali, Manojava, Sulohita, Sudhumravarna, Sphulingini, Vishvarupi. These have been spoken as seven tongues in the text.
Seven organs : Nose, tongue, eye, ear, skin, mind, intellect. These are called seven Rishis.
Seven Mansions (धाम) : जन्म, स्थान, नाम, धर्म, अर्थ, काम, मोक्ष ।
Seven priests : the seven organs of perception.
Sevenfold manner : Seven Rishis perform their duties in connection with the subject concerned, i.e., *eye* with seeing, ear with hearing, tongue with speaking etc.

81. Persons, who are excellent like God, noble like other good people, equal towards all, affectionate towards all, respectable, wellbalanced and possessors of worldly objects, succeed in life.

८२. ऋतश्च सत्यश्च ध्रुवश्च धरुणश्च । धर्ता च विधर्ता च विधारयः ॥

82. God is the Knower of truth, Most Excellent amongst the excellent, Resolute, the Support of all, the Sustainer, the Owner of all owners, and efficient Administrator.

८३. ऋतजिच्च सत्यजिच्च सेनजिच्च सुषेणश्च ।
अन्तिमित्रश्च दूरे अमित्रश्च गणः ॥

83. He, who is the advancer of knowledge, elevator of religion, Conqueror of armies, lord of goodly forces, keeper of friends near at hand; driver afar of foes, is worthy of estimation.

८४. ईदृक्षास एतादृक्षास ऊ षु णः सदृक्षासः प्रतिसदृक्षास एतन ।
मितासश्च सम्मितासो नो अद्य सभरसो मरुतो यज्ञे अस्मिन् ॥

84. O learned persons, the performers of seasonwise sacrifice (Yajna), well-qualified, resembling the aforesaid sacrificers, free from partiality, similar in nature to the highly learned, truthful and religious, come near unto us!
May the knowers of reality, discriminators of truth from untruth like a balance, the supporters and nourishers of their companions, protect us today in this sacrifice.

८५. स्वतवाँश्च प्रधासी च सान्तपनश्च गृहमेधी च ।
क्रीडी च शाकी चोज्जेषी ॥

85. He who exalts his men, feasts on dainty dishes, torments the foes, is an admirable householder, lover of games, and mighty, becomes a nice conqueror.

८६. इन्द्रं दैवीर्विशो मरुतोऽनुवर्तमानोऽभवन्यथेन्द्रं दैवीर्विशो मरुतोऽनुवर्तमानोऽभवन् ।
एवमिमं यजमानं दैवीश्च विशो मानषीश्चानुवर्तमानो भवन्तु ॥

86. O King, behave so that thy learned subjects regular performers of yajna, may become thy followers. Just as learned people, dear as breath, follow God, so should the literate and the illiterate persons follow this King, the giver of happiness through knowledge and teaching!

८७. इमꣳ स्तनमूर्जस्वन्तं धयापां प्रपीनमग्ने सरिरस्य मध्ये ।
उत्सं जषस्व मधमन्तमर्वन्त्समुद्रियꣳ सदनमा विशस्व ॥

87. O man resplendent like fire, drink as from a teat filled with milk, this invigorating juice of waters. In the midst of many welcome this well full of sweet water. Fast like a horse, enter thy oceanic dwellings.

[87]This text has also a spiritual meaning as follows :
O learned person, drink deep from the Vedas, God's teats, full of significant, forceful words, enjoy sweet, progressive devotion, and through contemplation, reach the spiritual home of knowledge.

८८. घृतं मिमिक्ष घृतमस्य योनिर्घृ ते श्रितो घृतम्वस्य धाम ।
अनुष्वधमा वह मादयस्व स्वाहाकृतं वृषभ वक्षि हव्यम् ॥

88. O sailor, wish thou to master water. Ghee is the home of fire. It rests in ghee. Ghee is its proper province. Utilise that fire for producing foodstuffs. O giver of pleasures; thou receivest the oblation consecrated through vedic incantations, hence gladden us!

८९. समुद्रादूर्मिमंधुमाँ२ उदारदुपाꣳशुना सममृतत्वमानट् ।
घृतस्य नाम गुह्यं यदस्ति जिह्वा देवानाममृतस्य नाभि: ॥

89. O men, know that forth from the ocean springs the watery wave of sweetness with rays of the sun. Being divine it is extremely pleasant in taste. The real cause of water is hidden. Salvation is the result of the teachings of the learned!

९०. वयं नाम प्र ब्रवामा घृतस्यास्मिन् यज्ञे धारायामा नमोभि: ।
उप ब्रह्मा शृणवच्छस्यमानं चतु:शृङ्गोऽवमीद्गौर एतत् ॥

90. He, whose knowledge of the four vedas is like four horns, who studies and enjoys the vedas, is perfectly well versed in them all, preaches them to humanity, and listens to their teachings from others, is the praiseworthy embodiment of knowledge. It is our duty to propagate it to others, and act upon it in our domestic life with words of veneration.

९१. चत्वारि शृङ्गा त्रयो अस्य पादा द्वे शीर्षे सप्त हस्तासो अस्य ।
त्रिधा बद्धो वृषभो रोरवीति महो देवो मर्त्याँ२ आ विवेश ॥

91. This yajna has got four horns, three feet, two heads, and seven hands, This mighty, attainable yajna, the giver of happiness, bound with a triple bond, roars loudly and enters into mortals.

९२. त्रिधा हितं पणिभिर्गुह्यमानं गवि देवासो घृतमन्वविन्दन् ।
इन्द्र एकꣳ सूर्य एकं जजान वेनादेकꣳ स्वधया निष्टतक्षु: ॥

[89]The real cause: Primordial matter the real cause of water is hidden, mysterious and unmanifested.

Professor Ludwig is unnecessarily furious over she explanations which Sayana gives. The sense of the text is not obscure as alleged by him.

[90]Professor Wilson following Sayana wrongly interprets the epithet 'four horned' as applying to God, who may be called a buffalo as a type of extraordinary strength. Mahidhar's interpretation of four horns as four officiating priests is also wide of the mark. 'Four horns' is a phrase used figuratively to denote the knowledge of the four vedas by a learned person. Horns are pillars of spiritual knowledge.

[91]Four horns : The four vedas.
Three feet : Morning, noon, and evening.
Two heads : The rising and setting times of the sun.
Seven hands : The seven metres of the veda like Gayatri etc.

92. The learned, masters of the worldly affairs, acquire after research the knowledge hidden in the vedas, and laid three-wise. Electricity exposes a part of that knowledge, sun another part, and the learned the third part by their wisdom and experience.

९३. एता अर्षन्ति हृद्यात्समुद्राच्छतव्रजा रिपुणा नावचक्षे ।
घृतस्य धारा अभि चाकशीमि हिरण्ययो वेतसो मध्य आसाम् ॥

93. These vedic speeches which flow from the inmost reservoir of the heart are incontrovertible by the thievish foe. I realise these speeches full of knowledge and see in their midst the Resplendent, Beautiful God.

९४. सम्यक् स्रवन्ति सरितो न धेना अन्तर्हृदा मनसा पूयमानाः ।
एते अर्षन्त्यूर्मयो घृतस्य मृगा इव क्षिपणोरीषमाणाः ॥

94. From the inmost recesses of the heart, purified by mind, flow together our speeches as streams flow to the ocean. These waves of knowledge pour swiftly like the deer running through the fear of a tiger.

९५. सिन्धोरिव प्राध्वने शूधनासो वातप्रमियः पतयन्ति यह्वाः ।
घृतस्य धारा अरुषो न वाजी काष्ठा भिन्दन्नूर्मिभिः पिन्वमानः ॥

95. Just as rushing down the rapids of a river, fall swifter than the wind the vigorous currents, just as the swift fleeting horse, breaking aside the battlefields, falls upon the enemy, watering the earth with perspiration arising out of his endeavour to kill the foe, so do the exalted speeches, full of knowledge, fall on the audience from the mouth of a preacher.

९६. अभि प्रवन्त समनेव योषाः कल्याण्यः समयमानासो अग्निम् ।
घृतस्य धाराः समिधो नसन्त ता जुषाणो हर्यति जातवेदाः ॥

96. Just as women of high character, of one mind, gently smiling, incline towards their husbands, so do the speeches of pure knowledge, glowing with apt use, meaning, and relation of words, reach a learned person, who enjoying them attains to brilliance.

Triple bond : The Mantra, Kalpa and Brahmana, prayer, ceremonial and rationale of the veda, or the three regions, Heaven, Firmament, and Earth.
Loud roaring is the sound of the recitation of the vedic verses.
Different explanations have been given by Mahidhar for these words.
Patanjali in his immortal work the Mahabhashya explains these words differently.
The verse can be applied to grammar (शब्द-शास्त्र).
Four horns are नाम (Noun) आख्यात (verb), उपसर्ग (a preposition prefixed to roots) and निपात (Indeclinable).
Three feet: Past, present and future.
Two heads: Nitya and कार्य (Effect).
Seven hands: Seven cases.
Triple bonds: Heart, Throat and Head.
[92]Laid threewise: placed in the earth, atmosphere and heaven, contemplation (Upasana) or in the form of knowledge (Jnan) and Action (Karma).
[96]One mind: Husband and wife should be of one agreeable mind, attached to each other.

६७. कन्या इव वहतुमेतवा उ अञ्ज्यञ्जाना अभि चाकशीमि ।
यत्र सोमः सूयते यत्र यज्ञो घृतस्य धारा अभि तत्पवन्ते ॥

97. As maidens deck themselves with gay adornments and exhibit their beauty to join their husbands, so, where prosperity reigns, where yajna is performed, there the intellectual speeches are sanctified on all sides, which I enjoy again and again.[97]

६८. अभ्यर्षत सुष्टुतिं गव्यमाजिमस्मासु भद्रा द्रविणानि धत्त ।
इमं यज्ञं नयत देवता नो घृतस्य धारा मधुमत्पवन्ते ॥

98. O married couple, welcome the laudable struggle for existence, procure the wisdom of speech, milk, curd and butter. May the learned bestow on us excellent possessions, and grant us this domestic life. The learned receive the instructive, sweet words of knowledge!

६९. धाम ते विश्वं भुवनमधि श्रितमन्तः समुद्रे हृद्यन्तरायुषि ।
अपामनीके समिथे य आभृतस्तमश्याम मधुमन्तं त ऊर्मिम् ॥

99. O God, this whole universe depends upon Thy power and might vast like the atmosphere. May we realise Thee!
O king may we acquire the strength that lies in thy breaths, thy heart, thy lively soldiers and thy battlefield, and thy wisdom full of admirable characteristics!

---

[97] I : a learned person.

CHAPTER XVIII

१. वाजश्च मे प्रसवश्च मे प्रयतिश्च मे प्रसितिश्च मे धीतिश्च मे क्रतुश्च मे स्वरश्च मे श्लोकश्च मे श्रवश्च मे श्रुतिश्च मे ज्योतिश्च मे स्वश्च मे यज्ञेन कल्पन्ताम् ॥

1. May my food and my prosperity, my exertion and my influence, my thought and my mental power, my independence and my speech, my hearing and my vedic knowledge, the light of my learning and my pleasure prosper through the contemplation of Adorable God, and the performance of philanthropic deeds for the good of humanity.

२. प्राणश्च मेऽपानश्च मे व्यानश्च मेऽसुश्च मे चित्तं च म आधीतं च मे वाक् च मे मनश्च मे चक्षुश्च मे श्रोत्रं च मे दक्षश्च मे बलं च मे यज्ञेन कल्पन्ताम् ॥

2. May my Pran and Apan, my Vyan and my Dhananjaya, my Nag breath and other breaths, my memory and my well defined knowledge, my voice and hearing, my mind and reflections, my eye and knowledge, my ear and vedic authority, my wisdom and honour, my strength and valour, prosper through the practice of religion.

३. ओजश्च मे सहश्च म आत्मा च मे तनूश्च मे शर्म च मे वर्म च मेऽङ्गानि च मेऽस्थीनि च मे परूँषि च मे शरीराणि च म आयुश्च मे जरा च मे यज्ञेन कल्पन्ताम् ॥

3. May my energy and my army, my soul and my body, my house and my armour, my limbs and my bones, my joints and my relatives' bodies, my life and my resources, my old age and youth prosper through the grace of God.

४. ज्यैष्ठ्यं च म आधिपत्यं च मे मन्युश्च मे भामश्च मेऽमश्च मेऽम्भश्च मे जेमा च मे महिमा च मे वरिमा च मे प्रथिमा च मे वर्षिमा च मे द्राघिमा च मे वृद्धं च मे वृद्धिश्च मे यज्ञेन कल्पन्ताम् ॥

4. May my preeminence and nice objects, my overlordship and property, my righteous indignation and tranquillity of mind, my angry passion and noble behaviour, my just possessions and acquirable objects, my coolness like water, and my milk, curd and butter, my victorious power and victory, my greatness and honour, my magnanimity and excellent conduct, my abundance and vast objects, my old age and youth, the continuity of my family and its smallness, my increase of riches and penury, my amelioration and consequent happiness prosper through religious practices.

*Pran : The breath that moves above the navel. Apan is the breath that moves down the navel. Vyan is the breath that moves throughout the body, and specially resides in the navel. Other breaths are Devdutt, Dhananjaya, etc.

५. सत्यं च मे श्रद्धा च मे जगच्च मे धनं च मे विश्वं च मे महश्च मे क्रीडा च मे मोदश्च मे जातं च मे जनिष्यमाणं च मे सूक्तं च मे सुकृतं च मे यज्ञेन कल्पन्ताम् ॥

5. May my truth and love for all, my faith and things that lead to its accomplishment, my progeny and their possessions, my wealth and food stuffs, my belongings and philanthropy, my beauty and honour, my play and sports materials, my enjoyment and extreme delight, my children born before and those born anew, my future children and my relation with them, my nice words and reflections, my pious acts and their aids prosper through true religious teachings.

६. ऋतं च मेऽमृतं च मे ऽयक्ष्मं च मे ऽनामयच्च मे जीवातुश्च मे दीर्घायुत्वं च मेऽनमित्रं च मे ऽभयं च मे सुखं च मे शयनं च मे सूषाश्च मे सुदिनं च मे यज्ञेन कल्पन्ताम् ॥

6. May my knowledge and its contributory cause, my immortality and juice worth drinking, my freedom from consumption and acts that remove sickness, my age free from disease and medicines that contribute to it, my life-strength and abstemiousness, my longevity and celibacy, my freedom from enemies and love for justice, my freedom from fear and valour, my happiness and its cause, my sleep and its contributory cause, my fair dawn and its cause, my fair day and useful deeds prosper through truthfulness.

७. यन्ता च मे धर्ता च मे क्षेमश्च मे धृतिश्च मे विश्वं च मे महश्च मे संविच्च मे ज्ञात्रं च मे सूश्च मे प्रसूश्च मे सीरं च मे लयश्च मे यज्ञेन कल्पन्ताम् ॥

7. May my leader and well-controlled possessions, my supporters and accepted truths, my protection and protector, my finances and toleration, my world and obedience to its laws, my mighty deeds and fair dealings, my determination and knowledge, my understanding and objects worth knowing, my impulses and thoughts, my propagation and eugenics, my plough and cultivators, my concentration and learning, prosper by following noble principles.

८. शं च मे मयश्च मे प्रियं च मेऽनुकामश्च मे कामश्च मे सौमनसश्च मे भगश्च मे द्रविणं च मे भद्रं च मे श्रेयश्च मे वसीयश्च मे यशश्च मे यज्ञेन कल्पन्ताम् ॥

8. May my welfare and its materials, my comfort and its means, my affection and its sources, my religious desire and its means, my purity of mind and its sources, my immense supremacy and its means my strength and its sources, my pleasure-giving comfort and its means, my pleasure of salvation and its sources, my excellent residence and its materials, my fame and its cause prosper through the grace of God.

९. उर्क् च मे सूनृता च मे पयश्च मे रसश्च मे घृतं च मे मधु च मे सग्धिश्च मे सपीतिश्च मे कृषिश्च मे वृष्टिश्च मे जैत्रं च म औद्भिद्यं च मे यज्ञेन कल्पन्ताम् ॥

9. May my well-cooked and fragrant food, my affectionate and truthful speech, my milk and prepared medicines, my sap and medicinal juices, my

butter and food cooked with it, my honey and sugar, my meals in company and means of enjoyment, my drinking in company and objects to be licked, my agriculture and foodgrains, my rain and purification of air through Homa, my impulse for conquest and trained army, my flowers and trees, flourish through the prayer of God.

१०. रयिश्च मे रायश्च मे पुष्टं च मे पुष्टिश्च मे विभु च मे प्रभु च मे पूर्णं च मे पूर्णतरं च मे कुयवं च मेऽक्षितं च मेऽन्न' च मेऽक्षुच्च मे यज्ञेन कल्पन्ताम् ॥

10. May the wealth of knowledge and enterprise, my property and cooked food, my prosperity and health, my mind the master of all topics and God's contemplation, my entire dealings and power, my accomplishment, cows, buffaloes, horses, and service of mankind, my pure foodgrains and rice, my freedom from hunger and thirst, my food and its spices, my satiety in food and thirst prosper through the kindness of God.

११. वित्तं च मे वेद्यं च मे भूतं च मे भविष्यच्च मे सुगं च मे सुपथ्यं च म ऋद्धं च म ऋद्धिश्च मे क्लृप्तं च मे क्लृप्तिश्च मे मतिश्च मे सुमतिश्च मे यज्ञेन कल्पन्ताम् ॥

11. May my well considered problems and my reflections, my topic worthy of consideration and thought, my past and present, my future and constant noble dealings, my good path and noble deeds, my wholesome diet and diagnosis, my prosperity and supernatural power, my achievement through yoga and contentment, my power and imagination, my ambition for strength and logic, my thought and investigation, my advanced intellect and steadiness prosper through the grace of God.

१२. व्रीहयश्च मे यवाश्च मे माषाश्च मे तिलाश्च मे मुद्गाश्च मे खल्वाश्च मे प्रियङ्गवश्च मेऽणवश्च मे श्यामाकाश्च मे नीवाराश्च मे गोधूमाश्च मे मसूराश्च मे यज्ञेन कल्पन्ताम् ॥

12. May my rice and my barley, my pulses and beans, my sesamum and grams, my kidney-beans and their cooking, my grams and their cooking, my millet and its cooking, my excellent rice and inferior corn, my rice of wild growth and their cooking, my wheat and its cooking, my lentils and other foodgrains prosper through the grace of God.

१३. अश्मा च मे मृत्तिका च मे गिरयश्च मे पर्वताश्च मे सिकताश्च मे वनस्पतयश्च मे हिरण्यं च मेऽयश्च मे श्यामं च मे लोहं च मे सीसं च मे त्रपु च मे यज्ञेन कल्पन्ताम् ॥

13. May my stone and ruby, my refined and rough clay, my clouds and corns, my mountains and their products, my sand thick and pulverised, my banyan trees and mango trees, my riches and silver, my iron and weapons, my sapphire and brilliant gem, my gold and precious stone, my lead and wax, my zinc and brass, multiply through governmental arrangements.

[12]Wild rice: which grow spontaneously without being sown.
[13]Government can work out the mines either directly or by giving licenses to the private individuals.

१४. अग्निश्च म आपश्च मे वीरुधश्च म ओषधयश्च मे कृष्टपच्याश्च मेऽकृष्टपच्याश्च मे ग्राम्याश्च मे पशव आरण्याश्च मे वित्तं च मे वित्तिश्च मे भूतं च मे भूतिश्च मे यज्ञेन कल्पन्ताम् ।

14. May my fire and lightning, my water and gems found in it, my creepers and vegetables, my plants and flowers, my corns ripened in fields and nice foodgrains, my corns ripened spontaneously in the jungles and those which ripen in the forest, my domestic animals and my wild forest animals, my substance and wealth, my gain and objects worth acquiring, my beauty and diverse possessions, my power and its source progress through skill and art.

१५. वसु च मे वसतिश्च मे कर्म च मे शक्तिश्च मे ऽर्थश्च म एमश्च म इत्या च मे गतिश्च मे यज्ञेन कल्पन्ताम् ॥

15. May my treasure and virtuous act, my dwelling and servants, my religious service and its doer, my ability and love, my collection of wealth and its collector, my noble effort and intellect, my way of knowing, my dealings and reason, my gait and muscular exercise prosper through exertion.

१६. अग्निश्च म इन्द्रश्च मे सोमश्च म इन्द्रश्च मे सविता च म इन्द्रश्च मे सरस्वती च म इन्द्रश्च मे पूषा च म इन्द्रश्च मे बृहस्पतिश्च म इन्द्रश्च मे यज्ञेन कल्पन्ताम् ॥

16. May my fiery sun and earthly fire, my lightning and air, my peace-affording articles and rain, my ruler the dispeller of injustice, and his ministers, my prosperous deed and its means, my teacher, the banisher of ignorance, and pupil, my instructive speech and the speaker of truth, my preacher, the remover of stupidity, and listeners, my nourisher and abstemiousness, my soul and physician, my guardian of vedic lore and King, my lord of supremacy and general of the army, prosper through the advancement of knowledge.

१७. मित्रश्च म इन्द्रश्च मे वरुणश्च म इन्द्रश्च मे धाता च म इन्द्रश्च मे त्वष्टा च म इन्द्रश्च मे मरुतश्च म इन्द्रश्च मे विश्वे च मे देवा इन्द्रश्च मे यज्ञेन कल्पन्ताम् ॥

17. May my breath residing in the heart and breath in the navel, my electrical fire and lustre, my breath in the throat and breath pervading the entire body, my sun and power of retention and attraction, my soul and patience, my bestower of supreme prosperity and just enterprise, my fire, the Consumer of substances and artisanship, my ruler, the extinguisher of foes, and craftsmanship, my airs and bodily humours, my ubiquitous lightning and its performances, may all belongings and riches, my beautiful forces of

---

16-17 In these two verses Griffith has not translated the twenty four words used, and put them as they are, which makes the sense unintelligible. The word Indra has been used twelve times in these two verses, which has in each case been translated differently by Swami Dayananda.

Giver of glory : Soul.

CHAPTER XVIII

nature, my giver of glory and its use, prosper through the knowledge of the science of air.

१८. पृथिवी च म इन्द्रश्च मेऽन्तरिक्षं च म इन्द्रश्च मे द्यौश्च म इन्द्रश्च मे समाश्च म इन्द्रश्च मे नक्षत्राणि च म इन्द्रश्च मे दिशश्च म इन्द्रश्च मे यज्ञेन कल्पन्ताम् ॥

18. May my earth and its substances, my electricity and physical exercise, my atmosphere and objects that reside in space, my support of supremacy and its use, my knowledge that leads to noble deeds and its contributory causes, my sun and substances diffused by it, my years and divisions of time, my apparent cause of the knowledge of time and the science of Arithmetic, my everlasting worlds and their inhabitants, my lightning, my regions and the substances residing therein, my teacher of the science of regions and Dhruva star prosper through the knowledge of Earth and Time.

१९. अ‍ंशुश्च मे रश्मिश्च मेऽदाभ्यश्च मेऽधिपतिश्च म उपा‍ंशुश्च मेऽन्तर्यामश्च म ऐन्द्रवायवश्च मे मैत्रावरुणश्च म आश्विनश्च मे प्रतिप्रस्थानश्च मे शुक्रश्च मे मन्थी च मे यज्ञेन कल्पन्ताम् ।

19. May my pervading sun and its heat, my method of eating and dainty dishes, my firm rule and protector, my master and his residence, my mental contemplation and solitude, my mid-breath and strength, my action dealing with electricity and air, and water, my Pran and Udan, and Vyan, my beauty like that of the sun and moon, and of mind, my gait and walks, my pure nature and semen, my spirit of investigation and milk-pot flourish through the proper use of fire.

२०. आग्रयणश्च मे वैश्वदेवश्च मे ध्रुवश्च मे वैश्वानरश्च म ऐन्द्राग्नश्च मे महावैश्वदेवश्च मे मरुत्वतीयाश्च मे निष्केवल्यश्च मे सावित्रश्च मे सारस्वतश्च मे पात्नीवतश्च मे हारियोजनश्च मे यज्ञेन कल्पन्ताम् ॥

20. May my yajna performed in November-December and its substances, my discourse with the learned and its result, my iron determination and its causes, my respect for all and respecter, my use of air and electricity and their sources, my spiritual enjoyment and its means, my lustre like the sun and its usefulness, my vows and their result, my performance of yajna in the company of my wife and its means, my procedure of yoking the horses in chariots and its materials prosper through skilful application of all substances.

२१. स्रुचश्च मे चमसाश्च मे वायव्यानि च मे द्रोणकलशश्च मे ग्रावाणश्च मेऽधिषवणे च मे पूतभृच्च म आधवनीयश्च मे वेदिश्च मे बर्हिश्च मेऽवभृथश्च मे स्वगाकारश्च मे यज्ञेन कल्पन्ताम् ।

21. May my ladles and their cleansing, my yajna cups and their contents,

my good substances in the air and its purifying acts, my Soma reservoir and its peculiar measurement, my pressing stones and mortar and pestle, my rod for pressing medicine, their pressing and grinding, my sauce and broom, my washing basin and telescope, my altar and its shape, my altar-grass and provisions for the yajna, my bath at the end of the yajna and smearing with fragrant sandal, my recitation of verses, and purifying oblations, prosper through the performance of Homa.

२२. अग्निश्च मे धर्मश्च मेऽर्कश्च मे सूर्यश्च मे प्राणश्च मेऽश्वमेधश्च मे पृथिवी च मेऽदितिश्च मे दितिश्च मे द्यौश्च मेऽङ्गुलयः शक्वरयो दिशश्च मे यज्ञेन कल्पन्ताम् ॥

22. May my fire and its use, my dignity and mental peace, my materials for worship and its purification, my sun and means of livelihood, my air, the cause of life and external air, my nation and national policy, my Earth and its trees, my uniform statesmanship and control of senses, my undecaying possessions and ephemeral body, my light of religion and day and night, my fingers, powers, four directions and sub-directions, be glorified through the grace of God.

२३. व्रतं च म ऋतवश्च मे तपश्च मे संवत्सरश्च मेऽहोरात्रे ऊर्वष्ठीवे बृहद्रथन्तरे च मे यज्ञेन कल्पन्ताम् ॥

23. May my sacred vow and speaking and preaching of truth, my inter seasons and progress of the sun to the North and solstices, my control of breath and heat and cold, my year and Kalpa and Mahakalpa, my thighs and knees, my big chariot, horses and bullocks prosper through religious practices.

२४. एका च मे तिस्रश्च मे तिस्रश्च मे पञ्च च मे पञ्च च मे सप्त च मे सप्त च मे नव च मे नव च म एकादश च म एकादश च मे त्रयोदश च मे त्रयोदश च मे पञ्चदश च मे पञ्चदश च मे सप्तदश च मे सप्तदश च मे नवदश च मे नवदश च म एकविꣳशतिश्च म एकविꣳशतिश्च मे त्रयोविꣳशतिश्च मे त्रयोविꣳशतिश्च मे पञ्चविꣳशतिश्च मे पञ्चविꣳशतिश्च मे सप्तविꣳशतिश्च मे सप्तविꣳशतिश्च मे नवविꣳशतिश्च मे नवविꣳशतिश्च म एकत्रिꣳशच्च म एकत्रिꣳशच्च मे त्रयस्त्रिꣳशच्च मे यज्ञेन कल्पन्ताम् ॥

---

[22] Fingers mean the armies, that catch hold of the foe, as fingers do an article.
Four directions : East, South, West and North.
Sub-Directions : Ishan (North East), Vayayya (North-West), Nairitya (South-West), Agneya (South-East).
[23] Solstices : Uttarayan and Dakshinayan.
Solstices : The time (21st June) at which the sun is farthest north, and is called the summer solstice, or about (22nd December) at which it is farthest south, is called the winter solstice. In the first case it touches the tropic of Cancer, and in the second that of Capricorn.

CHAPTER XVIII

24. May my One and my Three, and my Three and my Five, and my Five and my Seven, and my Seven and my Nine, and my Nine and my Eleven, and my Eleven and my Thirteen, and my Thirteen and my Fifteen, and my Fifteen and my Seventeen and my Seventeen and my Nineteen, and my Nineteen and my Twenty One, and my Twenty One and my Twenty Three, and my Twenty Three and my Twenty Five, and my Twenty Five and my Twenty Seven, and my Twenty Seven and my Twenty Nine, and my Twenty Nine and my Thirty One, and my Thirty One and my Thirty Three etcetera increase or decrease by addition or subtraction.

२५. चतस्रश्च मेऽष्टौ च मेऽष्टौ च मे द्वादश च मे द्वादश च मे षोडश च मे षोडश च मे विंशतिश्च मे विंशतिश्च मे चतुर्विंशतिश्च मे चतुर्विंशतिश्च मेऽष्टाविंशतिश्च मेऽष्टाविंशतिश्च मे द्वात्रिंशच्च मे द्वात्रिंशच्च मे षट्त्रिंशच्च मे षट्त्रिंशच्च मे चत्वारिंशच्च मे चत्वारिंशच्च मे चतुश्चत्वारिंशच्च मे चतुश्चत्वारिंशच्च मेऽष्टाचत्वारिंशच्च मे यज्ञेन कल्पन्ताम् ॥

25. May my Four and my Eight, and my Eight and my Twelve, and my Twelve and my Sixteen, and my Sixteen and my Twenty, and my Twenty and my Twenty Four, and my Twenty Four and my Twenty Eight, and my Twenty Eight and my Thirty Two, and my Thirty Two and my Thirty Six, and my Thirty Six and my Forty, and my Forty and my Forty Four, and my Forty Four and my Forty Eight etc. increase or decrease by addition and subtraction.

२६. त्र्यविश्च मे त्र्यवी च मे दित्यवाट् च मे दित्यौही च मे पञ्चाविश्च मे पञ्चावी च मे त्रिवत्सश्च मे त्रिवत्सा च मे तुर्यवाट् च मे तुर्यौही च मे यज्ञेन कल्पन्ताम् ॥

26. May my eighteen months bull and cow, my two years bull and cow, my thirty months bull and cow, my three years bull and cow, my four years bull and cow prosper through the science of rearing cattle.

२७. पष्ठवाट् च मे पष्ठौही च म उक्षा च मे वशा च म ऋषभश्च मे वेहच्च मेऽनड्वांश्च मे धेनुश्च मे यज्ञेन कल्पन्ताम् ॥

27. May my male beasts of burden like elephant and camel and similar beasts, my female beasts of burden like mare and she camel, and their loads,

---

[24] The odd digits of Arithmetic have been enumerated 1+2=3, 3+2=5, 5+2=7 and so on. So 33−2=31, 31−2=29, 29−2=27 etc. This verse teaches us addition and subtraction of Arithmetic from which are deduced multiplication, division, square, cube, square root, cube root, and reduction of fractions to a common denominator, described by Maharshi Dayananda in his commentary as योग (addition), बियोग (subtraction), गुणन (Multiplication), भाग (Division), वर्ग (Square), वर्गमूल (Squareroot), घन (cube), घनमूल (cuberoot) and भागजाति i.e., reduction of fractions to a common denominator.

The verse refers to Arithmetical progression with a common difference of two.

[25] In the last verse odd numbers were enumerated, whereas in this the even numbers are enumerated. The verse refers to Arithmetical progression with a common difference of four.

my powerful bull and cow, my impotent bull and barren cow, my young bull and strong cow, my calf-slipping and lean cow, my ox and cart-driver, my milch-cow and its milk-man prosper through proper training of cattle.

२८. वाजाय स्वाहा प्रसव।य स्वाहाऽपिजाय स्वाहा ऋतवे स्वाहा वसवे स्वाहाऽहर्पतये स्वाहाऽह्ने मुग्धाय स्वाहा मुग्धाय वेन॒ऽशिनाय स्वाहा विन॒ऽशिन श्रान्त्यायनाय स्वाहाऽन्त्याय भौवनाय स्वाहा भुवनस्य पतये स्वाहाधिपतये स्वाहा प्रजापतये स्वाहा ।
इयं ते राण्मित्राय यन्ताऽसि यमन ऊर्जे त्वा वृष्टचे त्वा प्रजानां त्वाऽऽधिपत्याय ॥

28. A learned man, who has got passion for battle, exertion for prosperity, tact for acquirement, practises yoga for knowledge, arranges for money for habitation, teaches the knowledge of time to the utilizer of days, practises non-attachment towards day and the stupid, uses truthful, friendly language for the confused and the master of decadent knowledge, renders sound advice to the vacillating and the most degraded, gives correct lead to the low-born and the friend of humanity, uses respectful language towards the leader of men, preaches the art of administration to the ruler, and reveals Kingly statesmanship to the guardian of his subjects, is an excellent politician.

Thou, the embodiment of noble qualities, art a guiding controller for the friend. Thee for vigour, thee for raining happiness, thee for the sovereign lordship of creatures do we accept.

२९. आयुर्यज्ञेन कल्पतां प्राणो यज्ञेन कल्पतां चक्षुर्यज्ञेन कल्पता॒ऽ श्रोत्रं यज्ञेन कल्पतां वाग्यज्ञेन कल्पतां मनो यज्ञेन कल्पतामात्मा यज्ञेन कल्पतां ब्रह्मा यज्ञेन कल्पतां ज्योतिर्यज्ञेन कल्पता॒ऽ स्वर्यज्ञेन कल्पतां पृष्ठं यज्ञेन कल्पतां यज्ञो यज्ञेन कल्पताम् ।
स्तोमश्च यजुश्च ऋक् च साम च बृहच्च रथन्तरं च ।
स्वर्देवा अगन्मामृता अ्भूम प्रजापते: प्रजा अ्भूम वेट् स्वाहा ॥

29. May life succeed through the service of God and the sages. May life breath thrive through union. May the eye thrive through the service of God and the sages. May the ear thrive through the service of God and the sages. May the voice thrive through the service of God and the sages.

May the mind thrive through the service of God and the sages. May the soul thrive through the service of God and the sages. May the knower of the four vedas thrive through the service of God and the sages. May the light of justice thrive through the service of God and the sages. May happiness thrive through the service of God and the sages. May passion for

---

[28]Utiliser of days: a labourer.
Thou: King.
[29]Through union: Through Pranayam and yoga, when we are united with God.
Eye thrive: When we look on humanity with love, and consider all high and low as brothers.
Ear thrive: By listening to the vedas and the sermons of the sages.
Voice thrive: Through the recitation of the vedas.
Brihat-Rathantra: Hymns of the Sama veda.

knowledge be satisfied through study. May desirable deed be performed through true behaviour. May the Atharva veda, the Yajur veda, the Rig veda, the Sama veda, and its Brihat, Rathantra, thrive through the grace of God and the sages. O sages, may we, freed from the pangs of birth and death attain to the happiness of final beatitude. May we become the true sons of God. May we be yoked to noble deeds and truthful speech!

३०. वाजस्य नु प्रसवे मातरं महीमदितिं नाम वचसा करामहे ।
यस्यामिदं विश्वं भुवनमाऽऽविवेश तस्यां नो देव: सविता धर्म सविषत् ॥

30. We, engaged in producing nice grain, sing the praises of adorable, immortal Mother the Earth, which envelops all these visible material worlds. May the Holy God, the Embodiment of glory, create of this Earth, in us, a desire for doing noble deeds.

३१. विश्वे अद्य मरुतो विश्व ऊती विश्वे भवन्त्वग्नय: समिद्धा: ।
विश्वे नो देवा अवसाऽऽगमन्तु विश्वमस्तु द्रविणं वाजो अस्मे ॥

31. Let all airs, all persons, like all thoroughly kindled fires be ready today for our protection. May all the learned persons come hither for protection. May we possess all riches and food.

३२. वाजो न: सप्त प्रदिशश्चतस्रो वा परावत: ।
वाजो नो विश्वदेवैर्धनसातविहावतु ॥

32. May our strength fill the seven regions and the four distant quarters. In this world may our knowledge of religious lore guard us with all the learned persons in the acquisition of wealth.

३३. वाजो नो अद्य प्र सुवाति दानं वाजो देवाँ२ ऋतुभि: कल्पयाति ।
वाजो हि मा सर्ववीरं जजान विश्वा आशा वाजपतिर्जयेयम् ॥

33. May food urge us today for charity. May food taken according to season strengthen our faculties, Yea, food hath made me rich in brave sons. As lord of food may I conquer all the regions.

३४. वाज: पुरस्तादुत मध्यतो नो वाजो देवान् हविषा वर्धयाति ।
वाजो हि मा सर्ववीरं चकार सर्वा आशा वाजपतिर्भवेयम् ॥

34. May food be before us, in the midst among us. May food eaten enhance our noble qualities. Yea, food hath made me rich in brave sons. As lord of food may I conquer all regions.

---

[30]Immortal Earth : Matter the cause of creation is unborn, indestructible, eternal, Here reference is to matter the primordial cause.

[32]Seven regions: Different worlds, as Sun, Moon, Mars, Mercury, Venus, Uranian Neptune. Some interpret the words as four directions, downward, upward and mid direction.

[33-34]Food is equivalent to strength.

३५. सं मा सृजामि पयसा पृथिव्याः सं मा सृजाम्यद्भिरोषधीभिः ।
सोऽहं वाज ꣳ सनेयमग्ने ॥

35. O learned person, I unite myself with the juices produced from the Earth. I unite myself with waters and with plants. As such may I gain strength!

३६. पयः पृथिव्यां पय ओषधीषु पयो दिव्यन्तरिक्षे पयो धाः ।
पयस्वती: प्रदिशः सन्तु मह्यम् ॥

36. O learned person, store milk in plants, water in the sky and water in the air. Teeming with milk for me be all the regions!

३७. देवस्य त्वा सवितुः प्रसवेऽश्विनोर्बाहुभ्यां पूष्णो हस्ताभ्याम् ।
सरस्वत्यै वाचो यन्तुर्यन्त्रेणाग्ने: साम्राज्येनाभिषिञ्चामि ॥

37. O King, I besprinkle thee with the arms (forces) of the sun's warmth and the moon's coolness, with the hands (powers) of attraction and retention of breath, with vedic speech, with the discipline of an administrator, and a ruler's sole dominion!

३८. ऋताषाड्ऋतधामाऽग्निर्गन्धर्वस्तस्यौषधयोऽप्सरसो मुदो नाम ।
स न इदं ब्रह्म क्षत्रं पातु तस्मै स्वाहा वाट् ताभ्यः स्वाहा ॥

38. A King is the maintainer of truth, practiser of truth, destroyer of foes like fire, guardian of the Earth; spreader of happiness like herbs born of water. May he protect this our Priesthood and Nobility. May he be entrusted with the responsibilities of the State, and may his subjects be honoured.

३९. स ꣳ हितो विश्वसामा सूर्यो गन्धर्वस्तस्य मरीचयोऽप्सरस आयुवो नाम ।
स न इदं ब्रह्म क्षत्रं पातु तस्मै स्वाहा वाट् ताभ्यः स्वाहा ॥

39. The sun is conjoined to all material objects and persons, is the sustainer of the Earth. Its rays that roam in air are well known as uniters and separators. Utilise those rays, thou Knower of the Sama Veda in full. Thou behavest rightly towards the sun. May thou protect this our Priesthood and Nobility and completion of our undertakings.

४०. सुषुम्णः सूर्यरश्मिश्चन्द्रमा गन्धर्वस्तस्य नक्षत्राण्यप्सरसो भेकुरयो नाम ।
स न इदं ब्रह्म क्षत्रं पातु तस्मै स्वाहा वाट् ताभ्यः स्वाहा ॥

---

[36] पय : milk or water.

[37] Besprinkle thee: Enthrone thee. Bestow on thee. A king is expected to possess the warmth of heart like the sun, and coolness of brain like the moon. He should be quick in making judgment, and slow to deliver it. These two qualities are his arms. He should have the power of control and subjugation like the breath. These qualities are his hands. He should have the knowledge of the vedas, be an efficient administrator, and protect his kingdom.

[39] Thou: A learned person.

CHAPTER XVIII

40. Moon is pleasant, receives light from the sun and imbibes its rays. Its Asterisms, and the rays present in the atmosphere, are full of lustre. May she protect this our Priesthood and Nobility. All Hail to the Moon, for completion of our undertakings. To those All-Hail.

४१. इषिरो विश्वव्यचा वातो गन्धर्वस्तस्यापो अप्सरस ऊर्जो नाम ।
स न इदं ब्रह्म क्षत्रं पातु तस्मै स्वाहा वाट् ताभ्य: स्वाहा ॥

41. Air is quick, pervades the whole universe, retains sound in the atmosphere. Its parts are well known as givers of vigour and movers in the atmospheric vapours. May it protect this our Priesthood and Nobility. All Hail to the air for success in our undertakings. To those All-Hail.

४२. भुज्यु: सुपर्णो यज्ञो गन्धर्वस्तस्य दक्षिणा अप्सरस स्तावा नाम ।
स न इदं ब्रह्म क्षत्रं पातु तस्मै स्वाहा वाट् ताभ्य: स्वाहा ॥

42. Sacrifice (yajna) is the bestower of delights, a nice nourisher, and the repository of vedic speech. Heartfelt famous prizes are its guerdons. May it protect this our Priesthood and Nobility. All-Hail to the Sacrifice for success in our undertakings. To those All-Hail.

४३. प्रजापतिर्विश्वकर्मा मनो गन्धर्वस्तस्य ऋक्सामान्यप्सरस एष्टयो नाम ।
स न इदं ब्रह्म क्षत्रं पातु तस्मै स्वाहा वाट् ताभ्य: स्वाहा ॥

43. He, who is the Lord of Creatures, Omnific, has a mind that possesses vedic speech. The famous verses of the Rigveda and Sama veda touch the innermost recesses of his heart, wherewith he honours the learned, loves truth and imparts knowledge. May he protect for us this veda and the Dhanur Veda. May he acquire truthful speech and realise religion. For these objects one should serve others in a righteous way.

४४. स नो भुवनस्य पते प्रजापते यस्य त उपरि गृहा यस्य वेह ।
अस्मै ब्रह्मणेऽस्मै क्षत्राय महि शर्म यच्छ स्वाहा ॥

44. O master of kingdom and protector of the subjects, in this world the householders and others depend upon thy support. Give great happiness in a nice way to the knower of God and the Veda and the Kshatriya trained in the art of administration!

४५. समुद्रोऽसि नभस्वानार्द्रदानु: शम्भूर्मयोभूरभि मा वाहि स्वाहा
मारुतोऽसि मरुतां गण: शम्भूर्मयोभूरभि मा वाहि स्वाहाऽवस्यूरसि दुवस्वाञ्छम्भूर्मयोभूरभि मा वाहि स्वाहा ॥

---

⁴⁰Those: Rays.
Asterism: Group of stars. Constellation.
⁴¹Those: Watery vapours.
Parts: Pran, Apan, Vyan, Udan and Saman.
⁴²Those: Guerdons, Dakshinas, sacrificial fees, priestly honoraria.
⁴³He: King.

45. O learned person thou art the master of voluminous water, the best-tower of calm nature, and deep like the ocean. Being the nice giver of happiness and blessings come unto me from all sides. O Knower of the science of air, thou art foremost amongst the group of the learned. Being the nice giver of happiness in this life and the life to come, come unto me from all sides!

Thou art worthy of laudable honour and desirous of self-protection. Being the nice giver of happiness and blessing, come unto me from all sides.

४६. यास्ते अग्ने सूर्ये रुचो दिवमातन्वन्ति रश्मिभिः ।
    ताभिर्नो अद्य सर्वाभी रुचे जनाय नस्कृधि ॥

46. O God, the lights in the sun, with their beams spread lustre all around. Unite us today with all those lights of thine. Make us worthy of love by every one!

४७. या वो देवाः सूर्ये रुचो गोष्वश्वेषु या रुचः ।
    इन्द्राग्नी ताभिः सर्वाभी रुचं नो धत्त बृहस्पते ॥

47. O God and learned persons whatever affection ye cherish for self and God, for kine and steeds, may lightning and fire, present in them, with all those affections vouchsafe us love!

४८. रुचं नो धेहि ब्राह्मणेषु रुचꣳ राजसु नस्कृधि ।
    रुचं विश्येषु शूद्रेषु मयि धेहि रुचा रुचम् ॥

48. O God grant love to our holy priests, set love in our ruling chiefs. Grant love to the Vaishyas and Shudras: give out of thy unbounded store of love, love unto me!

४९. तत्त्वा यामि ब्रह्मणा वन्दमानस्तदा शास्ते यजमानो हविर्भिः ।
    अहेडमानो वरुणेह बोध्युरुशꣳस मा न आयुः प्र मोषीः ॥

49. O Mighty God, through the veda, singing Thy praise, I pray unto Thee. The sacrificer through oblations and praises hankers after Thee. O God worshipped by many, never disrespected, give us in this world your knowledge. Steal not our life!

५०. स्वर्णं धर्मः स्वाहा
    स्वर्णार्कः स्वाहा
    स्वर्णं शुक्रः स्वाहा
    स्वर्णं ज्योतिः स्वाहा
    स्वर्णं सूर्यः स्वाहा ॥

[46] The text is the same as 13-22, but the interpretation is different in each verse.

[47] The text is the same as 13-23, but the interpretation in each verse is different. Learned persons cherish love for God and God cherishes love for his devotees. God gives us cows for milk and horses for use in the battle. Lightning and fire may mean the commander of the army and a highly learned man.

50. Properly utilised warmth conduces to happiness. Properly utilised fire conduces to happiness. Properly utilised air conduces to happiness. Properly utilised lustre of lightning conduces to happiness. Properly utilised sun conduces to happiness.

५१. अग्निं युनज्मि शवसा घृतेन दिव्य‍ࣳ सुपर्णं वयसा बृहन्तम् ।
तेन वयं गमेम ब्रध्नस्य विष्टप‍ࣳ स्वो रुहाणा अधि नाकमुत्तमम् ॥

51. I yoke with fulness of life and strength-giving butter, thee, fire, mighty, divine, and efficient in protection. Through that yajna-fire may we obtaining happiness, attain to the loftiest nature of God free from suffering and full of effulgence.

५२. इमौ ते पक्षावजरौ पतत्रिणौ याभ्या‍ࣳ रक्षा‍ࣳ स्यपह‍ࣳ स्यग्ने ।
ताभ्यां पतेम सुकृतामु लोकं यत्र ऋषयो जग्मुः प्रथमजाः पुराणाः ॥

52. O learned person, these cause and effect are thine two exalted immortal objects, wherewith thou drivest evils away!
May we with their aid fly to the regions of the pious, whither have gone the sages, well versed in the vedas, and masters of vedic lore.

५३. इन्दुर्दक्षः श्येन ऋतावा हिरण्यपक्षः शकुनो भुरण्युः ।
महान्त्सधस्थे ध्रुव आ निषत्तो नमस्ते अस्तु मा मा हि‍ࣳ सीः ॥

53. O learned ruler, thou art cool like the moon; full of wisdom, strong like a falcon, wedded to truth, fond of gold, impetuous, nourisher of all, great, settled in habitation, steadfast, to thee be reverence. Forbear to harm me!

५४. दिवो मूर्धासि पृथिव्या नाभिरूर्गपामोषधीनाम् ।
विश्वायुः शर्म सप्रथा नमस्पथे ॥

54. O learned person thou art the heaven's head, the Centre of earth, the essence of waters and plants. Thou art the enjoyer of full life of a hundred years, and full of glory. For right guidance be thou full of food and shelter !

५५. विश्वस्य मूर्धन्नधि तिष्ठसि श्रितः समुद्रे ते हृदयमप्स्वायुरपो दत्तोदधिं भिन्त ।
दिवस्पर्जन्यादन्तरिक्षात्पृथिव्यास्ततो नो वृष्ट्यावः ॥

---

[52] पक्षी may also mean according to Pt. Jaidev Vidyalankar God and soul. Rishi Dayananda interprets the word as Cause and Effect.

[53] The verse is applicable to God as well.

[54] Heaven's head: Just as the sun is topmost in the sky, so a learned person is foremost in an assembly of educated persons.

Centre of earth: A learned person is a central figure in managing the affairs of the State.

Essence of waters: Just as Soma is the essence of waters and plants, so a learned person is the commander, the head of the people.

55. O learned person, like the sun thou standest at the head of the whole world. Thy heart is fixed on God. Spend thy life for the betterment of the people. Preach noble deeds and knowledge. Advance irrigation by cutting canals out of rivers. Help us with rain sent from thy sky, cloud, firmament, earth or any other source of water!

५६. इष्टो यज्ञो भृगुभिराशीर्दा वसुभिः ।
तस्य न इष्टस्य प्रीतस्य द्रविणेहा गमेः ॥

56. O learned person, desire-fulfilling sacrifice (yajna) has been performed by highly learned persons and by Vasu Brahmcharis. With this well performed and beloved sacrifice accept thou our Dakshina!

५७. इष्टो अग्निराहुतः पिपर्तु न इष्टꣳ हविः ।
स्वगेदं देवेभ्यो नमः ।

57. May fire developed through Homa with oblations and purified substances, enhance our happiness. May this food acquired by us be offered to the sages.

५८. यदाकूतात्समसुस्रोढृदो वा मनसो वा सम्भृतं चक्षुषो वा ।
तदनु प्रेत सुकृतामु लोकं यत्र ऋषयो जग्मुः प्रथमजाः पुराणाः ॥

58. O discriminators between truth and untruth; hold fast the knowledge ye have gathered through exertion, soul-force, control of breath, mind, intellect, eyes, and ears. Follow the path of the aspirants after salvation where have gone the first-born ancient sages!

५९. एतꣳ सधस्थ परि ते ददामि यमावहाच्छेवधिं जातवेदाः ।
अन्वागन्ता यज्ञपतिर्वो अत्र तꣳस्म जानीत परमे व्योमन् ॥

59. Ye seekers after God, and common run of mankind, I, the knower of the meanings of the vedas, and guardian of sacrifice, having realised God, the treasure of happiness, preach unto ye, the true nature of God pervading this highest heaven. Know Him about Whom, I, the follower of religion, instruct thee!

६०. एतं जानाथ परमे व्योमन् देवाः सधस्था विद रूपमस्य ।
यदागच्छात्पथिभिर्देवयानैरिष्टापूर्त्तं कृणवाथाविरस्मै ॥

60. O learned persons living together, know this God spread in the highest heaven, and realise His true nature. He, who reaches Him through yogic paths of the sages, should reveal to Him pious acts pertaining to vedic injunctions and public utility!

⁵⁹I: A learned person.
⁶⁰इष्टापूर्त्तं: Acts enjoined by the vedas, say Yajna, charity, disinterested service, contemplation of God, and acts of public utility, say, construction of a well, tank, hospital and inn; and observance of chastity.

CHAPTER XVIII

६१. उद्बुध्यस्वाग्ने प्रति जागृहि त्वमिष्टापूर्ते सँ सृजेथामयं च ।
अस्मिन्त्सधस्थे अध्युत्तरस्मिन्विश्वे देवा यजमानश्च सीदत ॥

61. O learned priest, wake up, **attain to light**, expel the sleep of ignorance from your sacrificer (yajman) and bestow knowledge on him. Together with this sacrificer arrange for the yajna (sacrifice) and collect its materials!

Let all the learned priests and the sacrificer sit together in the yajna on nice seats.

६२. येन वहसि सहस्रं येनाग्ने सर्ववेदसम् ।
तेनेमं यज्ञं नो नय स्वर्देवेषु गन्तवे ॥

62. Through teaching one acquires vast knowledge. Through study the teacher and the taught acquire the knowledge of the vedas. Let this process of study and teaching be carried unto us for the attainment of happiness by the learned.

६३. प्रस्तरेण परिधिना स्रुचा वेधा च बर्हिषा ।
ऋचेमं यज्ञं नो नय स्वर्देवेषु गन्तवे ॥

63. With a handful of Darbha-grass, with the Yajur veda, with spoon, with altar, with nice execution, with the Rig Veda, O learned priest, conduct this sacrifice of ours with the support of the learned for acquiring worldly happiness!

६४. यद्दत्तं यत्परादानं यत्पूर्तं याश्च दक्षिणाः ।
तदग्निर्वैश्वकर्मणः स्वर्देवेषु नो दधत् ॥

64. Our gifts, our receiving of charitable grants, our pious works, our fees to priests, may the Omnific learned householder set all this for our happiness in religious usages.

६५. यत्र धारा अनपेता मधोर्घृतस्य च याः ।
तदग्निर्वैश्वकर्मणः स्वर्देवेषु नो दधत् ॥

65. There where all never-failing streams of honey and butter flow, may the learned knower of all actions grant us happiness for acquiring noble traits.

६६. अग्निरस्मि जन्मना जातवेदा घृतं मे चक्षुरमृतं म आसन् ।
अर्कस्त्रिधातू रजसो विमानोऽजस्रो धर्मो हविरस्मि नाम ॥

[61-62] The verses are the same as 15-54, 55, but with different interpretations.

[63] For the succes of a yajna the things mentioned in the verse are essential. The Darbha grass should be neat, clean, spoon, well washed, altar, well constructed, recitation of verses from the Yajur-Veda and the Rig-Veda should be done correctly.

[66] I : God.

Triple light: Satva, Rajas and Tamas.

Just as oblations are thrown into the blazing mouth of fire, so all souls having secured salvation go into the mouth of God and reside in Him.

66. I, the Revealer of the vedas, am Omniscient by nature. Sun is My eye, everlasting happiness of salvation is My mouth. I am Adorable, I am the Master of triple light; the Creator of regions, External, Lustrous, and Supplier of food at all places.

६७. ऋचो नामासि यजूँषि नामासि सामानि नागासि ।
ये अग्नयः पाञ्चजन्या अस्यां पृथिव्यामधि ।
तेषामसि त्वमुत्तमः प्र नो जीवातवे सुव ॥

67. O learned person I reveal the Rig-veda, the Yajur-veda, and the Sama-Veda. Learn from Me the vedic lore. O God, out of all the forces on the earth, that conduce to the welfare of humanity, Thou art the Foremost. Speed Thou us on to lengthened life!

६८. वार्त्रहत्याय शवसे पृतनाषाह्याय च ।
इन्द्र त्वाऽऽवर्तयामसि ॥

68. O Commander of the army, for the strength that slays the foes and conquers in the fight, and other resources, we turn thee hitherward to us!

६९. सहदानुं पुरुहूत क्षियन्तमहस्तमिन्द्र सं पिणक् कुणारुम् ।
अभि वृत्रं वर्धमानं पियारुमपादमिन्द्र तवसा जघन्थ ॥

69. O Commander, much invoked, kill thou the foes with thy strength, as the sun slays its companion the advancing cloud, that moves in the atmosphere, roars, is without hands, imbibes water and is without feet!

७०. वि न इन्द्र मृधो जहि नीचा यच्छ पृतन्यतः ।
यो अस्माँ२ अभिदासत्यधरं गमया तमः ॥

70. O Commander of the army, win battles, humble the men who challenge us, send down to nether darkness him who seeks to enslave us!

७१. मृगो न भीमः कुचरो गिरिष्ठाः परावत आ जगन्था परस्याः ।
सृकँ सँशाय पविमिन्द्र तिग्मं वि शत्रून् ताढि वि मृधो नुदस्व ॥

71. O Commander of the army, like a dreadful wild tiger roaming in the mountains with a crooked pace, encircle the distant foes. Crush thou the enemies, whetting thy sharp bolt, thou chastener of the wicked through punishment, and win battles!

७२. वैश्वानरो न ऊतय आ प्र यातु परावतः ।
अग्निर्नः सुष्टुतीरुप ॥

72. O ruler, just as the heat of the sun, being present in all creatures reaches the distant objects, so shouldst thou, come near us for our protection. Just as electricity being present in all objects lives near us, so shouldst thou listen to our eulogies!

७३. पृष्टो दिवि पृष्टो अग्निः पृथिव्यां पृष्टो विश्वा ओषधीरा विवेश ।
वैश्वानरः सहसा पृष्टो अग्निः स नो दिवा स रिषस्पातु नक्तम् ॥

73. Men should know fire in the brilliant sun, fire in the earth, air and water. The knowable fire in the shape of lightning, shining in the universe, has entered all the plants with vigour. Just as this fire preserves us by day and by night, so may thou the Commander preserve us always from a ferocious person.

७४. अश्याम तं काममग्ने तवोती अश्याम रयिं रयिवः सुवीरम् ।
अश्याम वाजमभि वाजयन्तोऽश्याम द्युम्नमजरारं ते ॥

74. O Commander of the army, may we fulfil our desires through thy protection. O Lord of wealth, may we get the riches which give us valiant sons. Waging fight may we succeed in battles. O Commander free from old age, with thy aid, may we win undecaying wealth and glory!

७५. वयं ते अद्य ररिमा हि काममुत्तानहस्ता नमसोपसद्य ।
यजिष्ठेन मनसा यक्षि देवानस्रेधता मन्मना विप्रो अग्ने ॥

75. O learned person, approaching with raised hands and adoration, we have this day fulfilled for thee thy longing!

O wise man, with undeviating fixed purpose, contemplative mood, and absolute restraint thou cultivatest good qualities!

७६. धामच्छदग्निरिन्द्रो ब्रह्मा देवो बृहस्पतिः ।
सचेतसो विश्वे देवा यज्ञं प्रावन्तु नः शुभे ॥

76. May the learned subduer of all places, the King, the knower of all the four vedas, the scholarly teacher, and the wise, guard our knowledge for our welfare.

७७. त्वं यविष्ठ दाशुषो नॄ: पाहि शृणुधी गिरः ।
रक्षा तोकमुत त्मना ॥

77. O most youthful king, guard the teachers who impart knowledge and listen to their sermons.

Protect with all thy force the offspring and the ladies of those who have died in war!

CHAPTER XIX

१. स्वाढ़ीं त्वा स्वादुना तीव्रां तीव्रेणामृताममृतेन ।
मधुमतीं मधुमता सृजामि सꣳ सोमेन ।
सोमोऽस्यश्विभ्यां पच्यस्व सरस्वत्यै पच्यस्वेन्द्राय सुत्राम्णे पच्यस्व ॥

1. O physician, thou art glorious like Soma. I fully instruct thee in the science of medicine. Just as I endow the sweet medicine with sweetness, bitter medicine with bitterness, the age-prolonging medicine with healing properties, the delicious medicine with delicious Soma, so shouldst thou dress up this medicine for husband and wife, dress it up for the learned lady, and dress it up for the dignified person, the deliverer of all from misery!

२. परीतो षिञ्चता सुतꣳ सोमो य उत्तमꣳ हवि: ।
दधन्वा यो नर्यो अप्स्वन्तरा सुषाव सोममद्रिभि: ॥

2. Soma is the best sacrificial food. It is useful for human body. It is produced in waters. Use well that Soma born of clouds.

३. वायो: पूत: पवित्रेण प्रत्यङ्क्सोमो अतिद्रुत: ।
इन्द्रस्य युज्य: सखा ।
वायो: पूत: पवित्रेण प्राङ्क्सोमो अतिद्रुत: ।
इन्द्रस्य युज्य: सखा ॥

3. Purified by the purifying process of the fast moving air, Soma is decidedly soul's fit friend. Purified by the purifying process of the fast moving air, Soma mixed with the organs of the body, is the king's proper friend.

४. पुनाति ते परिस्रुतꣳ सोमꣳ सूर्यस्य दुहिता ।
वारेण शश्वता तना ॥

4. O learned person, Sun's daughter (Dawn) doth with eternal excellent light, purify the Soma prepared by thee!

५. ब्रह्म क्षत्रं पवते तेज इन्द्रियꣳ सुरया सोम: सुत आसुतो मदाय ।
शुक्रेण देव देवता: पिपृग्धि रसेनान्नꣳ यजमानाय धेहि ॥

5. O learned person, the Soma (juice of medicines) prepared through purifying process and sacrifice (homa) for enjoyment, and taken for the removal of sickness, advances, the spiritual and temporal forces, brilliancy

---

¹Soma is the name of a medical herb, possessing efficacious healing properties. The word Soma has been used in the vedas in different senses of soul, king, milk, man, husband.

I :God.

CHAPTER XIX

237

and physical vigour. Give food with flavour to the sacrificer, and please the learned!

६. कुविदङ्ग यवमन्तो यवं चिद्यथा दान्त्यनुपूर्वं वियूय इहेहैषां कृणुहि भोजनानि ये बर्हिषो नम उक्तिं यजन्ति ।
उपयामगृहीतोऽस्यश्विभ्यां त्वा सरस्वत्यै त्वेन्द्राय त्वा सुत्राम्ण एष ते योनिस्तेजसे त्वा वीर्याय त्वा बलाय त्वा ॥

6. O Comrade, the agriculturists who produce food, instruct us how to grow more food. Protect and eat their produce in this world in a nice way. Just as these farmers reap in order the ripe barley and cleanse it by removing the chaff from it, so shouldst thou get strength by, sharing their corn, which is the cause of thy growth. The agriculturists accept thee for thy knowledge of Heaven and Earth, for thy nice speech expatiating on the science of agriculture, for thy being a good guardian and extirpator of foes, for thy boldness, for thy bravery and for thy strength!

७. नाना हि वां देवहितँ सदस्कृतं मा सँसृक्षाथां परमे व्योमन् ।
सुरा त्वमसि शुष्मिणी सोम एष मा मा हिँसी: स्वां योनिमाविशन्ती ॥

7. O king and subjects, each of ye has been allotted separate duty. May ye avail of the friendship of the learned. The Soma creeper, full of force, resides in its own place, rests in an open, elevated space. May ye both attain to it. Shun intoxicating objects. O learned person do not harm me and the Soma plants!

८. उपयामगृहीतोऽस्याश्विनं तेज: सारस्वतं वीर्यमैन्द्रं बलम् ।
एष ते योनिर्मदाय त्वाऽऽनन्दाय त्वा महसे त्वा ॥

8. O God, Thou art achieved through yamas and Niyamas. Thou hast got the splendour of the sun and moon, the vigour of vedic texts, and the might of lightning. My heart is Thy home. We all take Thee for enjoyment. We all take Thee for delight, and take Thee for greatness!

९. तेजोऽसि तेजो मयि धेहि
वीर्यमसि वीर्यं मयि धेहि
बलमसि बलं मयि धेह्यो-
जोऽस्योजो मयि धेहि
मन्युरसि मन्युं मयि धेहि
सहोऽसि सहो मयि धेहि ॥

9. O God, Thou art lustre; give me lustre. Thou art manly vigour; give me manly vigour. Thou art strength, give me strength. Thou art vitality; give me

---

[8]Yamas: Non-violence, Truthfulness, Abstaining from theft, Celibacy, self-Abnegation.
Niyamas: Cleanliness, Contentment, Austerity, Study, Trust in God.

vitality. Thou art righteous indignation; give me righteous indignation. Thou art forbearance; give me forbearance!

१०. या व्याघ्रं विषूचिकोभौ वृकं च रक्षति ।
श्येनं पतत्रिणꣳ सिꣳहꣳ सेमं पात्वꣳहस: ॥

10. The queen, who is the indicator of diverse worldly affairs, guards the subjects by killing both the tiger, and the wolf, the fast hawk and the lion, should prevent the King from wrongful conduct.

११. यदापिपेष मातरं पुत्र: प्रमुदितो धयन् ।
एतत्तदग्ने अनृणो भवाम्यहतौ पितरौ मया ।
सम्पृच स्थ सं मा भद्रेण पृङ्क्त विपृच स्थ वि मा पाप्मना पृङ्क्त ॥

11. O learned person, the delighted son teases the mother sucking her breast. With that son I become free from debt towards my parents. May my parents be unharmed and blissful by me!

O learned persons ye are my associates; unite me with good fortune. Ye are free from sin, keep me away from sin. Give me happiness in this life and the life to come!

१२. देवा यज्ञमतन्वत भेषजं भिषजाश्विना ।
वाचा सरस्वती भिषग्विन्द्रायेन्द्रियाणि दधत: ॥

12. O men, just as a lady doctor well versed in the science of medicine, with healthy organs of the body; physicians and surgeons, having mastery over the Ayurveda, and learned persons, stretch out the healing sacrifice, for prosperity with their speech, so shouldst ye do!

१३. दीक्षाये रूपꣳ शष्पाणि प्रायणीयस्य तोक्मानि ।
क्रयस्य रूपꣳ सोमस्य लाजा: सोमाꣳशवो मधु ॥

13. Grass buds are the symbols of consecration. Sprouts of corn are symbols of strengthening vital breaths. Fried grains are the symbols of equanimity of mind. Honey is the symbol of Soma-shoots.

१४. आतिथ्यरूपं मासरं महावीरस्य नग्नहु: ।
रूपमुपसदामेत्तिस्रो रात्री: सुराऽऽसुता ॥

14. Monthly presents to guests are the sign of hospitality. Clothing the naked is the symbol of a great warrior. The offer of medicinal elixir is the sign of honouring the guests.

[18]I become free : To maintain the family link, it is necessary to produce a son. If a householder is blessed with a son, he has discharged his debt towards his parents, by maintaining the succession of his family. To die without a son is to die without discharging the parental debt.

[12]The lessons taught by the physicians in the science of healing are a kind of yajna performed by them, for the betterment of the people.

Ayurveda: The science of medicine.

[13]Consecration: Diksha.

१५. सोमस्य रूपं क्रीतस्य परिस्रुत्परि षिच्यते ।
अश्विभ्यां दुग्धं भेषजमिन्द्रायेन्द्र ॐ सरस्वत्या ॥

15. O women, just as the juice of Soma medicine accepted by a learned lady is pleasant, as physicians and surgeons prepare the extracts of medicines, as an aspirant after prosperity master the science of lightning, so should ye!

१६. आसन्दी रूप ॐ राजासन्द्यां कुम्भी सुराधानी ।
अन्तर उत्तरवेद्या रूपं कारोतरो भिषक् ॥

16. O people, for the successful performance of a yajna make arrangement for these objects. Its nice execution, a seat for the king, a jar for corns in the altar, a pitcher for Soma, food that gives life placed in the northern altar, the priests and the physician!

१७. वेद्या वेदिः समाप्यते बर्हिषा बर्हिरिन्द्रियम् ।
यूपेन यूप आप्यते प्रणीतो अग्निरग्निना ॥

17. O people, just as the learned persons decorate the altar with materials for the yajna, obtain mighty riches through ceaseless effort, reap through the process of union and separation, the result of their effort at unity, produce well ordered light out of electricity, so should ye procure all kinds of happiness by properly using all resources!

१८. हविर्धानं यदश्विनाऽग्नीध्रं यत्सरस्वती ।
इन्द्रायेन्द्र ॐ सदस्कृतं पत्नीशालं गार्हपत्यः ॥

18. O householders, just as a learned man and woman collect materials for the yajna; a learned lady takes shelter with the priest, and the learned construct a house for the majestic husband to dwell in and impart happiness; this all is a householder's duty; which ye also should perform!

१९. प्रैषोभिः प्रैषानाप्नोत्याप्रीभिराप्रीयज्ञस्य ।
प्रयाजेभिरनुयाजान् वषट्कारैरिडाहुतीः ॥

19. He gets happiness, who has got servants to obey orders, maid-servants of pleasing manners, who perform their duty gracefully, necessary materials for the performance of yajna, and oblations to be put into the fire by sacrificial practices.

२०. पशुभिः पशूनाप्नोति पुरोडाशैर्हविं ॐ ष्या ।
छन्दोभिः सामिधेनीयज्याभिर्वषट्कारान् ॥

20. A householder gains cows from cows, sacrificial materials from ground rice-cakes, fire-kindling fuel from the knowledge of metres like Gayatri etc., and virtuous people from sacrificial practices.

---

[17]For the sake of unity or peace, sometimes separation or partition is a necessity.
[20]Fuel is burnt and put in the altar with the recitation of verses in Gayatri metre.

२१. धाना: करम्भ: सक्तव: परीवाप: पयो दधि ।
सोमस्य रूप ँ हविष आमिक्षा वाजिनं मधु ॥

21. Roasted grains, gruel, barley-meal, grains of roasted rice, milk, and curd, mingled milk, nice corns, and honey are the materials for Soma yajna.

२२. धानानाँ रूपं कुवलं परीवापस्य गोधूमा: ।
सक्तूनाँ रूपं बदरमुपवाका: करम्भस्य ॥

22. Jujube fruit is the type of parched corn. Wheat is the best product of agriculture. Jujube is the type of barley-meal. Barley is the type of gruel-groats.

२३. पयसो रूपं यद्वा दध्नो रूपं कर्कन्धूनि ।
सोमस्य रूपं वाजिन ँ सौम्यस्य रूपमामिक्षा ॥

23. Barley-grains are the symbol of milk. Ripe jujube fruits are the symbol of curd. The essence of corn is the symbol of Soma. The juices of Soma plants are like the mixture of milk and curd.

२४. आ श्रावयेति स्तोत्रिया: प्रत्याश्रावो अनुरूप: ।
यजेति धाय्यारूपं प्रगाथा येयजामहा: ॥

24. The students who are seekers after knowledge, should request the preceptor to instruct them in all branches of knowledge. The knowledge imparted to the pupils should be in consonance with their capacity, 'Pray grant' is the sign of receiving and assimilating knowledge. We, the performers of sacrifice are fit to sing praises.

२५. अर्ध-ऋचैरुक्थाना ँ रूपं पदैराप्नोति निविद: ।
प्रणवै: शस्त्राणा ँ रूपं पयसा सोम आप्यते ॥

25. A learned person gets songs of praise by verse-halves, short detached formulae by case-terminations. By Om exclamations he gets the mode of praise, prayer and contemplation. By water is got the soma juice.

२६. अश्विभ्यां प्रात: सवनमिन्द्रेणैन्द्रं माध्यंदिनम् ।
वैश्वदेव ँ सरस्वत्या तृतीयमाप्त ँ सवनम् ॥

26. They are the benefactors of humanity, who perform the morning yajna

---

[21] Mingled milk : a mixture of boiled milk, curd and sugar.
[22] Just as jujube fruit (बेर) is easily eaten by the goats, so parched corns (खीलां) are eaten conveniently.
Barley-meal (सत्तु)
Upvakas: seeds of the Wrightia Antidysenterica.
[23] Just as milk strengthens the body, so do the barley grains.
Just as curd produces semen so do jujube fruits produce strength.
[25] By water: Water is mixed with the Soma plant to extract its juice. Milk can also be used for the same purpose.
[26] Lightning means the heat of the sun at midday.

with the sun and moon, the glorious mid-day prosperity bringer yajna through lightning, the evening yajna, the giver of health, through true vedic speech, for reverence of the learned.

२७. वायव्यैर्वायव्यान्याप्नोति सतेन द्रोणकलशम् ।
कुम्भीभ्यामम्भृणौ सुते स्थालीभि स्थालीराप्नोति ॥

27. He is wealthy, who with the attributes of air gains the objects residing in air, by the process of separation gains the Drona and Kalash, vessels for Soma, by two jars of corn and water gains two cleansing vessels, and by the cooking pot gains the pots for cooking.

२८. यजुर्भिराप्यन्ते ग्रहा ग्रहै स्तोमाश्च विष्टुती: ।
छन्दोभिरुक्थाशस्त्राणि साम्नावभृथ आप्यते ॥

28. The recitation of the Yajur Veda gives us the knowledge of ceremonies (Sanskaras). The knowledge of ceremonies (Karma-Kanda) teaches us the attributes of objects and different praise-songs. Through Gayatri metres, and learned singers of the praise of fine traits are obtained the vedic verses worthy of recitation and weapons. The recitation of Sama veda gives us purification.

२९. इडाभिर्भक्षानाप्नोति सूक्तवाकेनाशिष: ।
शंयुना पत्नीसंयाजान्त्समिष्टयजुषा सँ‍उस्थाम् ॥

29. A learned person obtains eatable foodstuffs from parts of the earth, and fulfils desires by the utterance of true noble words. From a peaceful deed is derived good relation between husband and wife. Consummation is obtained by performing the ceremonies (Karma-kanda) of the Yajur Veda.

३०. व्रतेन दीक्षामाप्नोति दीक्षयाऽऽप्नोति दक्षिणाम् ।
दक्षिणा श्रद्धामाप्नोति श्रद्धया सत्यमाप्यते ॥

30. By the vow of celibacy one gains consecration, by consecration one gains wealth and position. By wealth and position one gains faith, by faith comes the knowledge of truth.

३१. एतावद्रूपं यज्ञस्य यद्देवेभ्र्‍हाणा कृतम् ।
तदेतत्सर्वमाप्नोति यज्ञे सौत्रामणी सुते ॥

31. He commences his second birth, who wearing the yajnopavit, joins a well arranged yajna, the nature of which has been explained by the learned, the vedas and God.

---

[27]Two cleansing vessels: पूनभृत and आधवनीय. In the latter the Soma in shaken, and the former receives the purified juice.

One who understands the science of air knows the science of measurement, and there by the science of cooking, which purifies food stuffs.

Avbrith: The expiatory bath of purification.

[30]Consecration: Devotion to a sacred use.

३२. सुरावन्तं बर्हिषदꣳ सुवीरं यज्ञꣳ हिन्वन्ति महिषा नमोभिः ।
दधानाः सोमं दिवि देवतासु मदेमेन्द्रꣳ यजमानाः स्वर्काः ॥

32. The exalted adorable sacrificers, equipped with food-stuffs, make prosperous with oblations the yajna, great like the sun in the sky, full of Soma juice, giver of heroes, the masters of physical and spiritual forces. May we be happy, doing noble deeds, befriending the dignified and learned persons, and gaining power.

३३. यस्ते रसः सम्भृत ओषधीषु सोमस्य शुष्मः सुरया सुतस्य ।
तेन जिन्व यजमानं मदेन सरस्वतीमश्विनाविन्द्रमग्निम् ॥

33. O learned person, the strong essence of Soma, duly collected by a charitable lady is drawn from plants. With that glanddening essence impel with joy, the sacrificer, the learned lady, the scholarly teachers and preachers, the supreme king and Commander, and the hero that burns the foe like fire!

३४. यमश्विना नमुचेरासुरादधि सरस्वत्यसुनोदिन्द्रियाय ।
इमं तꣳ शुक्रं मधुमन्तमिन्दुꣳ सोमꣳ राजानमिह भक्षयामि ॥

34. In this world, for wealth and physical strength, I drink and feed on Soma plant, producer of activity, brilliant, giver of glory, full of sweetness, highly invigorating, acquired by a learned lady and the King and Commander from clouds that do not release water.

३५. यदत्र रिप्तꣳ रसिनः सुतस्य यदिन्द्रो अपिबच्छचीभिः ।
अहं तदस्य मनसा शिवेन सोमꣳ राजानमिह भक्षयामि ॥

35. Whatever portion of this savoury fluid is clinging here, what the sun drank with his powers of attraction, I drink and feed on that brilliant Soma juice, with a pure mind.

३६. पितृभ्यः स्वधायिभ्यः स्वधा नमः ।
पितामहेभ्यः स्वधायिभ्यः स्वधा नमः ।
प्रपितामहेभ्यः स्वधायिभ्यः स्वधा नमः ।
अक्षन् पितरो ऽमीमदन्त पितरो ऽतीतृपन्त पितरः ।
पितरः शुन्धध्वम् ॥

36. We offer food and homage to our fathers who desire food and water. We offer food and homage to our grandfathers, who desire food and water. We offer food and homage to our great-grandfathers, who desire food and water. O parents eat the food we have prepared. O parents and teachers rejoice and make us full of joy. O preachers be satisfied and satisfy us. O learned persons be purified and purify us!

---

[33] According to Swami Dayananda there are twenty four kinds of Soma plants.
[35] Here means on the earth. A part has been drunk by the sun.

३७. पुनन्तु मा पितर: सोम्यास: पुनन्तु मा पितामहा:
पुनन्तु प्रपितामहा: । पवित्रेण शतायुषा ।
पुनन्तु मा पितामहा: पुनन्तु प्रपितामहा: ।
पवित्रेण शतायुषा विश्वमायुर्व्यश्नवै ॥

37. May fathers, full of glory and mental peace, purify me with a pure life of a hundred years. May grandfathers, purify me with a pure life of a hundred years. May great grandfathers purify me with a pure life of a hundred years. May learned and calm grandfathers purify me with a happy, pure life of a hundred years. May sedate great-grandfathers purify me with a pure life of a hundred years. May I obtain full length of life.

३८. अग्न आयूंषि पवस आ सुवोर्जमिषं च न: ।
आरे बाधस्व दुच्छुनाम् ॥

38. O learned parents, ye purify the age-prolonging foodgrains, send down upon us food and vigorous strength. Drive ye far away from us the company of evil persons!

३९. पुनन्तु मा देवजना: पुनन्तु मनसा धिय: ।
पुनन्तु विश्वा भूतानि जातवेद: पुनीहि मा ॥

39. O learned amongst the born, just as the wise purify me with knowledge and love, and purify our intellect, just as all material things purify me, so shouldst thou purify me!

४०. पवित्रेण पुनीहि मा शुक्रेण देव दीद्यत् ।
अग्ने क्रत्वा क्रतूंरनु ॥

40. O refulgent learned person, imparter of knowledge, first purify thyself with noble spiritual force, and then purify me. Purifying thyself with intellect and acts purify my intellect and acts again and again!

४१. यत्ते पवित्रमर्चिष्यग्ने विततमन्तरा ।
ब्रह्म तेन पुनातु मा ॥

41. O God purify me with Thy pure vedic knowledge diffused by Thy pure lustrous nature!

४२. पवमान: सो अद्य न: पवित्रेण विचर्षणि: ।
य: पोता स पुनातु मा ॥

42. God, Who in our midst, by His immaculate nature, is Pure and Giver of different sciences, is ever our Purifier and Preacher. My He, the Cleanser, make me clean.

४३. उभाभ्यां देव सवित: पवित्रेण सवेन च ।
मां पुनीहि विश्वत: ॥

43. O God, the Giver of happiness, Impeller for virtuous deeds, with true behaviour, full glory, knowledge and exertion, purify me on every side!

४४. वैश्वदेवी पुनती देव्यागाद्यस्यामिमा बह्वश्चस्तन्वो वीतपृष्ठा: ।
तया मदन्त: सधमादेषु वय ँ स्याम पतयो रयीणाम् ॥

44. Vedic speech, the benefactor of humanity and the repository of knowledge comes unto us and purifies us.
Through her may we in sacrificial banquets taking our pleasure be the lords of riches.

४५. ये समाना: समनस: पितरो यमराज्ये ।
तेषाँल्लोक: स्वधा नमो यज्ञो देवेषु कल्पताम् ॥

45. The officials, who in the realm of a just king, are equal in status and knowledge, have their dwelling place, food, reverence and sense of fairness approved by the learned.

४६. ये समाना: समनसो जीवा जीवेषु मामका: ।
तेषाँ श्रीर्मयि कल्पतामस्मिँल्लोके शत ँ समा: ॥

46. My folk yet living among those who live, are of one mind and similar attributes. On me be set their wealth through a hundred years in this world.

४७. द्वे सृती अश्रृणवं पितृणामहं देवानामुत मर्त्यानाम् ।
ताभ्यामिदं विश्वमेजत्समेति यदन्तरा पितरं मातरं च ॥

47. I have heard the mention of two pathways of birth and death, the ways of parents, the learned and the mortals. On these two roads each moving creature travels. Each soul leaves the present parents and assumes new ones.

४८. इद ँ हवि: प्रजननं मे अस्तु दशवीर ँ सर्वगण ँ स्वस्तये ।
आत्मसनि प्रजासनि पशुसनि लोकसन्यभयसनि ।
अग्नि: प्रजां बहुलां मे करोत्वन्नं पयो रेतो अस्मासु धत्त ॥

48. May my fiery husband make my progeny abundant. May this my married life bring me ten brave children, all good objects, physical strength, good progeny, cattle, spiritual force and fearlessness, for my welfare. O parents do ye confer on us food, milk, and manly vigour.

४९. उदीरतामवर उत्परास उन्मध्यमा: पितर: सोम्यास: ।
असुं य ईयुरवृका ऋतज्ञास्ते नोऽवन्तु पितरो हवेषु ॥

49. May our parents, who do not steal, know the truth, gain strength of battles, through control of breath, protect us well. May the lowest, highest, midmost elders calm and peaceful in nature, urge us on to battle.

⁴⁶Folk: Elders. Me: Their descendants.

५०. अङ्गिरसो न: पितरो नवग्वा अथर्वाणो भृगव: सोम्यास: ।
तेषां वयꣳ सुमतौ यज्ञियानामपि भद्रे सौमनसेॱ स्याम ॥

50. Our elders are masters of different principles of knowledge, preachers of new expositions on problems of learning, devotees of non-violence, highly learned, and deserving of supremacy.
May we follow the sound advice of these adorable elders, and enjoy their gracious loving-kindness.

५१. ये न: पूर्वे पितर: सोम्यासोॱनूहिरे सोमपीथं वसिष्ठा: ।
तेभिर्यम: सꣳ रराणो हविꣳष्युशन्न् शद्धि: प्रतिकाममत्तु ॥

51. Our aged learned parents, tranquil in mind, highly rich, come again and again to our Soma banquet.
Let just and self-controlled son, desiring for nice food, giver of pleasure, fulfil all his desires, with the aid of our parents desirous of our protection.

५२. त्वꣳ सोम प्र चिकितो मनीषा त्वꣳ रजिष्ठमनु नेषि पन्थाम् ।
तव प्रणीती पितरो न इन्दो देवेषु रत्नमभजन्त धीरा: ॥

52. O sedate learned fellow, thou art pre-eminent for wisdom. With thy wisdom, thou followest the straightest path of happiness. Make me also follow the same path. O learned fellow happy like the moon, the wise parents, with thy excellent guidance, make us enjoy riches amongst the learned!

५३. त्वया हि न: पितर: सोम पूर्वे कर्माणि चक्रु: पवमान धीरा: ।
वन्वन्नवात: परिधीꣳ रपोर्णु वीरेभिरश्वैर्मघवा भव न: ॥

53. O virtuous, glorious progeny, the religious deeds which our aged, wise and learned persons perform with thee, so shouldst we!
O non-violent, religious child remove our enemy from all sides with brave horsemen and bestow riches on us!

५४. त्वꣳ सोम पितृभि: संविदानोॱनु द्यावापृथिवी आ ततन्थ ।
तस्मै त इन्दो हविषा विधेम वयꣳ स्याम पतयो रयीणाम् ॥

54. O moon-like gladdening noble son, taking vow with thy learned fatherly teachers, spread pleasure, leading a religious life between the Earth and Heaven!
O beautiful son, may we offer thee gifts for thy pleasure, and may we become the lords of riches!

५५. बर्हिषद: पितर ऊत्यर्वागिमा वो हव्या चक्रमा जुषध्वम् ।
त आ गतावसा शन्तमेनाथा न: शं योररपो दधात् ॥

55. O justice loving fathers, who sit in an exalted assembly, come, help us. Accept these eatables we have prepared for ye!

Come to us with most auspicious favour, grant us happiness and purity of character, and keep miseries away from us.

५६. आ॒ऽहं पितृ॒न्त्सुवि॑दत्रा॒२ँ अवि॑त्सि॒ नपा॑तं च वि॒क्रम॑णं च॒ विष्णो॑: ।
बर्हिष॒दो ये स्व॒धया॑ सु॒तस्य॒ भज॑न्त पि॒त्वस्त इ॒हाग॑मिष्ठाः ॥

56. I know the elders, who impart sound knowledge. I know the eternal strength of God and His creation of the universe. May those visit our homes, who solely devoted to God, with their soul-force, and self-realisation, worship the Blissful Creator.

५७. उप॑हूताः॒ पित॑रः सो॒म्यासो॑ बर्हि॒ष्येषु॒ निधि॑षु प्रि॒येषु॑ ।
त आ ग॑मन्तु॒ त इ॒ह श्रु॑वन्त्वधि ब्रुवन्तु ते॑ऽवन्त्व॒स्मान् ॥

57. May they, the Fathers, worthy of homage, invited to their excellent, favourite wealth of oblations, come nigh unto us, listen to us. preach unto us, and afford us protection.

५८. आ यन्तु नः॑ पि॒तरः॑ सो॒म्यासोऽग्निष्वा॒त्ताः प॒थिभि॑र्दे॒वया॑नैः ।
अ॒स्मिन्य॒ज्ञे स्व॒धया॒ मद॑न्तोऽधि ब्रुवन्तु ते॑ऽवन्त्व॒स्मान् ॥

58. May they our fathers, having knowledge of the science of fire possessing mental peace, calmness and self-restraint come on Godward pathways, enjoying at this sacrifice their meals, may they teach and instruct us, and afford us protection.

५९. अग्निष्वा॒त्ताः पि॑तर॒ एह ग॑च्छत॒ सद॑ः-सद॒ः सद॑त सुप्रणीत॒यः ।
अ॒त्ता ह॒वीँषि॒ प्रय॑तानि ब॒र्हिष्यथा र॒यिँ सर्व॑वी॒रं द॑धातन ॥

59. May the learned persons, who know the science of fire and material objects, are well-versed in politics, come now for the spread of knowledge, visiting house to house, and staying there, eat the meals prepared carefully. Hence, being engaged in the noble work of spreading education, may they grant us riches with brave sons.

६०. ये अ॑ग्निष्वा॒त्ता ये अन॑ग्निष्वात्ता॒ मध्ये॑ दि॒वः स्व॒धया॒ माद॑यन्ते ।
तेभ्यः॑ स्व॒राडसु॑नीति॒मेतां य॑थाव॒शं त॒न्वं॑ कल्पयाति ॥

⁵⁶Prof. Ludwig and Prof. Grassman have not grasped the significance of the verse. Prof. Ludwig says Vikramanam is an unintelligible expression. Napatam has been translated as fire. Mahidhara takes Vishnu to mean 'of the sacrifice,' and napatam and Vikramanam as the two paths leading to the Gods and to the Fathers. Maharshi Dayananda interprets Vishnu 'of God'. Napatam as Eternal, Indestructible, Vikramanam as diverse creation of the universe. The verse is quite intelligible.

⁵⁷Fathers: The learned people.

⁵⁸Fathers: The teachers, the preachers and learned parents. Agnishwata has been translated by Mahidhara and Griffith as parents consumed by fire after death; whereas Rishi Dayananda interprets the word to refer to living persons who know full well the science of fire. The orthodox people generally quote this verse in support of Shradha ceremony of the dead, which is not corroborated by the text.

60. For those who know the science of fire, and are well-versed in sciences other than fire, and enjoy in the midst of knowledge with their own strength, may the Self Effulgent God, make long-lived this body endowed with vital breaths.

६१. अग्निष्वात्तानृतुमतो हवामहे नाराशꣳसे सोमपीथं य आशु: ॥
ते नो विप्रास: सुहवा भवन्तु वयꣳ स्याम पतयो रयीणाम् ॥

61. We invite for the good of humanity, the sages who know the science of fire, drink the medicinal juice of Soma, and are true to seasons. May they be charitable to us, and make us lords of wealth.

६२. आच्या जानु दक्षिणतो निषद्येमं यज्ञमभि गृणीत विश्वे ।
मा हिꣳसिष्ट पितर: केन चिन्नो यद्व आग: पुरुषता कराम ॥

62. O ye all learned people, injure us not for any sin which we through human frailty have committed!
Bowing with the bent knees and seated on the right we pay ye homage. Pray accept our respectful conduct.

६३. आसीनासो अरुणीनामुपस्थे रयिं धत्त दाशुषे मर्त्याय ।
पुत्रेभ्य: पितरस्तस्य वस्व: प्र यच्छत त इहोर्जं दधात ॥

63. Ye fathers grant riches to the charitably disposed persons and your sons sitting near their fascinating mothers!
Always give them a portion of your treasure, so that they may thereby gain energy.

६४. यमग्ने कव्यवाहन त्वं चिन्मन्यसे रयिम् ।
तन्नो गीर्भि: श्रवाय्यं देवत्रा पनया युजम् ॥

64. O learned person, brilliant like fire and bestower of nice objects on the wise, grant us the supremacy which thou through praise-worthy eloquence considerest fit to be granted to the learned!

६५. यो अग्नि: कव्यवाहन: पितॄन् यक्षदृतावृध: ।
प्रेदु हव्यानि वोचति देवेभ्यश्च पितृभ्य आ ॥

65. He, who persuades the learned to noble deeds, is resplendent like fire with the light of knowledge, and reveres the sages advanced in vedic lore, is fully fit to preach to the wise and the elders, the agreeable branches of knowledge.

६६. त्वमग्न ईडित: कव्यवाहनावाड्ढव्यानि सुरभीणि कृत्वी ।
प्रादा: पितृभ्य: स्वधया ते अक्षन्नद्धि त्वं देव प्रयता हवीꣳषि ॥

---

[63]They: mothers and their children.

66. O son, possessing the eloquence of the learned, pure like fire, praiseworthy, thou preparest fragrant meals. Offer them to the elders. Let them take them as food. O learned donor, eat thou the food prepared with effort!

६७. ये चेह पितरो ये च नेह याँश्च विद्य याँर् उ च न प्रविद्म ।
त्वं वेत्थ यति ते जातवेदः स्वधाभिर्यज्ञ ‍ॐ सुकृतं जुषस्व ॥

67. O sharp witted scholar, thou knowest well the number of fathers who are here and who are absent, whom we know and whom we know not. Thou knowest a large number of them and they know thee. Serve them with food and meritorious reverence!

६८. इदं पितृभ्यो नमो अस्त्वद्य ये पूर्वासो य उपरास ईयुः ।
ये पार्थिवे रजस्या निषत्ता ये वा नून ‍ॐ सुवृजनासु विक्षु ॥

68. Now let us offer food to the fathers who are more advanced than us in age and knowledge, who have taken to Banprastha and Sanyas Ashramas, who are engrossed in worldly affairs, and who work amongst the people of high character.

६९. श्रधा यथा नः पितरः परासः प्रत्नासो अग्न ऋतमाशुषाणाः ।
शुचीदयन् दीधितिमुक्थशासः क्षामा भिन्दन्तो अरुणीरप व्रन् ॥

69. O learned person, just as our noble, ancient elders, givers of sound instructions, pure, devotees of truth, spreading knowledge, acquire well-behaved wives and ground to dwell upon, remove ignorance, and cast away the coverings of darkness, so shouldst thou serve them!

७०. उशन्तस्त्वा नि धीमह्य ‍शन्तः समिधीमहि ।
उशन्न् ‍उशत आ वह पितृन् हविषे अत्तवे ॥

70. Right gladly do we make thee the store-house of knowledge. Right gladly do we educate thee. Gladly bring yearning fathers nigh to eat food.

७१. अपां फेनेन नमुचेः शिर इन्द्रोदवर्तयः ।
विश्वा यदजय स्पृधः ॥

71. O Commander of the army, just as the sun wrenches off the head of the cloud full of water but unwilling to release it, so do thou advance thy armies, and subdue all contending hosts!

७२. सोमो राजामृत ‍ॐ सुत ऋजीषेणाजहान्मृत्युम् ।
ऋतेन सत्यमिन्द्रयं विपान ‍ॐ शुक्रमन्धस इन्द्रस्येन्द्रियमिदं पयोऽमृतं मधु ॥

[67]Here: In the yajna.
Fathers: Elderly relatives, and aged learned persons.
[70]Thee: disciple or son.
We: Teachers or fathers.
[71]The word Namuchi is explained by Prof. Lanman as a waterspout in a lake, Rishi Dayananda has rightly interpreted it as a cloud that does not release water.

72. A renowned sage, through yoga, and religious practices, overcomes death and attains to salvation. Just as with food one gets strength, so he reaches the final beatitude on the strength of truth, realises his soul-force, manifests the supreme nature of his supreme soul, pure like milk, immortal like the Supreme Spirit, and sweet like honey.

७३. अन्ड्वच: क्षीरं व्यपिबत् कुङ्ङ्ङ्गिरसो धिया ।
ऋतेन सत्यमिन्द्रियं विपान॓ शुक्रमन्धस इन्द्रस्येन्द्रियमिदं पयोऽमृतं मधु ॥

73. Just as swan separates milk from water and drinks it, so a learned person, the embodiment of action, through yogic practices, strengthening his soul with pure food, acquires divine hearing, sweetness, healing medicine, pure love, and immaculate divine speech mingled with the eternal connection between word and its significance in all worldly objects.

७४. सोममङ्च्चो व्यमिबच्छन्दसा ह॓स: शुचिषत् ।
ऋतेन सत्यमिन्द्रियं विपान॓ शुक्रमन्धस इन्द्रस्येन्द्रियमिदं पयोऽमृतं मधु ॥

74. He, who enjoys the company of pure learned persons, is a discriminator, willingly drinks Soma juice out of waters, purifies food with vedic knowledge, is a cleanser of soul, equipped with the power of protection, knows God, is procurer of supremacy through the knowledge of yoga, acquires the happiness of soul, sweet like honey, salvation, and the apparent essence of knowledge.

७५. अन्नात्परिस्रुतो रसं ब्रह्मणा व्यपिबत् क्षत्रं पय: सोमं प्रजापति: ।
ऋतेन सत्यमिन्द्रियं विपान॓ शुक्रमन्धस इन्द्रस्येन्द्रियमिदं पयोऽमृतं मधु ॥

75. A king, who along with one knowing all the four vedas, enjoys his birth in a royal family and the milkwise invigorating essence of a well-cooked food, and with justice coupled with learning and decorum, administers his rule, the giver of glory, a gift from God, pre-eminent in all dealings, the remover of the darkness of injustice, the bestower of valour, and the source of diverse kinds of protection, always derives happiness from this his administration fit for enjoyment, imbued with justice, sweetness, and delightfulness.

७६. रेतो मूत्रं वि जहाति योनिं प्रविशदिन्द्रियम् ।
गर्भो जरायुणाऽऽवृत उल्वं जहाति जन्मना ।
ऋतेन सत्यमिन्द्रियं विपान॓ शुक्रमन्धस इन्द्रस्येन्द्रियमिदं पयोऽमृतं मधु ॥

76. The generative organ releases urine, but when it enters the womb, it releases semen. The caul-invested embryo leaves by its birth the covering folds. The child, by the removal of covering folds, in their contact with external air, acquires the wealth of soul, pure, excellent and enjoyable ; and is endowed with these eyes, sweet like juice, and source of everlasting knowledge.

७७. दृष्ट्वा रूपे व्याकरोत् सत्यानृते प्रजापति: ।
अश्रद्धामनृतेऽदधाच्छद्धाꣽ सत्ये प्रजापति: ।
ऋतेन सत्यमिन्द्रियं विपानꣽ शुक्रमन्धस इन्द्रस्येन्द्रियमिदं पयोऽमृतं मधु ॥

77. God through His pure knowledge, viewing both forms has explained truth and falsehood. He has assigned the lack of faith to falsehood, and faith to truth. He alone is worthy of worship by all, Who is the Abolisher of irreligiousness, Purifier, Sustainer, Truth personified, Path-indicator of mind, Revealer of manly vedic truth, Giver of salvation, Adorable, and source of knowledge.

७८. वेदेन रूपे व्यपिबत् सुतासुतौ प्रजापति: । ऋतेन सत्यमिन्द्रियं विपानꣽ शुक्रमन्धस इन्द्रस्येन्द्रियमिदं पयोऽमृतं मधु ॥

78. The soul, full of real knowledge, with the help of all the four vedas, realises the essence of Truth and Untruth. It acquires for itself foodstuffs as meals, riches, the givers of valour and righteous character, water, milk, imperishable knowledge, sweet delicious articles, and the knowledge bestowed by God.

७९. दृष्ट्वा परिस्रुतो रसꣽ शुक्रेण शुक्रं व्यपिबत् पय: सोमं प्रजापति: ।
ऋतेन सत्यमिन्द्रियं विपानꣽ शुक्रमन्धस इन्द्रस्येन्द्रियमिदं पयोऽमृतं मधु ॥

79. The king, who is easily accessible to all, and in a just manner, having carefully examined the juice of efficacious medicines, with pure intention, drinks the delight-giving, drinkable juice of medicines and enjoys the pleasure of knowledge, acquires God-given wealth, the procurer of pure food, and the giver of good drinks, the strength of a hero, and the sweet, disease-healing nectar of a glorious person.

८०. सीसेन तन्त्रं मनसा मनीषिण ऊर्णासूत्रेण कवयो वयन्ति ।
अश्विना यज्ञꣽ सविता सरस्वतीन्द्रस्य रुपं वरूणो भिषज्यन् ॥

80. Just as wise sages understand problems with mental force, prepare bullets with lead, and cloths with woollen thread, so do the learned, an educated wife, teachers and preachers perform sacrifice (yajna), and a skilled physician arranges for the elegance of affluence.

८१. तदस्य रूपममृतꣽ शचीभिस्तिस्रो दधुर्देवता: सꣽरराणा: ।
लोमानि शष्पैर्बहुधा न तोकमभिस्त्वगस्य माꣽ समभवन्न लाजा: ॥

81. Teacher, pupil and examiner, these three divine forces, impart and receive education.

With wisdom and deed, they with long hair, perform the sacrifice in diverse ways. We should understand the eternal nature of this sacrifice. Illiterate youths are not entitled to perform sacrifice (yajna). Hide, meat, parched grain should not be used in the yajna for oblation.

८२. तदश्विना भिषजा रुद्रवर्तनी सरस्वती वयति पेशो अन्तरम् ।
अस्थि मज्जानं मांसरैः कारोतरेण दधतो गवां त्वचि ॥

82. Whomsoever child, a good, intelligent mother gives birth to, that handsome baby with its internal organs, bones and marrow, should be protected on this earth with medicinal juices, like a well, by a physician and his wife, the infusers of life like vital airs.

८३. सरस्वती मनसा पेशलं वसु नासत्याभ्यां वयति दर्शतं वपुः ।
रसं परिस्रुता न रोहितं नग्नहुर्धीरस्तसरं न वेम ॥

83. The learned wife, with her knowledge, like birth, adorns her beautiful, well built body, and prepares meals, the removers of physical discomforts, available from all sides, ready at hand, the givers of delight like nectar. Her thoughtful husband receives pure ideas from his father and mother free from untruth.

८४. पयसा शुक्रममृतं जनित्र ॐ सुरया मूत्राज्जनयन्त रेतः ।
अपामर्ति दुर्मति बाधमाना ऊवध्यं वात ॐ सब्बं तदारात् ॥

84. Those learned persons get progeny, who chase afar folly and ill intention, generate near at hand, by milk and medicinal juices, through generative organ, pure, disease-destroying, children producing semen, that is present in all substances, and causes harm through excessive discharge.

८५. इन्द्रः सुत्रामा हृदयेन सत्यं पुरोडाशेन सविता जजान ।
यकृत् क्लोमानं वरुणो भिषज्यन् मतस्ने वायव्यें मिनाति पित्तम् ॥

85. A learned doctor, guarding the body against disease, giving us medical directions, removing sickness, realises through his soul the exact nature of disease, and with prescribed food, does not allow our lungs, liver, throat-artery, kidney and bile to be affected.

८६. आन्त्राणि स्थालीर्मधु पिन्वमाना गुदाः पात्राणि सुदुघा न धेनुः ।
श्येनस्य पत्रं न प्लीहा शचीभिरासन्दी नभिरुदरं न माता ॥

86. Entrails in the body are the cauldron for cooking food in which honey is mixed, bowels are the pans. This earth the bestower of glory is like a well-milking cow. A hawk's wing is the spleen. Navel, the centre of all strength is like the king's cushion. Belly is like a mother.

[82]Like a well: As well is taken care of, and protected so that its water is not contaminated, so should a child be kept healthy and free from disease by the use of medicines when necessary.
[83]Like birth: Just as a woman keeps the newly born child neat and clean, so does she keep her body clean.
[86]Just as belly digests what we eat, turns out the useless part of the meals, and utilises their essence, so does the mother teach a child to shun vice and imbibe virtue. Just as navel is the centre of the body, from which proceed arteries, so the king sitting on his cushion, i.e., gaddi is the centre of his government. Just as a hawk attacks the enemy and kills him, so the spleen remove all diseases and discomforts of the body.

८७. कुम्भो वनिष्ठुर्जनिता शचीभिर्यस्मिन्नग्रे योन्यां गर्भो अन्तः ।
प्लाशिर्व्यक्तः शतधार उत्सो दुहे न कुम्भी स्वधां पितृभ्यः ॥

87. A husband full of semen like a pitcher, enjoyer, progenitor of children, taker of good meals, full of nourishments, doer of noble deeds, master of hundreds of speeches, deep like a large pitcher, is like one who is engaged in the execution of his duty. A wife is a small jar of water. It is incumbent upon both to give food to their parents and protect the embryo in the womb.

८८. मुखँ सदस्य शिर इत् सतेन जिह्वा पवित्रमश्विनासन्त्सरस्वती ।
चष्पं न पार्युभिषगस्य वालो वस्तिनं शेपो हरसा तरस्वी ॥

88. Just as a wife, the recipient of semen, at the time of cohabitation keeps her head opposite to the head of the husband, and her face opposite to that of his, so should both husband and wife perform together their domestic duties. A husband is a protector like a physician. He lives happily like a child, and with tranquility produces progeny with penis keen with ardour.

८९. अश्विभ्यां चक्षुरमृतं ग्रहाभ्यां छागेन तेजो हविषा शृतेन ।
पक्ष्माणि गोधूमैः कुवलैरुतानि पेशो न शुक्रमसितं वसाते ॥

89. The immortal eyes are like the planets of the sun and moon. The goat's milk and cooked food give them keenness. Eyelashes are like wheat, and eyebrows are jujube. The white and black parts of the eye spread its beauty.

९०. अविनं मेषो नसि वीर्याय प्राणस्य पन्था अमृतो ग्रहाभ्याम् ।
सरस्वत्युपवाकैर्व्यानं नस्यानि बहिर्बदरैर्जजान ॥

90. Just as a learned lady with her husband, through mutual close relations, gives birth to a child, charming like jujubes, so for vigour in the nostril is made the immortal path of breath. The vyan breath goes through the body, guarding it and vying with other breaths, adds to the forces of the nostril.

९१. इन्द्रस्य रूपमृषभो बलाय कर्णाभ्याँ श्रोत्रममृतं ग्रहाभ्याम् ।
यवा न बहिर्भ्रुवि केसराणि कर्कन्धु जज्ञे मधु सारघं मुखात् ॥

91. A learned person acquires yoga, through acts of comprehension, like barley, hears with both ears, uses pure water, exercises of action, like sweet honey, performs acts of advancement, controls breath in Sushumna and concentrates thought in the midst of eyebrows, utters from his mouth God's knowledge. All this is the manifestation of His divine power.

---

[87] A husband possessing more force is compared to a Kumbh, a large pitcher and wife, with less strength to a Kumbhi, a small water jar.

[90] Control of breath: Pranayam protects a yogi from all afflictions, and being well practised advances his spiritual force, so does an educated mother with good instructions develop her children physically and spiritually.

[91] Sushumna: A particular artery of the human body, said to lie between Ida and Pingala, two of the vessels of the body. The comparison of barley and honey is not clear.

६२. आत्मन्न्पस्थ्ये न वृक्स्य लोम मुखे श्मश्रूणि न व्याघ्रलोम ।
केशा न शीर्षन्यशसे श्रियं शिखा सिꣳह्स्य लोम द्विषिरिन्द्रियाणि ॥

92. When a yogi visualises God in his soul at the time of Samadhi (concentration) his hair grow long like those of the wolf. His beard and moustache grow like the hair of a tiger. The hair of his head and tonsure grow like those of a lion. His organs are endowed with lustre, glory and royal power.

६३. अज्ञान्यात्मन् भिषजा तदश्विनात्मानमङ्ग्ङै: समधात् सरस्वती ।
इन्द्रस्य रूपꣳ शतमानमायुश्चन्द्रेण ज्योतिरमृतं दधाना: ॥

93. Just as a woman devoted to yoga, engrossed in deep meditation, practising the limbs of yoga puts her soul in contemplation, so should husband and wife free from disease like a good physician, practise the parts of yoga and attain to the beauty of supremacy. As men practising yoga live for a hundred years, so should we, full of happiness, realise the immortal nature of the soul.

६४. सरस्वती योन्यां गर्भमन्तरश्विभ्यां पत्नी सुकृतं विभर्ति ।
अपाꣳ रसेन वरुणो न साम्नेन्द्रꣳ श्रियं जनयन्नप्सु राजा ॥

94. O yogi, just as an educated wife bears in her womb the noblyfashioned infant, and an excellent king with the help of the teacher and preacher and the spiritual force of the self-abnegating, learned persons (Aptas) controlling the breaths, manifests his sovereignty for wealth, so shouldst thou do.

६५. तेज: पशूनाꣳ हविरिन्द्रियावत् परिस्रुता पयसा सारघं मधु ।
अश्विभ्यां दुग्धं भिषजा सरस्वत्या सुनासुताभ्याममृत: सोम इन्दु: ॥

95. The ghee of animals is eatable and giver of physical strength. The juice of medicines and delicious sugar mixed with milk also add to physical strength. The water yielded by two efficacious agencies, the sun and moon and lightning is also invigorating. The pressed and unpressed medicinal Soma juice acts like nectar.

---

⁹²A yogi generally lives in solitude of forests, where reside wolves, tigers and lions. Due to prolonged and deep concentration his hair grow like those of these animals who are his companions.

⁹⁴Just as mother safeguards the infant in her womb, and a king adds to royal power, so should a yogi attain to yoga-sidhis. There are eight limbs of yoga: Yam, Niyam, Aṣan, Pranayam, Pratyahar, Dharana, Dhyana, Samadhi,

CHAPTER XX

१. क्षत्रस्य योनिरसि क्षत्रस्य नाभिरसि ।
मा त्वा हिꣳसीन्मा मा हिꣳसीः ॥

1. O King, thou art the birth place of princely power, and centre of royal family. Let none harm thee, do not harm me!

२. नि षसाद धृतव्रतो वरुणः पस्त्यास्वा ।
साम्राज्याय सुक्रतुः ।
मृत्योः पाहि विद्योत्पाहि ॥

2. O King, endowed with wisdom and enterprise, imbiber of truth, good natured, sit thou in the midst of thy subjects in Legislatures for universal rule. Save us from death. Save us from fiery weapons!

३. देवस्य त्वा सवितुः प्रसवेऽश्विनोर्बाहुभ्यां पूष्णो हस्ताभ्याम् ।
अश्विनोर्भैषज्येन तेजसे ब्रह्मवर्चसायाभि षिञ्चामि ।
सरस्वत्यै भैषज्येन वीर्यायान्नाद्यायाभि षिञ्चामि—
न्द्रस्येन्द्रियेण बलाय श्रियै यशसेऽभि षिञ्चामि ॥

3. O King, in this world created by God, the Embodiment of glory, with the strength and valour of teachers and preachers, with the perseverance and enterprise of a heroic person, with the healing powers of a physician, for eloquence and study of the vedas, do I enthrone thee!
With the wealth of a magnate, for strength of body, riches and fame, do I enthrone thee.

४. कोऽसि कतमोऽसि कस्मै त्वा काय त्वा ।
सुश्लोक सुमङ्गल सत्यराजन् ॥

4. O famous and truthful king, doer of noble deeds, and dispenser of justice, thou art happy, thou art extremely happy, hence for God the Embodiment of happiness, for the advancement of Vedic knowledge, do I enthrone thee!

५. शिरो मे श्रीर्यशो मुखं त्विषिः केशाश्च श्मश्रूणि ।
राजा मे प्राणो अमृतꣳ सम्राट् चक्षुर्विराट् श्रोत्रम् ॥

5. May my head be full of grace, my mouth of fame, my hair and beard,

---

²Us: Soldiers, military generals.
³I: Adhvaryu, the master of the vedas, the representative of the King and the subjects who presides over the coronation ceremony.
⁵My: the enthroned King.

of brilliant sheen, my breath, of light and deathlessness, my eye, of even-handed love, my ear, of religious lore.

६. जिह्वा मे भद्रं वाङ्महो मनो मन्युः स्वराड् भामः ।
मोदाः प्रमोदा अङ्गुलीरङ्ग्रानि मित्रं मे सहः ॥

6. May my tongue taste invigorating food, my voice be full of adorable vedic lore, my mind be full of righteous indignation on the morally degraded, my intellect be self-illumined. Full of joy be my fingers, delightful my bodily organs, and conquering-strength my friend.

७. बाहू मे बलमिन्द्रियँ हस्तौ मे कर्म वीर्यम् ।
आत्मा क्षत्रमुरो मम ॥

7. Power and wealth are my arms, deed and heroism are my hands. Soul and heart are my shield against danger.

८. पृष्ठीमें राष्ट्रमुदरमँसौ ग्रीवाश्च श्रोणी ।
ऊरू अरत्नी जानुनी विशो मेऽङ्गानि सर्वतः ॥

8. My government is my back, my belly, shoulders, neck, hips, thighs, elbows, knees, and all other members of the body are my subjects.

९. नाभिमें चित्तं विज्ञानं पायुमेंऽपचितिर्भसत् ।
आनन्दनन्दावाण्डौ मे भगः सौभाग्यं पसः ।
जङ्घाभ्यां पद्भ्यां धर्मोऽस्मि विशि राजा प्रतिष्ठितः ॥

9. May my memory, navel, knowledge, anus, my wife's productive womb, my testicles, the givers of pleasure through cohabitation, my sovereignty and penis flourish. Standing on my legs and feet, in the midst of my subjects, free from favouritism, with even-handed justice, I rule as a king, with full fame.

१०. प्रति क्षत्रे प्रति तिष्ठामि राष्ट्रे प्रत्यश्वेषु प्रति तिष्ठामि गोषु ।
प्रत्यज्ञेषु प्रति तिष्ठाम्यात्मन् प्रति प्राणेषु प्रति तिष्ठामि पुष्टे प्रति द्यावापृथिव्योः प्रति तिष्ठामि यज्ञे ॥

10. I take my stand on princely power and kingship, on horses am I dependent, and on cows, on agencies of administration I depend, on my soul do I depend. On vital breaths am I dependent, and on invigorating cereals do I depend. I depend on justice like the sun and moon. I depend on the company of the learned, and on the spread of knowledge.

[9]A king should exercise control over all the organs of his body, and try to keep them healthy and efficient.
[10]I: King.

११ त्रया देवा एकादश त्रयस्त्रिꣳशाः सुराधसः ।
बृहस्पतिपुरोहिता देवस्य सवितुः सवे ।
देवा देवैरवन्तु मा ॥

11. There are three times eleven, i.e., thirty three fine objects imbued with attributes, duties and inherent properties, in this world created by God; of whom the sun is the most prominent, and which are serviceable to mankind. May the learned persons, with the help of these objects protect me.

१२. प्रथमा द्वितीयैर्द्वितीयास्तृतीयैस्तृतीयाः सत्येन सत्यं यज्ञेन यज्ञो यजुर्भिर्यजूꣳषि सामभिः सामान्यृग्भिभर्क्ऋ॑चः पुरोऽनुवाक्याभिः पुरोऽनुवाक्या याज्याभिर्याज्या वषट्कारैर्वषट्कारा आहुतिभिराहुतयो मे कामान्त्समर्धयन्तु भूः स्वाहा ॥

12. May the first Vasus with the second Rudras, the Rudras with the third Adityas (twelve months), the third Adityas with Truth, Truth with Sacrifice, Sacrifice with sacrificial texts of the Yajur veda, Yajur vedic texts with the knowledge of the Sama veda, Samans with praise-verses of the Rigveda, praise-verses with the texts of the Atharva veda, Atharva vedic texts with inviting texts pertaining to sacrifice (yajna), sacrificial texts with noble deeds, noble deeds with oblations, and oblations with truthful practices, fulfil my desires on this earth.

१३. लोमानि प्रयतिर्मम त्वग्म आनतिरागतिः ।
माꣳसं म उपनतिर्वंस्वस्थि मज्जा म आनतिः ॥

13. O teachers and preachers exert so that my hair be effort and attempt, my skin be reverence, my flesh be approach, wealth my inclination, my bone and marrow reverence!

१४. यद्देवा देवहेडनं देवासश्चकृमा वयम् ।
अग्निर्मा तस्मादेनसो विश्वान्मुञ्चत्वꣳहसः ॥

14. O learned persons, whatever disrespect we and other scholars show to the learned, may God set me free from all that iniquity and fault!

१५. यदि दिवा यदि नक्तमेनाꣳसि चकृमा वयम् ।
वायुर्मा तस्मादेनसो विश्वान्मुञ्चत्वꣳहसः ॥

---

[11]There are eight Vasus, eleven Rudras, and twelve Adityas, the twelve months, electricity and Yajna. These constitute thirty three devatas, fine objects, of whom the eleven Rudras form a part.

[12]All the 33 devatas, the forces of nature and the knowledge of all the four vedas, fulfil man's desires.

[13]Comparison is made between the parts of the body, and qualities of administration in a State. The joint effort of all in a state is like hair. The power of subduing the enemy is like my skin. Just as skin protects me so the spirit of reverence protects a state.

[14]We: Teachers and preachers.
Agni may also mean a learned person illumined like fire with the light of different branches of knowledge.

[15]Vaya may also mean, a learned Apta.

15. If in the day-time or at night, we have committed any act of sin, may God set me free from all that iniquity and fault.

१६. यदि जाग्रद्यदि स्वप्न एनाँसि चकृमा वयम् ।
सूर्यं मा तस्मादेनसो विश्वान्मुञ्चत्वँहस: ॥

16. If when awake or in our sleep we have committed acts of sin, May God set me free from all that iniquity and fault.

१७. यद्ग्रामे यदरण्ये यत्सभायां यदिन्द्रिये ।
यच्छूद्रे यद्यें यदेनश्चकृमा वयं यदेकस्याधि धर्मणि तस्यावयजनमसि ॥

17. Each fault in village or in forest, society or mind, each sinful act that we have done to Sudra or Vaishyas, or in preventing any body from religious performances, even of that sin, O God, Thou art the expiation!

१८. यदापो अघ्न्या इति वरुणेति शपामहे ततो वरुण नो मुञ्च ।
अवभृथ निचुम्पुण निचेरुरसि निचुम्पुण: ।
अव देवैर्देवकृतमेनोऽयक्ष्यव मर्त्यैर्मर्त्यकृतं पुरुराणो देव रिषस्पाहि ॥

18. O adorable God, The Giver of divine wisdom, Supreme of all, save me from the sin of taunting the vital breaths and inviolable cows!

O lord of celibacy and knowledge, thou art a slow-walker, giver of happiness, and full of delight, save us from distressing violence. Thou avertest the offence committed by the learned towards the learned and the ordinary mortals towards mortals!

१९. समुद्रे ते हृदयमप्स्वन्त: सं त्वा विशन्त्वोषधीरुतापः ।
सुमित्रिया न आप ओषधय: सन्तु दुर्मित्रियास्तस्मै सन्तु योऽस्मान्द्वेष्टि यं च वयं द्विष्म: ॥

19. O King, let thy heart be deep like the ocean. May thou obtain food, fruits, and drinkable juices. May water and medicinal herbs be pleasant for us like a friend. May these be inimical for those who dislike us and whom we dislike!

२०. द्रुपदादिव मुमुचान: स्विन्न: स्नातो मलादिव ।
पूतं पवित्रेणेवाज्यमाप: शुन्धन्तु मैनस: ॥

20. O learned persons pure like water and breath, purify me from sin, just as a ripe fruit is released from the tree, or as an exhausted person full of sweat is freed from dirt by bathing, or as ghee is purified by a sieve!

२१. उद्वयं तमसस्परि स्व: पश्यन्त उत्तरम् ।
देवं देवत्रा सूर्यमगन्म ज्योतिरुत्तमम् ॥

---

[16] Surya may also mean a learned person.
[17] Expiation: Means of atonement.
[18] See Yajur 6-22, 3-48.
[19] See Yajur 8-25, 6-22.

21. May we realising God from all sides, excellently attain to Him, far from darkness, full of Light, God among the gods, Embodiment of happiness, the Subtlest of all, and the Supreme Self Effulgent.

२२. अपो अद्यान्वचारिषँ॒ रसेन समसृक्ष्महि ।
पयस्वानग्न आगमं तं मा सँ॒सृज वर्चसा प्रजया च धनेन च ॥

22. O learned teacher, I, possessing the knowledge of the science of water, come unto thee. May I today heartily drink waters. Bestow on me the knowledge of the vedas, progeny and wealth, whereby I may get happiness!

२३. एधोऽस्येधिषीमहि समिदसि तेजोऽसि तेजो मयि धेहि ।
समावर्वति पृथिवी समुषाः समु सूर्यः ।
समु विश्वमिदं जगत् ।
वैश्वानरज्योतिभूँ॒यासं विभून् कामान् व्यश्नवै भूः स्वाहा ॥

23. O God, Thou conducest to our prosperity. Just as fuel illumines fire, so dost Thou illumine our souls. Thou art wisdom personified. Grant me the light of knowledge. Thou art omnipresent. Thou hast nicely created the Earth, Dawn, Sun, and this entire world. May we always prosper, having realized the Effulgent Lord, the Guide of the universe. May I achieve various big ambitions. May I realise God and Matter through truthful speech, and noble deeds!

२४. अभ्या दधामि समिधमग्ने व्रतपते त्वयि ।
व्रतं च श्रद्धां चोपैमीन्धे त्वा दीक्षितो ब्रह्म ॥

24. O God, the Fulfiller of vows, concentrating myself on Thee, I plunge in divine meditation like fuel in fire, whereby I acquire the vow of truth and faith!

Being initiated in celibacy and gaining knowledge, I kindle Thee.

२५. यत्र ब्रह्म च क्षत्रं च सम्यञ्चौ चरतः सह ।
तँल्लोकं पुण्यं प्रज्ञेषं यत्र देवाः सहाग्निना ॥

25. I consider that society or country to be the ideal, where the civil and military forces work together harmoniously, where the learned civil administrators cooperate with the commanders of the army.

२६. यत्रेन्द्रश्च वायुश्च सम्यञ्चौ चरतः सह ।
तँल्लोकं पुण्यं प्रज्ञेषं यत्र सेदिनं विद्यते ॥

26. Fain would I know that holy God, where birth and death unknown, where in complete accordance reside soul and God side by side.

---

[26]In the state of emancipation soul and God live together. There soul is free from the pangs of hunger and thirst, where the distress of birth and death is not felt.

२७. अंशुना ते अंशुः पृच्यतां परुषा परुः ।
गन्धस्ते सोममवतु मदाय रसो अच्युतः ॥

27. Let thy soul be united with God. Let each joint of thine be full of vigour. Let thy noble nature guard thy wealth. Let the imperishable sap of God's devotion be for thy joy.

२८. सिञ्चति परि षिञ्चन्त्युत्सिञ्चन्ति पुनन्ति च ।
सुरायै बभ्रवे मदे किन्त्वो वदति किन्त्वः ॥

28. Those who aspire after power, for delight pour in the stomach the sap of medicines, drink it, receive it excellently, and purify themselves, strengthen their body and soul. He who says 'What is this,' 'What is that,' gains nothing.

२९. धानावन्तं करम्भिणमपूपवन्तमुक्थिनम् ।
इन्द्र प्रातर्जुषस्व नः ॥

29. O learned person desirous of happiness, at morn accept our cake accompanied with grain and groats, with wheaten bread and hymns of praise!

३०. बृहदिन्द्राय गायत मरुतो वृत्रहन्तमम् ।
येन ज्योतिरजनयन्नृतावृधो देवं देवाय जागृवि ॥

30. O learned persons, advancers of truth, whereby ye create pleasant highly known spiritual power, for the attainment of Holy God, like sun the dispeller of cloud, chant the great Sama hymns in praise of God !

३१. अध्वर्यो अद्रिभिः सुतꣳ सोमं पवित्र आ नय ।
पुनाहीन्द्राय पातवे ॥

31. O Adhvaryu, bring into the sacred yajna, Soma, born of clouds. Purify it for king's drink !

३२. यो भूतानामधिपतिर्यस्मिँल्लोका अधि श्रिताः ।
य ईशे महतो महाँस्तेन गृह्णामि त्वामहं मयि गृह्णामि त्वामहम् ॥

32. He is the Lord of living beings, upon Whom the worlds depend. God is mighty. He is greater than space. Hence I realise Him, I realise Him in my heart.

३३. उपयामगृहीतोऽस्यश्विभ्यां त्वा सरस्वत्यै त्वेन्द्राय त्वा सुत्राम्ण एष ते योनिरश्विभ्यां त्वा सरस्वत्यै त्वेन्द्राय त्वा सुत्राम्णे ।

33. O learned person, thou art trained in nice rules of conduct, by the teacher and the preacher. Thou art educationally connected with them. I

---

[28] He who reviles the efficacy of medicines does not improve his body and soul.
[31] Adhvaryu: one of the four priests, Hota, Udgata. Adhvaryu and Brahma, who minister the yajna.

accept thee for didactic speech, for lofty supremacy, for effective guardianship, for thy possessing a noble, learned wife, for noble behaviour, and for full protection !

३४. प्राणपा मे अ्रपानपाश्चक्षुष्पा: श्रोत्रपाश्च मे ।
वाचो मे विश्वभेषजो मनसोऽसि विलायक: ॥

34. O God, Thou art the guardian of my inner breath and outward breath, the guardian of my eye and ear. All-healer of my voice, Thou art the Mollifier of my mind !

३५. अश्विनकृतस्य ते सरस्वतिकृतस्येन्द्रेण सुत्राम्णा कृतस्य ।
उपहूत उपहूतस्य भक्षयामि ॥

35. O learned person, invited, do I feed upon the food brought near, prepared by the experts and learned ladies, under instructions from the protecting king !

३६. समिद्ध इन्द्र उषसामनीके पुरोरुचा पूर्वकृद्धावृधान: ।
त्रिभिर्देवेस्त्रिꙪशता वज्रबाहुर्जघान वृत्रं वि दुरो ववार ।

36. O learned person, just as the sun kindled in forefront of Mornings, with forward light, long-active, waxing mighty, with thirty three supernatural powers of nature, the Thunder-wielder, smites dead the cloud, and throws light on the portals, so do thou with the help of warriors kill the foes, and open the doors of knowledge and religion!

३७. नराशꙪस: प्रति शूरो मिमानस्तनूनपात्प्रति यज्ञस्य धाम ।
गोभिर्वपावान् मधुना समञ्जन् हिरण्यैश्चन्द्री यजति प्रचेता: ॥

37. He, who is praised by the public, is the discoverer of different objects, is the master of just behaviour, is fearless, maintains the vitality of his body, is engaged in agriculture with oxen, is full of knowledge, is wealthy with gold, is extremely wise, and performs yajna, is fit for us to seek shelter under.

३८. ईडितो देवैर्हरिवाꙪ अ्रभिष्टिराजुह्वानो हविषा शर्धमान: ।
पुरन्दरो गोत्रभिद्वज्रबाहुरा यातु यज्ञमुप नो जुषाण: ॥

38. O Commander of the army may thou approach our sacrifice (yajna) rejoicing. Thou art lauded by the learned, lord of bay steeds, the performer of sacrifice, invited by the wise, advancest with giving and receiving knowledge. Fort-render, enjoyer of thy soldiers as the sun enjoys after rending asunder the cloud, and Thunder-wielder art thou!

३९. जुषाणो बर्हिर्हरिवान् न इन्द्र: प्राचीनꙪ सीदत् प्रदिशा पृथिव्या: ।
उरुप्रथा: प्रथमानꙪ स्योनमादित्यैरक्तं वसुभि: सजोषा: ॥

39. O learned person, just as the sun, residing in space, full of rays, vast in extent, accompanied by months and worlds like the Earth, stationed in an

intermediate quarter from the Earth, full of expanse, famous and ancient, is occupying its pleasant orbit, so shouldst thou be amongst us!

४०. इन्द्रं दुर: कवष्यो धावमाना वृषणं यन्तु जनय: सुपत्नी: ।
द्वारो देवीरभितो वि श्रयन्ताꣽ सुवीरा वीरं प्रथमाना महोभि: ॥

40. O people, just as glib-tongued, child-bearing ladies moving fast, reach the gates of lustrous, majestic and heroic husbands, and just as reputed, valiant, well-mannered, vigilant husbands, seek from all sides the asylum of wives, advanced in knowledge, so shouldst ye do!

४१. उषासानक्ता बृहती बृहन्तं पयस्वती सुदुघे शूरमिन्द्रम् ।
तन्तुं ततं पेशसा संवयन्ती देवानां देवं यजत: सुरुक्मे ॥

41. O people, just as Dawn and Night fair in appearance, coupled with the darkness of night, richly-yielding, with growing light, accompany the sun, long-extended, illuminator of worlds like the Earth, lofty, so should ye keep contact with an expressive heroic person!

४२. दैव्या मिमाना मनुष: पुरुत्रा होतारविन्द्रं प्रथमा सुवाचा ।
मूर्धन् यज्ञस्य मधुना दधाना प्राचीनं ज्योतिर्हविषा वृधात: ॥

42. Teacher and Preacher, companions of the learned, good organisers, charitable, pleasant-voiced, first to officiate on a yajna, leaders of multitude of people, who with sweet oblation increase the ancient light and glory, are fit to be adored by all.

४३. तिस्रो देवीर्हविषा वर्धमाना इन्द्रं जुषाणा जनयो न पत्नी: ।
अच्छिन्नं तन्तुं पयसा सरस्वतीडा देवी भारती विश्वतूर्ति: ॥

43. Vidya Sabha, Dharma Sabha and Rajya Sabha, all three bent on speedily solving problems, well-qualified and duly constituted, thriving through knowledge and authority, like wedded dames, taking charge of State's administration, with prowess, skill and affluence, preserve the government like the unbroken thread of progeny.

४४. त्वष्टा दधच्छुष्ममिन्द्राय वृष्णेऽपाकोऽचिष्टर्यशसे पुरूणि ।
वृषा यजन्वृषणं भूरिरेता मूर्धन् यज्ञस्य समनक्तु देवान् ॥

44. O learned person, just as an active scholar, full of vigour, gathers strength for a strong glorious Commander, being most famous, and adored throughout the land, masters various objects for glory, full of vitality, showering happiness like the cloud, acquires full might, and wishes for the sages in a well known place on the earth, so shouldst thou do!

[43]Vidya Sabha: Assembly of the learned.
 Dharma Sabha: Assembly of the religious.
 Rajya Sabha: Assembly of the Administrators.
 These are three Assemblies, which should run efficiently the administration of a country.

४५. वनस्पतिरवसृष्टो न पाशैस्तमन्या समञ्जञ्छमिता न देवः ।
इन्द्रस्य हव्यैर्जेठरं पृणानः स्वदाति यज्ञं मधुना घृतेन ॥

45. He, who rears the trees by erecting strong barriers round them, creating contact with the soul, like one under orders, conduces to our happiness, fills the treasure of fame, as one fills the belly with sacrifice, performs sacrifice with edible objects like honey and butter, and tastes them well, remains immune from disease.

४६. स्तोकानामिन्दु प्रति शूर इन्द्रो वृषायमाणो वृषभस्तुराषाट् ।
घृतप्रुषा मनसा मोदमानाः स्वाहा देवा अमृता मादयन्ताम् ॥

46. Just as a strong, exalted, heroic person, overpowers the violent foe, but is pleased with an upright, straight-forward man with little merit, so with brilliant knowledge, and truthful deeds, let the immortal sages, full of joy and contentment contribute to our happiness.

४७. आ यात्विन्द्रोऽवस उप न इह स्तुतः सधमदस्तु शूरः ।
वावृधानस्तविषीर्यस्य पूर्वीर्द्यौर्न क्षत्रमभिभूति पुष्यात् ॥

47. May the mighty ruler, applauded at present, being fearless and heroic, augmenting his forces, well trained by past commanders, whose sovereignty, competent to subdue the foes shines like the sun, strengthen us, and come to us for our protection, and may he occupy a dignified position.

४८. आ न इन्द्रो दूराद आ आसादभिष्टिकृदवसे यासदुग्रः ।
ओजिष्ठेभिर्नृपतिर्वज्रबाहुः सङ्गे समत्सु तुर्वणिः पृतन्यून् ॥

48. May the foe-subduing Commander, acquiring desired happiness with arms, nourisher of men, accompanied by valiant warriors, full of righteous indignation on the wicked, and swift killer of foes, come to us from far or near for our protection in battles, and guard and honour our men.

४९. आ न इन्द्रो हरिभिर्यात्वच्छावर्चीनोऽवसे राधसे च ।
तिष्ठाति वज्री मघवा विरप्शीं यज्ञमनु नो वाजसातौ ॥

49. May the Commander of the army, mighty, facing the enemy with the force of his knowledge, well-trained in the use of arms, with disciplined cavalry, stand in combat to guard and enrich us. May he nicely share our this administrative business based on truth and justice.

५०. त्रातारमिन्द्रमवितारमिन्द्रꣳ हवे-हवे सुहवꣳ शूरमिन्द्रम् ।
ह्वयामि शक्रं पुरुहूतमिन्द्रꣳ स्वस्ति नो मघवा धात्विन्द्रः ॥

50. O Commander, in each battle I invite thee, the rescuer, the destroyer of the ignoble, affable, the giver of glory, deserving of invocation, the Subduer of the foes, the preserver of administration, quick in action, adored by the multitude, and the castigator of the enemy's army. O Bounteous Lord, may thou give us happiness!

५१. इन्द्रः सुत्रामा स्ववाँ२ अवोभिः सुमृडीको भवतु विश्ववेदाः ।
बाधतां द्वेषो अभयं कृणोतु सुवीर्यस्य पतयः स्याम ॥

51. The ruler, a good protector, accompanied by his excellent assistants, full of wealth, diffuser of happiness, should protect his subjects by administering justice, remove the opponents, render all free from fear, and himself be fearless, whereby we may be the lords of vigour.

५२. तस्य वयंꣶ सुमतौ यज्ञियस्यापि भद्रे सौमनसे स्याम ।
स सुत्रामा स्ववाँ२ इन्द्रो अस्मे आराच्चिद् द्वेषः सनुतर्युयोतु ॥

52. May the ruler, our good preserver, with his noble family members, a father unto us, drive from us away, even from far and near, our foemen.
May we dwell in the auspicious favour of and obey the orders of the ruler, who is fit to perform acts of sacrifice.

५३. आ मन्द्रैरिन्द्र हरिभिर्याहि मयूररोमभिः ।
मा त्वा के चिन्नि यमन् विं न पाशिनोऽति धन्वेव ताँ२ इहि ॥

53. O Mighty Commander, go forth, with excellent steeds having tails like peacock plumes, to conquer thy foes. Let none check thy course, as fowlers capture the bird. Come unto us like a skilful archer!

५४. एवेदिन्द्रं वृषणं वज्रबाहुं वसिष्ठासो अभ्यचंन्त्यर्कैः ।
स न स्तुतो वीरवद्धातु गोमद्यूयं पात स्वस्तिभिः सदा नः ॥

54. O wealthy citizens, just as learned persons laud the slayer of foes, who is powerful, whose arms wield weapons, so should ye. Thus praised may he guard our wealth in men and cattle. Ye heroes, preserve us evermore with blessings!

५५. समिद्धो अग्निरश्विना तप्तो घर्मो विराट् सुतः ।
दुहे धेनुः सरस्वती सोमꣶ शुक्रमिहेन्द्रियम् ॥

55. Just as in this world, vedic text, like the milch-cow, multiplies our pure glory and wealth, so should I perfect it. O men and women just as heated, radiant, impelled, burning, unified fire protects the world, so should I protect it!

५६. तनूपा भिषजा सुतेऽश्विनोभा सरस्वती ।
मध्वा रजाꣳ सीन्द्रियमिन्द्राय पथिभिर्वहान् ॥

56. O people, just as both husband and wife, conversant with medical science, guardians of the body, accomplished with noble nature and good dealings, possessing vedic knowledge and sweetness in speech in this world, preserve by different devices wealth and the people for the king, so ye should contact them!

५७. इन्द्रायेन्दु꣡ सरस्वती नराश꣡सेन नग्नहुम् ।
अधातामश्विना मधु भेषजं भिषजा सुते ॥

57. Both kinds of physicians, well versed in the science of medicine, for the removal of ailment, in this world, prescribe medicine skilfully and with a sweet voice. May speech full of commendable learning, coupled with words of praise from men, lead to affluence, conducive to happiness.

५८. आजुह्वाना सरस्वतीन्द्रायेन्द्रियाणि वीर्यम् ।
इडाभिरश्विनाविष꣡ समू꣡र्जं꣡ स꣡ रियं꣡ दधुः ॥

58. An educated wife, praised on all sides, for her prosperous husband, acquires gold, strong organs, and butter that builds the body.

Physicians with their medical knowledge resplendent like the sun and moon, with efficacious medicines, acquire foodstuffs, good might and nice religious wealth.

५९. अश्विना नमुचेः सुत꣡ सोम꣡ शुक्रं परिस्रुता ।
सरस्वती तमा ऽभरद्द्रहिषेन्द्राय पातवे ॥

59. Laudable man and woman, who moving freely, imbued with noble qualities, deeds, and characteristics, with acts conducive to happiness, for the attainment of supreme power, delivery from an incurable disease, and for safety, use the juice of well-prepared, strength-infusing medicines, always remain happy.

६०. कवष्यो न व्यचस्वतीरश्विभ्यां न दुरो दिशः ।
इन्द्रो न रोदसी उभे दुहे कामान्त्सरस्वती ॥

60. Just as highly applauded lightning pervading the sun and moon, illumines directions and gates, and engulfs the Earth and Heaven, so do I an educated woman accomplish my desires.

६१. उषासानक्तमश्विना दिवेन्द्र꣡ सायमिन्द्रियैः ।
सञ्जानाने सुपेशसा समञ्जाते सरस्वत्या ॥

61. O learned persons, just as the sun and moon, of fair hue, at dawn and night, by day and in the evening, are adorned by manifesting lightning, so should ye adorn yourselves with the noble qualities of soul and well disciplined speech!

६२. पातं नो अश्विना दिवा पाहि नक्त꣡ सरस्वति ।
दैव्या होतारा भिषजा पातमिन्द्र꣡ सचा सुते ॥

---

[57]There are two kinds of physicians: one who treats the physical ailments, and the other who deals with mental maladies. The word Nagnahu (नग्नहु) in the verse has been translated by Griffith as the drug used for fermenting the sura (सुरा), Rishi Dayananda translates it as 'conducive to happiness.'

62. O virtuous teachers and preachers, guard us in day and night, O highly educated mother guard us. O health-giving physician, according well, protect the juice of medicines!

६३. तिस्रस्त्रेधा सरस्वत्यश्विना भारतीडा ।
तीव्रं परिस्रुता सोममिन्द्राय सुषुवुर्मंदम् ॥

63. Well-disciplined speech, protecting mother, laudable preachress, these three, and two good physicians, should produce differently the strong, gladdening, well-begotten juice of medicines.

६४. अश्विना भेषजं मधु भेषजं नः सरस्वती ।
इन्द्रे त्वष्टा यशः श्रियʘ रूपʘ रूपमधुः सुते ॥

64. May the teacher and preacher, imparters of knowledge, a highly educated mother, a skilled workman, give us glory, fame, and divers beautiful objects for the consummation of our affluence.

६५. ऋतुथेन्द्रो वनस्पतिः शशमानः परिस्रुता ।
कीलालमश्विभ्यां मधु दुहे धेनुः सरस्वती ॥

65. Just as didactic speech through free use fulfils our desires like a milch-cow, and just at a mighty tree growing with the passage of seasons, with its sweet juice and edible products fulfils our desires under the advice of physicians, so may I fulfil my desires.

६६. गोभिनं सोममश्विना मासरेण परिस्रुता ।
समधातʘ सरस्वत्या स्वाहेन्द्रे सुतं मधु ॥

66. O physicians, just as we attain to supremacy, with measured rice diet, with speech full of instruction, knowledge and sweetness, with cows' milk and its products, so should ye use the juice of medicines, highly efficacious and well prepared!

६७. अश्विना हविरिन्द्रियं नमुचेर्धिया सरस्वती ।
आ शुक्रमासुराद्वसु मघमिन्द्राय जभ्रिरे ॥

67. Good physicians and an educated lady, with their wisdom, through the use of material objects resulting from indestructible matter, should cultivate an acceptable mind, and acquire from cloud strength, brilliant treasure, and ample wealth.

[63]Disciplined speech: the instructions of a physician.
Differently: In three ways, each working independently.
Two physicians: Healers of physical and mental ills.
[66]Physicians means two physicians as stated in verse 63.
[67]Clouds give us timely rain, which enriches our agricultural land, and adds to our wealth by bumper harvests.

६८. यमश्विना सरस्वती हविषेन्द्रमवर्धयन् ।
स बिभेद बलं मघं नमुचावासुरे सचा ॥

68. Teacher and preacher united together, and an educated woman, with oblations made of material provisions, whose home is in clouds born of indestructible matter, strengthen their might, which shatters to pieces even the splendid force of the enemy.

६९. तमिन्द्रं पशवः सचाश्विनोभा सरस्वती ।
दधाना अभ्यनूषत हविषा यज्ञ इन्द्रियैः ॥

69. O people, use nicely Soma, imbued with strength-giving quality, in yajna's oblations, just as two learned teacher and preacher, experts in the science of medicine utilise it, or just as an educated lady avails of it, or just as cattle use it !

७०. य इन्द्र इन्द्रियं दधुः सविता वरुणो भगः ।
स सुत्रामा हविष्पतिर्यजमानाय सश्चत ॥

70. They who acquire wealth for supremacy, attain to happiness. He becomes dignified, who imbued with the spirit of service, full of excellence, desirous of advancement, good guardian, protector of yajna's oblations, enjoys wealth through the sacrificer.

७१. सविता वरुणो दधद्यजमानाय दाशुषे ।
आदत्त नमुचेर्वसु सुत्रामा बलमिन्द्रियम् ॥

71. An excellent urger, a good guardian bestowing gifts on the liberal offerer, should attract the force and well-trained mind of a sacrificer, who abandons not the path of virtue.

७२. वरुणः क्षत्रमिन्द्रियं भगेन सविता श्रियम् ।
सुत्रामा यशसा बलं दधाना यज्ञमाशत ॥

72. O men, just as a noble soul, striving for affluence, speaker of the Assembly, a good guardian, full of prosperity, acquires sovereignty, a just mind, worldly wealth and philanthropic deeds, so should ye acquire them, possessing renown and strength!

७३. अश्विना गोभिरिन्द्रियमश्वेभिर्वीर्यं बलम् ।
हविषेन्द्रं सरस्वती यजमानमवर्धयन् ॥

[68]Whose refers to oblations, which rise up and reside in clouds.
[70]He : Priest.
A sacrificer (yajman) adds to the wealth of the priest (Purohit), just as the priest advances the fame and glory of the sacrificer.
[71]An excellent urger, a good guardian means the king or a noble soul.
[72]A good guardian: The speaker of the Assembly is the guardian of the rights and privileges of its members.

73. Teacher, preacher, and an educated lady, with disciplined speech, well trained horses, and enterprise, should augment wealth, prowess, strength, and enhance a mighty devotee of truth.

७४. ता नासत्या सुपेशसा हिरण्यवर्तनी नरा ।
सरस्वती हविष्मतीन्द्र कर्मसु नोऽवत ॥

74. May both teacher and preacher, fair of form, rolling in wealth, an educated wife, possessing serviceable objects, and thou a learned fellow, help us in all our acts.

७५. ता भिषजा सुकर्मणा सा सुदुघा सरस्वती ।
स वृत्रहा शतक्रतुरिन्द्राय दधुरिन्द्रियम् ॥

75. May both the healers of the body and soul, righteous in their deeds, an educated woman, who imparts knowledge just as a cow yields milk, and a highly sagacious person, like the sun that tears asunder the cloud, possess riches for the sake of prosperity.

७६. युवं सुराममश्विना नमुचावासुरे सचा ।
विपिपाना: सरस्वतीन्द्रं कर्मस्वावत ॥

76. O teacher and preacher, ye both, co-operating together, and learned subjects, like the uninterrupted eternal cloud, behave most beautifully in sovereign deeds, and so act as our protectors in diverse ways!

७७. पुत्रमिव पितरावश्विनोभेन्द्रावथु: काव्यैर्दंसनाभि: ।
यत्सुरामं व्यपिव: शचीभि: सरस्वती त्वा मघवन्नभिष्णक् ॥

77. O learned person, full of wealth, knowledge and affluence, thou wisely drinkest the juice of efficacious medicines, thou art served by thy educated wife, may thou be protected by the teacher and preacher with the works of the poets, just as father and mother rear their son !

७८. यस्मिन्नश्वास ऋषभास उक्षणो वशा मेषा अवसृष्टास आहुता: ।
कीलालपे सोमपृष्ठाय वेधसे हृदा मतिं जनय चारुमग्नये ॥

78. He, who collects, trains and takes useful service from horses, bulls, oxen, barren cows and rams, is the protector of foodgrains, is imbued with an amiable disposition, and is a wise, brilliant person, deserves hearty respect.

७९. अहाव्यग्ने हविरास्ये ते स्रुचीव घृतं चम्वीव सोम: ।
वाजसनिं रयिमस्मे सुवीरं प्रशस्तं धेहि यशसं बृहन्तम् ॥

79. O learned person, within thy mouth is poured the offering, as Soma into cup, ghee into ladle.

[78]We should respect the persons who train animals for useful service.

Vouchsafe us wealth, strength-winning, blest with heroes, and wealth, lofty praised by men, and full of splendour.

८०. अश्विना तेजसा चक्षुः प्राणेन सरस्वती वीर्यम् ।
वाचेन्द्रो बलेनेन्द्राय दधुरिन्द्रियम् ॥

80. Teacher and preacher, an educated lady, the leader of the Assembly give to the soul, sight with lustre, manly strength with breath, vigorous power with voice and might.

८१. गोमद्दू पु णासत्याश्वावद्यातमश्विना ।
वर्ती रुद्रा नृपाय्यम् ॥

81. O highly educated people, wedded to truth, chastisers of the wicked, equipped with horses and pasture-land for cows, just as ye command respect from men, so should we!

८२. न यत्परो नान्तर आदधर्षद्दृषण्वसू ।
दुःशँसो मर्त्यो रिपुः ॥

82. O head of the State and Chief of the Staff administer the State in a way that no internal or external malicious mortal foe be able to harm it !

८३. ता न आ वोढमश्विना रियं पिशङ्गसन्दृशम् ।
धिष्ण्या वरिवोविदम् ॥

83. O wise Head of the State and Chief of the Staff lead us on to wealth, glittering like gold, and highly serviceable!

८४. पावका नः सरस्वती वाजेभिर्वाजिनीवती ।
यज्ञं वष्टु धियावसुः ॥

84. May vedic speech, our purifier, powerful through the force of diverse forms of knowledge, with wisdom and riches acquired through enterprise, beautify our yajna.

८५. चोदयित्री सूनृतानां चेतन्ती सुमतीनाम् ।
यज्ञं दधे सरस्वती ॥

85. Vedic text, the impeller of truthful speeches, the inspirer of perceptions, expatiates on God.

८६. महो अर्णः सरस्वती प्र चेतयति केतुना ।
धियो विश्वा वि राजति ॥

[81]Educated people refers to two persons, the teacher and preacher.
[84]Yajna: Sacrifice, or an act of public service of utility.
[85]This verse can also be thus interpreted:
O soul full of knowledge and supremacy, urged by intellect, served by the wise, learn the vedic truth, from a highly intellectual and wise sage.

86. Vedic text, with its store of knowledge, illuminates the vast ocean of words, and brightens all pious thoughts.

८७. इन्द्रा याहि चित्रभानो सुता इमे त्वायव: ।
अण्वीभिस्तना पूतास: ॥

87. O king, marvellously bright, enjoy these fine objects, full of qualities, prepared and purified by fingers for thee!

८८. इन्द्रा याहि धियेषितो विप्रजूत: सुतावत: ।
उप ब्रह्माणि वाघत: ॥

88. O learned and renowned king, well urged and taught by the wise, impelled by intellect, enjoy food-grains and riches prepared with skill and wisdom!

८९. इन्द्रा याहि तूतुजान उप ब्रह्माणि हरिव: ।
सुते दधिष्व नश्चन: ॥

89. O vital soul, expeditious in action, attain to vedic knowledge. For our thriving transaction produce edible corn!

९०. अश्विना पिबतां मधु सरस्वत्या सजोषसा ।
इन्द्र: सुत्रामा वृत्रहा जुषन्ताꣳ सोम्यं मधु ॥

90. O people, just as loving teacher and preacher, with chastened speech, enjoy sweet knowledge, and as a glorious king, good guardian, slayer of foes as the sun is of clouds, eats the sweet corn grown in the midst of Soma herbs, so should ye do.

CHAPTER XXI

१. इमं मे वरुण श्रुधी हवमद्या च मृडय ।
त्वामवस्युरा चके ॥

1. O God, hear this prayer of mine, be ever gracious unto us. Longing for help I yearn for Thee !

२. तत्त्वा यामि ब्रह्मणा वन्दमानस्तदा शास्ते यजमानो हविर्भिः ।
अहेडमानो वरुणेह बोध्युरुशंस मा न आयुः प्र मोषीः ॥

2. O Worshipful God, with my prayer, I attain unto Thee through vedic knowledge. A worshipper longs to realise Thee with his oblations. O praiseworthy God, worthy of respect, give us Thy knowledge in this world, steal not our life from us !

३. त्वं नो अग्ने वरुणस्य विद्वान् देवस्य हेडो अव यासिसीष्ठाः ।
यजिष्ठो वह्नितमः शोशुचानो विश्वा द्वेषांसि प्र मुमुग्ध्यस्मत् ॥

3. O Omnicient God, Thou art the Master of all branches of knowledge, put far away from us disrespect to a learned person. Extremely venerable, Effulgent and Purifier, remove Thou far from us all feelings of hatred !

४. स त्वं नो अग्नेऽवमो भवोती नेदिष्ठो अस्या उषसो व्युष्टौ ।
अव यक्ष्व नो वरुणं ररणो वीहि मृडीकं सुहवो न एधि ॥

4. O God, be thou the nearest unto us. Protect us with Thy power of protection, while now this Morn is breaking. Reconcile the learned to us; be Bounteous, give us happiness and nice charity !

५. महीमू षु मातरं सुव्रतानामृतस्य पत्नीमवसे हुवेम ।
तुविक्षत्रामजरन्तीमुरूचीं सुशर्माणमदितिं सुप्रणीतिम् ॥

5. We call to protect us, this unimpaired Earth, the mother of those who stick steadfastly to their vow, the rearer of truth, full of wealth, free from decay, the giver of various objects, equipped with excellent houses and pleasureable politics.

६. सुत्रामाणं पृथिवीं द्यामनेहसं सुशर्माणमदितिं सुप्रणीतिम् ।
दैवीं नावं स्वरित्रामनागसमस्रवन्तीमा रुहेमा स्वस्तये ॥

6. May we ascend, for weal, this vessel, affording protection, vast in size, well renowned, flawless, highly accommodating, complete in construction, used by the king and his subjects for political purposes, rowed with good rudders, comfortable, free from leakage, and built by skilled architects.

७. सुनावमा रहेयमस्रवन्तीमनागसम् ।
शतारित्राऽ स्वस्तये ॥

7. May I ascend for welfare the goodly ship, free from defect in construction, that leaketh not, and is equipped with manifold anchors.

८. आ नो मित्रावरुणा घृतैर्गव्यूतिमुक्षतम् ।
मध्वा रजाऽ सि सुक्रतू ॥

8. O intellectual and industrious pair of artisans, behaving like Pran and Udan, sprinkle with water our walking-path for two miles, and provide all places with sweet water!

९. प्र बाहवा सिसृतं जीवसे न आ नो गव्यूतिमुक्षतं घृतेन ।
आ मा जने श्रवयतं युवाना श्रुतं मे मित्रावरुणा हवेमा ।

9. O teacher and preacher, ye, uniters and disuniters like both the arms, come unto me for improving my life. Arrange water to be sprinkled for us for two miles. Give us the nice lessons of glory, and hear our mutual discussions!

१०. शं नो भवन्तु वाजिनो हवेषु देवताता मितद्रव: स्वर्का: ।
जम्भयन्तोऽहिं वृकऽ रक्षाऽसि सनेम्यस्मद्युयवन्नमीवा: ॥

10. O highly learned person, possessing arms and foodstuffs, slow mover, behaving like scholars, worldly wise, crushing the thief and ignoble souls, as sun crushes the cloud, become for us an ancient pleasure-giver, and completely banish our afflictions!

११. वाजे-वाजेऽवत वाजिनो नो धनेषु विप्रा अमृता ऋतज्ञा: ।
अस्य मध्व: पिबत मादयध्वं तृप्ता यात पथिभिर्देवयानै: ॥

11. O immortal, truth-knowing, learned and wise people, help us in each fray, and our efforts to earn wealth. Drink deep the essence of knowledge, be joyful, be satisfied : then follow the paths which the sages are wont to tread!

१२. समिद्धो अग्नि: समिधा सुसमिद्धो वरेण्य: ।
गायत्री छन्द इन्द्रियं त्र्यविगौर्वंयो दधु: ॥

⁸Just as Pran and Udan, the ingoing and outgoing breaths work together, so should the gracious pair of artisans work.
 Roads outside the city should be sprinkled with water for walking and suppressing dust. Pt. Jaidev, Vidyalankar, translates the verse, that Government should make arrangements for drinking-booths and schools for the spread of knowledge at a distance of every two miles.
 The Lucknow Vedic Sansthan translators interpret the verse as: O learned people, fill our temple of knowledge with your fine teachings. Spread your sweet instructions to distant places as well.
⁹Unite and disunite : A teacher and preacher ask the students to unite and work in cooperation. They ask us to shun the company of the wicked and the evil-minded and remain away from them,

12. Just as kindled fire, the Sun highly illumined with its light, an excellent person, the Gayatri metre please the mind, and just as a person protecting the body, its organs and soul, singing the praise of God attains to longevity, so should the learned do.

१३. तनूनपाच्छुचिव्रतस्तनूपाश्च सरस्वती ।
उष्णिहा छन्द इन्द्रियं दित्यवाङ्गौर्वंयो दधुः ॥

13. Just as a religious-minded person, who lets not the body decay, who preserves his physical strength, vedic speech, and Ushniha metre, realises the significance of soul, and just as a devotee, creating love for worldly destructible objects expands his desires, so should the learned do.

१४. इडाभिरग्निरीड्यः सोमो देवो अमर्त्यः ।
अनुष्टुप्छन्द इन्द्रियं पञ्चाविगौर्वंयो दधुः ॥

14. Just as a learned person, lustrous like fire, immortal by nature, supreme, fit for eulogy and research, divine, guarded by five vital breaths, laudable for his knowledge, and just as Anushtup-metre with praises, attain to self satisfaction and intellectual mind, so should all do.

१५. सुबर्हिरग्निः पूषण्वान्त्स्तीर्णबर्हिरमर्त्यः ।
बृहती छन्द इन्द्रियं त्रिवत्सो गौर्वंयो दधुः ॥

15. Just as a learned person, brilliant like fire, air-minded, immortal by nature, gracing the space, and Brihati-metre, realise the significance of soul, and just as persons docile like a cow, control their bodies, organs and minds, so should we all do.

१६. दुरो देवीर्दिशो महीर्ब्रह्मा देवो बृहस्पतिः ।
पङ्क्तिश्छन्द इहेन्द्रियं तुर्यंवाङ्गौर्वंयो दधुः ॥

16. O people, just as glittering doors, mighty regions, air in space, resplendent sun, Pankti-metre, and a learned person in the fourth Ashrama, gain power and life in this world so should ye acquire life and power!

१७. उषे यह्वी सुपेशसा विश्वे देवा अमर्त्याः ।
त्रिष्टुप्छन्द इहेन्द्रियं पष्ठवाङ्गौर्वंयो दधुः ॥

---

[13]Ushniha metre: A person who remains celibate, and increases his physical, mental and spiritual strength for 28 years, like the 28 syllables of the Ushniha metre.

[14]Anushtup-metre: A Brahmchari who observes celibacy and improves his body and soul for 32 years, like 32 syllables of the Anushtap metre.

[15]Brihati-metre : A Brahmchari who observes celibacy and strengthens his body and soul for 36 years, like 36 syllables of the Brihati metre Mahidhar interprets त्रिवत्स as a steer of 3 years age, whereas Rishi Dayananda interprets it as a learned person, who controls the body, organs and mind.

[16]Pankti-metre: A Brahmchari who observes celibacy for 40 years, like 40 syllables of of the Pankti-metre तुर्यंवाड् गौ may also mean a yajna supervised by four priests, Hota, Adhvarya, Udgata and Brahma.

[17]Trishtup-metre: A Brahmchari who leads a life of celibacy up to fortyfour years like the fortyfour syllables of the Trishtup metre.

17. O people, just as in this world, the female teacher and preacher of lovely form, like two dawns of great brilliance, all the immortal bright forces of nature, the Trishtup metre and the bull that carries burden on its back, give us wealth and life, so should ye all acquire them!

१८. दैव्या होतारा भिषजेन्द्रेण सयुजा युजा ।
जगती छन्द इन्द्रियमनड्वान्गौर्वयो दधुः ॥

18. O people, just as good physicians, the correct dispensers of medicine with skill, with mind awakened, shrewd amongst the learned, bestowers of knowledge, ox and cow, and Jagati metre give us good wealth, so should ye all acquire the same!

१९. तिस्र इडा सरस्वती भारती मरुतो विशः ।
विराट् छन्द इहेन्द्रियं धेनुगौर्नं वयो दधुः ॥

19. O people, just as the Earth, speech and intellect, all three, air-folk, subjects, illuminating strength of various kinds, like the milchcow, in this world, give wealth and attainable objects, so should ye all acquire these!

२०. त्वष्टा तुरीपो अद्भुत इन्द्राग्नी पुष्टिवर्धना ।
द्विपदा छन्द इन्द्रियमुक्षा गौर्नं वयो दधुः ॥

20. O people, wonderful, speedy, subtle, invigorating air and fire, human beings who stand on two feet like the metre having two quarters, and like a vigorous bull give life and physical strength, know ye them!

२१. शमिता नो वनस्पतिः सविता प्रसुवन् भगम् ।
ककुप्छन्द इहेन्द्रियं वशा वेहद्वयो दधुः ॥

21. O people, just as the sun, the giver of tranquility, and nourisher of trees, produces wealth and a Brahmchari observing celibacy for twentyeight years, like the Kakup metre of twentyeight syllables, the Assembly that controls the State, and the statesmanship of the ruler that nips in the bud the machinations of the wicked, give us life and power, so should ye do!

२२. स्वाहा यज्ञं वरुणः सुक्षत्रो भेषजं करत् ।
अतिच्छन्दा इन्द्रियं बृहद्दृष्भो गौर्वयो दधुः ॥

22. O people, just as a noble, wealthy person, correctly uses an efficacious medicine, as a man more advanced than the others, like the Ati metre, and an excellent bull attain to supremacy and perform their personal duty, so should ye all do!

[18] Jagati metre : A Brahmchari who observes celibacy up to forty-eight years like the forty-eight syllables of Jagati metre.
[23] There are four metres with which Ati(अति) is prefixed. i.e., Ati Dhriti, Ati Ashti, Ati Shakwari, Ati Jagati. In each of these metres there are four syllables more than in the ordinary metres.

२३. वसन्तेन ऋतुना देवा वसवस्त्रिवृता स्तुताः ।
रथन्तरेण तेजसा हविरिन्द्रे वयो दधुः ॥

23. O people, eight vasus, full of divine qualities, extolled by humanity, present in past, present and future, where people move in conveyances, afford pleasure in the spring. The learned acquire with dignity, in light of the sun, longevity, through offering oblations!

२४. ग्रीष्मेण ऋतुना देवा रुद्राः पञ्चदशे स्तुताः ॥
बृहता यशसा बलँ हविरिन्द्रे वयो दधुः ॥

24. O people, know the highly extolled Rudra Brahmcharis, who in Summer season, with the recitation of Panchdash stoma of fifteen verses, give strength and life to the soul, with fame and sacrifice!

२५. वर्षाभिऋतुनाऽऽदित्या स्तोमे सप्तदशे स्तुताः ।
वैरूपेण विशौजसा हविरिन्द्रे वयो दधुः ॥

25. O people know ye the Aditya Brahmcharis, who endowed with many qualities, living in the midst of people, in the rainy season, praised with the recitation of Saptdasha stoma of seventeen verses, give life to the soul with strength and sacrifice!

२६. शारदेन ऋतुना देवा एकविँश ऋभव स्तुताः ।
वैराजेन श्रिया श्रियँ हविरिन्द्रे वयो दधुः ॥

26. O people, serve those wise and divine persons, who praised with a hymn of twentyone verses, in the Autumn season, give to the soul grace, life and sacrifice, with riches and the significance conveyed in virat verses!

२७. हेमन्तेन ऋतुना देवास्त्रिणवे मरुत स्तुताः ।
वलेन शक्वरीः सहो हविरिन्द्रे वयो दधः ॥

27. O men, serve those learned persons, who in winter, praised with a hymn of twentyseven verses, give might, sacrifice and pleasure to the soul with cloud and cows, the source of strength!

---

[23]Eight Vasus: Sun, Moon, Earth, Space, etc. Vasu also means Brahmchari who observes celibacy for 24 years.

[24]Rudra Brahmcharis: Those who observe the vow of celibacy for 36 years.
Rudras also mean ten vital breaths (Pran) and soul.
Panchdasha: a recitation of 15 verses, known as Panchdasha Stoma occurring in the Atharva Veda.

[25]Aditya Brahmchari : Those who observe the vow of celibacy and study the vedas for fortyeight years.
Adityas also mean twelve months of the year, forming a part of 33 devatas along with 8 vasus and 11 Rudras.
Saptdasha Stoma: A hymn of 17 verses in the Atharva veda.

[26]Virat verses occur in the Sama Veda. A hymn of 21 verses means a Sukta with this number of verses.

[27]Trinava: A hymn of 27 verses.

२८. शशिरेण ऋतुना देवास्त्रयस्त्रिंशेशमृता स्तुता: ।
सत्येन रेवती: क्षत्रं हविरिन्द्रे वयो दधु: ॥

28. O men acquire knowledge of material objects from those immortal, laudable learned persons, who in Dew-time, possessing the knowledge of thirty-three gods, with the force of truth and strength of subjects that overcome the armies of wealthy foes, give power, sacrifice, and pleasure to the soul!

२९. होता यक्षत्समिधाऽग्निमिडस्पदेशिवनेन्द्रं सरस्वतीमजो धूम्रो न गोधूमै: कुवलैर्भेषजं मधु शष्पैर्नं तेज इन्द्रियं पय: सोम: परिस्रुता घृतं मधु व्यन्त्वाज्यस्य होतर्यज ॥

29. Just as a Hota, on this earth in a place of oblations, with fuel, burns the fire, and like the sun and moon, acquires supremacy and instructive speech, and just as a person uses wheat purple coloured like a he-goat, and jujube fruit as medicine, so, thou, sacrificer, perform Homa with eloquence, sweet water, precious substances, milk, corn, well pressed medicinal herbs, ghee and honey.

३०. होता यक्षत्नूनपात्सरस्वतीमविमेषो न भेषजं पथा मधुमता भरन्नशिवनेन्द्राय वीर्यं बदरैरुपवाकाभिर्भेषजं तोक्मभि: पय: सोम: परिस्रुता घृतं मधु व्यन्त्वाज्यस्य होतर्यज ॥

30. Just as a Hota, the remover of physical imperfections, imbibes instructive speech, and like a sheep and a ram, obtains medicine from a watery path, and utilises the Sun, Moon, and valour for acquiring supremacy, and avails of jujube fruits and didactic instructions as healing medicine, or just as one acquires with his sons, water, well pressed medicinal herbs, ghee, and honey, so shouldst thou sacrificer give butter offerings.

३१. होता यक्षत्नराशंसं न नग्नहुं पतिं सुरया भेषजं मेष: सरस्वती भिषग्रथो न चन्द्रयशिवनोर्वपा इन्द्रस्य वीर्यं बदरैरुपवाकाभिर्भेषजं तोक्मभि: पय: सोम: परिस्रुता घृतं मधु व्यन्त्वाज्यस्य होतर्यज ॥

31. Just as a Hota worships the Lord who sends to jail the wicked persons and is praised by the subjects, uses medicine with water, solidifies the force of the warriors of a general who rends asunder the ignoble foes, or just as a preacher is a mental healer, or a speech full of knowledge acts like a physician, or just as a conveyance helps us in reaching our destination, so does a wealthy person help us for success in life. Just as the strength of a foe-killing king, manages the air flights between the earth and heaven, or just as an intelligent person uses well received moral instructions as medicine

[28] Immortal: Persons of deathless fame.
  Thirtythree gods: Eight Vasus, Eleven Rudras, Twelve months, Lightning and Yajna, the 3 forces of nature.
[29] Hota: one of the four guardians of a yajna.
  Jujube fruit: बदर, बेर.

like the jujube fruit, so shouldst a sacrificer along with children, offer butter oblations, full of milk, well pressed juice of medicines, ghee and honey.

३२. होता यक्षदिडेडित आजुह्वान: सरस्वतीमिन्द्रं बलेन वर्धयन्नृषभेण गवेन्द्रियमश्विनेन्द्राय भेषजं यवै: कर्कन्धुभिर्मधु लाजैर्नं मासरं पय: सोम: परिस्तुता घृतं मधु व्यन्त्वाज्यस्य होतर्यज ॥

32. Just as a laudable person, invoked with honour, and praised in a eulogistic language, acquires supremacy and fine speech, by dint of exertion, increases wealth by fast moving bull, understands the significance of Heaven and Earth, uses barley as medicine for acquiring might, eats boiled rice sweet like jujube fruit and parched grains; so shouldst thou, O sacrificer offer butter oblations, with the juice of well-prepared medicinal herbs, milk, ghee and honey!

३३. होता यक्षद्धिरण्यंम्रदा भिषङ् नासत्या भिषजाश्विनाश्वा शिशुमती भिषग्धेनु: सरस्वती भिषग्दुह इन्द्राय भेषजं पय: सोम: परिस्तुता घृतं मधु व्यन्त्वाज्यस्य होतर्यज ॥

33. Just as a learned person acts as a physician for removing our doubts, like a woollen cloth which pressed removes cold; just as a mare with nice foals, runs so fast, as if it flies to heaven, just as two physicians, true to their profession, proficient in the science of medicine confer together; Just as a disease-killing and milk-yielding cow acts as a physician, or a speech full of knowledge plays the part of a physician for purifying the soul, so, O sacrificer, shouldst thou offer butter oblations with water, milk, Soma juice, ghee and honey procured by thee!

३४. होता यक्षददुरो दिश: कवष्यो न व्यचस्वतीरश्विभ्यां न दुरो दिश इन्द्रो न रोदसी दुघे दुहे धेनु: सरस्वत्यश्विनेन्द्राय भेषज शुक्रं न ज्योतिरिन्द्रयं पय: सोम: परिस्तुता घृतं मधु व्यन्त्वाज्यस्य होतर्यज ॥

34. Just as a learned person, like perforated objects, provides for the doors of the sacrificial hall, spacious like the regions; just as he protects its doors and regions from rain and fire, and fully masters the Earth and space like lightning; just as he makes the knowledge full speech useful for the soul like a cow; just as the Sun and Moon, like life-infusing water, mature medicinal herbs, just as he contacts the illuminating mind for its perfection, so shouldst thou, O sacrificer offer butter oblations with milk, soma juice, ghee and honey procured by thee!

३५. होता यक्षत्सुपेशसोषे नक्तं दिवाश्विना समञ्जाते सरस्वत्या त्विषिमिन्द्रे न भेषज श्येनो न रजसा हृदा श्रिया न मासरं पय: सोम: परिस्तुता घृतं मध व्यन्त्वाज्यस्य होतर्यज ।

[34]Perforated objects: Just as pegs are nailed in perforated objects to make them fixed and strong, so a learned person should arrange to make the doors of the yajnashala strong and durable.

35. Just as beautiful wives, with control over passions, serve their husbands, and the Sun and Moon spread light during the day and night, and learned persons give splendour and coolness to the soul; as a good cook like a learned person with the knowledge of planets, devotedly prepares nice, dainty meals; so shouldst thou, O sacrificer offer butter oblations with well prepared medicinal herbs and their juices, water and honey procured by thee!

३६. होता यक्षद्दैव्या होतारा भिषजाऽश्विनेन्द्रं न जागृवि दिवा नक्तं न भेषजै:
शूष॑सरस्वती भिषक् सीसेन दुह इन्द्रियं पय: सोम: परिस्तुता घृतं मधु व्यन्त्वाज्यस्य होतर्यज ॥

36. God, the organiser of this yajna of the universe, has created the earthly fire, and atmospheric air, the Sun and Moon as healing physicians and the lightning. The animating lightning like a physician, with balms and lead-dust, yields strength and physical power. O sacrificer offer butter oblations, with well prepared juice, milk, medicinal herbs, ghee and honey procured by thee!

३७. होता यक्षत्तिस्रो देवीर्न भेषजं त्रयस्त्रिधातवोऽपसो रूपमिन्द्रे हरिण्ययमश्विनेडा न भारती वाचा सरस्वती मह इन्द्राय दुह इन्द्रियं पय: सोम: परिस्तुता घृतं मधु व्यन्त्वाज्यस्य होतर्यज ॥

37. Just as a learned person uses the three Assemblies as a remedy for uprooting the ills of administration; or as an active soul possessing truth, spirit, liability to err, and spoken of in the first, second and third persons, perceives the light of eye in the lightning. Just as the Sun and Moon are the instructors of all like laudable receptive intelligence; or just as a highly learned woman, with her scholarly and instructive eloquence amasses great wealth for her famous husband, so shouldst thou O learned person perform Havan with well prepared juices, milk, medicinal herbs, butter and honey acquired by thee!

३८. होता यक्षत् सुरेतसमृषभं नर्यापसं त्वष्टारमिन्द्रमश्विना भिषज न सरस्वतीमोजो न जूतिरिन्द्रियं वृको न रभसो भिषग् यश: सुरया भेषज॑ श्रिया न मासरं पय: सोम: परिस्तुता घृतं मधु व्यन्त्वाज्यस्य होतर्यज ॥

38. Just as a learned person utilises a powerful bull, and a noble person, the remover of miseries, and doer of good deeds amongst his fellows, avails of air and lightning as a physician, and didactic speech for strength, just as an intelligent person acquires vigour, mental force, and speed like a destructive weapon, derives wealth and corn from water, considers medicine as a

---

[37]Three Assemblies: Raj Sabha, Vidya Sabha, Dharma Sabha. Soul possesses the qualities of Satva, Rajas, Tamas.

It is spoken of as we, you and they in the plural, or I, thou, he, she or it in the singular.

Thou: The sacrificer yajman.

valuable thing, and receives well cooked meals, so shouldst thou acquire with exertion, juices worth drinking, supremacy, butter and honey, and perform Havan with them and specially butter.

३९. होता यक्षद्वनस्पतिᳪ शमितारᳪ शतक्रतुं भीमं न मन्युᳪ राजानं व्याघ्रं नमसा-श्विना भामᳪ सरस्वती भिषगिन्द्राय दुह इन्द्रियं पय: सोम: परिस्रुता घृतं मधु व्यन्त्वाज्यस्य होतर्यज ॥

39. Just as an intelligent physician for the acquisition of wealth like the Sun, the protector of its rays, welcomes a man, the advocate of peace, full of wisdom and doer of diverse deeds; cultivates anger to inspire awe, respects a king for killing the tiger with a deadly weapon; just as a learned lady, the Speaker of the Assembly and Chief of the Staff are filled with anger, so shouldst thou acquire with exertion wealth, juices, medicinal herbs, ghee, and honey, and perform Homa with them and mainly butter.

४०. होता यक्षदग्निᳪ स्वाहाऽऽज्यस्य स्तोकानांᳪ स्वाहा मेदसां पृथक् स्वाहा छागमश्विभ्यांᳪ स्वाहा मेषंᳪ सरस्वत्यैᳪ स्वाहाऋषभमिन्द्राय सिंᳪहाय सहस इन्द्रियंᳪ स्वाहाऽग्निं न भेषजंᳪ स्वाहा सोममिन्द्रियंᳪ स्वाहेन्द्रंᳪ सुत्रामाणंᳪ सवितारं वरुणं भिषजां पतिंᳪ स्वाहा वनस्पति प्रियं पाथो न भेषजंᳪ स्वाहा देवा आज्यपा जुषाणो अग्निर्भेषजं पय: सोम: परिस्रुता घृतं मधु व्यन्त्वाज्यस्य होतर्यज ॥

40. Just as a learned person makes the best use of ghee, takes due care of minor unctuous objects, uses fire in diverse nice ways, takes the help of state officials and cattle-breeders for the removal of suffering through cultured speech; properly utilises a well built person for acquiring supremacy, avails of enterprise and strength for helping the slayer of foes, amasses wealth by honest means, treats fire as a healer like medicine, pacifies mind with tranquillity and knowledge, cures through pathology the army general, a good guardian; and a wealthy person, a patron of physicians; instructs with his knowledge the protectors of forests, and endears like corn a lovable medicine; and just as learned devotees of science, brilliant like fire, serve and consult a physician, so shouldst thou O sacrificer, procure juices, milk, medicinal herbs, ghee and honey, and perform Havan with them and chiefly butter!

४१. होता यक्षदश्विनौ छागस्य वपाया मेदसो जुषेतांᳪ हविर्होतर्यज ।
होता यक्षत्सरस्वतीं मेषस्य वपाया मदसो जुषतांᳪ हविर्होतर्यज ।
होता यक्षदिन्द्रमृषभस्य वपाया मेदसो जुषतांᳪ हविर्होतर्यज ॥

41. Just as a learned person deals in various trades, avails of oily oblations, rears cattle and uses goat, bull, buffalo for purposes of cultivation, for sowing seeds, and growing cotton for making clothes thereof, so shouldst thou O sacrificer do. Just as a learned person enhances the power of discussion of rival disputants; puts greasy oblations in the fire, and cultivates scholarly speech, and rightly utilises all these things, so shouldst thou O sacrificer do!

CHAPTER XXI

Just as a learned person resorts to a device that enhances the strength of the bull, puts into fire oily oblations, and elevates his soul, rightly uses all these substances, so shouldst thou, O sacrificer do!

४२. होता यक्षदश्विनौ सरस्वतीमिन्द्रᳪ सुत्रामाणमिमे सोमा: सुरामाणश्छागैनं मेषैर्ऋषभै: सुता: शष्पैनं तोक्मभिर्लाजैर्मंहस्वन्तो मदा मासरेण परिष्कृता: शुक्रा: पयस्वन्तोऽमृता: प्रस्थिता वो मधुश्चुतस्तानश्विना सरस्वतीन्द्र: सुत्रामा बृत्रहा जुषन्ताᳪ सोम्यं मधु पिबन्तु मदन्तु व्यन्तु होतर्यज ।

42. Just as a learned person duly respects the teacher and the preacher, the scholarly speech, and the king, the guardian of his subjects; just as these learned, duly elected, charitably disposed member of the Assembly, save us from explosive substances and beasts of prey, and grant us beautiful and fascinating articles; just as honourable persons respected by their progeny with parched grains, pure and gracious, joyfully eat the cooked rice with milk, and nice water; just as aged spiritual people, full of sweet qualities, who travel from one place to the other, accept the offerings made by the people and just as honoured persons, a learned lady and a famous person, affording protection like the Sun, the slayer of clouds, accept sweet Soma juice, drink it, derive pleasure, and master all branches of knowledge, so shouldst thou, O sacrificer make full use of all objects!

४३. होता यक्षदश्विनौ छागस्य हविष आत्तामद्य मध्यतो मेद उद्भृतं पुरा द्वेषोभ्य: पुरा पौरुषेय्या गृभो घस्तान्नूनं घासे अञ्जानां यवसप्रथमानाᳪ सुमत्क्षराणाᳪ शतरुद्रियाणा- मनिष्वात्तानां पीवोपवसनानां पार्श्वत: श्रोणित: शितामत उत्सादतोऽङ्गादङ्गादवत्तानां करत एवाश्विना जुषेताᳪ हविर्होतर्यज ॥

43. Just as a learned person keeps company with the teacher and the preacher, who ever derive in a nice manner the useful things like milk and greasy butter from a goat, and surely eat them before they are snatched by the wicked, and asked for by a chaste beggar women; just as they utilise rough and refined meals, chiefly of barley, delicious, chasers of hundreds of ailments, prepared in fire, just as good physicians remove ills from the sides, from the thighs, from the stomach, from each limb causing pain, and from vital organs of the patients, and partake of eatable foods, so shouldst thou, O sacrificer, use all these substances!

४४. होता यक्षत् सरस्वतीं मेषस्य हविष आवयदद्य मध्यतो मेद उद्भृतं पुरा द्वेषोभ्य: पुरा पौरुषेय्या गृभो घसन्नूनं घासे अञ्जानां यवसप्रथमानाᳪ सुमत्क्षराणाᳪ शतरुद्रियाणाम्- निष्वात्तानां पीवोपवसनानां पार्श्वत: श्रोणित: शितामत उत्सादतोऽङ्गादङ्गादवत्तानां करदेवᳪ सरस्वती जुषताᳪ हविर्होतर्यज ॥

44. Just as a learned person, with the good nature of an instructed person, having extracted out of oblation the greasy substance, ever acquires it, develops

---

[44]Extraction of greasy substance refers to the yajna Shesh (remnant) which should be eaten by the performers of the yajna.

speech, holds it in veneration, and surely eats it before enemies snatch it or a respectable married woman asks for it; just as persons beautiful to sit for dinner, individually or collectively, showerers of happiness, wearers of ungaudy clothes, having knowledge of electricity, conveyers of the opinion of the learned to the masses are freed by a skilled physician from physical ills from the sides, from the things, from the stomach, and from each limb causing pain, so shouldst an educated lady cherish him, so shouldst thou, O sacrificer perform yajna!

४५. होता यक्षदिन्द्रमृषभस्य हविष श्रावयदद्य मध्यतो मेद उद्भृतं पुरा द्वेषोभ्य: पुरा पौरुषेय्या गृभो घसन्नूनं घासे अज्ञानां यवसप्रथमाना ॐ सुमत्क्षराणा ॐ शतरुद्रियाणाम्- ग्निष्वात्तानां पीवोपवसनानां पार्श्वत: श्रोणित: शितामत उत्सादतोऽङ्गादङ्गादवत्ता- नां करदेवमिन्द्रो जुषता ॐ हविहोर्तयज ॥

45. Just as a learned person, attains to supremacy, and uses a medicine which cures ills of the sides, of the thighs, of a limb suffering acute pain, of excretory organ, nay of each organ, of persons, beautiful to sit for dinner, cultivators of barley, showerers of happiness, digesters of meals, wearers of rough, ungaudy clothes, chastisers of hundreds of the wicked, magnanimous in spirit and which the king uses, and just as the king daily acquires well protected nice greasy substance derived out of oblation, certainly respects and eats it before it is snatched by the enemies or a respectable woman asks for it, so shouldst thou, O sacrificer be conversant with all dealings!

४६. होता यक्षद्वनस्पतिमभि हि पिष्टतमया रभिष्ठया रशनयाधित । यत्राश्विनोश्छागस्य हविष: प्रिया धामानि यत्र सरस्वत्या मेषस्य हविष: प्रिया धामानि यत्रेन्द्रस्य ऋषभस्य हविष: प्रिया धामानि यत्राग्ने: प्रिया धामानि यत्र सोमस्य प्रिया धामानि यत्रेन्द्रस्य सुत्राम्ण: प्रिया धामानि यत्र सवितु: प्रिया धामानि यत्र वरुणस्य प्रिया धामानि यत्र वनस्पते: प्रिया पाथा ॐ सि यत्र देवानामाज्यपानां प्रिया धामानि यत्राग्नेर्होतु: प्रिया धामानि तत्रैतान्प्रस्तुत्येवोपस्तुत्येवोपावस्रक्षद्रभीयस इव कृत्वी करदेवं देवो वनस्पतिर्जुषता ॐ हविहोर्तयज ॥

46. A learned person performs deeds with his excellent, speedy power of commencement. Where the cattle eat the grass nourished by the Sun and Moon, where oblations reach fascinating places, where there are streams for rams to roam about, and where oblations reach fascinating stations, where there are found dignified persons, and oblations reach fascinating places, where there are good stations of fire and electricity, where there grow efficacious medicines in good places, where abide excellent people, the protectors of humanity, where there arise and blow charming and attractive zephyrs, where there are the birth places of greatmen, where there are fruits of trees, where the planets revolve in their orbits and afford protection to the souls in their beautiful stations, where there are the abodes of learned persons

---

[45] Which means medicine.

CHAPTER XXI

who spread knowledge and give us comforts ; there shouldst thou praise these substances at opportune times, and having praised them from near, make their fullest use according to their merits, attributes and nature. Making their collection, thou shouldst use them in practical works, like undertakings begun in right earnest.

Just as fire, the fosterer of sun's rays, enjoys oblations, and reaches the trees and protects them, so shouldst thou O sacrificer be conversant with all dealings!

४७. होता यक्षदग्निꣳ स्विष्टकृतमयाङ्ग्निरश्विनोश्छागस्य हविष: प्रिया धामान्ययाट् सरस्व-त्या मेषस्य हविष: प्रिया धामान्ययाडिन्द्रस्य ऋषभस्य हविष: प्रिया धामान्ययाङ्ग्ने: प्रिया धामान्ययाट् सोमस्य प्रिया धामान्ययाडिन्द्रस्य सुत्राम्ण: प्रिया धामान्ययाट् सवितु: प्रिया धामान्ययाड् वरुणस्य प्रिया धामान्ययाड् वनस्पते: प्रिया पाथाꣳ स्ययाड् देवानामाज्यपानां प्रिया धामानि यक्षदग्नेर्होतु: प्रिया धामानि यक्षत् स्वं महिमानमाय-जतामेज्या इष: कृणोतु सो अध्वरा जातवेदा जषताꣳ हविर्होर्तर्यज ॥

47. Just as a learned person acquires the desired fire, and just as the fire, acquires the fascinating stations of air, lightning, and healing oblations; just as he praises the fascinating stations of oblations, speech, and persons desirous of victory; just as he praises the fascinating positions of a dignified king possessing noble traits and oblations ; just as he praises the fascinating powers of electricity, just as he praises the fascinating powers of sovereignty; just as he praises the charming forces of a protecting commander of the army; just as he praises the bewildering discoveries of wealth producing science; just as he admires the places of fine water and men, and acquires the fruits of charming trees; just as he praises the habitations of the learned who drink fruit juices and protect knowable objects: just as he praises the majestic rays of the sun that draws water and emits light; just as he realises his greatness; just as a highly intellectual person cherishes noble aspirations; performs deeds of mutual cooperation, and uninterrupted yajnas, and enjoys all useful substances, so shouldst thou, O sacrificer, be conversant with all dealings!

४८. देवं बर्हि: सरस्वती सुदेवमिन्द्रꣳ अश्विना ।
तेजो न चक्षुरक्ष्योर्बर्हिषा दधुरिन्द्रियं वसुवने वसुधेयस्य व्यन्तु यज ॥

48. O learned person, just as a highly intellectual wife praises her noble, educated husband, the space and the teacher and preacher, like brilliance of the eyes and just as educated persons, for the acquisition of wealth, use devices to accumulate riches, acquire and possess wealth testing it with the sight of their eyes, so shouldst thou acquire and possess it!

---

[48]It : wealth.
Thou : Sacrificer-Performer of the yajna.

४९. देवीद्वारो अश्विना भिषजेन्द्रे सरस्वती ।
प्राणं न वीर्यं नसि द्वारो दधुरिन्द्रियं वसुवने वसुधेयस्य व्यन्तु यज ॥

49. O learned person, just as Air and the Sun, an educated wife, and physicians, for gain of wealth having secured the bright gates meant for going in and coming out, like breath in the nostril, gain strength, and master nine gates of the body, and for enjoying wealth, the wise gain the treasure of riches, so shouldst thou be conversant with all dealings!

५०. देवी उषासावश्विना सुत्रामेन्द्रे सरस्वती ।
बलं न वाचमास्य उषाभ्यां दधुरिन्द्रियं वसुवने वसुधेयस्य व्यन्तु यज ॥

50. O learned person, just as lustrous morning and evening, protection-affording sun, moon and an educated wife, for one aspiring after the acquisition of wealth, for his acquiring the treasure of riches, like speech in the mouth, grant him strength and wealth morning and evening, and behave likewise unto all, so shouldst thou be conversant with all dealings!

५१. देवी जोष्ट्री सरस्वत्यश्विनेन्द्रमवर्धयन् ।
श्रोत्रं न कर्णयोर्यशो जोष्ट्रीभ्यां दधुरिन्द्रियं वसुवने वसुधेयस्य व्यन्तु यज ॥

51. O learned person, just as lustrous, adorable morning and evening, the bestowers of knowledge, air and lightning magnify the Sun, and men acquire fame, just as ears give us the power to hear, and grant wealth to him who aspires after riches, and wants to amass wealth, so shouldst thou be conversant with all dealings !

५२. देवी ऊर्जाहुती दुघे सुदुघेन्द्रे सरस्वत्यश्विना भिषजाऽवतः ।
शुक्रं न ज्योति स्तनयोराहुती धत्त इन्द्रियं वसुवने वसुधेयस्य व्यन्तु यज ॥

52. O learned persons, just as beautiful and grand morning and evening, corn oblation, a woman-educator, healing physicians, teacher and preacher guard light pure like water, so should ye strengthen the body as breasts strengthen themselves with milk, and in this world full of riches, give money to him who yearns for it, so that all persons may become rich. O seeker after virtue, so shouldst thou be conversant with all dealings!

५३. देवा देवानां भिषजा होतारविन्द्रमश्विना ।
वषट्कारैः सरस्वती त्विषि न हृदये मतिं होतृभ्यां दधुरिन्द्रियं वसुवने वसुधेयस्य व्यन्तु यज ॥

---

⁴⁹Gates: The gates of a well-ventilated house, in which air and sun's rays enter, and people go in and come out like breath in the nostril.
Nine gates. Nine parts of the body which are its gates, i. e., two eyes, two ears, two nostrils, mouth, the penis and the anus.
⁵⁰Thou: Learned person.
⁵¹Thou: Learned person.
⁵³They: Physicians.

53. O learned persons, just as amongst the educated persons, good physicians, the givers of ease to the body, well advanced in the science of medicine, with noble deeds, attain to supreme glory, and a woman with her admirable learning and didactic speech, plants wisdom like light in her heart, and they, along with the charitably disposed, cultivate a pure mind for the distributor of the treasure's wealth and accumulate riches, so should ye be conversant with all dealings!

५४. देवीस्तिस्रस्तिस्रो देवीरश्विनेडा सरस्वती ।
शूषं न मध्ये नाभ्यामिन्द्राय दधुरिन्द्रियं वसुवने वसुधेयस्य व्यन्तु यज ॥

54. O student, just as mother, mistress, preachress, these three ladies full of glow with knowledge, in this world full of wealth, for the soul aspiring after wealth, accept as their pupils, the three girls, superior, medium and low in intellect, and just as teacher and preacher, laudable and learned ladies, like energy and power in the middle of navel, cultivate the mind, and just as all these procure these things, so shouldst thou be conversant with all transactions!

५५. देव इन्द्रो नराशꣳसस्त्रिववरूथः सरस्वत्यश्विभ्यामीयते रथः ।
रेतो न रूपममृतं जनित्रमिन्द्राय त्वष्टा दधदिन्द्रियाणि वसुवने वसुधेयस्य व्यन्तु यज ॥

55. O learned person, just as a highly intellectual, educated man; who has his abode underneath the ground, on the earth and in the space, with his instructive speech, leads the instructors of humanity on the path of virtue, just as a conveyance propelled by fire and steam takes us to destination, and just as God, the Dispeller of misery, like pleasure-giving water and semen-virile, invests in this world the soul, aspirant after wealth, with physical beauty and limbs like ear, eye, etc., and just as these procure all these things, so shouldst thou be conversant with all dealings!

५६. देवो देववनस्पतिर्हिरण्यपर्णो अश्विभ्याꣳ सरस्वत्या सुपिप्पल इन्द्राय पच्यते मधु ।
ओजो न जूतिऋषभो न भामं वनस्पतिनों दधदिन्द्रियाणि वसुवने वसुधेयस्य व्यन्तु यज ॥

56. O learned person, just as water and heat, the brilliant rays of the resplendent and lustrous sun, and advanced skill, ripen the sweet fruits of the fig tree for man, just as water possesses velocity, and a strong man controls wrath, so trees in this world, the mainstay of humanity, produce wealth for us and for him who aspires after wealth; just as all these acquire these substances, so shouldst thou be conversant with all dealings!

५७. देवं बर्हिर्वारितीनामधवरे स्तीर्णमश्विभ्यामूर्णम्रदाः सरस्वत्या स्योनमिन्द्र ते सदः ।
ईशायै मन्युꣳ राजानं बर्हिषा दधुरिन्द्रियं वसुवने वसुधेयस्य व्यन्तु यज ॥

---
[54] Thou: Student.
[55] Thou: Learned person.

57. O soul, master of physical organs, thou hast fine speech, pleasure and restful peace. Thou art soft like the wool. Skilled engineers, with the use of air and electricity, through their useful workmanship prepare conveyances that move in water, overshadowed by the beautiful space. Just as learned persons amass wealth for the soul, that roams in space between the earth and sky, is brilliant, contemplative and eager for supremacy; and obtain these good things, so shouldst thou O sacrificer be conversant with all dealings!

५८. देवो अग्नि: स्विष्टकृद्देवान्यक्षद्यथायथ ॐ होताराविन्द्रमश्विना वाचा वाच ॐ सरस्वती-मग्नि ॐ सोम ॐ स्विष्टकृत् स्विष्ट इन्द्र: सुत्रामा सविता वरुणो भिषगिष्टो देवो वनस्पति: स्विष्टा देवा आज्यपा: स्विष्टो अग्निरग्निना होता होत्रे स्विष्टकृद्यशो न दधदिन्द्रियमूर्ज-मपचिति ॐ स्वधां वसुवने वसुधेयस्य व्यन्तु यज ॥

58. O learned person, just as in this world, for a person aspiring after wealth, beautiful fire, the giver of desired happiness rightly diffuses itself on planets like the Earth etc; just as sacrificers with the aid of air, electricity, sun, speech and learned discourse derive benefit from fire and moon ; just as a benign ruler, giver of happiness, liked by all, a nice protector, the sun, the storer of water, a physician, the desired, beautiful banyan tree give us desired happiness; just as handsome lovable scholars, drinkers of drinkable juice, worshippers, and fire the accomplisher of desired act, like wealth the bringer of fame, bring for the sacrificer physical strength, energy, honour and food ; just as these obtain these things, so shouldst thou be conversant with all dealings!

५९. अग्निमद्य होतारमवृणीतायं यजमान: पचन् पक्ती: पचन् पुरोडाशान् बध्नन्नश्विभ्यां छाग ॐ सरस्वत्यै मेषमिन्द्राय ऋषभ ॐ सुन्वन्नश्विभ्या ॐ सरस्वत्या इन्द्राय सुत्राम्णे सुरासोमान् ॥

59. O men, just as this sacrificer, mastering the science of cooking and preparing sacrificial oblations resorts to fire, the giver of comforts; and just as he uses goat's milk for strengthening vital breaths, sheep's milk for invigorating his voice, and cow's milk for supremacy, and just as sacrificers press the essence of medicinal herbs for the protecting ruler, and for developing instructive speech, so should ye ever do!

६०. सूपस्था अद्य देवो वनस्पतिरभवदश्विभ्यां छागेन सरस्वत्यै मेषेणेन्द्राय ऋषभेणाक्षँस्तान् मेदस: प्रति पचतागृभीषतावीवृधन्त पुरोडाशँरपुरश्विना सरस्वतीन्द्र: सुत्रामा सुरासोमान् ॥

60. O men, just as our neighbours and a well-mannered person, like the fig tree affording shelter under its shade, use the goat's milk that kills all germs

---

⁵⁸Thou: Learned person.
⁵⁹Ye: Men.
⁶⁰Ye: Men.
Oil means clarified butter derived from the milk of these animals.

for strengthening vital breaths, sheep's milk for invigorating voice and cow's milk for supremacy, and eat the greasy digestible oils of those cattle, and gain vitality by eating well-prepared rice-cakes; just as vital breaths, praiseworthy tongue, and the majestic ruler that affords us protection drink the essence of the juices of medicinal herbs, so should ye do!

६१. त्वामद्य ऋष आर्षेय ऋषीणां नपादवृणीतायं यजमानो बहुभ्य आ सञ्जतेभ्य एष मे देवेषु वसु वार्यायक्ष्यत इति ता या देवा देव दानान्यदुस्तान्यस्मा आ च शास्वा च गुरुस्वेपितश्च होतरसि भद्रवाच्याय प्रेषितो मानुषः सूक्तवाकाय सूक्ता ब्रूहि ॥

61. O Rishi (Seer), foremost amongst the Rishis, descendant of Rishis, this sacrificer hath chosen thee today, of all the learned persons assembled together. He knows thou shalt win for him choice-worthy treasure, and all good serviceable objects, amongst the sages; hence he chooses thee!

O learned person, beloved of all, preach unto this sacrificer all the gifts of knowledge the sages impart, and being well trained remain active!

O Hota, thou hast been sent as the man, selected for good speech, and for preaching the vedic doctrines. Preach thou the vedic verses!

---

[61]Rishi: One who knows and understands the significance of vedic texts.
Hota: A learned person who imparts knowledge of humanity.

CHAPTER XXII

१. तेजोऽसि शुक्रममृतमायुष्पा आयुर्मे पाहि ।
देवस्य त्वा सवितुः प्रसवेऽश्विनोर्बाहुभ्यां पूष्णो हस्ताभ्यामा ददे ॥

1. O learned person, in this world created by the Resplendent God, I take thee with arms strong like air and lightning and with hands powerful like the rays of the Sun. Thou art immortal by nature, virile and bright. Thou art the protector of life. Extend thy life and protect mine!

२. इमामगृभ्णन् रशनामृतस्य पूर्व आयुषि विदथेषु कव्या ।
सा नो अस्मिन्त्सुत आ बभूव ऋतस्य सामन्त्सरमारपन्ती ॥

2. We realise in this created world the Omnipresence of God, which clearly describes from the beginning to the end, the relation between the primordial causes, God and matter. The sages in the beginning of creation, know through the vedas this power of God's Omnipresence.

३. अभिधा असि भुवनमसि यन्तासि धर्त्ता ।
स त्वमग्निं वैश्वानरꣳ सप्रथसं गच्छ स्वाहाकृतः ॥

3. O learned person thou art cool like water, thou art a preacher, thou art controller, thou being eulogised, art the upholder of all transactions. Know thou fire, wide in fame and guide of all things!

४. स्वगा त्वा देवेभ्यः प्रजापतये ब्रह्मणश्वं मन्त्स्यामि देवेभ्यः प्रजापतये तेन राध्यासम् ।
तं बधान देवेभ्यः प्रजापतये तेन राध्नुहि ॥

4. O learned person, I will place this fire in the yajna, for thee, independent in actions, for the wise and the householder. Through that sacrificial fire may I, accomplished with noble traits, succeed as a householder. Use that fire in the yajna!
Make me fit to act as a good householder, endowed with noble traits.

५. प्रजापतये त्वा जुष्टं प्रोक्षामीन्द्राग्निभ्यां त्वा जुष्टं प्रोक्षामि वायवे त्वा जुष्टं प्रोक्षामि विश्वेभ्यस्त्वा देवेभ्यो जुष्टं प्रोक्षामि सर्वेभ्यस्त्वा देवेभ्यो जुष्टं प्रोक्षामि ।
यो अर्वन्तं जिघाꣳसति तमभ्यामीति वरुणः । परो मर्त्यः परः श्वा ॥

5. O learned person, he, who wishes to kill a horse, should be punished by a noble person. Such a person is an enemy. He, low in character like a dog is an enemy and must be checked by thee. I sprinkle thee loved by all

---

[3] Just as water and fire are the source of life for all, so should a learned person be considered as our guide and controller.
[5] Useful animals like horse should not be destroyed.
I means Priest or Purohit.

as protector of the people. I anoint thee loved by all, for the protection of soul and fire. I anoint thee loved by all for the protection of air. I anoint thee loved by all, for the protection of all the educated persons. I anoint thee loved by all, for protecting beautiful physical objects like the Earth!

६. अग्नये स्वाहा सोमाय स्वाहा ऽपां मोदाय स्वाहा सवित्रे स्वाहा वायवे स्वाहा विष्णवे स्वाहेन्द्राय स्वाहा बृहस्पतये स्वाहा मित्राय स्वाहा वरुणाय स्वाहा ॥

6. Make the best use of fire. Take medicines. Derive joy by drinking water. Enjoy well the warmth and light of the Sun. Have knowledge of air and vital breaths. Perform yajna in fire. Meditate on God, the Guardian of all great objects. Respect and love your friends. Pay homage to noble souls.

७. हिङ्काराय स्वाहा हिङ्कृताय स्वाहा क्रन्दते स्वाहा ऽवक्रन्दाय स्वाहा प्रोथते स्वाहा प्रप्रोथाय स्वाहा गन्धाय स्वाहा घ्राताय स्वाहा निविष्टाय स्वाहोपविष्टाय स्वाहा सन्दिताय स्वाहा वल्गते स्वाहा ऽऽसीनाय स्वाहा शयानाय स्वाहा स्वपते स्वाहा जाग्रते स्वाहा कूजते स्वाहा प्रबुद्धाय स्वाहा विजृम्भमाणाय स्वाहा विचृताय स्वाहा सव्हानाय स्वाहोपस्थिताय स्वाहा ऽऽयनाय स्वाहा प्रायणाय स्वाहा ॥

7. Reverence for him who recites the Sama Veda. Reverence for him who has recited the Sama Veda. Reverence for the warrior who challenges the foe. Reverence for the victor who welcomes the learned. Reverence for him accomplished in all actions. Reverence for the most accomplished. Reverence for him food of perfume. Reverence for the perfumed. Reverence for him who builds a cantonment and resides therein. Reverence for him who sits in a yogic posture. Reverence for him who tears asunder the foes. Reverence for the learned guest who keeps moving. Reverence for the elders while sitting and sleeping. Reverence for the elders fast asleep, waking and warbling. Reverence for a man of knowledge. Reverence for the elder yawning. Reverence for the architect. Reverence for him who makes a collection of curiosities. Reverence for the neighbours. Reverence for supreme knowledge. Reverence for him who imparts knowledge.

८. यते स्वाहा धावते स्वाहोद्द्रावाय स्वाहोद्द्रुताय स्वाहा शूकाराय स्वाहा शूकृताय स्वाहा निषण्णाय स्वाहोत्थिताय स्वाहा जवाय स्वाहा बलाय स्वाहा विवर्तमानाय स्वाहा विवृत्ताय स्वाहा विधून्वानाय स्वाहा विधूताय स्वाहा शुश्रूषमाणाय स्वाहा शृण्वते स्वाहेक्षमाणाय स्वाहेक्षिताय स्वाहा वीक्षिताय स्वाहा निमेषाय स्वाहा यदत्ति तस्मै स्वाहा यत् पिबति तस्मै स्वाहा यन्मूत्रं करोति तस्मै स्वाहा कुर्वते स्वाहा कृताय स्वाहा ॥

[7]Yogic posture: Asana.
Learned guest: अतिथि, Atithi.
A person who respects the persons and topics mentioned in the verse will always remain happy.
[8]Due care of urine: The learned people should take special care of their urine to keep it free from sugar, albumen and phosphates, so that kidneys may work in order.
Drinks means water, milk and curd.

8. Reverence to the soul that exerts, and is fleeting. Reverence to the warrior that jumps and moves fast. Reverence to him who performs duty promptly and is full of agility. Reverence to him who is sitting peacefully, and him who is up and doing. Reverence to him who is speedminded, and is physically stout. Reverence to him who behaves prominently. Reverence to him who is respected extraordinarily. Reverence to him who controls his mental cravings, and him who is free from sin. Reverence to him who longs to hear the sermons of the learned, and him who listens to the word of knowledge. Reverence to the seer. Reverence to him whom others want to look at, and who is closely looked at. Reverence to him who closes his eyes in contemplation, reverence to him who takes food in time, reverence to him who drinks when needed, and takes due care of his urine. Reverence to him in action, and reverence for his accomplishments.

६. तत्सवितुर्वरेण्यं भर्गो देवस्य धीमहि ।
धियो यो नः प्रचोदयात् ॥

9. O Creator of the Universe! O All holy and worthy of adoration! May we contemplate Thy adorable Self. May thou guide our understanding!

१०. हिरण्यपाणिमूतये सवितारमुप ह्वये ।
स चेत्ता देवता पदम् ॥

10. I invoke for aid, God, the Controller of luminous planets like the Sun, etc. worthy of attainment, and the Bestower of perfect glory. He, the Embodiment of knowledge, tells us how to distinguish between truth and untruth. He is worthy of adoration.

११. देवस्य चेततो मही प्र सवितुर्हवामहे ।
सुमतिꣳ सत्यराधसम् ॥

11. Having meditated on the Adorable God, the Creator of the universe, the Sentient, we acquire excellent, supreme intellect wherewith we arrive at truth.

१२. सुष्टुतिꣳ सुमतीवृधो रातिꣳ सवितुरीमहे ।
प्र देवाय मतीविदे ॥

12. Having eulogised God, the Creator of the universe, and the Developer of intellect, we seek His gift for the seeker after wisdom, and aspirant after knowledge.

१३. रातिꣳ सत्पतिं महे सवितारमुप ह्वये ।
आसवं देववीतये ॥

13. For the attainment of high noble qualities, in a contemplative mood,

---

⁹This is the Gayatri Mantra. It occurs also in 3-35, 30-2, 36-3.

CHAPTER XXII

I eulogise the Giver, the Protector of souls Devoted to truth, the Creator of the universe, and Effulgent in nature.

१४. देवस्य सवितुर्मतिमासवं विश्वदेव्यम् ।
धिया भगं मनामहे ॥

14. In proximity to the Giver of happiness and the Creator of the universe, we acquire intellect and supremacy, with that intellect we pray for excellent glory, the benefactor of the learned.

१५. अग्निꣳ स्तोमेन बोधय समिधानो अमर्त्यम् ।
हव्या देवेषु नो दधत् ॥

15. Well kindled fire carries our offerings to divine objects like air etc. Burn with fuel such a fire indestructible in nature.

१६. स हव्यवाडमर्त्य उशिग्दूतश्चनोहितः ।
अग्निर्धिया समृण्वति ॥

16. Oblation-bearer, immortal, resplendent, eager messenger, giver of food-grains, fire is utilised in mechanical arts and crafts.

१७. अग्निं दूतं पुरो दधे हव्यवाहमुप ब्रुवे ।
देवाꣳ२ आ सादयादिह ॥

17. I place in front the fire, that acts like an envoy in making our mechanical works successful, that gives us food to eat, and brings us enjoyments in this world, I instruct the learned to make its full use.

१८. अजीजनो हि पवमान सूर्यं विधारे शक्मना पयः ।
गोजीरया रꣳहमाणः पुरन्ध्या ॥

18. O purifying, pervading fire, thou hast verily manifested the sun, moving with the force that gives life to earth and cows, and sustains all; and retains waters with its strength!

१९. विभूर्मात्रा प्रभूः पित्राऽडवोऽसि ह्योऽस्यत्योऽसि मयोऽस्यर्वाऽसि सप्तिरसि वाज्यसि
वृषाऽसि नृमणा असि ।
ययुर्नामाऽसि शिशुर्नामाऽस्यादित्यानां पत्वाऽन्विहि
देवा आशापाला एतं देवेभ्योऽश्वं मेधाय प्रोक्षितꣳ रक्षतेह रन्तिरिह रमतामिह
धृतिरिह स्वधृतिः स्वाहा ॥

19. O learned persons, the fulfillers of our desires, ye are mighty like the

---

[15] Fire is indestructible in its atomic state.
[17] I refers to Purohit.
[18] Force refers to the sun, rain from the sun sustains cows and earth, and retains waters.
[19] Bringers of rain: Through the performance of yajnas.
Here: in this world.
Moistened: Water is used to extinguish fire.

mother Earth, eminent like the father air, ye are the accomplishers of journey, fast movers like the horse, constant travellers, acquirers of happiness, friendly towards all, utilisers of material objects, speedy in action, bringers of rain, sharp realisers of all things with an intelligent mind, marchers on the foes for victory, possessors of speech that simplifies subtle subjects, follow the path of the wise. Protect nicely this pervading fire, moistened with water, for the enjoyment of pleasures, for developing intellect and chastising the wicked. Here is delight. Here enjoy pleasure. Here is contentment. Here is self-satisfaction.

२०. काय स्वाहा कस्मै स्वाहा कतमस्मै स्वाहा स्वाहाऽधिमाधीताय स्वाहा मन: प्रजापतये स्वाहा चित्तं विज्ञातायादित्यै स्वाहा अदित्यै मह्यै स्वाहा अदित्यै सुमृडीकायै स्वाहा सरस्वत्यै स्वाहा सरस्वत्यै पावकायै स्वाहा सरस्वत्यै बृहत्यै स्वाहा पूष्णे स्वाहा पूष्णे प्रपथ्याय स्वाहा पूष्णे नरन्धिषाय स्वाहा त्वष्ट्रे स्वाहा त्वष्ट्रे तुरीपाय स्वाहा त्वष्ट्रे पुरुरूपाय स्वाहा विष्णवे स्वाहा विष्णवे निभूयपाय स्वाहा विष्णवे शिपिविष्टाय स्वाहा ॥

20. Reverence for him who brings happiness, reverence for God the Embodiment of joy, reverence for the king who is foremost amongst the many. Show respect to him who makes a collection of objects, and him who studies different sciences. Have respect for the deep-thinker, and the protector of the subjects. Show respect to him whose mind is contemplative, who is the master of knowledge. Have respect for the mother Earth, for the mighty, immortal word of God, for the mother, the supplier of happiness. Make full use of the streams. Revere the speech full of knowledge which purifies us. Respect the noble sayings of the learned. Respect a strong man. Respect him who takes hygienic meals for the maintenance of his vitality. Respect the preacher who sermonises and makes us spiritually strong. Have respect for the diffuser of light, for the builder of boats, for him who spreads education. Worship God, Who creates objects of variegated forms. Pray unto the All-pervading Providence. Meditate on Universal God, Who Self-protected, protects others. Contemplate upon Him Who is present in every sentient being.

२१. विश्वो देवस्य नेतुर्मर्तो वुरीत सख्यम् ।
विश्वो राय इषुध्यति द्युम्नं वृणीत पुष्यसे स्वाहा ॥

21. May every mortal man contract the friendship of the guiding God. Each one solicits Him for wealth, and for strength, aspires after fame and riches through noble deeds.

२२. आ ब्रह्मन् ब्राह्मणो ब्रह्मवर्चसी जायतामा राष्ट्रे राजन्य: शूर इषव्योऽतिव्याधी महारथो जायतां दोग्ध्री धेनुर्वोढानड्वानाशु: सप्ति: पुरन्धिर्योषा जिष्णू रथेष्ठा: सभेयो युवास्य यजमानस्य वीरो जायतां निकामे-निकामे न: पर्जन्यो वर्षतु फलवत्यो न ओषधय: पच्यन्तां योगक्षेमो न: कल्पताम् ॥

22. O God let there be born in our country the Brahmana, illustrious for the knowledge of the vedas; let there be born the prince, heroic, skilled

archer, piercing the foe with shafts, mighty warrior; the cow giving abundant milk, the ox good at carring burden; the swift courser; the woman skilled in domestic affairs. May this sacrificer be blessed, with sons, conquering, equipped with conveyances, civilised, young, and heroic. May cloud send rain according to our desire; may our fruitbearing trees ripen; may acquisition and preservation of property be secured to us.

२३. प्राणाय स्वाहा ऽपानाय स्वाहा व्यानाय स्वाहा चक्षुषे स्वाहा श्रोत्राय स्वाहा वाचे स्वाहा मनसे स्वाहा ॥

23. Control the out-going, in-going and diffusive breaths through yogic practices. Take care of your eyesight. Enhance your power of hearing. Use your speech nicely. Concentrate your mind.

२४. प्राच्यै दिशे स्वाहा ऽर्वाच्यै दिशे स्वाहा दक्षिणायै दिशे स्वाहा ऽर्वाच्यै दिशे स्वाहा प्रतीच्यै दिशे स्वाहा ऽर्वाच्यै दिशे स्वाहोदीच्यै दिशे स्वाहा ऽर्वाच्यै दिशे स्वाहोर्ध्वायै दिशे स्वाहाऽर्वाच्यै दिशे स्वाहा ऽर्वाच्यै दिशे स्वाहा ऽर्वाच्यै दिशे स्वाहा ॥

24. Have scientific knowledge and make use of the Eastern Region, and its hitherward Region; the Southern Region, and its hitherward Region; the Western Region and its hitherward Region; the Northern Region and its hitherward Region; the Upward Region and its hitherward Region; the Downward Region and its hitherward Region.

२५. श्रद्भ्यः स्वाहा वार्भ्यः स्वाहोदकाय स्वाहा तिष्ठन्तीभ्यः स्वाहा स्त्रवन्तीभ्यः स्वाहा स्यन्दमानाभ्यः स्वाहा कूप्याभ्यः स्वाहा सूद्याभ्यः स्वाहा धार्याभ्यः स्वाहा ऽर्णवाय स्वाहा समुद्राय स्वाहा सरिराय स्वाहा ॥

25. Purify, utilise, and use ordinary waters, excellent healing waters, waters rising above in vapours through sun's heat; standing waters, fast flowing waters, slowly moving waters; well-waters, rain-waters; tank-waters, sea-waters, waters in the ocean; and charming and beautiful waters.

२६. वाताय स्वाहा धूमाय स्वाहा ऽभ्राय स्वाहा मेघाय स्वाहा विद्योतमानाय स्वाहा स्तनयते स्वाहा ऽवस्फूर्जते स्वाहा वर्षते स्वाहा ऽववर्षते स्वाहोग्रं वर्षते स्वाहा शीघ्रं वर्षते स्वाहोद्गृह्णते स्वाहोद्गृहीताय स्वाहा प्रुष्णते स्वाहा शीकायते स्वाहा प्रुष्वाभ्यः स्वाहा ह्रादुनीभ्यः स्वाहा नीहाराय स्वाहा ॥

26. Perform yajna for the purification of air; for the purification of misty air, for purifying fine cloud; for purifying the cloud; for purifying the dense shining cloud; for purifying the thundering lightning; for purifying the bursting cloud; for purifying the raining cloud, for purifying the pouring cloud; for purifying the violently raining cloud; for purifying the high cloud that has held water; for purifying the sprinkling cloud, for purifying the drizzling cloud; for purifying the clouds that rain cats and dogs; for purifying the thundering clouds; and for purifying the hoar-frost.

---

[24]Each region has got उपदिशा which is called hitherward region.

२७. अग्नये स्वाहा सोमाय स्वाहेन्द्राय स्वाहा पृथिव्यै स्वाहा ऽन्तरिक्षाय स्वाहा दिवेस्वाहा दिग्भ्यः स्वाहा ऽऽशाभ्यः स्वाहोर्ध्वायै दिशेस्वाहा ऽर्वाच्यै दिशे स्वाहा ॥

27. Improve your digestive faculty; make full use of efficacious juices. Elevate your soul. Till the soil. Enjoy the firmament, and light in the sky. Utilise the quarters and subquarters. Understand the significance of the upward region, and the downward region.

२८. नक्षत्रेभ्यः स्वाहा नक्षत्रियेभ्यः स्वाहा ऽहोरात्रेभ्यः स्वाहा ऽर्धमासेभ्यः स्वाहा मासेभ्यः स्वाह ऋतुभ्यः स्वाहा ऽऽर्तवेभ्यः स्वाहा संवत्सराय स्वाहा द्यावापृथिवीभ्यां स्वाहा चन्द्राय स्वाहा सूर्याय स्वाहा रश्मिभ्यः स्वाहा वसुभ्यः स्वाहा रुद्रेभ्यः स्वाहा ऽऽदित्येभ्यः स्वाहा मरुद्भ्यः स्वाहा विश्वेभ्यो देवेभ्यः स्वाहा मूलेभ्यः स्वाहा शाखाभ्यः स्वाहा वनस्पतिभ्यः स्वाहा पुष्पेभ्यः स्वाहा फलेभ्यः स्वाहौषधीभ्यः स्वाहा ॥

28. Perform yajna for indestructible objects and for their assemblage; for day and night, for the half months; for the months; for the seasons and for the objects produced in them and for the year to derive happiness. Perform yajna for the purification of Heaven and Earth; for the Moon, for the Sun, and his rays. Perform yajna for the betterment of the Vasus, the Rudras and the Adityas. Perform yajna for purifying the airs; for the acquisition of noble qualities, for improving the roots and branches of forest trees, flowers, fruits and herbs.

२९. पृथिव्यै स्वाहा ऽन्तरिक्षाय स्वाहा दिवे स्वाहा सूर्याय स्वाहा चन्द्राय स्वाहा नक्षत्रेभ्यः स्वाहा ऽद्भ्यः स्वाहौषधीभ्यः स्वाहा वनस्पतिभ्यः स्वाहा परिप्लवेभ्यः स्वाहा चराचरेभ्यः स्वाहा सरीसृपेभ्यः स्वाहा ॥

29. Perform yajna for the improvement of the Earth, the Firmament, the sky, the Sun, the Moon and the Stars.
Perform yajna for the improvement of waters, herbs and forest trees. Perform yajna for meteors, animate and inanimate things, and things that creep and crawl for our comfort.

३०. असवे स्वाहा वसवे स्वाहा विभुवे स्वाहा विवस्वते स्वाहा गणश्रिये स्वाहा गणपतये स्वाहा ऽभिभुवे स्वाहा ऽधिपतये स्वाहा शूषाय स्वाहा सँसर्पाय स्वाहा चन्द्राय स्वाहा ज्योतिषे स्वाहा मलिम्लुचाय स्वाहा दिवा पतयते स्वाहा ॥

30. Perform yajna for the purification of vital breaths; the soul that resides in the body, the pervading air, the Sun, the lightning, the air that protects multitude of objects, for the hero chastises the wicked, for the king, for

---

28Vasus: Eight forces of nature or Vasu Brahmcharis observing celibacy for 24 years.
  Rudras: Ten vital breaths, and soul, or Rudra Brahmcharis observing celibacy for 36 years.
  Adityas : Twelve months of the year, or Aditya Brahmcharis observing celibacy for 48 years.
  Assemblage : Collectively. All indestructible objects taken together.

acquiring strength, for the reptiles, for gold, for light of the Sun, Moon and stars; for keeping the thieves under control, and for the Sun that nourishes the day.

३१. मधवे स्वाहा माधवाय स्वाहा शुक्राय स्वाहा शुचये स्वाहा नभसे स्वाहा नभस्याय स्वाहेषाय स्वाहोर्जाय स्वाहा सहसे स्वाहा सहस्याय स्वाहा तपसे स्वाहा तपस्याय स्वाहा ॐहंसस्पतये स्वाहा ॥

31. Perform yajna to make comfortable and pleasant the month Chetra (March-April), the Baisakh (April-May), the Jeshtha (May-June), the Asharh (June-July), the Shravan (July-August), the Bhadra (August-September), the Aswin (September-October), the Kartika (October-November), the Margshish (November-December), the Paush (December-January), the Magh (January-February), the Phalgun (February-March), the thirteenth or intercalary month.

३२. वाजाय स्वाहा प्रसवाय स्वाहा ऽपिजाय स्वाहा क्रतवे स्वाहा स्वः स्वाहा मूर्ध्ने स्वाहा व्यश्नुविने स्वाहा अन्त्याय स्वाहा अन्त्याय भौवनाय स्वाहा भुवनस्य पतये स्वाहा अधिपतये स्वाहा प्रजापतये स्वाहा ॥

32. Produce good foodstuffs. Manufacture articles. Protect the foodstuffs produced. Develop intellect and perform noble deeds. Arrange for comforts. Purify your head. Don't waste your semen. Exert for final beatitude. Worship God, the final living entity in the universe. Adore God, the Protector of the world. Serve God, the Preacher of the Vedas to humanity. Pray to God, the Protector of all created beings.

३३. आयुर्यज्ञेन कल्पताꣳ स्वाहा प्राणो यज्ञेन कल्पताꣳ स्वाहा ऽपानो यज्ञेन कल्पताꣳ स्वाहा व्यानो यज्ञेन कल्पताꣳ स्वाहोदानो यज्ञेन कल्पताꣳ स्वाहा समानो यज्ञेन कल्पताꣳ स्वाहा चक्षुर्यज्ञेन कल्पताꣳ स्वाहा श्रोत्रं यज्ञेन कल्पताꣳ स्वाहा वाग्यज्ञेन कल्पताꣳ स्वाहा मनो यज्ञेन कल्पताꣳ स्वाहा ऽऽत्मा यज्ञेन कल्पताꣳ स्वाहा ब्रह्मा यज्ञेन कल्पताꣳ स्वाहा ज्योतिर्यज्ञेन कल्पताꣳ स्वाहा स्वर्यज्ञेन कल्पताꣳ स्वाहा पृष्ठं यज्ञेन कल्पताꣳ स्वाहा यज्ञो यज्ञेन कल्पताꣳ स्वाहा ॥

33. May life be devoted to the service of God, the learned and the spread of knowledge in a noble manner. May breath improve through yoga and physical practices. May downward breath, diffusive breath, upward breath, digestive breath, improve through necessary precautions. May vision, hearing, speech, mind, soul, the master of the four Vedas, light of knowledge and happiness, and questionings advance through sacrifice performed in a right way.

---

[31]Intercalary month : मल मास Inserted in the twelve months, so called because during that month religious ceremonies are not performed.

[33]ऋतवो वै पृष्ठानि । शत० 13-3-2-1.
Prishtha may mean season as well. Swami Dayananda has translated the word as **subtle questionings.**

May God be pleased with us through sacrifice performed in a spirit of devotion.

३४. एकस्मै स्वाहा द्वाभ्याꣳ स्वाहा शताय स्वाहैकशताय स्वाहा व्युष्टयै स्वाहा स्वर्गाय स्वाहा ॥

34. Worship one God. Have knowledge of Cause and Effect, Please hundreds of souls. Practise hundred and one trades. Acquire the power to burn down sins. Attain to final beatitude full of happiness.

CHAPTER XXIII

१. हिरण्यगर्भः समवर्तताग्रे भूतस्य जातः पतिरेक आसीत् ।
स दाधार पृथिवीं द्यामुतेमां कस्मै देवाय हविषा विधेम ॥

1. God is the Creator of the universe, its one Lord, the Sustainer of luminous objects like the sun. He was present before the creation of the world. He sustains this Earth and the Sun in past, present and future. Let us worship with self dedication of our soul, Him, the Embodiment of happiness.

२. उपयामगृहीतोऽसि प्रजापतये त्वा जुष्टं गृह्णाम्येष ते योनिः सूर्यस्ते महिमा ।
यस्तेऽहन्त्संवत्सरे महिमा सम्बभूव यस्ते वायावन्तरिक्षे महिमा सम्बभूव यस्ते दिवि सूर्ये महिमा सम्बभूव तस्मै ते महिम्ने प्रजापतये स्वाहा देवेभ्यः ॥

2. O God, Thou art realisable through yoga. I serve Thee and accept Thee as Protector of the King who takes care of his subjects. This primordial matter and the Sun testify to Thy Greatness. Thy Majesty is discernible in the day and year. Thy Majesty is seen in the wind and firmament. Thy Majesty is traceable in the luminous Sun. For all that, for Thy protecting greatness and for the learned persons, we always sing praises!

३. यः प्राणतो निमिषतो महित्वैक इद्राजा जगतो बभूव ।
य ईशे अस्य द्विपदश्चतुष्पदः कस्मै देवाय हविषा विधेम ॥

3. God by His grandeur is the sole Ruler of the moving world that breathes and slumbers. He is the Sovereign Lord of these men and cattle. Let us worship with devotion, Him, the Embodiment of happiness.

४. उपयामगृहीतोऽसि प्रजापतये त्वा जुष्टं गृह्णाम्येष ते योनिश्चन्द्रमास्ते महिमा ।
यस्ते रात्रौ संवत्सरे महिमा सम्बभूव यस्ते पृथिव्यामग्नौ महिमा सम्बभूव यस्ते नक्षत्रेषु चन्द्रमसि महिमा सम्बभूव तस्मै ते महिम्ने प्रजापतये देवेभ्यः स्वाहा ॥

4. O God, Thou art realisable through yoga. I serve Thee and accept Thee as Protector of the king who takes care of his subjects. This water and moon testify to Thy greatness. Thy Majesty is seen in the night and year. Thy Majesty is found in the Earth and fire. Thy Majesty is discernible in the immortal worlds and the moon. For all that, for Thy protecting greatness and for the learned persons, we always sing praises!

५. युञ्जन्ति ब्रध्नमरुषं चरन्तं परि तस्थुषः ।
रोचन्ते रोचना दिवि ॥

5. They, who unite their souls with God, Who pervades all stationary

---

*Day and year : The regularity of time, the rising and setting of the sun in time all the year round, indicate the Majesty of God.

objects, and protects the vital parts of our body, shine in Him like beams in the Sun.

६. युञ्जन्त्यस्य काम्या हरी विपक्षसा रथे ।
शोणा धृष्णू नृवाहसा ॥

6. Just as experts yoke to the chariot two beautiful horses, controlled with difficulty and through diverse devices; tawny, stout, our bearers from one place to the other, so do the yogis yoke their organs of sense, mind, and vital breaths to God.

७. यद्वातो अपो अग्निनीग्निप्रियामिन्द्रस्य तन्वम् ।
एतꣳ स्तोत्रनेन पथा पुनरश्वमावर्तयासि नः ॥

7. O laudable learned person, just as artisans control the beautiful diffused form of electricity, swift like the wind, and erect electrical contrivances worked with water, so do ye prepare with the aid of electricity a fast moving machine, that takes us from one place to the other!

८. वसवस्त्वाञ्जन्तु गायत्रेण छन्दसा रुद्रास्त्वाञ्जन्तु त्रैष्टुभेन छन्दसा ऽऽदित्यास्त्वाञ्जन्तु जागतेन छन्दसा ।
भूर्भुवः स्वर्लाजी ३ ऽच्छाची ३ न्यव्ये गव्य एतदन्नमत्त देवा एतदन्नमद्धि प्रजापते ॥

8. O king, the protector of his subjects, the Vasus approach thee with Vedic verses in Gayatri Metre, Rudras approach thee with verses in Trishtup metre, Adityas approach thee with verses in Jagati metre, eat thou this food, O learned people eat ye this food prepared from barley and cow's milk and its products, and move on Earth, Ether, Heaven, and distinct planets moving in their orbits!

९. कः स्विदेकाकी चरति क उ स्विज्जायते पुनः ।
किꣳ स्विद्धिमस्य भेषजं किम्वावपनं महत् ॥

9. Who moveth singly and alone? Who is brought forth to life again? What is the remedy of cold. What is the vast field for production?

१०. सूर्य एकाकी चरति चन्द्रमा जायते पुनः ।
अग्निर्हिमस्य भेषजं भूमिरावपनं महत् ॥

10. The Sun moves singly and alone. The Moon is brought to life again. Fire is the remedy of cold. The Earth is the vast field for production.

११. का स्विदासीत्पूर्वंचित्तिः किꣳ स्विदासीद् बृहद्वयः ।
का स्विदासीत्पिलिप्पिला का स्विदासीत्पिशङ्गिला ॥

11. What is the primary thought? What is the bird of mighty size? What is the majestic beautiful thing? What absorbs light?

[8]Vasus, Rudras and Adityas are the learned persons observing celibacy for 24, 36 and 48 years.

[9-12]In 9th and 10th, and 11th, 12th verses there are questions and answers.

१२. द्यौरासीत्पूर्वंचित्तिरश्व आसीद् बृहद्दयः ।
अविरासीत्पिलिप्पिला रात्रिरासीत्पिशङ्गिला ॥

12. Rain is the primary thought. Fire is like the mighty bird, Earth is the majestic, beautiful object that protects us with corn. Night absorbs light.

१३. वायुष्ट्वा पचतैरवत्वसितग्रीवश्छागैर्न्यग्रोधश्चमसैः शल्मलिर्वृद्धया ।
एष स्य राध्यो वृषा पड्भिश्चतुर्भिरेदगन्ब्रह्मा कृष्णश्च नोऽवतु नमोऽग्नये ॥

13. O student, may air help thee with cooked viands black-necked fire with powers of digestion, fig tree with clouds, Shalmali tree with its increase. May the stallion, that moves on the roads the chariot, bestower of happiness come unto thee on his four feet. May the learned scholar of the four Vedas, free from the darkness of ignorance fill us with virtues. May we offer him food!

१४. सꣳशितो रश्मिना रथः सꣳशितो रश्मिना हयः ।
सꣳशितो अप्स्वप्सुजा ब्रह्मा सोमपुरोगवः ॥

14. Body is strengthened through penance, warm like the sun's rays. Organs are also strengthened through penance. Vital breaths are invigorated through penance. A learned yogi advances spiritually through the attainment of love for God.

१५. स्वयं वाजिꣳस्तन्वं कल्पयस्व स्वयं यजस्व स्वयं जुषस्व ।
महिमा तेऽन्येन न सन्नशे ॥

15. O seeker after knowledge, thyself strengthen the body, thyself walk in the company of the learned, and thyself serve them. Let not thy greatness be marred by any one!

१६. न वा उ एतन्म्रियसे न रिष्यसि देवाꣳ2 इदेषि पथिभिः सुगेभिः ।
यत्रासते सुकृतो यत्र ते ययुस्तत्र त्वा देवः सविता दधातु ॥

16. O Soul, thou art immortal and indestructible. By fair paths thou cultivatest noble qualities. May the resplendent God place thee in that place, where the godly yogis dwell, and derive pleasure!

१७. अग्निः पशुरासीत्तेनायजन्त स एतँल्लोकमजयद्यस्मिन्नग्निः स ते लोको भविष्यति तं जेष्यसि पिबैता अपः ।
वायुः पशुरासीत्तेनायजन्त स एतँल्लोकमजयद्यस्मिन्वायुः स ते लोको भविष्यति तं जेष्यसि पिबैता अपः ।
सूर्यः पशुरासीत्तेनायजन्त स एतँल्लोकमजयद्यस्मिन्त्सूर्यः स ते लोको भविष्यति तं जेष्यसि पिबैता अपः ॥

---

[13]Shalmali : The silk-cotton tree. A lofty and thorny tree with red flowers. It is called सेमर tree.

Black-necked : Fire with its dark smoke.

Four feet : with full speed.

17. O seeker after knowledge, in this world, fire is a thing of beauty. Just as learned persons perform yajnas with it, so shouldst thou do. Just as a learned person masters this beautiful place of sacrifice, so shouldst thou do. If thou wilt properly manage the place of yajna, fire will manifest itself as a thing worth seeing. Drink thou the waters purified by the yajna!

Air is a thing of beauty. Just as learned persons perform yajnas with it, so shouldst thou do. Just as a learned person masters the atmosphere, the home of air, so shouldst thou do. If thou wilt master the atmosphere, air will look as a beautiful thing. Breathe thou the air purified by the yajna. Sun is a thing of beauty. The learned perform yajnas with its aid. Just as a learned person acquires full knowledge about the sun, so shouldst thou do. If thou wilt do it, sun will appear as a beautiful thing unto thee. Enjoy thou the beams of the sun purified through the yajna, and reigning of the universe.

१८. प्राणय स्वाहा ऽपानाय स्वाहा व्यानाय स्वाहा ।
अम्बे अम्बिकेऽम्बालिके न मा नयति कश्चन ।
ससस्त्यश्वक: सुभद्रिकां काम्पीलवासिनीम् ॥

18. O mother, grandmother, great-grandmother, I cannot be subdued by a man, who, though he be quick like a horse, and in full possession of wealth, the bringer of good fortune, and sustainer of an easeloving person, but lies in idle slumber. I utter truthful speech for the sustenance of vital breath. I use instructive speech for warding off misery. I speak the truth for the preservation of my soul that pervades the body!

१६. गणानां त्वा गणपतिꣳ हवामहे प्रियाणां त्वा प्रियपतिꣳ हवामहे निधीनां त्वा निधिपतिꣳ हवामहे वसो मम ।
आहमजानि गर्भधमा त्वमजासि गर्भधम् ॥

19. O God, we invoke Thee, the troop-lord of troops. We invoke Thee, the Lord of the beloved ones. We invoke Thee, the Lord of the treasure of knowledge. O God, all beings reside in Thee. Thou art my judge. I know Thee full well free from birth, the Sustainer of Matter that keeps the universe in its womb. Thou knowest Matter!

२०. ता उभौ चतुर: पद: संप्रसारयाव स्वर्गे लोके प्रोर्णुवाथां वृषा वाजी रेतोधा रेतो दधातु ॥
20. The King and his subjects in unison, magnify the four stages of

---

[18]One should never lapse into idleness, though he be the master of wealth. A wealthy person should be active and enterprising.

[20]Dharma: Law, custom, piety, duty, justice, merit, character, the soul.
Artha: Worldly prosperity.
Kama: Affection, object of desire.
Moksha: Liberation, deliverance.

Griffith has not translated the 10 verses 20-29 saying that these stanzas are not reproducible even in the semi-obscurity of a learned European language; and stanzas 30, 31 would be unintelligible without them.

Ubbat and Mahidhar have translated these stanzas in an obscene language unfit for reproduction. Swami Dayananda has given to the world their correct interpretation.

Dharma, Arth, Kama, Moksha, wherewith they reside happily in their country. The King, the chastiser of the wicked, full of knowledge, the possessor of strength and prowess, lends valour to his subjects.

२१. उत्सक्थ्या अव गुदं धेहि समञ्जिं चारया वृषन् ।
य स्त्रीणां जीवभोजनः ॥

21. O powerful King, punish the immoral person residing amongst women, and the degraded woman living amongst men, with feet upwards, and head downwards; spread happiness amongst your people, and establish your well established reign of justice!

२२. यकासकौ शकुन्तिकाऽऽह्लगिति वञ्चति ।
आह्रन्ति गभे पसो निगल्गलीति धारका ॥

22. The King establishes his rule over his subjects, which aspiring after happiness, acquire it bit by bit. His subjects are weak like the tiny sparrow, realises land revenue from the people to be spent on their advancement.

२३. यकोऽसकौ शकुन्तक आह्रलगिति वञ्चति ।
विवक्षत इव ते मुखमध्वर्यो मा नस्त्वमभि भाषथाः ॥

23. O harmless King, don't utter untruth before us. Let not thy tongue utter meaningless words like a prattler. A King who has got no control over his tongue will be extirpated like a weak sparrow, and defrauded by his subjects!

२४. माता च ते पिता च तेऽग्रं वृक्षस्य रोहतः ।
प्रतिलामीति ते पिता गभे मुष्टिमतँसयत् ॥

24. O king, thy forbearing and loving mother, and thy father brilliant and nourishing like the sun, rule over the prosperity and riches of the sovereignty of this mundane universe. Thy father has beautified his rule for his subjects. I, as his subject, do love him dearly!

२५. माता च ते पिता च तेऽग्रे वृक्षस्य क्रीडतः ।
विवक्षत इव ते मुखं ब्रह्मन्मा त्वं वदो बहु ॥

25. O master of all the four vedas, thy mother patient like the Earth, and thy father shining like the Sun, enjoy with knowledge and grandeur the mastery of the universe. Thy mouth is eager to speak, but thou shouldst not talk much.

२६. ऊर्ध्वमिनामुच्छापय गिरौ भारँ हरन्निव ।
अथास्यै मध्यमेधता शीते वाते पुनन्निव ॥

[26]A learned person should not talk much without purpose. He should follow the maxim 'Speech is silver, silence is gold". Too much talking is not a sign of wisdom.

26. O King, like the man taking a load up to the mountain, always lift up these excellent subjects of thine full of sovereign wealth!

Having acquired these precious subjects attain to prosperity, just as an agriculturist in a cool breeze separates corn from the chaff and improves physically by its use.

२७. उर्ध्वेनमुच्छ्रयतादिगिरौ भारꣳ हरन्निव ।
अथास्य मध्यमेजतु शीते वाते पुनन्निव ॥

27. O learned persons among the subjects, elevate this king in all administrative designs, as a labourer takes a load up to the mountain. Having thus contributed to the prosperity of the State, aspire after pure deeds, like the corn purified in a cool breeze!

२८. यदस्या अꣳ हुभेद्याः कृधु स्थूलमुपातसत् ।
मुष्काविदस्य एजतो गोशफे शकुलाविव ॥

28. The king and officials, who contribute to the grandeur of their subjects in part or full, and both make them energetic, tremble when they unjustly realise taxes from them, just as tiny fishes tremble in the water below the cow's hooves.

२९. यद्देवासो ललामगुं प्र विष्टीमिनमाविषुः ।
सक्थ्ना देदिश्यते नारी सत्यस्याक्षिभुवो यथा ॥

29. Just as we distinguish between man and woman from their organs, so we realise truth from visible evidence. Learned persons with the help of truth acquire humility and their desired objects.

३०. यद्धरिणो यवमत्ति न पुष्टं पशु मन्यते ।
शूद्रा यदर्येजारा न पोषाय धनायति ॥

30. A licentious king who squeezes money out of his subjects, like the deer who destroys the barley field, cannot see his people thrive. A Shudra maid-servant who has got illicit connection with her master, does not desire the progress of her family.

३१. यद्धरिणो यवमत्ति न पुष्टं बहु मन्यते ।
शूद्रो यदर्ये जारो न पोषमनु मन्यते ॥

31. A King, who destroys his subjects, like the deer the barley field, cannot see his people thrive.

A Shudra servant who has got illicit connection with his mistress, does not desire the progress of his family.

[31] A king who plunders and teases his subjects, is like the deer who eats barley in the field, and doesn't allow it grow.

Similarly the King who impoverishes and destroys his subjects is like the male servant who violates the chastity of his mistress, and thereby nullifies her dignity, fame and wealth.

३२. दधिक्राव्णो अकारिषं जिष्णोरश्वस्य वाजिनः ।
सुरभि नो मुखा करत्प्र ण आयूँषि तारिषत् ॥

32. I sing the praise of God, obtainable by him who deeply meditates upon Him, the Remover of miseries, and full of splendour. May He strengthen our vital breaths, and prolong the days we have to live.

३३. गायत्री त्रिष्टुब्जगत्यनुष्टुप्पङ्क्तया सह ।
बृहद्युष्णिहा ककुप्सूचीभिः शम्यन्तु त्वा ॥

33. O King, may the vedic verses in Gayatri, Trishtup, Jagati, Anushtup, Pankti, Brihati, Ushnik and Kakup metres uttered by the subjects, pacify thee!

३४. द्विपदा याश्चतुष्पदास्त्रिपदा याश्च षट्पदाः ।
विच्छन्दा याश्च सच्छन्दाः सूचीभिः शम्यन्तु त्वा ॥

34. O King, may the two-footed, four-footed, three-footed, six-footed metrical divisions, with different metres or one uniform metre, uttered by the subjects pacify thee!

३५. महानाम्न्यो रेवत्यो विश्वा आशाः प्रभूवरीः ।
मेघीर्विद्युतो वाचः सूचीभिः शम्यन्तु त्वा ॥

35. May the Mahanamni and Revati vedic verses, all far spread Supreme Regions, the lightning in the clouds, and the voices uttered by the subjects, satisfy the king.

[33]Gayatri: that protects the singer.
Trishtup: that protects us from mental, material and natural afflictions.
Jagati: Diffused like the earth.
Anushtup: Whereby worldly afflictions are warded off.
Ushnik: Whereby we sing early in the morning.
Brihati: Full of deep significance.
Kakup: Full with the meaning of elegant stanzas.
विशो वै सूच्यः । शत० 13-2-10-2.
Suchi means subjects. Suchi means needle. Just as a needle sews and joins together the broken parts of a cloth, so do these verses concentrate the mind of seeker after knowledge on God.

[34]Dvipada: Brahmcharis. Chatushpada: Grihasthis.
Tripada: Vanprasthis.
Shatpada: Seekers after emancipation, Moksha.
Vichhanda: Self sacrificing.
Satchhanda: Equipped with special spiritual resources.
The verse may also mean: May the Brahmcharis, Grihasthis, Vanprasthis, Sanyasis, the aspirers after Moksha, self sacrificing persons and those equipped with special spiritual resources pacify thee.

[35]Mahanamnis: Whose name is great: nine verses of the Samaveda in Sakvari metre.
Revatis: Verses from which the Raivata Saman is formed, so named from Rigveda 1.30.13 in which the word revati, splendid, or wealthy, occurs.

३६. नार्यस्ते पत्न्यो लोम विचिन्वन्तु मनीषया ।
देवानां पत्न्यो दिशः सूचीभिः शम्यन्तु त्वा ॥

36. O learned teachress, the girls, who with sharp intellect, obey thy order, become the wives of learned persons. O unmarried girl, the wives of learned persons, who through careful inspection learn the art of cooking, pure like the regions, grant thee knowledge and peace!

३७. रजता हरिणीः सीसा युजो युज्यन्ते कर्मभिः ।
अश्वस्य वाजिनस्त्वचि सिमाः शम्यन्तु शम्यन्तीः ॥

37. Affectionate, fascinating, amorous wives, well trained in domestic economy, according to religious rites, are united for life with powerful husbands full of noble qualities, and placed under their protection. May they tranquil and peaceful, bound by the ties of affection, enjoy life.

३८. कुविदङ्ग यवमन्तो यवच्चिद्यथा दान्त्यनुपूर्वं वियूय ।
इहेहैषां कृणुहि भोजनानि ये बर्हिषो नम उक्तिं यजन्ति ॥

38. O king, just as farmers reap the barley-corn, winnow and protect it; so shouldst thou arrange for food for those engaged in the contemplation of God!

३९. कस्त्वा छ्यति कस्त्वा विशास्ति कस्ते गात्राणि शम्यति ।
क उ ते शमिता कविः ॥

39. O student, who admonishes thee? Who imparts thee sound instruction? Who pacifies thy organs? Who is thy teacher who is well versed in religious lore and performs the yajnas?

४०. ऋतवस्त ऋतुथा पर्व शमितारो वि शासतु ।
संवत्सरस्य तेजसा शमीभिः शम्यन्तु त्वा ॥

40. May the truly learned persons, bestowers of peace, give necessary instructions for rearing the subjects. O people, may they pacify ye by means of King's dignity, and peaceful expedients!

४१. अर्धमासाः परूँषि ते मासा आ च्छ्यन्तु शम्यन्तः ।
अहोरात्राणि मरुतो विलिष्टꣳ सूदयन्तु ते ॥

41. O King, may day and night, half months and months, affording felicity, adorn the different periods of thy life. May the learned remove thy doubt!

४२. दैव्या अध्वर्यवस्त्वा च्छ्यन्तु वि च शासतु ।
गात्राणि पर्वशस्ते सिमाः कृण्वन्तु शम्यन्तीः ॥

42. O male and female students, may the learned teachers and preachers give ye special instructions; and thereby eliminate your weaknesses. May

CHAPTER XXIII

they examine each joint of your limbs. May your mother and other female relations bound in the ties of affection, give ye similar instructions!

४३. द्यौस्ते पृथिव्यन्तरिक्षं वायुश्छिद्रं पृणातु ते ।
सूर्यस्ते नक्षत्रैः सह लोकं कृणोतु साधुया ॥

43. O female student or mistress, may Sky, Earth Space, Air, Sun and Moon with the stars of heaven, appease each organ of thine, grant success to thy undertaking; and prepare a nice, true, beautiful world for thee!

४४. शं ते परेभ्यो गात्रेभ्यः शमस्त्ववरेभ्यः ।
शमस्थभ्यो मज्जभ्यः शम्वस्तु तन्वै तव ॥

44. O student, just as the Earth contributes to the welfare of vital and minor organs of thy body, thy bones and marrow, so thy teachers with their qualities, actions and noble nature add to thy pleasure!

४५. कः स्विदेकाकी चरति क उ स्विज्जायते पुनः ।
किं॒ स्विद्धिमस्य भेषजं किम्वावपनं महत् ॥

45. Who moveth singly and alone? Who is brought forth to life again? What is the remedy of cold? What is the vast field for production.

४६. सूर्य एकाकी चरति चन्द्रमा जायते पुनः ।
अग्निर्हिमस्य भेषजं भूमिरावपनं महत् ॥

46. The sun moves singly and alone. The moon is brought to life again. Fire is the remedy of cold. Earth is the vast field for production.

४७. किं॒ स्वित्सूर्यसमं ज्योतिः किं॒ समुद्रसमं॒ सरः ।
किं॒ स्वित्पृथिव्यै वर्षीयः कस्य मात्रा न विद्यते ॥

47. What lustre is like the sun's light? What lake is equal to the sea? What is more spacious than the Earth? What thing is that which is beyond measure.

४८. ब्रह्म सूर्यसमं ज्योतिर्द्यौः समुद्रसमं॒ सरः ।
इन्द्रः पृथिव्यै वर्षीयान् गोस्तु मात्रा न विद्यते ॥

48. God is lustre like the sun. Heaven is a flood to match the sea. Sun is vaster than the Earth. Beyond all measure is speech.

४९. पृच्छामि त्वा चितये देवसख यदि त्वमत्र मनसा जगन्थ ।
येषु विष्णुस्त्रिषु पदेष्वेष्टस्तेषु विश्वं भुवनमा विवेशा३ ॥

49. O God, Friend of the learned, I ask, for information, if Thou in spirit

---

⁴⁵⁻⁴⁶See 23-9,10 The repetition of these verses in not clear. No commentator has explained it.
⁴⁹Vishnu: God who permeates all objects.
Three steps: Creation, sustenance, and Dissolution or Earth, Space, and Sky, or name, birth and place.

hast pervaded the universe! Is this created world contained in the three steps in which Vishnu is worshipped?

५०. अपि तेषु त्रिषु पदेष्वस्मि येषु विश्वं भुवनमा विवेश ।
सद्यः पर्येमि पृथिवीमुत द्यामेकेनाङ्गेन दिवो अस्य पृष्ठम् ॥

50. I pervade those three steps in which resides the whole of this universe. This Earth and Heaven I encircle in a moment with a part of My might. Even beyond Heaven am I.

५१. केश्वन्तः पुरुष आ विवेश कान्यन्तः पुरुषे अर्पितानि ।
एतद्ब्रह्मन्नुप वल्हामसि त्वा किँ स्विन्नः प्रति वोचास्यत्र ॥

51. What are the things which God hath entered in? What are the things which God hath contained within Him? This riddle we propose to thee, O knower of the vedas; whereby we become great. Pray tell us what mystery lies in it.

५२. पञ्चस्वन्तः पुरुष आ विवेश तान्यन्तः पुरुषे अर्पितानि ।
एतत्त्वात्र प्रतिमन्वानो अस्मि न मायया भवस्युत्तरो मत् ।

52. Within five things hath God found entrance. These things hath God within Him established. O questioner, this is the thought which I return in answer. Though thou art wise, yet thou art not my superior in wisdom.

५३. का स्विदासीत्पूर्वचित्तिः किँ स्विदासीद् बृहद्वयः ।
का स्विदासीतिपिलिप्पिला का स्विदासीतिपिशङ्गिला ॥

53. O learned person, I ask of thee.
What is accumulated in time without beginning? What is the great source of creation? What is the majestic thing?
What absorbs the bodies!

५४. द्यौरासीत्पूर्वचित्तिरश्व आसीद् बृहद्वयः ।
अविरासीतिपिलिप्पिला रात्रिरासीतिपिशङ्गिला ॥

54. O questioner, know that, lightning is accumulated in the beginning. Intellect is the source of creation. Matter is the majestic thing. Dissolution absorbs all bodies!

५५. का ईमरे पिशङ्गिला का ईं कुरुपिशङ्गिला ।
क ईमास्कन्दमर्षति क ईं पन्थां वि सर्पति ॥

⁵⁰I: God.
Theer steps: Birth, name and place.
⁵¹Whereby: with the knowledge or solution of which riddle.
⁵²Five Things: Five elements, Water, Air, Fire, Earth, and space.
⁵³The verse is the same as 23-11 but the interpretation is different.
⁵⁴Intellect महतत्त्व
Dissolution: प्रलय
The verse is the same as 23-12 but the interpretation is different.

55. O learned person! what appears and disappears again and again? Who eats the corn-fields again and again? What moves with rapid spring and bounds again and again? What glides and winds along the path of water?

५६. अजारे पिशङ्गिला श्वावित्कुरुपिशङ्गिला ।
शश आस्कन्दमर्षत्यहिः पन्थां वि सर्पति ॥

56. O questioner know, that eternal matter resolves the world in itself at the time of dissolution, Porcupine destroys the corn-fields. Like hare the air moves with leaps and bounds. Cloud creeps winding on the path.

५७. कत्यस्य विष्ठाः कत्यक्षराणि कति होमासः कतिधा समिद्धः ।
यज्ञस्य त्वा विदथा पृच्छमत्र कति होतार ऋतुशो यजन्ति ॥

57. How many supports hath this world got? How many are the means of its creation? How many things are worth bartering? How many things kindle knowledge? How many Hotas worship in due season? O learned fellow, here I ask thee of the knowledge of these subjects!

५८. षडस्य विष्ठाः शतमक्षराण्यशीतिर्हॊमाः समिधो ह तिस्रः ।
यज्ञस्य ते विदथा प्र ब्रवीमि सप्त होतार ऋतुशो यजन्ति ॥

58. This world has got six seasons as its supports. Hundreds of things like water etc. are the means of its creation. Countless things are worth using and bartering. Three things kindle knowledge. Seven Hotas perform yajan in due season.
O questioner I explain to thee these different topics of knowledge!

५९. को अस्य वेद भुवनस्य नाभिं को द्यावापृथिवी अन्तरिक्षम् ।
कः सूर्यस्य वेद बृहतो जनित्रं को वेद चन्द्रमसं यतोजाः ॥

59. Who knoweth the paramount lord of this world?
Who knoweth the Heaven, the Earth, and the wide space between them! Who knoweth the creator of the mighty Sun? Who knoweth the Moon, and whence she was generated?

६०. वेदाहमस्य भुवनस्य नाभिं वेद द्यावापृथिवी अन्तरिक्षम् ।
वेद सूर्यस्य बृहतो जनित्रमथो वेद चन्द्रमसं यतोजाः ॥

60. O questioner I know the paramount Lord of this world. I know the

---

[57] This world has been described as a king of yajna.
[58] Three things : Spiritual, physical and natural objects (Dayananda); or childhood, manhood and old age ; or fire, lightning and sun; or summer, winter, and rainy season.
  Seven Hotas : Five breaths, mind and soul according to Swami Dayananda's interpretation. Some consider seven rays of the sun as seven Hotas, some commentators interpret seven breaths is the head as seven Hotas.
  I : a learned person.
[60] Matter is the material and God the efficient cause of the universe. God has created the Sun and the Moon.

Heaven, the Earth, and the wide space between them. I know the efficient and physical causes of the mighty Sun. I know the Moon, and her Creator!

६१. पृच्छामि त्वा परमन्तं पृथिव्या: पृच्छामि यत्र भुवनस्य नाभि: ।
पृच्छामि त्वा वृष्णो अश्वस्य रेत: पृच्छामि वाच: परमं व्योम ॥

61. I ask thee of Earth's extremest limit, Where is the centre of the world, I ask thee? I ask thee of the strength of the powerful stout person. I ask of the highest space where speech abideth.

६२. इयं वेदि: परो अन्त: पृथिव्या अयं यज्ञो भुवनस्य नाभि: ।
अयँ सोमो वृष्णो अश्वस्य रेतो ब्रह्मायं वाच: परमं व्योम ॥

62. This equator is the Earth's extremest limit. This Adorable God imbued with qualities is the controller of the world. This efficacious Soma, the King of medicines is the strength of a stout person. This master of all the four vedas is the highest abode for vedic speech.

६३. सुभू: स्वयम्भू: प्रथमोऽन्तर्महत्यर्णवे ।
दधे ह गर्भमृत्वियं यतो जात: प्रजापति: ॥

63. God, Who has produced the Sun, is Excellent, and Self-Existent, the First within the mighty world. He lays down the timely embryo. All should worship Him.

६४. होता यक्षत्प्रजापतिँ सोमस्य महिम्न: ।
जुषतां पिबतु सोमँ होतर्यज ॥

64. O charitably disposed person, just as a learned recipient, with the grandeur of his supremacy, worships the Lord of the Universe, pleases Him through service, and drinks the essence of medicinal herbs, so shouldst thou worship Him and drink the juice of medicinal herbs!

६५. प्रजापते न त्वदेतान्यन्यो विश्वा रूपाणि परि ता बभूव ।
यत्कामास्ते जुहुमस्तन्नो अस्तु वयँ स्याम पतयो रयीणाम् ॥

65. O God, none besides Thee, comprehendest all these created forms. Give us our heart's desire when we invoke Thee. May we be lords of rich possessions and knowledge!

---

⁶²Pt. Jaidev Vidyalankar interprets Soma as the forces of nature like the sun, fire, air, lightning, etc. which constitute the strength of the Mighty, Omnipresent God. He interprets वृष्ण: as Mighty, and अश्व as Omnipresent God. Rishi Dayananda translates वेदि: as equator but Pt. Jaidev Vidyalankar and Griffith translate the word as altar.

CHAPTER XXIV

१. अश्वस्तूपरो गोमृगस्ते प्राजापत्याः कृष्णग्रीव आग्नेयो रराटे पुरस्तात्सारस्वती मेध्यघस्ताद्न्वोराश्विनावधोरामौ बाह्वो: सौमापौष्ण: श्यामो नाभ्यां सौर्यामी श्वेतश्च कृष्णश्च पार्श्वयोस्त्वाष्ट्रो लोमशस्सक्थ्योर्वाय्यव्य: श्वेत. पुच्छ इन्द्राय स्वपस्याय वेहद्दैष्ण्वो वामन: ॥

1. Horse, violent goat, forest cow possess the qualities of the sun. A black-necked beast, excellent amongst the beasts, has the qualities of fire.

An ewe possesses the qualities of speech and lives amongst the beasts, like tongue between the jaws. Two goats white-coloured in the lower parts of the body, resembling two arms possess the qualities of day and night.

A dark-coloured beast possesses the qualities of the sun and moon, and is considered as a navel amongst the beasts.

White and dark-coloured beasts, possess the qualities of the sun and air. They act as sides amongst the beasts.

Beasts with abundance of hair possess the qualities of Twashta. They are like thighs amongst the beasts. A white beast possesses the qualities of air, and is like tail amongst the beasts.

A cow that slips her calf is imbued with the qualities of Indra, the doer of noble deeds.

A beast dwarfish in size belongs to Vishnu.

२. रोहितो धूम्ररोहित: कर्केन्धुरोहितस्ते सौम्या बभ्रुरुणबभ्रु: शुकबभ्रुस्ते वारुणा: शितिरन्ध्रोऽन्यत: शितिरन्ध्र: समन्तशितिरन्ध्रस्ते सावित्रा: शितिबाहु रन्यत: शितिबाहु: समन्तशितिबाहुस्ते बाहस्पत्या: पृषती क्षुद्रपृषती स्थूलपृषती ता मैत्रावरुण्य: ॥

2. The red goat, the smoky red, the jujube-red, these belong to Soma.

The brown, the ruddy brown, the parrot-brown, these beasts belong to Varuna. One with white ear holes, one with partly white, one with wholly white, belong to Savita. Beasts with white, partly white, wholly white arms belong to Brihaspati. Beasts speckled with spots, with small spots, with big spots, belong to Pran and Udan.

३. शुद्धवाल: सर्वशुद्धवालो मणिवालस्त आश्विना: श्वेत: श्येताक्षोऽरुणस्ते रुद्राय पशुपतये कर्णा यामा अवलिप्ता रौद्रा नभोरूपा: पार्जन्या: ॥

Vishnu : One occupying a high position.
[1]The exact significance of these animals being attached to the forces of nature is not clear to me.
Twashta : Who kills the enemy's forces with warlike instruments.
[2]Belong to : Possess the qualities of.
Brihaspati : विद्युत्, lightning.
Belong to Varuna : Are excellent.
Savita : Sun. Those animals possess the qualities of the sun.

3. The bright haired, the wholly bright haired, the jewel-haired beasts possess the qualities of the sun and moon. The white, the white-eyed, the reddish beasts, possess the qualities of fire, the protector of cattle. Beasts of burden possess the qualities of air. Beasts with heavy limbs possess the qualities of vital breaths. Sky-coloured beasts belong to the cloud.

४. पृश्निस्तिरश्चीनपृश्निरूर्ध्वपृश्निस्ते मारुता: फल्गूलोंहितोर्णी पलक्षी ता: सारस्वत्य: प्लीहाकर्ण: शुण्ठाकर्णोऽध्यालोहकर्णस्ते त्वाष्ट्रा: कृष्णग्रीव: शितिकक्षोऽञ्जिसक्थस्त ऐन्द्राग्ना: कृष्णाञ्जिरलपाञ्जिर्मंहाञ्जिस्त उपस्या: ॥

4. Speckled, transversely speckled, upward speckled beasts belong to the Marutas. The beasts fond of fruits, red-haired, sharp-eyed belong to Saraswati. The beasts having ears like spleen, dry ears, golden ears belong to Twashta. The black-necked, the white-flanked, the bulky-thighed beasts belong to Indra and Agni. Beasts with faltering, feeble, fast gaits belong to the Dawn.

५. शिल्पा वैश्वदेव्यो रोहिण्यस्त्र्यवयो वाचेऽविज्ञाता अदित्यै सरूपा धात्रे वत्सतर्यो देवानां पत्नीभ्य: ॥

5. The beautiful beasts useful in arts, belong to the all-gods. Beasts used for riding and protected by three agencies belong to vak. The unknown beasts belong to Aditi. Beasts of the same colour belong to their Protector. Tender-aged goats and sheep possess the qualities of consorts of the gods.

६. कृष्णग्रीवा आग्नेया: शितिभ्रवो वसूनाꣵ रोहिता रुद्राणाꣵ श्वेता अवरोकिण आदित्यानां नभोरूपा: पार्जन्या: ॥

6. Black necked animals possess the qualities of fire. White browed animals possess the qualities of Vasus. Red coloured animals possess the qualities of Rudras. Bright animals who prevent others from going astray possess the qualities of Adityas. Water coloured animals possess the qualities of clouds.

७. उन्नत ऋषभो वामनस्त ऐन्द्रावैष्णवा उन्नत: शितिबाहु: शितिपृष्ठस्त ऐन्द्राबाहंस्पत्या: शुक्ररूपा वाजिना: कल्माषा आग्निमारुता: श्यामा: पौष्णा: ॥

7. The tall, the sturdy, the animals with distorted organs possess the qualities of electricity and air. Animals possessing the strength of arms that cut and shear things, and delicate back, possess the qualities of air and sun.

[4]Marutas : Air.
Saraswati : Speech.
Twashta : Sun.
Indra, Agni : Air and lightning.
[5]Three agencies : Father, mother and instructor.
Aditi : The Earth.
Vak : speech.
[6]Vasus eight in number, eleven Rudras, and Adityas, the twelve months have already been explained. Vasus, Rudras, and Adityas also mean Brahmcharis.

The parrot-coloured, fast, variegated animals possess the qualities of fire and air. Dark-coloured possess the qualities of a cloud.

८. एता ऐन्द्राग्ना द्विरूपा अग्नीषोमीया वामना अनड्वाह आग्नावैष्णवा वशा मैत्रावरुण्योऽन्यत एन्यो मैत्र्यः ॥

8. These two-coloured animals possess the qualities of air and lightning. Animals with distorted organs and the oxen possess the qualities of Soma and fire, and fire and air. Barren cows possess the qualities of Pran and Udan. Partly variegated animals possess the qualities of a friend.

९. कृष्णग्रीवा आग्नेया बभ्रवः सौम्याः श्वेता वायव्या अविज्ञाता आदित्यं सरूपा धात्रे वत्सतर्यो देवानां पत्नीभ्यः ॥

9. Black-necked animals possess the qualities of fire. Animals with brown colour like that of an ichneumon possess the qualities of Soma. White animals belong to air. The undistinguished animals possess the qualities of Earth. Animals of the same colour, possess the qualities of air. Tender-aged calves belong to the protective forces of the Sun.

१०. कृष्णा भौमा धूम्रा आन्तरिक्षा बृहन्तो दिव्याः शबला वैद्युताः सिध्मास्तारकाः ॥

10. Black animals used for ploughing the land belong to the Earth. Smoke coloured animals belong to the Firmament. Animals with good nature, actions, and habits, tall in size, and whitish belong to the Lightning. Animals conducive to bliss alleviate our sufferings.

११. धूम्रान्वसन्तायालभते श्वेतान्ग्रीष्माय कृष्णान्वर्षाभ्योऽरुणाञ्छरदे पृषतो हेमन्ताय पिशङ्गाञ्छिशिराय ॥

11. Man should wear smoke-coloured clothes in Spring, white in Summer; black in the Rains; red in Autumn; bulky in Winter; reddish-yellow in the Dewy Season.

१२. त्र्यवयो गायत्र्यै पञ्चावयस्त्रिष्टुभे दित्यवाहो जगत्यै त्रिवत्सा अनुष्टुभे तुर्यवाह उष्णिहे ॥

12. Animals protected in the three stages of life belong to the Gayatri metre. Animals well protected with five vital breaths belong to the Trishtup, Beasts of burden belong to Jagati. Grown up animals belong to the Anushtup. The aged beasts belong to Ushnih.

---

[12]Three stages : childhood, youth and old age.

Gayatri, Trishtup, Jagati, Anushtup and Ushnih are names of Metres. Their connection with animals is not clear to me.

१३. पष्ठवाहो विराज उक्षाणो बृहत्या ऋषभाः ककुभेऽनड्वाहः पङ्क्त्यैं धेनवोऽतिच्छन्दसे ॥

13. Animals who carry burden on the back belong to the virat. Full grown bulls belong to the Brihati. Strong bulls belong to the Kakup. Bulls who carry the cart belong to the Pankti. Milch cows belong to the Atichhand.

१४. कृष्णग्रीवा आग्नेया बभ्रवः सौम्या उपध्वस्ताः सावित्रा वत्सतर्यः सारस्वत्यः श्यामाः पौष्णा पृश्नयो मारुता बहुरूपा वैश्वदेवा वशा द्यावापृथिवीया ॥

14. Black-necked animals belong to Agni. Brown animals are calm by nature. Mixed-coloured belong to Savita. Weaned she-kids belong to Saraswati. Dark-coloured belong to cloud which brings rain. Cows full of milk belong to the agriculturists. Many coloured animals belong to the learned. All glittering substances belong to the Heaven and Earth.

१५. उक्ताः सञ्चरा एता ऐन्द्राग्नाः कृष्णा वारुणा पृश्नयो मारुताः कायास्तूपराः ॥

15. These animals who move nicely, have been described. They belong to Indra and Agni, The animals who plough the land and pull carts belong to Varuna. The speckled animals resemble man in nature. The violent animals belong to Prajapati.

१६. अग्नयेऽनीकवते प्रथमजानालभते मरुद्भ्यः सान्तपनेभ्यः सवार्त्यान्मरुद्भ्यो गृहमेधिभ्यो बर्षिकहान्मरुद्भ्यः क्रीडिभ्यः सँँसृष्टान्मरुद्भ्यः स्वतवद्भ्योऽनुसृष्टान् ॥

16. A learned person should secure first class high souled, highly educated persons for the commander of the army. For persons who observe celibacy and are affectionate, he should secure men born in virtuous surrounding. For wise householders, he should secure aged persons. For laudable, sportive pleasure-loving persons, he should secure well-merited associates. For the self-strong independent persons, he should secure willing followers.

१७. उक्ताः सञ्चरा एता ऐन्द्राग्नाः प्राशृङ्गा माहेन्द्रा बहुरूपा वैश्वकर्मणाः ॥

17. These paths have been mentioned in which roam the animals belonging to air and lightning; those with beautiful horns belonging to Mahendra, the many-coloured belonging to Vishvakarma.

१८. धूम्रा बभ्रुनीकाशाः पितॄणाँँसोमवतां बभ्रवो धूम्रनीकाशाः । पितॄणां बर्हिषदां कृष्णा बभ्रुनीकाशाः पितॄणामग्निष्वात्तानां कृष्णाः पृश्नतस्त्र्यम्बकाः ॥

18. The animals of peace-loving parents are smoke-coloured and of brow-

---
¹³Belong to : are like.
Virat, Brihati, Kakup, Pankti, Atichhand are the names of metres.
¹⁴Saraswati : Goddess of speech.
¹⁷Mahendra : Animals possessing the qualities of a powerful King.
Vishvakarma : An expert engineer.
¹⁸Three forces : God, Soul, Matter.

nish hue. The animals of parents who sit in the assembly for performing yajnas are brown and smoky-looking. The animals of parents who know the science of fire are black and brownish-looking.

The animals of the learned who know the three forces are black and bulky.

१९. उक्ता: सञ्चरा एता: शुनासीरीया: श्वेता वायव्या: श्वेता: सौर्या: ॥

19. O men, bring into use the pre-mentioned agricultural animals, and white animals possessing the qualities of air, and white animals shining like the sun!

२०. वसन्ताय कपिञ्जलानालभते ग्रीष्माय कलविङ्कान्वर्षभ्यस्तित्तिरीञ्छरदे वर्तिका हेमन्ताय ककराञ्छिशिराय विककरान् ॥

20. An expert in the knowledge of animals finds Kapinjalas in spring; sparrows in summer; partridges in the Rains; quails in Autumn; Kakras in Winter; Vikakras in the Dewy season.

२१. समुद्राय शिशुमारानालभते पर्जन्याय मण्डूकान्द्भ्यो मत्स्यान्मित्राय कुलीपयान्वरुणाय नाक्रान् ॥

21. An expert in the knowledge of watery beings, finds porpoises in the sea, frogs after rains, fishes in water, ducks outside water for sunshine, crocodiles in deep water.

२२. सोमाय हंसानालभते वायवे बलाका इन्द्राग्निभ्यां क्रुञ्चान्मित्राय मद्गून्वरुणाय चक्रवाकान् ॥

22. An expert in the knowledge of birds finds geese revelling in moonshine; female cranes near fire; water-crows in the sun; ruddy geese loving each other.

२३. अग्नये कुटरूनालभते वनस्पतिभ्य उलूकानग्नीषोमाभ्यां चाषान्शिवभ्यां मयूरान्मित्रावरुणाभ्यां कपोतान् ॥

23. An expert in the knowledge of birds finds cocks enjoying the warmth of fire; owls sitting on fruitless trees; blue jays enjoying the sun and Soma; peacocks sun and moon; pigeons fond of affection and mutual liking.

२४. सोमाय लबानालभते त्वष्ट्रे कौलीकान्गोषादीर्देवानां पत्नीभ्य: कुलीका देवजामिभ्योऽग्नये गृहपतये पारुष्णान् ॥

24. An expert in the science of birds finds quails for affluence; Kaulikas

---

[20]Kapinjalas : Health-cocks, or francolins.
Kakras, Vikakras : Special unidentified birds.
Birds have connection with seasons, in which they revel and enjoy.
[22]Chakravakas : chakwa, chackwi, well-known for mutual love.
[24]Kaulikas, Kulikas, Parushnas are unidentified birds.
Gaushadis : Birds who sit on the backs of the cows and eat the germs which destroy the cows, and thus protect them.

for fame; Goshadis for the Consorts of the learned; Kulikas for the sisters of learned; Parushnas for Lord of the Homestead, behaving like fire.

२५. ब्रह्णे पारावतानालभते राज्ये. सीचापूरहोरात्रयोः सन्धिभ्यो जतूमसिभ्यो दात्यौहान्त्सं-वत्सराय महतः सुपर्णान् ॥

25. An expert in the science of time should study pigeons in the beginning of the day; sichapus in the night; bats in the morning and evening, gallinules for the knowledge of months, birds with beautiful feathers for realizing the beauty of the year.

२६. भूम्या आखूनालभतेऽन्तरिक्षाय पाङ्क्त्रान्दिवे कशान्दिग्भ्यो नकुलान्बभ्रुकानवान्तर-दिशाभ्यः ॥

26. An expert in the science of Earth should study rats for understanding the nature of ground; birds who fly in groups, for firmament; voles for light; mungooses for the quarters; brownish ichneumons for the intermediate spaces.

२७. वसुभ्य ऋश्यानालभते रुद्रेभ्यो रुरूनादित्येभ्यो न्यङ्कून्विश्वेभ्यो देवेभ्यः पृषतान्त्साध्येभ्यः कुलुङ्गान् ॥

27. An expert in the knowledge of animals should secure blackbucks for Vasu Brahmcharis; stags for Rudra Brahmcharis : Nayanku deer for Aditya Brahmcharis; spotted deer for all the learned; Kulinga antelopes for yogis engrossed in meditation.

२८. ईशानाय परस्वत आलभते मित्राय गौरान्वरुणाय महिषान्बृहस्पतये गवयाँस्त्वष्ट्र उष्ट्रान् ॥

28. Praswan deer should be secured for the wealthy; Gaur deer for the friend; buffaloes for the most prosperous; forest cows for the guardian of the virtuous; camels for the artisans.

२९. प्रजापतये पुरुषान्हस्तिन आलभते वाचे प्लुषीश्चक्षुषे मशकाञ्छ्रोत्राय भृङ्गाः ॥

29. For the service of the king valiant soldiers and elephants should be secured; white ants for eloquence; mosquitoes for sight, black bees for hearing.

---

²⁵Sichapus : unidentified bird.
A bat sees more vividly and eats in the joints of Day and Night. For the rest of time it is rather blind.
²⁷Five different kinds of deer are mentioned in the verse. Their skins serve as seats (Asan) for the Brahmcharis, the learned and the yogis.
²⁸Camels are beasts of burden. They carry loads in the desert where no other conveyance is serviceable.

३०. प्रजापतये च वायवे च गोमृगो वरुणायारण्यो मेषो यमाय कृष्णो मनुष्यराजाय मर्कटः शार्दूलाय रोहिद्दृषभाय गवयी क्षिप्रश्येनाय वर्तिका नीलङ्गोः कृमिः समुद्राय शिशुमारो हिमवते हस्ती ॥

30. For swiftness like a king and air Gomriga should be known; a wild ram for an excellent person; a black deer for the Lord of Justice; a monkey for the king; a red doe for the tiger; a female Goyal for a civilized person, a quail for the swift falcon; a worm for the Nilangu, a porpoise for the sea; an elephant for the snowy mountain.

३१. मयुः प्राजापत्य उलो हलिक्ष्णो वृषद्ँशस्ते धात्रे दिशां कङ्को धुङ्क्षाग्नेयी कलविङ्को लोहिताहिः पुष्करसादस्ते त्वाष्ट्रा वाचे क्रुञ्चः ॥

31. A despicable person belongs to the king; the tiny worm, the lion, the cat belong to one given to mental abstraction; the heron belongs to the quarters; the female bird named Dhunksha possesses the qualities of fire; sparrow, red snake, and the bird residing in the tank belong to Twashta (sun), the curlew belongs to speech.

३२. सोमाय कुलुङ्ग आरण्योऽजो नकुलः शाका ते पौष्णाः कोष्टा मायोरिन्द्रस्य गौरमृगः पिद्वो न्यङ्कुः कक्कटस्तेऽनुमत्यै प्रतिश्रुत्कायै चक्रवाकः ॥

32. An antelope should be had for prosperity; wild goat, mungoose, saka (a strong animal) are meant for the powerful; an ordinary jackal is subservient to a superior jackal; white deer is meant for a wealthy person, Pidva; Nayanku, Kakkat are for Anumati; the chakravaka (ruddy goose) is for the Echo.

३३. सौरी बलाका शार्गः सृजयः शयाण्डकस्ते मैत्राः सरस्वत्यै शारिः पुरुषवाक् श्वाविद्भौमी शार्दूलो वृकः पृदाकुस्ते मन्यवे सरस्वते शुकः पुरुषवाक् ॥

33. The female crane belongs to the sun; Sarga, Srijaya, Sayandaka, these three belong to breath, the human-voiced female parrot belongs to the stream; the porcupine belongs to the ground; tiger, wolf, viper belong to anger; the human voiced parrot belongs to the sea.

---

[30]In some cases connection between the animals and other animate and inanimate objects mentioned in this verse and previous verses is not clear.
A king is compared to a monkey, as he is irascible and rash in nature like a monkey.
Nilangu : said to be a species of worm; perhaps a tape worm.
Gomriga : an animal that purifies the earth.
Goyal : Female Nilgaya (नीलगाय).

[32]Saka: variously explained as bird, fly, long eared beast. Pidva, Nayanku, Kakkat are the names of different kinds of deer.
Anumati : Divine favour personified.
Echo : because the male and female chakravakas are condemned to pass the night on the opposite banks of a river, incessantly calling to each other.

[33]Saarga (चातक) the bird Cucculus melanolencous said to subsist on rain drops.

३४. सुपर्णः पार्जन्य आतिर्वाहसो दर्विदा ते वायवे बृहस्पतये वाचस्पतये पैङ्गराजोऽलज आन्तरिक्ष: प्लवो मद्गुर्मेत्स्यस्ते नदीपतये द्यावापृथिवीयः कूर्मः ॥

34. The eagle belongs to the cloud; the Aati, the serpent, the woodpecker, these are for air; the Paingraja is for Brihaspati; the Alaja belongs to the Firmament; pelican, cormorant, fish, these belong to the ocean; the tortoise belongs to the Heaven and Earth.

३५. पुरुषमृगश्चन्द्रमसो गोधा कालका दार्वाघाटस्ते वनस्पतीनां कृकवाकुः सावित्रो हँसो वातस्य नाक्रो मकरः कुलीपयस्तेऽकूपारस्य ह्रियै शल्यकः ॥

35. The buck that purifies men belongs to the moon; iguana, kaalakaa, wood pecker, these belong to the trees; the cock belongs to the sun; the swan belongs to air; crocodile, dolphin, and watery birds, these belong to the sea; the porcupine to modesty.

३६. एण्यह्नो मण्डूको मूषिका तित्तिरिस्ते सर्पाणां लोपाश आश्विनः कृष्णो रात्र्या ऋक्षो जतुः सुषिलीका त इतरजनानां जहका वैष्णवी ॥

36. The black-doe belongs to the day; frog, female-rat, partridge, these belong to the serpents; the jackal belongs to the Aswins, the black buck to the night; bear, bat, sushilikaa, these belong to the other folk; the pole-cat belongs to vishnu.

३७. अन्यवापोऽर्धमासानामृश्यो मयूरः सुपर्णस्ते गन्धर्वाणामपामुद्रो मासां कश्यपो रोहित्कुण्ड्नाची गोलत्तिका तेऽप्सरसां मृत्यवेऽसितः ॥

37. The cuckoo belongs to the Half Months; antelope, peacock, swan are meant for the musicians; the otter is an aquatic being; the tortoise belongs to the Months; doe-antelope kundrirachi, Golattikaa belong to the beam of the sun; the black snake belongs to death.

३८. वर्षाहृऋतूनामाखुः कशो मान्थालस्ते पितॄणां बलायाजगरो वसूनां कपिञ्जलः कपोत उलूकः शशस्ते निऋत्यै वरुणायारण्यो मेघः ॥

---

[34]Brihaspati : Thundering lightning. The birds and beasts whose names are left untranslated in this and the following Verses are unidentified.
[35]Belongs to : possesses the qualities of, is related to.
Kaalakaa : A black bird.
Iguana means lizard.
[36]Aswins: Agni and Soma.
Other Folk : Low despicable people, besides the noble and virtuous. Bear is cruel in nature and being a beast is without tail. Bat is neither a bird nor a beast. Sushilikaa being a bird, lives in a den. These beasts and birds, being low are like the degraded people.
[37]Kundrinachi : a forest femalebeast.
Golattikaa : a special female beast.
The voice of an antelope is Rishbha, of peacock Shataja, of Swan Panchma, Musicians follow the voices of these animals and learn music.

CHAPTER XXIV

38. The frog belongs to the seasons; the rat, the kasha, the Manthal, these are the guardians; the python is for strength; Kapinjala is for the Vasus; pigeon, owl, hare are the harbingers of adversity; the wild ram serves as an example for the person trying to remove the foe.

३९. शिवत्र आदित्यानामुष्ट्रो घृणीवान्वार्ध्रीनसस्ते मत्या अरण्याय सूमरो रुरु रौद्र: क्वयि: कुटरुदर्तियौहस्ते वाजिनां कामाय पिक: ॥

39. The diverse coloured animal belongs to the Adityas (months) the camel, the Ghriniwan, the big goat are for thought; Nil-Gaya is for the forest; the Ruru named deer is Rudra's Kvayi, cock, gallinule possess the qualities of horses; the cuckoo belongs to Passion.

४०. खड्गो वैश्वदेव: श्वा कृष्ण: कर्णो गर्दभस्तरक्षुस्ते रक्षसामिन्द्राय सूकर: सिंहो मारुत: कृकलास: पिप्पका शकुनिस्ते शरव्यायै विश्वेषां देवानां पृषत: ॥

40. Rhinoceros serves all warriors in preparing their shield; the black dog, the long-eared ass, the hyena are used fot protection, against the demons; the boar is for the king who wants to tear asunder the foes, the lion is swift like air; the chameleon, the Pippaka, the vultures are used for making arrows; the spotted antelope is used for preparing mrigshalas (seats of the deer's skin) for all the learned people.

---

[38] A wild ram gives a severe fight to the opponent, so a brave man should give fight to the foe and extirpate him. Where owl, pigeon and hare reside, that place soon becomes deserted and dilapidated.

Kapinjala : A white bird.

[39] Ghriniwan : a strong animal of a special species, Cuckoo is the favourite bird of cupid, the God of love. Her voice (supposed to say Pi Kahan, Where is my darling?) is chiefly heard in spring.

[40] Hippaka : A female bird. Chameleon means lizard. In this chapter mention has been made of beasts, birds, reptiles, forest animals, watery beings and worms. Learned persons should study their qualities and make the best possible use of them.

CHAPTER XXV

१. शादं दद्भिरवकां दन्तमूलैर्मृदं बर्स्वेस्तेगान्द ॐष्ट्राभ्याॐ सरस्वत्या अग्रजिह्वं जिह्वाया उत्सादमवक्रन्देन तालु वाज ॐ हनुभ्यामप ग्रास्येन वृषणमाण्डाभ्यामादित्याँ श्मश्रुभिः पन्थानं भ्रूभ्यां द्यावापृथिवी वर्तोभ्यां विद्युतं कनीनकाभ्या ॐ शुक्लाय स्वाहा कृष्णाय स्वाहा पार्याणि पक्ष्माण्यवार्या पक्ष्माणि पार्या इक्षवः ॥

1. Learn from teeth the act of biting; from gums the method of protection; from tooth-sockets the way of pounding; sharpness from fangs. Use the tongue-tip for a learned utterance; learn the act of uprooting from the tongue, the use of palate by crying slowly; chew food with both the jaws; drink waters with the mouth. Acquire the knowledge of oozing semen from testicles. Recognise the Aditya Brahmcharis from their beard; know the path from eyebrows; know the Sun and Earth from their motion; lightning from the pupils of eyes. Observe celibacy for the protection of semen, acquire knowledge through high character. Objects worth acceptance are worthy of preservation. Objects after one's desire should not be resisted. Don't show disrespect to your own men. Friends and relatives should be fostered.

२. वातं प्राणेनापानेन नासिके उपयाममधरेणोष्ठेन सदुत्तरेण प्रकाशेनान्तरमनुकाशेन बाह्यं निवेश्यं मूर्धनि स्तनयित्नुं निर्बाधेनाशनिं मस्तिष्केण विद्युतं कनीनकाभ्यां कर्णाभ्यां श्रोत्र ॐ श्रोत्राभ्यां कर्णौ तेदनीमधरकण्ठेनापः शुष्ककण्ठेन चित्तं मन्याभिरदिति ॐ शीर्ष्णा निऋॅतिं निर्जंजल्पेन शीर्ष्णा संक्रोशैः प्राणान् रेष्माण ॐ स्तुपेन ॥

2. Fill air with thy Pran; empty the nostrils with Apan; with upper and lower lips observe restraint, silence and control; with the light of knowledge purify thy soul; with the practice of cleanliness purify the exterior body; reflect upon God with thy head; by constant thinking create your doubt to know the truth; understand with thy brain the internal fire; receive full light with the pupils of thy eyes; advance hearing with thy ears; strengthen thy external ears with the internal organs of hearing; eat food with thy lower throat; drink water with thirsty throat; strengthen thy mind with practices of knowledge; develop indestructible wisdom with thy head; attain to mother Earth through death, with your ragged head; improve your vital breaths through loud roaring; remove the disease of ignorance with full might.

²Pran : Ingoing breath.
Apan : Outgoing breath.
Ragged head : When one's head loses vitality and consciousness, he dies, and is reduced to earth through cremation.
The words (रेष्माण ॐ स्तुपेन) have been interpreted as 'Kill the violent enemy with violence, by Pt. Jaidev Vidyalankar. Vedic religion generally preaches non-violence or Ahinsa, but on certain occasions for self-preservation and protecting the chastity of womenfolk it sanctions the use of violence. This interpretation is in keeping with the spirit of the vedas.

CHAPTER XXV

३. मशकान् केशेरिन्द्र॒ स्वपसा वहेन बृहस्पति॒ शकुनिसादेन कूर्मञ्छफैराक्रमण॒ स्थूरा-
भ्यामृक्षलाभि: कपिञ्जलाञ्जवं जङ्घाभ्यामध्वानं बाहुभ्यां जाम्बीलेनारण्यमग्निमतिरुभ्यां
पूषणं दोर्भ्यामशिवनाव॒साभ्या॒रुद्र॒ रोराभ्याम् ॥

3. Keep mosquitoes away with the whisk of hair. Realise soul and God through noble deeds. Approach the learned preceptor in a conveyance. Utilise the services of the learned with the allurement of money.

Make an attack with full force. Finish journey with stout thighs. Get learned preachers by arranging for their livelihood. Develop speed with arms. Grow fruitful thorny jambir trees in the forest. Kindle fire with care and desire. Get strength through the exercise of arms. Serve the king and subjects with arms and shoulders. Honour a preacher by patient hearing of his sermons.

४. अग्ने: पक्षतिर्वायोर्निपक्षतिरिन्द्रस्य तृतीया सोमस्य चतुर्थ्यादित्ये पञ्चमीन्द्राण्यै षष्ठी
मरुता॒ सप्तमी बृहस्पतेरष्टम्यर्यम्णो नवमी धातुर्दशमीन्द्रस्यैकादशी वरुणस्य द्वादशी
यमस्य त्रयोदशी ॥

4. The first rib of the right side of the chest is like fire; the second like air; the third like sun; the fourth like moon; the fifth like sky; the sixth like the flash of lightning; the seventh like mind; the eighth like Mahat-Tatva; the ninth like a servant who honours his master; the tenth like the creator of the world; the eleventh like a glorious person; the twelfth like a noble person; the thirteenth like a just ruler.

५. इन्द्राग्न्यो: पक्षति: सरस्वत्यै निपक्षतिर्मित्रस्य तृतीयापां चतुर्थी निर्ऋत्यै पञ्चम्यग्नीषोमयो:
षष्ठी सर्पाणा॒ सप्तमी विष्णोरष्टमी पूष्णो नवमी त्वष्टुर्दशमीन्द्रस्यैकादशी वरुणस्य
द्वादशी यम्ये त्रयोदशी द्यावापृथिव्योर्दक्षिणं पार्श्वं विश्वेषां देवानामुत्तरम् ॥

5. On the left side of the chest, the first rib is like air and fire; the second like speech; the third like a friend; the fourth like water, the fifth like earth; the sixth like fire and water; the seventh like serpents; the eighth like the All-pervading God; the ninth like the supporter; the tenth like a luminary; the eleventh like the soul; the twelfth like a noble person; the thirteenth like the wife of a judge. The right flank is like the Sun and Earth, the left like all the learned persons.

६. मरुता॒ स्कन्धा विश्वेषां देवानां प्रथमा कीकसा रुद्राणां द्वितीयाऽऽदित्यानां तृतीया
वायो: पुच्छमग्नीषोमयोर्भासदौ कुञ्चौ श्रोणिभ्यामिन्द्राबृहस्पती ऊरुभ्यां मित्रावरुणावल्गा-
भ्यामाक्रमण॒ स्थूराभ्यां बलं कुष्ठाभ्याम् ॥

---

³Just as fisherman catch tortoises with a net offering them some bait; so the services of the learned should be acquired by offering them tempting remuneration.
As with hoofs attack animals, so an enemy should be attacked with full force.
Just as fishermen catch with fetters small watery birds like kapinjalas, so the learned persons should be acquired by arranging for their livelihood.
⁴The thirteen ribs of the right side of the chest are compared to thirteen objects.
Mahat-Tatva : Intellect.

6. The shoulders of men are like the cantonments in a State. The foremost function of all learned persons is to preach. To punish the wicked is the second act of awe-inspiring learned persons. To do justice is the third act of justice loving celibate learned persons. The tail of an animal is an instrument of airing. Fire and water give light. Two learned persons of discrimination like two swans are like the buttocks of the state. Air and sun are like thighs. Pran and Udan are like persons walking at full pace. Attack should be made with full certainty. Gain strength from powerful objects.

७. पूषणं वनिष्ठुनाऽन्धाहीन्त्स्थूलगुदया सर्पान्गुदाभिर्विहृ॒त आन्त्रैरपो वस्तिना वृषणमाण्डाभ्यां वाजिनꣳशेपेन प्रजाꣳरेतसा चाषान् पित्तेन प्रदरान् पायुना कूष्माꣳच्छकपिण्डै: ॥

7. Beg for alms from the wealthy. Catch blind serpents from large intestines; serpents from the entrails and subdue them. Overpower the crooked serpents from the guts. Discharge water through the bladder. Strengthen scrotum with the testicles. Examine the strength of a horse from his penis. Produce progeny with semen. Digest meals with the force of bile. Strengthen your belly by free discharge of digested food through anus. Obtain the strength of administration through forces.

८. इन्द्रस्य क्रोडोऽदित्यै पाजस्यं दिशां जत्रवोऽदित्यै भसज्जीमूतान् हृदयौपशेनान्तरिक्षं पुरीतता नभ उदर्येण चक्रवाकौ मतस्नाभ्यां दिवं वृक्काभ्यां गिरीन् प्लाशिभिरुपलान् प्लीह्ना वल्मीकान् क्लोमभिग्लौंभिर्गुल्मान् हिराभि: स्त्रवन्तीर्हृदान् कुक्षिभ्याꣳ समुद्रमुदरेण वैश्वानरं भस्मना ॥

8. People should know the working of the lightning; the best foodgrain for the earth; the union of the quarters; the continual filling of space with light by the sun. Clouds are like the soul that sleeps in the heart. Pericardium is vast like the atmosphere. Entrails of the belly are like water. Both parts of the neck are like a lovely pair of male and female goose. Sky is like kidneys. Mountains are like the belly's ducts which receive the meals. Clouds are like the spleen. Paths are refreshing like water. The arteries on the right side of the belly are like pain, pleasure and sorrow. Streams are known for inundation. Both flanks are like lakes. The Sea is like the belly. The gastric fluid is like the ashes.

९. विधृतिं नाभ्या घृतꣳ रसेनापो यूष्णा मरीचीर्विप्रुड्भिर्नीहारमूष्मणा शीनं वसया पृष्वा

[8]Just as sky rains water, so kidneys discharge urine. Just as lakes are full of water, so flanks are full of blood.

Just as waters rise from the sea, rain on the Earth and produce medicinal herbs and foodstuffs, so the essence of meals rises from the belly, reaches each and every part of the body, and strengthens our skin-hair and flesh.

Gastric fluid : The digestive fire of the stomach, Just as this fire digests the food, and converts it into blood, so ordinary fire burns timber and reduces it to ashes.

Sea is like : Just as all rivers run into sea, so all meals go into the belly.

अश्रुभिर्हादिनीर्दूषीकाभिरस्ना रक्षाꣳसि चित्राण्यङ्गैनक्षत्राणि रूपेण पृथिवीं त्वचा जुम्बकाय स्वाहा ॥

9. Know steady abstraction of the mind from the navel; ghee from curd; waters from decocted juice; sunbeams from fat that strengthens the organs; hoar-frost from bodily heat; coagulated ghee from life that prevails in the body; water-fountain from tears; thunderbolt from the rheum of eyes; objects worth protection from blood; marvellous things from limbs; stars from their beauty; earth from skin that covers the blood and flesh. Use truthful language for an energetic person.

१०. हिरण्यगर्भः समवर्तताग्रे भूतस्य जातः पतिरेक आसीत् ।
स दाधार पृथिवीं द्यामुतेमां कस्मै देवाय हविषा विधेम ॥

10. God, the possessor of resplendent planets, existed before the creation of the world. He is the One Lord of all created beings. He sustains the Earth, the Sun and the created world. May we worship with devotion, Him, the Illuminator and Giver of pleasure.

११. यः प्राणतो निमिषतो महित्वैक इद्राजा जगतो बभूव ।
य ईशे अस्य द्विपदश्चतुष्पदः कस्मै देवाय हविषा विधेम ॥

11. God by his grandeur is the sole Ruler of the moving world that breathes and slumbers. He is the Lord of men and cattle. May we worship with devotion, Him the Illuminator and Giver of happiness.

१२. यस्येमे हिमवन्तो महित्वा यस्य समुद्रꣳ रसया सहाहुः ।
यस्येमाः प्रदिशो यस्य बाहू कस्मै देवाय हविषा विधेम ॥

12. By Whose might, are these snow-clad mountains standing, and men call the atmosphere filled with water, His possession? Whose arms are these heavenly regions? May we worship with devotion, Him the Illuminator and Giver of happiness.

१३. य आत्मदा बलदा यस्य विश्व उपासते प्रशिषं यस्य देवाः ।
यस्य च्छायामृतं यस्य मृत्युः कस्मै देवाय हविषा विधेम ॥

13. God is the Giver of spiritual force, and physical strength. His Commandments all the learned persons acknowledge. He is the maker of all laws. His support is life immortal and transgression of His Law is death. May we worship with devotion, Him, the Illuminator and Giver of happiness.

१४. आ नो भद्राः क्रतवो यन्तु विश्वतोऽदब्धासो अपरीतास उद्भिदः ।
देवा नो यथा सदमिद् वृधे असन्नप्रायुवो रक्षितारो दिवे-दिवे ॥

---

[9] Just as the heat of the body enlivens all organs, so the medicinal herbs grow through frost.
[10] cf 13-4, 23-1.
[11] cf 23-3.

14. May auspicious force of wisdom come to us from the every side, continual, unhindered, and as remover of afflictions. May thereby the learned persons, our guardians, advanced in age, attend our assembly day by day for our gain.

१५. देवानां भद्रा सुमतिर्ॠजूयतां देवानाँ रातिरभि नो निवर्तताम् ।
देवानाँ सख्युपसेदिमा वयं देवा न आयुः प्रतिरन्तु जीवसे ॥

15. May the auspicious favour of the learned be ours. May the bounty of the righteous fill us with virtues. May we devoutly seek the friendship of the learned. May they extend our life that we may live.

१६. तान्पूर्वया निविदा हूमहे वयं भगं मित्रमदितिं दक्षमस्त्रिधम् ।
अर्यमणं वरुणँ सोममश्विना सरस्वती नः सुभगा मयस्करत् ॥

16. We, through vedic speech, accepted by our ancestors; long through mutual emulation for a teacher and a preacher, honest, guardian of the people, inviolable, giver of prosperity, friendly, completely wise, noble, and affluent. May auspicious vedic speech grant us all felicity.

१७. तन्नो वातो मयोभु वातु भेषजं तन्माता पृथिवी तत्पिता द्यौः ।
तद् ग्रावाणः सोमसुतो मयोभुवस्तदश्विना श्रृणुतं धिष्ण्या युवम् ॥

17. O teachers and preachers, firm like the Earth, ye both hear from us what we have read. May the wind waft to us that pleasant medicine. May respectable Earth and fostering Sun secure it for us. May clouds the producers of herb and givers of joy secure us that medicine!

१८. तमीशानं जगतस्तस्थुषस्पतिं धियञ्जिन्वमवसे हूमहे वयम् ।
पूषा नो यथा वेदसामसद् वृधे रक्षिता पायुरदब्धः स्वस्तये ॥

18. Him we invoke for aid Who reigns supreme, the Lord of all that stands or moves, and Inspirer of wisdom. May He, the Nourisher of all our Keeper and our Guard Non-violent, promote, the increase of our wealth for our good.

१९. स्वस्ति न इन्द्रो वृद्धश्रवाः स्वस्ति नः पूषा विश्ववेदाः ।
स्वस्ति नस्ताक्ष्यों अरिष्टनेमिः स्वस्ति नो बृहस्पतिर्दधातु ॥

19. May the Master of vast knowledge, may Mighty God prosper us. May the Nourisher of all, the Author of all the vedas prosper us.

May He the Giver of all comforts like the horse prosper us. May God the Lord of all the elements of Nature vouchsafe us prosperity.

---

[16] Students acquire knowledge from teachers through mutual competition and emulation, We-students.

[19] Just as a horse takes us from one place to the other and gives us pleasure, so does God give us happiness by fulfilling our wants.

२०. पृषदश्वा मरुतः पृश्निमातरः शुभंयावानो विदथेषु जग्मयः ।
अग्निजिह्वा मनवः सूरचक्षसो विश्वे नो देवा अवसागमन्निह ॥

20. Let all the learned persons, stout in body, followers of the mother veda, moving in glory, visitors of battle-fields, fire-tongued, contemplative, brilliant in knowledge like the Sun, come hither for our protection.

२१. भद्रं कर्णेभिः श्रृणुयाम देवा भद्रं पश्येमाक्षभिर्यजत्राः ।
स्थिरैरङ्गैस्तुष्टुवाँसस्तनूभिर्व्यशेमहि देवहितं यदायुः ॥

21. O sociable learned persons, may we with our ears listen to what is good, and with our eyes see what is good!
With limbs and bodies firm may we extolling God lead a life conducive to the good of the sages.

२२. शतमिन्नु शरदो अन्ति देवा यत्रा नश्चक्रा जरसं तनूनाम् ।
पुत्रासो यत्र पितरो भवन्ति मा नो मध्या रीरिषतायुर्गन्तोः ॥

22. O learned persons, may we live in your company for a hundred years. Let not our bodies decay before that period, in which old age our sons become fathers in turn. Break ye not in the midst our course of fleeting life!

२३. अदितिर्द्यौरदितिरन्तरिक्षमदितिर्माता स पिता स पुत्रः ।
विश्वे देवा अदितिः पञ्च जना अदितिर्जातमदितिर्जनित्वम् ॥

23. Immortal is the heaven, Immortal is the atmosphere, Matter the mother of all is immortal. Immortal is Father God.
Immortal is the soul that nourishes the body. All divine objects like the Earth are immortal. Five vital breaths are immortal. All that is born and shall be born is immortal because of its immortal cause.

२४. मा नो मित्रो वरुणो अर्यमायुरिन्द्र ऋभुक्षा मरुतः परिख्यन् ।
यद्वाजिनो देवजातस्य सप्तेः प्रवक्ष्यामो विदथे वीर्याणि ॥

24. May not the friendly, glorious, and just king; nor the noble souls shorten our life; so that we may display our valour in war, like a fleeting, efficient horse.

२५. यन्निर्णिजा रेक्णसा प्रावृतस्य रातिं गृभीतां मुखतो नयन्ति ।
सुप्राङजो मेम्यद्विश्वरूप इन्द्रापूष्णोः प्रियमप्येति पाथः ॥

[20]Hither : In our country or yajna.
[21]Ayu may also mean full age of one hundred years.
[23]God, soul, matter are by nature eternal and immortal.
Other created things are immortal as they are created again and again, and their cause कारण is also immortal. Panch Jana may also mean Brahmanas, Kshatriyas, Vaishas, Shudras and Nishadas the barbarians. Panch Jana may also mean the five elements, air, water, fire, earth and Akash (space).

25. Those who gladly accept the substances offered in charity by a virtuous wealthy person; and the eternal soul, worthy of attainment, a nice questioner, beauty of the world, who eats the charming food prepared through fire and air; derive full enjoyment.

२६. एष: छाग: पुरो अश्वेन वाजिना पूष्णो भागो नीयते विश्वदेव्य: ।
अभिप्रियं यत्पुरोडाशमर्वता त्वष्टेदेनᳪ सौश्रवसाय जिन्वति ॥

26. This perishable body made of earth, the home of all organs is created for the enjoyment of the soul. God, for the excellent enjoyment of this active soul, grants this enjoyable object.

२७. यद्धविष्यमृतुशो देवयानं त्रिर्मानुषा: पर्यश्वं नयन्ति ।
अत्रा पूष्ण: प्रथमो भाग एति यज्ञं देवेभ्य: प्रतिवेदयन्नज: ॥

27. Thoughtful persons strengthen this excellent embodied soul, at times in three different stages.
Soul enters this body, the foremost part of the Earth, for doing noble deeds for the sake of spiritual enjoyment.

२८. होताध्वर्युरावया अग्निमिन्धो ग्रावग्राभ उत शᳪस्ता सुविप्र: ।
तेन यज्ञेन स्वरंकृतेन स्विष्टेन वक्षणा आ पृणध्वम् ॥

28. Invoker, atoner, fire-kindler, bringer of rain, sage, scholar-encircled, thou ministering priest, with this well ordered, well-desired sacrifice, fill full the channels of the rivers.

२९. यूपव्रस्का उत ये यूपवाहाश्चषालं ये अश्वयूपाय तक्षति ।
ये चार्वते पचनᳪ सम्भरन्त्युतो तेषामभिगूर्त्तिनं इन्वतु ॥

29. The hewers of the yajna's post and those who carry it, and those who carve the knob to deck the horse's stake; and those who prepare the cooking utensils for the steed and those who strive hard, may their perseverance be attained to by us.

३०. उप प्रागात्सुमन्मेऽधायि मन्म देवानामाशा उप वीतपृष्ठ: ।
अन्वेनं विप्रा ऋषयो मदन्ति देवानां पुष्टे चकृमा सुबन्धुम् ॥

30. He, who, competent to afford shelter to all, himself comes to me for my welfare, and who fulfils the desires of the learned, is the source of delight on sight to the learned and sages. May we produce amongst the learned such a strong man, having beautiful brothers.

---

[26]Enjoyable object : Body.
[27]Three different stages : Jagrit-waking, swapan-dreaming, sushupti-profound sleep or repose.
[28]Through yajna, an Adhvaryu, the ministering priest gets rain which fills the rivers.

CHAPTER XXV

३१. यद्वाजिनो दाम सन्दानमर्वतो या शीर्षण्या रशना रज्जुरस्य ।
यद्वा घास्य प्रभृतमास्ये तृण᳖ सर्वा ता ते ग्रपि देवेष्वस्तु ॥

31. Just as the fleet courser is controlled by halter and his feetropes, the head stall, the bridle and the cords about him, and the grass is put within his mouth to bait him, so should the learned people control their organs and eat nourishing diet.

३२. यदश्वस्य क्रविषो मक्षिकाश यद्वा स्वरौ स्वधितौ रिप्तमस्ति ।
यद्धस्तयो: शमितुर्यन्नखेषु सर्वा ता ते ग्रपि देवेष्वस्तु ॥

32. O men, the fly eateth the flesh and blood of a fast-running horse. The vedic utterances in a yajna are like thunderbolts, part of the oblation adhereth to the sacrificer's hands and nails. May all this be with ye and the learned !

३३. यदूवध्यमुदरस्याववाति य ग्रामस्य क्रविषो गन्धो ग्रस्ति ।
सुकृता तच्छमितार: कृण्वन्तूत मेघ᳖ श्रृतपाकं पचन्तु ॥

33. Food undigested that comes out of the belly, and the bad odour rising from the raw half-cooked food should be removed by skilled cooks. Let the digestive powers of ours digest the nice well-cooked food.

३४. यत्ते गात्रादग्निना पच्यमानादभि शूलं निहतस्यावधावति ।
मा तद्भूम्यामाश्रिषन्मा तृणेषु देवेभ्यस्तदुशद्भ्रयो रातमस्तु ॥

34. Whatever word of quick wisdom, comes with certainty and exertion out of thy mouth, seasoned with thy mental fire, waste not that on earth or grass, but give it as instruction to the noble, learned persons.

३५. ये वाजिनं परिपश्यन्ति पक्वं या ईमाहु: सुरभिनिर्हरेति ।
ये चार्वतो मा᳖ सभिक्षामुपासत उतो तेषामभिगूर्तिनं इन्वतु ॥

35. They who crave for the meat of a horse, and declare the horse fit to be killed should be exterminated.
They who keep the fast horse well trained and disciplined, deserve to be praised by us for the strength of their character and perseverance.

३६. यन्नीक्षणं मांस्पचन्या उखाया या पात्राणि यूष्ण ग्रासेचनानि ।
ऊष्मण्यापिधाना चरूणामङ्का: सूना: परि भूषन्त्यश्वम् ॥

36. Realisation of soul-force, that ripens our knowledge, the organs of perception which accomplish our knowledge, the Pranas (vital breaths) which

---

[32] The learned people should keep horses in sheds where flies may not bite them. They should perform yajnas with the loud recitation of vedic verse. Just as the hands and nails of the performer of a yajna are washed with water to clear the particles of oblation so should the horses be washed to remove the dirt sticking to their body.

[35] Eating the meat of a horse and other animals is prohibited in this verse. They who eat the meat of animals should be exterminated. They who train and make the animals useful deserve praise.

[36] Organs of perception : There are five called (ज्ञानेन्द्रिय) the skin, tongue, eye, ear and nose.

serve as a cloak for our life; the signs of exalted character and the rays of knowledge jointly adorn a strong soul.

३७. मा त्वाऽग्निर्ध्वनयीद्धूमगन्धिर्मोखा भ्राजन्त्यभि विक्त जघ्रि: ।
इष्टं वीतमभिगूर्तं वषट्कृतं तं देवास: प्रति गृभ्णन्त्यश्वम् ॥

37. O men, just as the intelligent persons accept with favour the beloved, offered, persevering, and consecrated horse, so should ye know them in all respects!

Let not the smoke-scented fire make the animal crackle with pain; nor the glowing caldron-smell break him to pieces.

३८. निक्रमणं निषदनं विवर्तनं यच्च पड्वीशमर्वत: ।
यच्च पपौ यच्च घासिं जघास सर्वा ता ते अपि देवेष्वस्तु ॥

38. The starting, sitting, rolling and fastening of the horse, his drinking and eating, should all be controlled by intelligent keepers.

३९. यदश्वाय वास उपस्तृणन्त्यधीवासं या हिरण्यान्यस्मै ।
सन्दानमर्वन्तं पड्वीशं प्रिया देवेष्वा यामयन्ति ॥

39. The robe they spread upon the horse to clothe him, the uppercovering and the golden trappings; the halters which restrain the steed, and the heel-ropes, all these are pleasing to the learned.

४०. यत्ते सादे महसा शूकृतस्य पार्ष्ण्या वा कशया वा तुतोद ।
स्रुचेव ता हविषो अध्वरेषु सर्वा ता ते ब्रह्मणा सूदयामि ॥

40. If one, when seated, with excessive urging with his heel or with his whip distresses a horse; all these woes, as with oblation's ladle at sacrifices, with my might I banish.

४१. चतुस्त्रिंश॑द्वाजिनो देवबन्धोर्वङ्क्रीरश्वस्य स्वधिति: समेति ।
अच्छिद्रा गात्रा वयुना कृणोत परुष्परुरनुघुष्या विशस्त ॥

41. O people, just as a horse-breaker, whom the wise befriend, understands the thirty four gaits of a horse, and a veterinary assistant with his knowledge renders his organs free from flaw, and fully examines each and every part of his body; so should ye keep away all maladies powerful like a thunderbolt !

---

[37] Useful animals like horses should not be killed, nor their meat cooked for eating. They should be protected against fire.

[38] The verse may also allude to the Brahmcharis (students) whose walking, sitting, lying, eating and drinking should be supervised by their learned preceptors (gurus).

[39] The verse may also allude to a Brahmchari student at the time of his departure from the Guru.

[40] One : A rider.
    I : Priest.

४२. एकस्त्वष्टुरश्वस्या विशस्ता द्वा यन्तारा भवतस्तथ ऋतुः ।
या ते गात्राणामृतुथा कृणोमि ता-ता पिण्डानां प्र जुहोम्यग्नौ ॥

42. O people, just as spring alone gives beauty to a graceful horse, or two seasons control him; so do I control your organs and livelihood, and give you various objects in different seasons, and place all these under the custody of a learned person!

४३. मा त्वा तपत्प्रिय आत्माऽपियन्तं मा स्वधितिस्तन्व आ तिष्ठिपत्तं ।
मा ते गृध्नुरविशस्ताऽतिहाय छिद्रा गात्राण्यसिना मिथू कः ॥

43. Let not thy God-loving soul torment thee, as it departs from thy body. Let not the hatchet linger in thy body. Let not a greedy, clumsy immolator, cut unduly with sword thy vulnerable limbs.

४४. न वा उ एतन्म्रियसे न रिष्यसि देवाँ२ इदेषि पथिभिः सुगेभिः ।
हरी ते युञ्जा पृषती अभूतामुपस्थादा‌ऽजी धुरि रासभस्य ॥

44. Soul dieth not, not is it injured. Performing noble acts it attains to godhead. May thy powerful Pran and Apan be yoked through Yoga. May a learned person take up the duty of preaching.

४५. सुगव्यं नो वाजी स्वश्व्यं पुंसः पुत्राँ२ उत विश्वापुषं रयिम् ।
अनागास्त्वं नो अदितिः कृणोतु क्षत्रं नो अश्वो वनतां हविष्मान् ॥

45. May this learned person bring us all-sustaining riches, wealth in good kine, good horses, and manly offspring. Freedom from sin may Earth vouchsafe us. May this noble soul, the giver of commendable pleasures rule over us.

४६. इमा नु कं भुवना सीषधामेन्द्रश्च विश्वे च देवाः ।
आदित्यैरिन्द्रः सगणो मरुद्भिरस्मभ्यं भेषजा करत् ।
यज्ञं च नस्तन्वं च प्रजां चादित्यैरिन्द्रः सह सीषधाति ॥

46. Just as the glorious king and all learned persons hold under control these worlds, so should we speedily gain happiness.
Just as the Sun with his satellites, and twelve months manifests all worlds, so should a physician helped by other persons give us medicines. May the king with learned persons regulate our sacrifice, our bodies and our progeny.

४७. अग्ने त्वं नो अन्तम उत त्राता शिवो भवा वरूथ्यः ।
वसुरग्निर्वसुश्रवा अच्छा नक्षि द्युमत्तमं रयिं दाः ॥

---

⁴²Just as horse-breakers train horses according to seasons, so do the preceptors teach the pupils how to behave. Just as air is purified by oblations in fire, so ignorant superstitions are put in the fire of knowledge, whereby our souls are purified.
⁴⁶Sacrifice : Our respect and reverence for the learned.

47. O teacher and preacher, with mastery over the vedas, become near us our protectors, welfarers, givers of knowledge and wealth in our homes. Give us wealth most splendidly renowned. Come nigh unto us, so that we may express reverence unto ye!

४८. तं त्वा शोचिष्ठ दीदिवः सुम्नाय नूनमीमहे सखिभ्यः ।
स नो बोधि श्रुधी हवमुरुष्या णो ऽ अघायतः समस्मात् ॥

48. O virtuous learned person, grant us knowledge. We pray unto thee for our happiness and the good of our friends. Listen to our call; and protect us from evil-minded and sinful persons!

CHAPTER XXVI

१. अग्निश्च पृथिवी च सन्नते ते मे सं नमतामदो वायुश्चान्तरिक्षं च सन्नते ते मे सं नमतामद
आदित्यश्च द्यौश्च सन्नते ते मे सं नमतामद आपश्च वरुणश्च सन्नते ते मे सं नमतामद: ।
सप्त स॒सदो अष्टमी भूतसाधनी ।
सकामाँ२ अध्वनस्कुरु संज्ञानमस्तु मे॒मुना ॥

1. Fire and Earth are favourable to me; may they be subservient to me in the accomplishment of that aim of mine.

Air and firmament are favourable to me; may they be subservient to me in the accomplishment of that aim of mine. Sun and his light are favourable to me; may they be subservient to me in the accomplishment of that aim of mine. Waters and clouds are favourable to me, may they be subservient to me in the accomplishment of that aim of mine. Out of these seven forces are the mainstay of all beings, the eighth is Earth which keeps every one under its sway. O God make all our paths pleasant and comfortable!

May I thus obtain true knowledge from these forces.

२. यथेमां वाचं कल्याणीमावदानि जनेभ्य: ।
ब्रह्मराजन्याभ्या॒ शूद्राय चार्याय च स्वाय चारणाय च ।
प्रियो देवानां दक्षिणायै दातुरिह भूयासमयं मे कामः समृध्यतामुप मादो नमतु ॥

2. I do hereby address this salutary speech for the benefit of humanity, for the Brahmanas, the Kshatriyas, the Shudras, the Vaishas, the kinsfolk and the men of lowest position in society.

Dear may I be to the learned and the guerdon-giver in this world, Fulfilled be this desire of mine. May I achieve my aim.

३. बृहस्पते अति यदर्यो अर्हाद् द्युमद्विभाति क्रतुमज्जनेषु ।
यद्दीदयच्छवस ऋतप्रजात तदस्मासु द्रविणं धेहि चित्रम् ।
उपयामगृहीतोऽसि बृहस्पतये त्वैष ते योनिर्बृहस्पतये त्वा ॥

3. O God, the guardian of mighty material objects and souls, Thou art realised through the practice of yoga. We accept Thee as the Protector of

---

[1] Fire, air, firmament, sun, water, cloud and sky are seven Sansdas (forces). All beings exist on their support. Bhutaddhni is Earth that keeps under its arms all human beings.
Man should make full use of the forces of nature and fulfil the aim of his life.
[2] I : God.
Salutary speech : All the four vedas. The vedas are meant for the good of all, high or low. Those who restrict their study to the high castes and deprive the Shudras and the untouchable from reading or hearing them read, disobey the mandate of God and thus commit sin.
I in the second para refers to the king.

the vedas, which symbolise The authority, and as the Nourisher of selfless scholars!

O God, Truth is nobly born of Thee. O God Thou adequately kindlest in men splendid refulgent mind, laudable wisdom and effectual active mind!

Thou existest as a highly resplendent entity through self-force.

Grant us marvellous knowledge, riches and fame.

४. इन्द्र गोमन्निहा याहि पिबा सोम꣡ शतक्रतो । विद्यद्विर्ग्रविभि: सुतम् ।
उपयामगृहीतोऽसीन्द्राय त्वा गोमत एष ते योनिरिन्द्राय त्वा गोमते ॥

4. O learned person, possessing vast wisdom and knowledge of the vedas, come here, and drink the juice of medicines ripened by clouds. Thou hast controlled thy senses through yamas and niyamas. We accept thee as the master of worldly kingship and grand supremacy. This is thy home of knowledge. We accept thee as protector of vedic speech, and as full of glory!

५. इन्द्रा याहि वृत्रहन्पिबा सोम꣡ शतक्रतो ।
गोमद्विर्ग्रविभि: सुतम् ।
उपयामगृहीतोऽसीन्द्राय त्वा गोमत एष ते योनिरिन्द्राय त्वा गोमते ॥

5. O exalted learned person, full of wisdom and deeds, slayer of foes like the cloud-dispeller sun, come, and drink deep the essence of knowledge produced by the knowers of the vedas. Thou hast controlled thy soul by yogic practices. We accept thee as the master of milk-yielding kine and grand supremacy. This is thy home of knowledge. We accept thee as the master of worldly possessions, and desirous of glory!

६. ऋतावानं वैश्वानरमृतस्य ज्योतिषस्पतिम् ।
अजस्रं धर्ममीमहे ।
उपयामगृहीतोऽसि वैश्वानराय त्वैष ते योनिवैश्वानराय त्वा ॥

6. We daily pray for the light of knowledge, unto God, the Lord of learning, the Leader of humanity, and the Embodiment of Truth. Thou art realised through yogic practices. I accept Thee as the Leader of humanity! This heart is Thy home.

I accept Thee as being the Lover of all people.

७. वैश्वानरस्य सुमतौ स्याम राजा हि कं भुवनानामभिश्री: ।
इतो जातो विश्वमिदं वि चष्टे वैश्वानरो यतते सूर्येण ।
उपयामगृहीतोऽसि वैश्वानराय त्वैष ते योनिवैश्वानराय त्वा ।

⁴Here : In this world.

Yamas : Mental restraints. They are five. Ahinsa (Non-violence), Satya (Truth), Asteya (Avoidance of theft). Brahmcharya (celibacy), Aprigraha (Renunciation).

Niyamas : शौच (Purity of body and mind),संतोष(contentment),तप (Penance), स्वाध्याय (Religious study) ईश्वरप्रणिधान (Resignation to the will of God).

7. Just as the Sun, filled with the lustre of grandeur, in the midst of illuminated worlds, gives us pleasure, and therefore illuminates this world with his light, just as lightning exerts with the Sun, so should we continue in God's grace.

O learned person thou art acceptable through beautiful restraints. I respect thee for thy knowledge of electricity. This is thy home. I respect Thee for thy accomplishing electrical projects!

८. वैश्वानरो न ऊतय आ प्र यातु परावतः ।
अग्निरुक्थेन वाहसा ।
उपयामगृहीतोऽसि वैश्वानराय त्वैष ते योनिर्वैश्वानराय त्वा ॥

8. Just as a learned person foremost amongst the leaders comes for our protection from far away, so should a person brilliant like fire come in a commendable conveyance.

We accept thee full of literary thought for a learned person. We accept thee, whose this house is meant for the leader of the learned.

९. अग्निऋषिः पवमानः पाञ्चजन्यः पुरोहितः ।
तमीमहे महागयम् ।
उपयामगृहीतोऽस्यग्नये त्वा वर्चस एष ते योनिरग्नये त्वा वर्चसे ॥

9. We pray to him, the master of five senses and lover of five castes, affectionate to all, pure, the knower of the significance of vedic texts, glowing like fire with the warmth of knowledge; the lord of wealth, offspring and palatial buildings. Thou art imbued with religious laws. I accept thee as a dignified literary person. This is thy home of knowledge. I accept thee as a dignified, literary, religious person.

१०. महाँ २ इन्द्रो वज्रहस्तः षोडशी शर्म यच्छतु ।
हन्तु पाप्मानं योऽस्मान्द्वेष्टि ।
उपयामगृहीतोऽसि महेन्द्राय त्वैष ते योनिर्महेन्द्राय त्वा ॥

10. May the mighty, thunder-armed, perfectly virtuous king grant us a comfortable home, may he slay the wicked man who hates us.

Thou art equipped with justice and statesmanship. We accept thee for the extreme supremacy. This is thy kingly palace. We accept thee as a paramount sovereign.

११. तं वो दस्ममृतीषहं वसोर्मन्दानमन्धसः ।
अभि वत्सं न स्वसरेषु धेनव इन्द्रं गीर्भिर्नवामहे ॥

11. O people, just as cows low to their calves all the day long, so with our songs we glorify for ye, this king, the dispeller of affliction, the checker of assault, and the enjoyer of riches and foodgrains!

⁹Five castes : Brahmana, Kshatriya, Vaisha, Shudra and Nishada.
¹¹Thou : King.

१२. यद्द्राहिष्ठं तदग्नये बृहदर्चं विभावसो ।
महीषीव त्वद्रयिस्त्वद्राजा उदीरते ॥

12. O learned people honour the king who is great and giver of extreme comfort. Like the queen, riches and foodstuffs proceed from the king!

१३. एह्यू षु ब्रवाणि तेऽग्न इत्थेतरा गिरः ।
एभिर्वर्धास इन्दुभिः ।

13. O wise, learned person, come, here I sing verily other songs to thee, With these praises shalt thou grow strong!

१४. ऋतवस्ते यज्ञं वि तन्वन्तु मासा रक्षन्तु ते हविः ।
संवत्सरस्ते यज्ञं दधातु नः प्रजां च परि पातु नः ॥

14. O learned person, the seasons spread thy yajna, the months protect thy offering. May our year strengthen thy yajna. May thou keep our children safe in every way!

१५. उपह्वरे गिरीणाꣳ सङ्गमे च नदीनाम् ।
धिया विप्रो अजायत् ॥

15. In the solitude of mountains and confluence of streams a sage develops his spiritual force, contemplating on God through yoga.

१६. उच्चा ते जातमन्धसो दिवि सद्भूम्या ददे ।
उग्रꣳ शर्म महि श्रवः ॥

16. O learned person, I admire thy house, high in altitude, full of foodstuffs, well ventilated and airy, grand in sight and extremely commendable. May it be durable like the Earth!

१७. स न इन्द्राय यज्यवे वरुणाय मरुद्भ्यः ।
वरिवोवित्परि स्रव ॥

17. O amiable scholar, fully knowing the duty of service, flow the juice of learning for the king, respectable sacrificer and us mortals!

१८. एना विश्वान्यर्यꣳ आ द्युम्नानि मानुषाणाम् ।
सिषासन्तो वनामहे ॥

18. God gives instruction for all these graceful glories of men. Willing to serve God, we pray for pleasures.

१९. अनु वीरैरनु पुष्यास्म गोभिरन्वश्वैरनु सर्वेण पुष्टैः ।
अनु द्विपदाऽनु चतुष्पदा वयं देवा नो यज्ञमृतुथा नयन्तु ॥

---

[13]Other : Which thou dost not know or hast not heard before and are new.

19. May we be prosperous with strong, brave sons, strong kine, strong horses, the strength of all, strong quadrupeds and strong men about us. May the learned guide our sacrifice (yajna) season-wise.

२०. अग्ने पत्नीरिहा वह देवानामुशतीरुप ।
त्वष्टारꣳ सोमपीतये ॥

20. O teachress bring thou near thee in this domestic life, for drinking the juice of medicines, husbands full of attributes like thee, and consorts of the learned; and may thy husband invite near him the lustrous scholars!

२१. अभि यज्ञं गृणीहि नो ग्नावो नेष्टः पिब ऋतुना ।
त्वꣳ हि रत्नधा असि ॥

21. O eloquent leader, make our fair dealings worthy of praise. Thou art the giver of wealth. Drink the juice of medicines!

२२. द्रविणोदाः पिपीषति जुहोत प्र च तिष्ठत ।
नेष्ट्रादृतुभिरिष्यत ॥

22. O men, just as the giver of wealth and fame, according to seasons, humbly desires to drink the juice, so should ye procure this juice, perform havan, and attain to glory!

२३. तवायꣳ सोमस्त्वमेह्यर्वाङ् शश्वत्तमꣳसुमना अस्य पाहि ।
अस्मिन् यज्ञे बर्हिष्या निषद्या दधिष्वेमं जठर इन्दुमिन्द्र ॥

23. O learned person desirous of supremacy, secure well thy contact with power. In the performance of religious deeds, with a tranquil mind, protect this eternal soul of thine. Sitting steadfastly in this yajna, take into thy belly this efficacious medicinal juice!

२४. अ्रमेव नः सुहवा आ हि गन्तन नि बर्हिषि सदतना रणिष्टन ।
अथा मदस्व जुजुषाणो अन्धसस्त्वष्टर्देवेभिर्जनिभिः सुमद्गणः ॥

24. O majestic scholar, serving gladly thy preceptor, in gladsome company, with noble qualities, and with thy mother, sister and wife, be happy in the acquisition of nice foodstuffs!
Afterwards make others happy like a comfortable house. O learned people, well invoked, establish us in fair dealings, sit near us at ease, and give us good instructions!

२५. स्वादिष्ठया मदिष्ठया पवस्व सोम धारया ।
इन्द्राय पातवे सुतः ॥

[19] पुत्रो वै वीरः शत॰ 3-3-1-12.

25. O mighty learned fellow, for thee is this juice pressed, for the protection of riches. Purify thyself with its sweetest and most gladdening flow!

२६. रक्षोहा विश्वचर्षणिरभि योनिमपोहते ।
द्रोणे सधस्थमासदत् ॥

26. The fiend-queller, and the friend of all, in his country attains to reverence and a dignified position, and lives happily in his house filled with gold.

CHAPTER XXVII

१. समास्त्वाग्न ऋतवो वर्धयन्तु संवत्सरा ऋषयो यानि सत्या ।
सं दिव्येन दीदिहि रोचनेन विश्वा आ भाहि प्रदिशश्चतस्रः ॥

1. O learned person, may years, seasons, knowers of vedic interpretation and all the verities strengthen thee!
Just as the sun with celestial effulgence illumines all the four efficacious regions so should thou long for knowledge, and manifest justice.

२. सं चेध्यस्वाग्ने प्र च बोधयैनमुच्च तिष्ठ महते सौभगाय ।
मा च रिषदुपसत्ता ते अग्ने ब्रह्माणस्ते यशसः सन्तु मान्ये ॥

2. Shine thou, O learned person lustrous like fire, make this seeker after knowledge, rise up erect for great and happy fortune. Be those uninjured who adore thee. Let not thy priests, the knowers of all the four vedas, turn against thee. Don't spoil thy glory and progress!

३. त्वामग्ने वृणते ब्राह्मणा इमे शिवो अग्ने संवरणे भवा नः ।
सपत्नहा नो अभिमातिजिज्च्च स्वे गये जागृह्यप्रयुच्छन् ॥

3. O learned person, these masters of the vedas elect thee as their leader. Be thou propitious unto them in this election. Remove thou the errors of our foes. O learned person being free from sloth and pride, watch in thy house, and keep us also conscious!

४. इहैवाग्ने अधि धारया रयिं मा त्वा नि कन्पूर्वंचितो निकारिणः ।
क्षत्रमग्ने सुयममस्तु तुभ्यमुपसत्ता वर्धतां ते अनिष्वृत् ॥

4. O learned person, amass wealth in this world. Let not the old, exalted, learned persons, ever devoted to action, tolerate thy moral degradation!
O ruler, famous for thy humility, let thy administration be run by just laws. May thy adorers, following non-violence make thee strong. May the State riches make thee happy!

५. क्षत्रेणाग्ने स्वायुः सꣳरभस्व मित्रेणाग्ने मित्रधेये यतस्व ।
सजातानां मध्यमस्था एधि राजामग्ने विहव्यो दीदिहीह ॥

5. O learned person commence thy youth with wealth in this world!
O king, flowing with knowledge and humility, exert to maintain friendship with the religious, learned friends!
O justice-loving head of the state, act as an umpire in the midst of your coequal virtuous kings. Be renowned as worthy of praise!

---

³Watch in thy house : Remain slothless doing the household duties.

६. अति निहो अति स्रिधोऽत्यचित्तिमत्यराऽतिमग्ने ।
विश्वा ह्यग्ने दुरिता सहस्वाथाऽस्मभ्यᳪ सहवीराᳪ रयिं दाः ॥

6. O king, renouncing untruth, suppress fully the wicked persons, overcome spiritual ignorance, and banish miserliness. O learned person, drive away all sins; vouchsafe us opulence with an army of heroic soldiers!

७. अनाधृष्यो जातवेदा अनिष्टृतो विराडग्ने क्षत्रभृद्दीदिहीह ।
विश्वा आशाः प्रमुञ्चन्मानुषीभियः शिवेभिरद्य परि पाहि नो वृधे ॥

7. O king, invincible, full of knowledge, free from misery, refulgent, and an able administrator, be dear to us in this task of government. Illumine all regions. Chase human ills and griefs with the help of philanthropic persons. Guard us for prosperity!

८. बृहस्पते सवितर्बोधयैनᳪ सᳪशितं चित्सन्तराᳪसᳪशिशाधि ।
वर्धयैनं महते सौभगाय विश्व एनमनु मदन्तु देवाः ॥

8. O learned fellow, the guardian of big persons, excellent preacher of learning, sharpening the intellect of this king, give him knowledge; instruct him well, instruct thoroughly his subjects. Exalt him to great and high felicity. Let all the learned persons rejoice following his good will!

९. अमुत्रभूयादध यदमस्य बृहस्पते अभिशस्तेरमुञ्च ।
प्रत्यौहतामश्विना मृत्युमस्माद्देवानामग्ने भिषजा शचीभिः ॥

9. O learned fellow, the guardian of big persons, be free from the fruit of sins in the next birth. Chase death far from him who follows the instructions of the religious and law-abiding persons!

O skilled physician, just as the teacher and preacher achieve their aim by dint of deeds and wisdom, so shouldst thou skilfully prepare efficacious medicines, whereby thou preservest the health of the people!

१०. उद्वयं तमसस्परि स्वः पश्यन्त उत्तरम् ।
देवं देवत्रा सूर्यमगन्म ज्योतिरुत्तमम् ॥

10. Looking upon the sun's light free from darkness, we fully realise God, the Giver of happiness, the Saviour of humanity, Omnipresent, Excellent, the Soul of animate and inanimate objects, and Self-Effulgent.

११. ऊर्ध्वा अस्य समिधो भवन्त्यूर्ध्वा शुक्रा शोचीᳪष्यग्ने ।
द्युमत्तमा सुप्रतीकस्य सूनोः ॥

11. This fire, the accomplisher of many mighty deeds, the discharger of children from wombs, has splendid faggots as its fuel; and unlifted, lofty and brilliant flames.

१२. तनूनपादसुरो विश्ववेदा देवो देवेषु देवः ।
पथो अनक्तु मध्वा घृतेन ॥

12. O men, know air as an object of usefulness amongst the useful objects, devoid of lustre, all-possessing, the protector of bodies, highly desirable, and the sprinkler of paths with sweet water through rain!

१३. मध्वा यज्ञं नक्षसे प्रीणानो नराशँसो अग्ने ।
सुक्रदेवः सविता विश्ववारः ॥

13. O learned person, thou art the admirer of persons, doer of noble deeds, worthy of praise, full of ambition, desirous of supremacy, wise in dealings; and a comer to this sacrifice with sweet words!

१४. अच्छायमेति शवसा घृतेनेदानो बर्हिर्नमसा ।
अग्निँसुचो अध्वरेषु प्रयत्सु ॥

14. This extolling learned person, the carrier of knowledge, in non-violent sacrifices attainable through exertion, nicely procures ladles and fire accompanied by corn, water and power.

१५. स यक्षदस्य महिमानमग्नेः स ई मन्द्रा सुप्रयसः ।
वसुश्चेतिष्ठो वसुधातमश्च ॥

15. That learned person, daintily fed, realises the greatness of this fire. He is the best wealth-giver, and wisest protector. He gets water and enjoyable oblations.

१६. द्वारो देवीरन्वस्य विश्वे व्रता ददन्ते अग्ने ।
उरुव्यचसो धाम्ना पत्यमाना ॥

16. The learned persons, lording over all, with the splendour of that widely expansive fire, expound the vows of truthfulness, and the bright sources of the knowledge of fire.

१७. ते अस्य योषणे दिव्ये न योना उषासानक्ता ।
इमं यज्ञमवतामध्वरं नः ॥

17. May Dawn and Night, like two beautiful consorts, protect in our home this non-violent sacrificial worship of ours.

---

[13] This verse has been interpreted by Pt. Jaidev Vidyalankar, as applying to soul as well. Soul is the preserver of the body, lover of breaths (pranas), infuser of strength, seer of knowledge, and lord of organs. May the soul illumine the paths of its existence with knowledge and light.

[14] The fire used in locomotives accompanied with water and fuel, moves fast with great force. We should make use of fire in yajnas and fast-moving locomotives.

[15] The learned persons who realise the greatness of fire become wealthy.

१८. दैव्या होतारा ऊर्ध्वमध्वरं नोऽग्नेर्जिह्वामभि गृणीतम् ।
कृणुतं नः स्विष्टम् ॥

18. Ye two learned persons, givers of pleasure, greet with praises this lofty non-violent sacrifice of ours. Conduct well the flame of fire in connection with our beautiful sacrifice.

१९. तिस्रो देवीर्बर्हिरेदꣳ सदन्त्विडा सरस्वती भारती ।
मही गृणाना ॥

19. May Ida, Saraswati, Bharati, three mighty forms of eulogy fill this atmosphere.

२०. तन्नस्तुरीपमद्भुतं पुरुक्षु त्वष्टा सुवीर्यम् ।
रायस्पोषं वि ष्यतु नाभिमस्मे ॥

20. May God grant us wealth and strength, eagerly obtainable, possessing wondrous merits, powers and qualities; residing in various objects, beautifully mighty; and relieve us of misery.

२१. वनस्पतेऽव सृजा ररानस्तमना देवेषु ।
अग्निर्हव्यꣳ शमिता सूदयाति ॥

21. O investigator, the guardian of religious lore, just as sacrificial fire renders subtle the oblations and diffuses them in the air, so shouldst thou rejoicing thyself in the midst of the learned, explore objects worth acquisition!

२२. अग्ने स्वाहा कृणुहि जातवेद इन्द्राय हव्यम् ।
विश्वे देवा हविरिदं जुषन्ताम् ॥

22. O learned person, well-versed in knowledge, for the sake of supremacy, use truthful speech and perform yajna. May all the learned people be benefited with this yajna!

२३. पीवो अन्ना रयिवृधः सुमेधाः श्वेतः सिषक्ति नियुतामभिश्रीः ।
ते वायवे समनसो वि तस्थुर्विश्वेन्नरः स्वपत्यानि चक्रुः ॥

23. Persons equally learned, increases of wealth, exceedingly wise, eaters of invigorating diet, exert to develop their progeny. May they stand firm to acquire the knowledge of air, which being active and developing, full of grace, purifies the men steadfast in their religious path.

२४. राये नु यं जज्ञतू रोदसीमे राये देवो धिषणा धाति देवम् ।
अध वायुं नियुतः सश्चत स्वा उत श्वेतं वसुधिर्ति निरेके ॥

---

[19]Ida : praiseworthy speech.
Saraswati : A speech full of knowledge.
Bharati : A speech replete with vedic lore.

CHAPTER XXVII

24. Whomsoever the Firmament and Earth give birth for the acquisition of wealth, and whom the wife accepts eagerly as a husband for wealth's sake; they, in a solitary place, unite and disunite their souls with and from God, and enjoy the vast air, the sustainer of the Earth and heavenly bodies.

२५. आपो ह यद्बृहतीर्विश्वमायन् गर्भं दधाना जनयन्तीरग्निम् ।
ततो देवानाꣳ समवर्ततासुरेकः कस्मै देवाय हविषा विधेम ॥

25. When the subtle and primary elements containing the All-prevading matter, the primordial cause of the universe, came into being producing the fiery Sun, there was one God present in all the forces of nature. Let us adore with our devotion the pleasure-giving God.

२६. यश्चिदापो महिना पर्यपश्यद्दक्षं दधाना जनयन्तीर्यज्ञम् ।
यो देवेष्वधि देव एक आसीत् कस्मै देवाय हविषा विधेम ॥

26. God with His Might sees fully the subtle and primary elements, full of potency, and generators of the universe. He amongst all souls and material objects is the one supreme Lord. Let us adore with knowledge and yoga, Him, Who is the Embodiment and Giver of pleasure.

२७. प्र यांभिर्यासि दाश्वाꣳ समच्छा नियुद्भिर्वायविष्टये दुरोणे ।
नि नो रयिꣳ सुभोजसं युवस्व नि वीरं गव्यमश्व्यं च राधः ॥

27. O learned person, powerful like the air, we carefully seek thee, full of desirable, noble qualities. Send in our home wealth, worthy of enjoyment and giver of pleasure. Give us a heroic son, and gifts of kine and horses!

२८. आ नो नियुद्भिः शतिनीभिरध्वरꣳ सहस्रिणीभिरुप याहि यज्ञम् ।
वायो अस्मिन्त्सवने मादयस्व यूयं पात स्वस्तिभिः सदा नः ॥

28. O learned person, powerful like the air, come to our non-violent sacrifice with thy hundreds and thousands of instructions. Gladden us in this world. O sages, preserve us evermore with propitious advice!

२९. नियुत्वान्वायवा गह्यꣳ शुक्रो अयामि ते ।
गन्तासि सुन्वतो गृहम् ॥

29. O God, the Ordainer of Law, just as this purifying, fast moving air, visits the sacrificer's house, so come upto me. Thou art Providence, hence I realise Thy Nature!

३०. वायो शुक्रो अयामि ते मध्वो अग्रं दिविष्टिषु ।
आ याहि सोमपीतये स्पार्हो देव नियुत्वता ॥

30. O learned person, powerful like the air, purifier art thou. I imbibe the excellent essence of thy speech in the assemblies of the learned. O well merited scholar, the scion of a lovely father, come thou with grand glory, to drink the Soma juice!

३१. वायुरग्रेगा यज्ञप्री: साकं गन्मनसा यज्ञम् ।
शिवो नियुद्भि: शिवाभि: ॥

31. O learned person, just as air, with definite propitious motions, comes to the sacrifice, so with noble intentions, as a leader, and nice performer of the yajna, come thou to the yajnashala with a concentrated mind!

३२. वायो ये ते सहस्रिणो रथासस्तेभिरा गहि ।
नियुत्वान्त्सोमपीतये ॥

32. O learned person, come thou to us to drink the Soma juice, with full force, accompanied by thousands of thy admirers in chariots!

३३. एकया च दशभिश्च स्वभूते द्वाभ्यामिष्टये विꣳशती च ।
तिसृभिश्च वहसे त्रिꣳशता नियुद्भिर्वायविह ता वि मुञ्च ॥

33. O learned person, resplendent with thy glory, just as air in this world, under set rules comes to the sacrifice (yajna) with one, ten, two, twenty three and thirty motions, so with knowledge and action, for the applicability of learning expound thou those laws unto us!

३४. तव वायवृतस्पते त्वष्टुर्जामातरद्भुत ।
अवाꣳस्या वृणीमहे ॥

34. O powerful learned person, Lord of Truth, beloved like a son-in-law, wonderful in deeds, renowned for learning, we welcome thy efforts for our protection!

३५. अभि त्वा शूर नोनुमोऽदुग्धा इव धेनव: ।
ईशानमस्य जगत: स्वदृशमीशानमिन्द्र तस्थुष: ॥

35. O fearless king, like unmilked kine, we sing thy praise, as we do unto God, the Lord of all animate and inanimate beings, and most beautiful to look at!

३६. न त्वावाꣳ अन्यो दिव्यो न पार्थिवो न जातो न जनिष्यते ।
अश्वायन्तो मघवन्निन्द्र वाजिनो गव्यन्तस्त्वा हवामहे ॥

36. O Bounteous Lord, none other pure like Thee, hath been or ever will be born on earth. Desiring enterprise and using nice speech, as men of might we call on Thee!

[31] Yajnashala: Place of worship, where the yajna is performed.

[33] The Lucknow Vedic Sons than interprets eleven, as ten breaths and soul; twenty two as ten organs of sense, mind and eleven rudras; and thirty three as 8 vasus, 11 rudras, 12 adityas, Prajapati and yajna.

Swami Dayananda explains two as learning and activity. The different forms of air's motions are not clear.

[35] Unmilked kine: Just as kine, who have not been milked, bow to give milk to the calf, so we bow unto the king and God.

३७. त्वामिद्धि हवामहे सातौ वाजस्य कारव: ।
त्वां वृत्रेष्विन्द्र सत्पतिं नरस्त्वां काष्ठास्वर्वत: ॥

37. O King, the protector of the people, we, the scholars and scientists invoke the alone in war. Just as the Sun is seen after it dispels the clouds, so we see thee in the army active and swift like a horse. We invoke thee in all directions!

३८. स त्वं नश्चित्र वज्रहस्त धृष्णुया मह स्तवानो अद्रिव: ।
गामश्वं रथ्यमिन्द्र सं किर सत्रा वाजं न जिग्युषे ॥

38. O wonderful learned person, whose hand holds thunderbolt, praised as mighty, possessing a lofty position like the mountain, grant unto us and the conqueror, kine and chariot steeds and even knowledge of truth!

३९. कया नश्चित्र आ भुवदूती सदावृध: सखा ।
कया शचिष्ठया वृता ॥

39. O wonderful learned person, befriend the ever prospering person. Protect us with thy succour. Yoke us to noble deeds with thy powerful protection!

४०. कस्त्वा सत्यो मदानां मंहिष्ठो मत्सदन्धस: ।
दृढा चिदारुजे वसु ॥

40. O learned person, the giver of happiness, lover of truth, highly dignified, he, who pleases thee with delightful foods; collects medicines for the elimination of disease, and amasses wealth, deserves our adoration!

४१. अभी षु ण: सखीनामविता जरितृणाम् ।
शतं भवास्यूतये ॥

41. O learned person, thou art the protector of our friends and admirers. For affection's sake approach us with hundred aids. Thou art worthy of our reverence!

४२. यज्ञा-यज्ञा वो अग्नये गिरा-गिरा च दक्षसे ।
प्र-प्र वयममृतं जातवेदसं प्रियं मित्रं न शंसिषम् ॥

42. At every sacrifice, sing the glory of God, for the acquisition of strength. Let us praise the Wise and Everlasting God again and again as a well-beloved Friend.

४३. पाहि नो अग्न एकया पाह्युत द्वितीयया ।
पाहि गीर्भिस्तिसृभिरूर्जां पते पाहि चतसृभिर्वसो ॥

43. O learned person, bestower of beautiful habitation, and refulgent like

---

[43]This verse may also mean, O God the Lord of Power, protect us with Rigveda, with Rig and Yajur, with Rig, Yajur and Sama, with Rig, Yajur, Sama and Atharva. Pt. Jaidev Vidyalankar, Mahidhar, and Vedic Sansthan have thus translated this verse. I have given the interpretation of Maharshi Dayananda Saraswati.

fire, protect us with sound advice. Protect us with thy teaching. Protect us with three instructions of action, contemplation, and knowledge. O Lord of power and might, protect us with four counsels of religion, worldly prosperity, affection and final emancipation of soul!

४४. ऊर्जो नपात् ॐ स हिनायमस्मयुदर्शिम हव्यदातये ।
भुवद्वाजेष्वविता भुवद्वृध उत त्राता तनूनाम् ॥

44. O student, advance knowledge, the preserver of thy enterprise. Thou art our well-wisher, and helper in battles; the saviour of our bodies for progress. We select thee as a fit recipient of precious objects!

४५. संवत्सरोऽसि परिवत्सरोऽसीदावत्सरोऽसीद्वत्सरोऽसि वत्सरोऽसि ।
उषसस्ते कल्पन्तामहोरात्रास्ते कल्पन्तामर्धमासास्ते कल्पन्तां मासास्ते कल्पन्तामृतवस्ते कल्पन्ताॐ संवत्सरस्ते कल्पताम् ।
प्रेत्या एत्यै सं चाञ्च प्र च सारय ।
सुपर्णचिदसि तया देवतयाऽङ्गिरस्वद् ध्रुवः सीद ॥

45. O aspirant after knowledge, thou art the follower or law like the year, renouncer of immorality like the relinquished year, definite like the year, steadfast like the year, and active like the year. Prosper thy Dawns! Prosper thy Days and Nights! Prosper thy Half-months (months, Seasons and Years)!

Combine them for their going and coming, and send them forward on their ordered courses.

Thou art the collector of the sources of protection. With that divinity lie steady like the vital breath.

---

[45] The words Samvatsar, Parivatsar, Idavatsar, and Vatsar are the names given to the years of the five-year cycle, intended with the aid of an intercalary month, to adjust the difference between the lunar and the solar year.

CHAPTER XXVIII

१. होता यक्षत्समिधेन्द्रमिडस्पदे नाभा पृथिव्या अधि ।
दिवो वर्ष्मन्त्समिध्यत ओजिष्ठश्चर्षणीसहां वेत्वाज्यस्य होतर्यज ॥

1. O sacrificer, just as the master of noble qualities, with the display of knowledge, concerning the laudable art of speech, on the earth's centre, and on the height of heaven, in the midst of thundering clouds, kindles and perceives the fire and electricity, and as the mightiest of the lords of men, properly manifests himself and enjoys the butter, so shouldst thou keep company with him!

२. होता यक्षत्तनूनपातमूतिभिर्जेतारमपराजितम् ।
इन्द्रं देवꣳ स्वविदं पथिभिर्मधुमत्तमैर्नराशꣳसेन तेजसा वेत्वाज्यस्य होतर्यज ॥

2. O sacrificer, just as the pleasure-giving person, with due protections and religious paths, rich in valuable advice like sweet water, befriends the mighty king, the guardian of our bodies, the conqueror, unconquered, full of delight, adorned with knowledge and humility, and understands all knowable topics with his well-praised spiritual and moral power; so shouldst thou cultivate friendly intercourse with him!

३. होता यक्षदिडाभिरिन्द्रमीडितमाजुह्वानममर्त्यम् ।
देवो देवै: सवीर्या वज्रहस्त: पुरन्दरो वेत्वाज्यस्य होतर्यज ॥

3. O sacrificer, just as the pleasure-giving person, with well-trained modes of speech, wins the king equipped with knowledge and supremacy, above the ordinary run of mankind, full of rivalry against foes, praised and just as he, the thunder-wielder, the breaker-down of the enemies, cities, full of power, learned, performs with the help of the learned, the duties of a ruler, so shouldst thou cultivate friendly inter-course with him!

४. होता यक्षद्बर्हिषीन्द्रꣳ निषद्वरं वृषभं नर्यापसम् ।
वसुभी रुद्रैरादित्यै: सयुग्भिर्बर्हिरासद्वेत्वाज्यस्य होतर्यज ॥

4. O giver of charity, just as a person desirous of happiness, with Vasus, Rudras and Adityas for companions, in the Assembly of the learned, wins the favour of the king, adorned with statesmanship, near whom are seated noble learned advisers, full of power, who appreciates the noble deeds of men, and sits in the court to administer justice, and acquires happiness, so shouldst thou be happy!

---

[1]Earth's centre: the altar. A learned person kindles fire in the altar.
Sacrificer: Yajman.

[4]Vasus, Rudras and Adityas are Brahmcharis who respectively observe the vow of celibacy for 24, 36 and 48 years.

५. होता यक्षदोजो न वीर्यꣳ सहो द्वार इन्द्रमवर्धयन् ।
सुप्रायणा अस्मिन्यज्ञे वि श्रयन्तामृतावृधो द्वार इन्द्राय मीढुषे व्यन्त्वाज्यस्य होतर्यज ॥

5. O sacrificer, just as spacious gates, like the fast flow of water, enhance power, lustre and dignity; so should the learned have access to the expedients of knowledge and humility in this sociable world, for the kind, heroic and mighty king. They should learn the art of administration. Hota should perform the yajna, so shouldst thou do!

६. होता यक्षदुषे इन्द्रस्य धेनू सुदुघे मातरा मही ।
सवातरौ न तेजसा वत्समिन्द्रमवर्धतां वीतामाज्यस्य होतर्यज ॥

6. O giver of happiness, just as two cows living in the open air, the fulfillers of our noble desires, behaving mother-like, nourish the highly developed calf, like material fire and sun's heart, the two aspects of lightning, and just as Hota performs the yajna with oblations, so shouldst thou do!

७. होता यक्षद्दैव्या होतारा भिषजा सखाया हविषेन्द्रं भिषज्यतः ।
कवी देवौ प्रचेतसाविन्द्राय दत्त इन्द्रियं वीतामाज्यस्य होतर्यज ॥

7. O physician, regular in thy meals and recreation, just as two physicians, givers of happiness, expert in the diagnosis of physical ills, excellent amongst the learned, dispellers of disease, friendly to each other, wise, full of the knowledge of medical science, experienced in the art of medicine, adepts in medical treatment, treat the ills of the soul, amass wealth for worldly progress, and attain to longevity, so shouldst thou do!

८. होता यक्षत्तिस्रो देवीर्नं भेषजं त्रयस्त्रिधातवोऽपस इडा सरस्वती भारती मही: ।
इन्द्रपत्नीर्हविष्मतीर्व्यन्त्वाज्यस्य होतर्यज ॥

8. O aspirant after happiness, just as a teacher, the imparter and recipient of learning, performs the duty of reading and teaching; just as a teacher, a preacher and a physician, developing the three humours, i.e., bone, marrow and semen, engrossed in actions, imbibe Ida, Saraswati and Bharati, the three efficacious and highly venerable speeches, the illuminators of knowledge, full of instructions and protectors of the soul, so shouldst thou cultivate them!

९. होता यक्षत्त्वष्टारमिन्द्रं देवं भिषजꣳ सुयजं घृतश्रियम् ।
पुरुरूपꣳ सुरेतसं मघोनमिन्द्राय त्वष्टा दधदिन्द्रियाणि वेत्वाज्यस्य होतर्यज ॥

9. Inculcator of good virtues, just as an abstemious person, befriends a physician, the remover of physical maladies, the possessor of riches, full of

---

⁸Indrapatni: Just as a wife serves and protects the husband, so do these three kinds of speech protect the soul.
Ida: the speech worthy of praise.
Saraswati: the speech full of knowledge.
Bharati: the speech, the preserver and developer of beautiful knowledge.
Them: the three kinds of speech.

many qualities, physically strong, highly social, brilliant, and supreme, and in obedience to the soul, the urger of knowledge, controlling his senses, gains power, so shouldst thou do!

१०. होता यक्षद्वनस्पतिꣳ शमितारꣳ शतक्रतुं धियो जोष्टारमिन्द्रियम् । मध्वा समञ्जन्पथिभिः सुगेभिः स्वदाति यज्ञं मधुना घृतेन वेत्वाज्यस्य होतर्यज ॥

10. O charitably disposed person, just as a performer of yajna, associates with a sacrificer, the provider of shelter like the sun, the master of manifold wisdom, the doer of deeds; and with practical rules of conduct, enjoys the wealth of the world, displayed by him, and performs yajna with savoury butter, so shouldst thou do!

११. होता यक्षदिन्द्रꣳ स्वाहाऽऽज्यस्य स्वाहा मेदसः स्वाहा स्तोकानाꣳ स्वाहा स्वाहाकृतीनाꣳ स्वाहा हव्यसूक्तीनाम् । स्वाहा देवा आज्यपा जुषाणा इन्द्र आज्यस्य व्यन्तु होतर्यज ॥

11. O imparter of knowledge, just as a person who acquires learning and prosperity, and grants us affluence, studies the truthful sayings of religious lore, understands the working of oily substances, listens to the excellent lovely words of little children, attends the performance of Homa by persons who speak the truth and act upon it, acquires the active, mighty supremacy of wisdom that emanates from the beautiful teachings of religious books; and just as learned persons, delighted with kind words of truth, and drinking clarified butter attain to greatness, so shouldst thou perform yajna!

१२. देव बर्हिरिन्द्रꣳ सुदेवं देवैर्वीरवत्स्तीर्णं वेद्यामवर्धयत् । वस्तोर्वंतं प्राक्तोभृंतꣳ राया बर्हिष्मतोऽत्यगाद्ऽसुवने वसुधेयस्य वेतु यज ॥

12. O learned person, just as an oblation in Homa, performed in the day and at night, transgressing the air and water in the atmosphere, adds to the wealth of the world, and protected in the altar by ghee and fuel, contributes to health, and increases our happiness, so shouldst thou associate with a heroic, dignified man of learning, who is accompanied by well-mannered learned persons possessing riches vast like the space!

१३. देवीर्द्वार इन्द्रꣳ सङ्वाते वीड्वीर्यामन्नवर्धयन् । आ वत्सेन तरुणेन कुमारेण च मीवतापावर्णꣳ रेणुक्काटं नुदन्तां वसुवने वसुधेयस्य व्यन्तु यज ॥

13. O learned person, just as excellent, brilliant doors, and a praiseworthy, young, heroic boy, making the horse march on a path leaving aside

---

[10]Enjoys refers to the performer of yajna.
Him refers to the sacrificer, the priest.
[13]Blind Well: Well which is filled with earth, and does not look like a well : and is likely to deceive a rider.

the blind well, add to our prestige, so shouldst thou acquiring wealth, and removing all impediments, enjoy this rich world and perform sacrifice!

१४. देवी उषासानक्तेन्द्रं यज्ञे प्रयत्यह्वेताम् ।
देवीर्विश: प्रायासिष्टाꣳ सुप्रीते सुधिते वसुधेयस्य वीतां यज ॥

14. O learned person, just as pleasant, lovely and lustrous day and night, goad the sacrificer to action in a yajna, and just as they for proper use of wealth, approach the just and educated persons, nay the whole world, so shouldst thou perform yajna!

१५. देवी जोष्ट्री वसुधिती देवमिन्द्रमवर्धताम् ।
अयाव्यन्याचा द्वेषाꣳस्यान्या वक्षद्वसु वार्याणि यजमानाय शिक्षिते वसुने वसुधेयस्य वीतां यज ॥

15. O learned person, just as lustrous day and night, wealth-givers, engulfing all objects, heighten the radiant sun, and one of them the night drives away hatreds and sins; the other, the Dawn brings boons and treasures; and just as day and night in which men receive education, under the sky on this earth a part of the world, comprehend the active sacrificer, so shouldst thou perform yajna!

१६. देवी ऊर्जाहुती दुघे सुदुघे पयसेन्द्रमवर्धताम् ।
इषमूर्जमन्या वक्षत्सग्धिꣳ सपीतिमन्या नवेन पूर्वं दयमाने पुराणेन नवमधातामूर्जमूर्जाहुती ऊर्जयमाने वसु वार्याणि यजमानाय शिक्षिते वसुने वसुधेयस्य वीतां यज ॥

16. O learned person, just as educated persons, in this world, the creation of God, in day and night, comprehend the soul intent upon the acquisition of spiritual knowledge; and just as day and night the retainers of strength and breath, the givers of happiness, gladden us with water, impel our noble ambitions and add to our prosperity, one of which brings food and energy, the other feast and drinks, and just as the outgoing and in-coming nights blend the old energy with the new and new with the old, and day and night, the decreasers of life and dissipators of strength, preserve our existence so shouldst thou perform yajna!

१७. देवा दैव्या होतारा देवमिन्द्रमवर्धताम् ।
हताघशꣳसावाभाष्टी वसु वार्याणि यजमानाय शिक्षितौ वसुने वसुधेयस्य वीतां यज ॥

17. O learned person, just as pleasant air and fire, celebrated for their excellent attributes, the sustainers of the world heighten the radiant sun's might, exterminate the diseases that kill the sinful thieves, and acting as monitors to the soul, procure us riches and drinkable water in God's world, so shouldst thou perform yajan!

---

[15] Boons: Fresh waters etc.

१८. देवीस्तित्रस्तिस्रो देवी: पतिमिन्द्रमवर्धयन् ।
अस्पृक्षद्द्वारती दिव॑ हृद्वैर्यज्ञ॒ँसरस्वतीडा वसुमती गृहान् वसुवने वसुधेयस्य
व्यन्तु यज ॥

18. O learned person, Bharati, the speech, uttered through breath, Saraswati, the speech full of wisdom, and Ida, the speech enriched with wealth, and the performer of yajna, occupy the householders. These three divine forms of speech, heighten the might of the lustrous and protecting soul. For gain of wealth they are cherished by the householders. Aspire after them and may thou master them!

१६. देव इन्द्रो नराश॑ँसस्त्रिवरूथस्त्रिबन्धुरो देवमिन्द्रमवर्धयत् ।
शतेन शितिपृष्ठानामाहित: सहस्त्रेण प्र वर्तते मित्रावरुणेदस्य होत्रमर्हतो बृहस्पति स्तो-
त्रमश्विनाध्वर्य्वं वसुवने वसुधेयस्य वेतु यज ॥

19. O learned person, just as the soul hankering after eminence, praised by men, master of various houses comfortable in all times, the past, present and future, develops brilliant electricity with hundred devices, and seated on the back of fast-moving animals engages himself in the thousand forms of activities; and just as the pran and udan, the companions of the soul fit to earn living, electricity, the guardian of great projects of the world, laudable sun and moon, and the man willing to perform yajna, are all made serviceable by the soul for helping the aspirant after riches; so shouldst thou perform yajna!

२०. देवो देव॑र्वनस्पतिर्हिरण्यपर्णो मधुशाख: सुपिप्पलो देवमिन्द्रमवर्धयत् ।
दिवमग्रेणास्पृक्षदान्तरिक्षं पृथिवीमदृ॑ँहीद्वसुवने वसुधेयस्य वेतु यज ॥

20. O learned person, just as Vanaspati, imbued with fine qualities, with leaves shining like gold, sweet boughs, fair fruit, bestower of praiseworthy benefits, heightens the cloud, the remover of poverty, and full of nice attributes; and being highly important desires light, establishes the Earth and space and grows for the soul, the diffuser of wealth in the world, so shouldst thou perform yajna!

२१. देवं बर्हिर्वारितीनां देवमिन्द्रमवर्धयत् ।
स्वासस्थमिन्द्रेणासन्नमन्या बर्हि॑ँष्यभ्यभूद्वसुवने वसुधेयस्य वेतु यज ॥

21. O learned person, just as the beautiful atmosphere, residing in the laudable universe, enjoying the imminence of God, the Mainstay of all, heightens the celestial lightning, is ubiquitous, and engages the attention of a scientist in this precious world, so shouldst thou do!

२२. देवो अग्नि: स्विष्टकृद्देवमिन्द्रमवर्धयत् ।
स्विष्टं कुर्वन्त्स्विष्टकृत्स्विष्टमद्य करोतु नो वसुवने वसुधेयस्य वेतु यज ॥

---
[18]तिस्रो देवी: The repetition of these words is meant to show their importance.
[20]Vanaspati: The herb that rears the rays of the sun.
Earth and Space: The herbs suck sustenance from the Earth and fill the space with water drawn by the rays of the Sun out of them.

22. O learned person, just as efficacious fire, with diverse uses, heightens the noble soul, and just as fire accomplishing the desired ambition, being highly serviceable, fulfils our cherished aim, so shouldst thou ever contribute to our happiness, amass wealth, and give monetary help to the scientist in this precious world!

२३. अग्निमद्य होतारमवृणीतायं यजमान: पचन्पक्ती: पचन्पुरोडाशं वधन्त्रिन्द्राय छागम् ।
सुपस्था अद्य देवो वनस्पतिरभवदिन्द्राय छागेन ।
अद्यत्तं मेदस्त: प्रति पचताग्रभीदवीवृधत्पुरोडाशेन त्वामद्य ऋषे ॥

23. O learned person, the knower of the significance of vedic hymns, just as this sacrificer, for the sake of supremacy, now cooks foods and special preparations for Homa, keeps a goat, for the removal of diseases, and honours a learned priest, expert in the performance of yajna; and just as the shining Sun, protector of its rays, for grandeur's sake, becomes eminent at the time of sacrifice, by cutting into pieces and absorbing the oily and wet oblations, which come into contact with it, the ripener of all objects; and just as the Sun accepts all substances put into the fire and grows thereby, so do I exert to make thee prosperous!

२४. होता यक्षत्समिधानं महद्यश: सुसमिद्धं वरेण्यमग्निमिन्द्रं वयोधसम् ।
गायत्रीं छन्द इन्द्रियं त्र्यवि गां वयो दधद्वेत्वाज्यस्य होतर्यज ॥

24. O seeker after knowledge, just as a charitably disposed learned person, performs Havan, and preserves the Gayatri verse, brilliant like fire, splendidly graceful, venerable, highly glorious, bestower of beautiful life, bringer of supremacy, expounder of true significance; and retains freedom, wealth, three-fold protecting vedic speech, and longevity, and enjoys the essence of knowledge, so shouldst thou perform yajna!

२५. होता यक्षत्तनूनपातमुद्भिदं यं गर्भमदितिर्दधे शुचिमिन्द्रं वयोधसम् ।
उष्णिहं छन्द इन्द्रियं दित्यवाहं गां वयो दधद्वेत्वाज्यस्य होतर्यज ॥

25. O seeker after knowledge, just as the preserver of noble qualities, preserves him, like a mother preserving the embryo, the protector of the body, the comer-out after splitting the mother's womb, and sends Homa's oblations to the pure Sun, the prolonger of life, and preserving through the divine Ushnik verse, the powerful organs of the soul like ear etc., preaching practical wisdom, and rearing handsome birds, enjoys all these nature's gifts, so shouldst thou enjoy them!

[23]I: The Purohit, the priest.
[24]Three-fold protecting: Vedic speech protects our body, mind and tongue. The learned teacher should teach the people, the Gayatri Mantra, self-control, observance of Brahmcharya, and the art of enjoying long life.
[25]Preserves him: rears, guards, and protects the pupil.

२६. होता यक्षदीड़ेन्यमीडितं वृत्रहन्तममिडाभिरीड्यꣶ सह: सोममिन्द्रं वयोधसम् ।
अनुष्टुभं छन्द इन्द्रियं पञ्चाविं गां वयो दधद्वेत्वाज्यस्य होतर्यज ॥

26. O sacrificer, just as a man possessing noble qualities, comes in contact with the Sun, the slayer of clouds, so should he come with instructive words, in contact with adorable, adored power, laudable medicinal herbs, and the soul, the sustainer of beautiful breaths. He enjoys all nature's gifts, the organs like ear, sustainable freedom, the Earth, the protector of five breaths and desirable objects in this knowable world, so shouldst thou enjoy them all!

२७. होता यक्षत्सुबर्हिषं पूषण्वन्तममर्त्यꣶ सीदन्तं बर्हिषि प्रियेऽमृतेन्द्रं वयोधसम् ।
बृहतीं छन्द इन्द्रियं त्रिवत्सं गां वयो दधद्वेत्वाज्यस्य होतर्यज ॥

27. O charitably disposed person, just as a virtuous person, becomes united with the soul immortal, vast like space, immersed in the contemplation of the Beautiful God, deathless in its purity, full of strength, enjoyer of space and pure water, extending over all; and attains to happiness preserving celibacy for 36 years like the 36 syllables of Brihati metre, full of knowledge, physical organs, vedic lore, having action, worship and knowledge as its sons, and enjoys nice pleasure, so shouldst thou do!

२८. होता यक्षद्द्वचस्वती: सुप्रायणा ऋतावृधो द्वारो देवीर्हिरण्ययीर्ब्रह्माणमिन्द्रं वयोधसम् ।
पङ्क्तिं छन्द इहेन्द्रियं तुर्यवाहं गां वयो दधद्दचन्त्वाज्यस्य होतर्यज ॥

28. O sacrificer, just as in this world, a virtuous person, possesses wide-opening portals, easy to pass through, Yajna strengthening, electroplated and beautiful; and just as he associates with a learned person, full of knowledge and wisdom, with mastery over the four vedas; and observes Brahmcharya for forty years like the forty syllables of the Pankti metre, has got wealth, strong bulls able to carry, four times the luggage, and vital vigour; and just as he performs Homa with these oblations mixed with ghee, and just as other persons resort to yajna, so shouldst thou perform sacrifice with these oblations!

२९. होता यक्षत्सुपेशसा सुशिल्पे बृहती उभे नक्तोषासा न दर्शते विश्वमिन्द्रं वयोधसम् ।
त्रिष्टुभं छन्द इहेन्द्रियं पष्ठवाहं गां वयो दधद्वीतामाज्यस्य होतर्यज ॥

29. O sacrificer, just as in this world, like two lofty Day and Night, lovely to look at, in which beautiful works of art and industry are performed; the

---

[27]Brihati metre: It consists of 36 syllables, so a virtuous man should observe celibacy for 36 years.

त्रिवत्सम्: This word has been translated by Mahidhar, Ubbat and Griffith as 3 years old steer, whereas Maharshi Dayananda translates it as vedic lore having action, worship, and knowledge as its sons, i.e., subjects dealt with.

[28]Sacrificer: One who performs yajna.

A learned person should construct houses, with wide, electroplated gates, with open space for performing yajnas and beautiful in appearance.

beautiful teacher and preacher; acquire excellent supremacy, the support of ambition, and celibacy of forty four years like 44 syllables of the Trishtup metre, vitality, longevity, strength of physical organs, and possess bullocks fit to carry luggage on the back, and just as a virtuous person, uses oblations mixed with ghee, so shouldst thou perform Havan!

३०. होता यक्षत्प्रचेतसा देवानामुत्तमं यशो होतारा दैव्या कवी सयुजेन्द्रं वयोधसम् ।
जगतीं छन्द इन्द्रियमनड्वाहं गां वयो दधद्धीतामाज्यस्य होतर्यज ॥

30. O charitably disposed person, just an intelligent teacher and pupil, highly educated amongst the learned, sociable, doers of good deeds, givers of knowledge, masters of great fame, and desired happiness, acquire grandeur, celibacy of 48 years like the 48 syllables of the Jagati metre, learning, wealth, and bullocks to carry the cart, and just as a virtuous person, offers oblations mixed with ghee, so shouldst thou. perform Homa!

३१. होता यक्षत्पेशस्वतीस्तिस्रो देवीर्हिरण्ययीर्भारतीबृंहती मंही: पतिमिन्द्रं वयोधसम् ।
विराजं छन्द इहेन्द्रियं धेनुं गां न वयो दधद्वचन्त्वाज्यस्य होतर्यज ॥

31. O sacrificer, just as in this world, a virtuous person acquires three kinds of speech precious like gold, and beautiful, namely Bharati, Brihati, Mahi; an aged protecting ruler, a Brahmchari observing vow of celibacy for 33 years, like 33 syllables of the Virat metre, the expositor of various subjects, desired object, and happiness enjoyed by souls and comes in contact with us like a milch cow, so shouldst thou, attaining to all these objects acquire the desirable fruit of knowledge!

३२. होता यक्षत्सुरेतसं त्वष्टारं पुष्टिवर्धनं रूपाणि बिभ्रत् पृथक् पुष्टिमिन्द्रं वयोधसम् ।
द्विपदं छन्द इन्द्रियमुक्षाणं गां न वयो दधद्रेत्वाज्यस्य होतर्यज ॥

32. O charitably disposed person, just a virtuous persons protects a man full of glory and vigour, advanced in age, maintaining varied beautiful qualities, strengthener of growth, brilliant, and heroic, and sustains two-footed human beings, liberty, vigour of physical organs, and maintains strength like a full-grown ox, and performs Homa with vedic texts, understanding their significance, so shouldst thou perform Homa!

३३. होता यक्षद्वनस्पतिं शमितारं शतक्रतुं हिरण्यपर्णमुक्षिथनं रशनां बिभ्रत् वशिं भगमिन्द्रं वयोधसम् ।
ककुभं छन्द इहेन्द्रियं वशां वेहतं गां वयो दधद्रेत्वाज्यस्य होतर्यज ॥

33. O charitably disposed person, just as in this world, a performer of

---

[31]Bharati: Worthy of assimilation.
Brihati: Deep and meditative.
Mahi: Resorted to by great men.

[33]Just as a barren cow being mated with powerful bulls produces nothing and keeps their semen under her control, so as performer of yajna controls all those who attempt to disturb the yajna. Just as a calf-slipping cow, being pregnant destroys embryo through miscarriage, so a strong sacrificer destroys the enemies and intruders in his yajna.

yajna with ghee, like the Sun, the giver of tranquillity, the protector with its light and beams; masters the soul, full of wisdom, uttering commendable words with finger, worthy of control, full of grace, giver of the strength of life; and acquires wealth, the prop of worldly prosperity and giver of felicity, and performs yajna with gladness possessing desired object, and qualities of a barren and calf-slipping cow; so shouldst thou perform yajna!

३४. होता यक्षत्स्वाहाकृतीरग्निं गृहपतिं पृथग्वरुणं भेषजं कविं क्षत्रमिन्द्रं वयोधसम् । अतिच्छन्दसं छन्द इन्द्रियं बृहद्दृषभं गां वयो दधद्चन्त्वाज्यस्य होतर्यज ॥

34. O sacrificer, just as a virtuous person, preserves a householder, brilliant like fire, in which oblations are put with vedic recitations; and associates severally with a noble person, an experienced physician, a sagacious, aged king, and his government; and observes prolonged Brahmcharya like the syllables of Atichhandas and Gayatri metres, and possesses the strength of a strong bull, enjoys long life; and performs? Homa with ghee oblations, liked by all ; so shouldst thou perform yajna!

३५. देवं बर्हिर्वयोधसं देवमिन्द्रमवर्धयत् । गायत्र्या छन्दसेन्द्रियं चक्षुरिन्द्रे वयो दधद्सुवने वसुधेयस्य वेतु यज ॥

35. O learned person, just as well-merited space develops the beautiful, life-infusing Sun, and just as a yogi through Gayatri metre establishes in the soul, the power of perceive like an eye, and enjoy long life, and befriends a man, who makes the best use of the riches of this world, the source of all wealth, so shouldst thou perform yajna!

३६. देवीद्वारो वयोधसः शुचिमिन्द्रमवर्धयन् । उष्णिहा छन्दसेन्द्रियं प्राणमिन्द्रे वयो दधद्सुवने वसुधेयस्य व्यन्तु यज ॥

36. O learned person, just as the lustrous doors of our houses, allow full and free entry of life-infusing, pure air, and develop the breath in the soul, conducive to its welfare, residence in which increases the treasure of one aspiring after riches, and thus they become graceful, so shouldst thou with vedic verses in Ushnik metre secure these lovely objects and perform Havan!

३७. देवी उषासानक्ता देवमिन्द्रं वयोधसं देवी देवमवर्धताम् । अनुष्टुभा छन्दसेन्द्रियं बलमिन्द्रे वयो दधद्सुवने वसुधेयस्य वीतां यज ॥

37. O learned person just as like Day and Night two ladies, the teachress and the taught, develop the strength-giving and virtuous soul, and just as a wife advances the noble husband, and bears children from one aspiring after

---

[34]Atichhandas: Ati Dhriti, Ati Ashti, Ati Shakvari, and Ati jagati are called Atichhandas with 76, 68, 60 and 48 syllables. A learned virtuous person is ordained to remain celibate even upto 60, 68, 76, years like the syllables of Atichhandas.

[36]Residence in houses with wide open doors which admit air from all sides increases age, strength, health, wealth and mental peace.

treasure and riches; so shouldst thou with vedic verses in Anushtup metre, acquire the strength of soul enjoyed by it throughout life!

३८. देवी जोष्ट्री वसुधिती देवमिन्द्रं वयोधसं देवी देवमवर्धताम् ।
ब्रुहत्या छन्दसेन्द्रिय ॐ श्रोत्रमिन्द्रे वयो दधद्वसुवने वसुधेयस्य वीतां यज ॥

38. O learned person, just as dignified, affectionate ladies, fond of knowledge, advance their virtuous children, the givers of sustenance and preservers of life, and just as a noble wife glorifies her noble husband, and cultivates with vedic verses in Brihati metre, in the soul, the power of hearing created by God, so shouldst thou enjoying happiness, resulting from the due use of wealth, perform Havan!

३६. देवी ऊर्जाहुती दुघे सुदुघे पयसेन्द्रं वयोधसं देवी देवमवर्धताम् ।
पङ्क्त्या छन्दसेन्द्रिय ॐ शुक्रमिन्द्रे वयो दधद्वसुवने वसुधेयस्य वीतां यज ॥

39. O learned person, just as oblations of purified cereals, fillers of objects with juice, accomplishers of aims, full of fragrance, advance through rain water the soul, preserving life, as a devoted, educated wife advances her husband of high moral character; and with the aid of Pankti verses fill the soul with heroism and affluence, so shouldst thou enjoying happiness, resulting from the proper use of wealth, perform Havan!

४०. देवा द॑व्या होतारा देवमिन्द्रं वयोधसं देवौ देवमवर्धताम् ।
त्रिष्टुभा छन्दसेन्द्रियं त्विषिमिन्द्रे वयो दधद्वसुवने वसुधेयस्य वीतां यज ॥

40. O charitably disposed teacher and preacher, just as lovely learned persons, fulfillers of our ambitions, develop the wishful and life-preserving soul, as parents develop their son; so should ye associate with a person aspiring after wealth. O learned person, so shouldst thou, with the aid of Trishtup verses, developing the soul's power of hearing and enjoying happiness, perform noble deeds like the yajna!

४१. देवीस्तिस्रस्तिस्रो देवीर्वयोधसं पतिमिन्द्रमवर्धयन्
जगत्या छन्दसेन्द्रिय ॐ शूष्मिन्द्रे वयो दधद्वसुवने वसुधेयस्य व्यन्तु यज ॥

41. O learned person, just as Goddesses three, three Goddesses, heighten the king, the protector and possessor of vital force, and pervade everywhere, so shouldst thou with Jagati verses, developing in thy soul the strength of overpowering the enemy's force, and enhancing the vitality of thy physical

---

[38]Ladies: Teachress and her girl students.
[39]According to Pt. Jaidev Vidyalankar, 'Pankti Chhandas' means the act of cooking meals.
[40]Trishtup verse: The military force, according to Pt. Jaidev Vidyalankar.
[41]Three goddesses: Teacher, Preacher, Examiner, three learned ladies. These words have been repeated for the sake of emphasis.

organs, perform yajna like the sacrificer, who gives away his treasure and wealth in charity!

४२. देवो नराशँसो देवमिन्द्र ँवयोधसं देवो देववर्धयत् ।
विराजा छन्दसेन्द्रियँ ँरूपमिन्द्रे वयो दधद्ध्रुसुवने वसुधेयस्य वेतु यज ॥

42. O learned person, just as a person, praised by all, strengthens the king, advanced in age, and endowed with noble qualities, actions and nature, as an educated person strengthens a pupil hankering after knowledge, and develops in the soul, beauty and power, with verses in virat metre, so shouldst thou, enjoying the desired happiness, perform yajna for one who uses properly his treasure and wealth!

४३. देवो वनस्पतिर्देवमिन्द्रं वयोधसं देवो देववर्धयत् ।
द्विपदा छन्दसेन्द्रियं भगमिन्द्रे वयो दधद्ध्रुसुवने वसुधेयस्य वेतु यज ॥

43. O learned person, just as the nice fig-tree, the Forest Sovereign, enhances long-lived, excellent prosperity, like a cultured person conducing to the welfare of another well mannered educated man; so with Dwipada verses, thou shouldst establish fortune and strength in the soul, and enjoying the desired happiness perform yajna for him who gives his treasure in charity!

४४. देवं बर्हिर्वारितीनां देवमिन्द्रं वयोधसं देवं देववर्धयत् ।
ककुभा छन्दसेन्द्रियं यश इन्द्रे वयो दधद्ध्रुसुवने वसुधेयस्य वेतु यज ॥

44. O learned person, just as nice water in the atmospheric ocean, contributes to the welfare of an aged, good ruler, and a developed soul develops another soul, so shouldst thou with Kakup verses, for full prosperity, acquire fame and vital strength, and enjoying the wished for happiness, perform yajna for him who makes proper use of his riches!

४५. देवो अग्निः स्विष्टकृद्देवमिन्द्रं वयोधसं देवो देववर्धयत् ।
अतिच्छन्दसा छन्दसेन्द्रियं क्षत्रमिन्द्रे वयो दधद्ध्रुसुवने वसुधेयस्य वेतु यज ॥

45. O learned person, just as the Omniscient God, the Fulfiller of our desires and aims, strengthens the long-lived, virtuous soul, as a teacher strengthens the pupil, so shouldst thou with the pleasant Ati Jagati verses perform yajna, so that thou possessing sway, vital strength, fascinating nature, mayest improve the king full of learning and humility, and giver of charity from his treasure!

[43]Dwipada: with the strength of the two-footed servants according to Pt. Jaidev Vidyalankar.
[44]Kakup: a metre of 3 padas 8+12+8 syllables.
[45]Atichhandas: hypermeter; any metre of more than forty-eight syllables.

४६. अग्निमद्य होतारमवृणीतायं यजमान: पचन्पक्ती: पचन्पुरोडाशं बधन्त्रिन्द्राय वयोधसे छागम् ।
सूपस्था अद्य देवो वनस्पतिरभवदिन्द्राय वयोधसे छागेन । अघत्तं मेदस्त: प्रतिपचताग्रभी-
दवीवृधत्पुरोडाशेन त्वामद्य ऋषे ॥

46. O learned person, the knower of the significance of vedic hymns, just as this sacrificer, cooking different kinds of meals and making special preparations for Homa, honours today a learned priest expert in the performance of yajna, so for the sake of longevity and supremacy, shouldst thou keep a goat, the remover of diseases!

Just as a learned person, the protector of forests, becomes ready with the help of a scholar, the remover of doubts, for serving the king, the advancer of our life and the extirpator of foes, so should all people live together peacefully. Just as the sacrificer, feeds thee with the yajna preparations and greasy substances, and develops thee physically, so should you, the sacrificer and the priest eat yajna remnants.

⁴⁶This verse is the same as 23rd in this chapter, but with a different interpretation.

CHAPTER XXIX

१. समिद्धो अञ्जन् कृदरं मतीनां घृतमग्ने मधुमत्पिन्वमान: ।
वाजी वहन् वाजिनं जातवेदो देवानां वक्षि प्रियमा सधस्थम् ॥

1. O learned person, brilliant like fire, famous for sagacity, just as fire enkindled, manifesting itself, strengthens the belly of men, and enjoying the highly efficacious butter, achieves stability through educated priests, as a skilled rider makes the horse move fast; so shouldst thou attain to the desired abode of pleasure.

२. घृतेनाऽञ्जन्त्सं पथो देवयानान् प्रजानन् वाज्यपेतु देवान् ।
अनु त्वा सप्ते प्रदिश: सचन्ताꣳ स्वधामस्मै यजमानाय धेहि ॥

2. O learned person, active like the horse, just as fast electricity, being produced from water, illuminates the paths wherein tread the learned, wielding mastery over it, enjoy thou the company of the wise, whereby thou mayest control all quarters and directions. Bestow thou food on this sacrificer!

३. ईड्यश्चासि वन्द्यश्च वाजिन्नाशुश्चासि मेध्यश्च सप्ते ।
अग्निष्ट्वा देवेर्वसुभि: सजोषा: प्रीतं वहि वहतु जातवेदा: ॥

3. O active, enterprising, educated artisan, as thou, full of enjoyments and kindness, utilisest adorable fire, by mixing it with serviceable material objects, which takes thee to distant places, hence thou art worthy of praise, veneration, swiftness, and companionship!

४. स्तीर्णं बर्हि: सुष्टरीमा जुषाणोरु पृथु प्रथमानं पृथिव्याम् ।
देवेभिर्युक्तमदिति: सजोषा: स्योनं कृण्वाना सुविते दधातु ॥

4. O learned person, just as we nicely expand electricity widely diffused on the earth, famous, pervading all parts of conveyances, water and space, enjoyed by the people, present in heavenly bodies, giver of comfort, indestructible, affording seat to all in electric planes, so shouldst thou do!

५. एता उ व: सुभगा विश्वरूपा वि पक्षोभि: श्रयमाणा उदाते: ।
ऋष्वा: सती: कवष: शुम्भमाना द्वारो देवी: सुप्रायणा भवन्तु ॥

5. May these your doors, beautiful, wearing different colours, lofty, sonorous, lovely, rich in adornment, offer easy passage into houses both right and left, like two rows of birds.

²It: Electricity.

६. अन्तरा मित्रावरुणा चरन्ती मुखं यज्ञानामभि संविदाने ।
उषासा वा𝄇 सुहिरण्ये सुशिल्पे ऋतस्य योनाविह सादयामि ॥

6. Just as in the body Pran and Udan regulate all its functions, so, both morning and evening tell us of the time of commencement of the yajna. They are beautiful and full of light. I establish them in this house for the sake of truth.

७. प्रथमा वा𝄇 सरथिना सुवर्णा देवौ पश्यन्तौ भुवनानि विश्वा ।
अपिप्रयं चोदना वां मिमाना होतारा ज्योतिः प्रदिशा दिशन्ता ॥

7. O teacher and preacher, ye both, excellent amongst all, borne on one car, bright coloured, beholding all creatures, ye charitable, seers, and spreaders of light!

I always keep ye happy and contented. Ye both, knowing the vedic rules and ordinances, charitable in disposition, preach the light of knowledge, with your supreme intellect.

८. आदित्यैर्नो भारती वष्टु यज्ञ𝄇 सरस्वती सह रुद्रैर्न आवीत् ।
इडोपहूता वसुभिः सजोषा यज्ञं नो देवीरमृतेषु धत्त ॥

8. May Bharati, the speech of the Adityas, illuminate your yajna. May Saraswati, the speech of the Rudras, be our helper. May Ida, the speech invoked in accord by the Vasus give us happiness. May these three Goddesses place us amongst the immortals.

९. त्वष्टा वीरं देवकामं जजान त्वष्टुर्वा जायत आशुरश्वः ।
त्वष्टेदं विश्वं भुवनं जजान बहोः कर्तारमिह यक्षि होतः ॥

9. Just as a learned person, produces a brave son devoted to scholars; just as a horse learns through instruction how to run fast and remain active; just as Self-Effulgent God brings to life this universe; so shouldst thou Priest worship God, the Creator of the world!

१०. अश्वो घृतेन त्मन्या समक्त उप देवाँ२ ऋतुशः पाथ एतु ।
वनस्पतिर्देवलोकं प्रजानन्नग्निना हव्या स्वदितानि वक्षत् ॥

10. O learned person, knowing well the path of the sages, the benefactors of humanity; just as fast-moving fire, coupled with water, itself, in different seasons, performing useful deeds, gives us food, and just as the Sun, the protector of rays, carries away our sweet oblations, so shouldst thou deal properly with thy soul!

*Adityas: Persons having first class knowledge, after observing celibacy for 48 years.
Rudras: Those who observe celibacy for 36 years, and possess good knowledge.
Vasus: Who observe celibacy for 24 years, and possess ordinary knowledge.
Bharati: Speech full of information and vigour.
Saraswati: Speech full of knowledge.
Ida: Speech full of praise.

११. प्रजापतेस्तपसा वावृधानः सद्यो जातो दधिषे यज्ञमग्ने ।
स्वाहाकृतेन हविषा पुरोगा याहि साध्या हविरदन्तु देवाः ॥

11. O learned person, brilliant like fire, progressing and soon attaining to fame, through God's grace, thou guardest the sacrifice with consecrated offering. Go unto those leading sages, who, achieving success through their accomplishments, eat our oblations!

१२. यदक्रन्दः प्रथमं जायमान उद्यन्त्समुद्रादुत वा पुरीषात् ।
श्येनस्य पक्षा हरिणस्य बाहू उपस्तुत्यं महि जातं ते अर्वन् ॥

12. O learned person, active like a horse, when thou roarest with full splendour, like air created in the beginning by God from the atmosphere, and the arms of thy hero become strong like eagle-pinions, thou deservest applause for this glaring great deed!

१३. यमेन दत्तं त्रित एनमायुनगिन्द्र एणं प्रथमो अध्यतिष्ठत् ।
गन्धर्वो अस्य रशनामगृभ्णात् सूरादश्वं वसवो निरतष्ट ॥

13. O learned persons, air creates electricity from the Earth, water and space, and yokes it to useful ends. In conjunction with air, diffused, renowned electricity, assumes sway everywhere. It receives the rays of the Sun, the protector of the earth; and makes subtle with the Sun, the fast moving air!

१४. असि यमो अस्यादित्यो अर्वन्नसि त्रितो गुह्येन व्रतेन ।
असि सोमेन समया विपृक्त आहुस्ते त्रीणि दिवि बन्धनानि ॥

14. O man, full of force like fire, by mysterious nature; thou art coupled with action, contemplation and knowledge; thou art disciplined like a just ruler; thou art resplendent with knowledge like the Sun; thou art like a learned person; thou art specially united with grandeur. They say there are three bonds in the spread of knowledge that hold thee.

१५. त्रीणि त आहुर्दिवि बन्धनानि त्रीण्यप्सु त्रीयन्तः समुद्रे ।
उतेव मे वरुणश्छन्त्स्यर्वन् यत्रा त आहुः परमं जनित्रम् ॥

15. O learned person, the sages say, there are three bonds in the spread of knowledge that hold thee; three bonds in the control of breath, three bonds in the atmosphere that cause rain; they speak of thy sublimest birth, and thou payest homage to those noble learned souls; may they all be connected with me through deliberation!

[13]It: Electricity.
[14]Three bonds: Three debts one owes to the sages, the parents and the learned, called Rishi ऋण, Pitri ऋण, and Deva ऋण.
[15]Bonds of breath: food, seed and tillage.
Bonds of atmosphere: cloud, lightning and thunder.

१६. इमा ते वाजिन्नवमार्जनानीमा शफानाꣳ सनितुर्निधाना ।
अत्रा ते भद्रा रशना अपश्यमृतस्य या अभिरक्षन्ति गोपाः ॥

16. O enterprising commander of the army, just as I look after the bathing procedures of these horses of yours, and the places for the protection of their hooves; just as in this army, I see the auspicious reins of the horses, which save us from misfortune, and direct their right usage, so shouldst thou see!

१७. आत्मानं ते मनसारादजानामवो दिवा पतयन्तं पतङ्गम् ।
शिरो अपश्यं पथिभिः सुगेभिररेणुभिर्जेहमानं पतत्रि ॥

17. O learned person I recognise thy soul going high up from below, like the Sun in heaven. Just as I see the aeroplanes from far, and round like the head, soaring, striving upward by paths unsoiled by dust, and pleasant to travel, so shouldst thou see!

१८. अत्रा ते रूपमुत्तममपश्यं जिगीषमाणमिष आ पदे गोः ।
यदा ते मर्त्तो अनु भोगमानडादिद् ग्रसिष्ठ ओषधीरजीगः ॥

18. O brave person, I behold thy form matchless in beauty, eager to win foes and the food produced here from the Earth. Whenever a man brings thee thy eatables, thou, then, being the most voracious eater, swallowest medicines!

१९. अनु त्वा रथो अनु मर्यो अर्वन्ननु गावोऽनु भगः कनीनाम् ।
अनु व्रातासस्तव सख्यमीयुरनु देवा ममिरे वीर्यं ते ॥

19. O learned person, when the learned amongst the graceful persons, long for thy friendship, and educated persons favourably measure thy vigour, the aeroplanes, ordinary run of mankind, kine and supremacy follow thee!

२०. हिरण्यशृङ्गोऽयो अस्य पादा मनोजवा अवर इन्द्र आसीत् ।
देवा इदस्य हविरद्यमायन् यो अर्वन्तं प्रथमो अध्यतिष्ठत् ॥

20. O people, know that the head of the state should be sharp and brilliant like horns, and lustrous like lightning. Like a horse marching on his path, the king should be the first lord of fire and gold. His feet should possess the velocity of mind. The members of his Cabinet should receive their maintenance allowance from him!

[16]I: King.
   Which: Reins.
   Their: Horses.
[17]I: King.
[20]Lord of fire: The king should possess planes for travelling.
   Velocity of mind: The king should generally fly in air with the velocity of mind, to save time.

२१. ईमन्तास: शिलिकमध्यमास: स॒ शूरणासो दिव्यासो अत्या: ।
हँसा इव श्रेणिशो यतन्ते यदाक्षिषुर्दिव्यमज्ममश्वा: ॥

21. O men possess horses fiery in spirit, with attractive places to sit on, thin bellied, quick conquerors of battles, well trained, fast in motion, putting forth their strength like swans in lengthened order, and treading on pure paths!

२२. तव शरीरं पतयिष्णुर्वर्तन्तव चित्तं वात इव ध्रजीमान् ।
तव श्रृङ्गाणि विष्ठिता पुरुत्रारण्येषु जर्भुराणा चरन्ति ॥

22. O brave person, thy body is mortal, but thy spirit is swift like the wind in motion. Thy soldiers are spread abroad in all directions, and being stout and strong move about in many wildernesses; follow thou the path of virtue!

२३. उप प्रागाच्छसनं वाज्यर्वा देवद्रीचा मनसा दीध्यान: ।
अज: पुरो नीयते नाभिरस्यानु पश्चात्कवयो यन्ति रेभा: ॥

23. The beautiful, lustrous, active, fast, dexterous horse, in the company of the learned, merrily goes to the battle-field. The valiant ride on its back, and the wise singing the praise of knowledge follow it.

२४. उप प्रागात्परमं यत्सधस्थमर्वाँ२ अच्छा पितरं मातरं च ।
अद्या देवाञ्जुष्टतमो हि गम्या अथा शास्ते दाशुषे वार्याणि ॥

24. The learned person, who being highly respected, longs for the eminent position of friends, educated father and mother and the sages, and exceedingly acquires eatables for the donor, deserves to be loved by all.

२५. समिद्धो अद्य मनुषो दुरोणे देवो देवान् यजसि जातवेद: ।
आ च वह मित्रमहश्चिकित्वान्त्वं दूत: कविरसि प्रचेता: ॥

25. O wise person, respecter of friends, thou, this day, kindled like the illuminated fire, walkest in their company, as a reflective, literary person. Rich in intellect, tormentor of the wicked, highly conscious, possessing unobstructed knowledge of all subjects, cultivate fully noble virtues in the house!

२६. तनूनपात्पथ ऋतस्य यानान्मध्वा समञ्जन्त्स्वदया सुजिह्व ।
मन्मानि धीभिरुत यज्ञमृन्धन् देवत्रा च कृणुह्यध्वरं न: ॥

26. O fair-tongued, preserver of various objects, make pleasant for all, the commendable paths of rectitude, with thy sweet sermon and excellent

---

[23]Excellent horses are helpful in gaining victory in a battle.

exposition. Develop the society and philosophical subjects with thy holy thoughts, and strengthen our innocuous worship through learned persons!

२७. नराशꣳसस्य महिमानमेषामुप स्तोषाम यजतस्य यज्ञैः ।
ये सुक्रतवः शुचयो धियन्धाः स्वदन्ति देवा उभयानि हव्या ॥

27. To these the pure, the most wise, the thought-inspiring learned persons, who enjoy food conducive both to body and soul, who are worthy of veneration, respected by the people, and full of greatness, we offer admiration with deeds of devotion.

२८. आजुह्वान ईड्यो वन्द्यश्चा याह्यग्ने वसुभिः सजोषाः ।
त्वं देवानामसि यह्व होता स एनान्यक्षीषितो यजीयान् ॥

28. O learned person, full of noble qualities, amongst scholars, thou art charitable and companionable. Walk in the company of these prompt scholars. Being lovely towards the learned, deserving praise and adoration, go near them!

२९. प्राचीनं बर्हिः प्रदिशा पृथिव्या वस्तोरस्या वृज्यते अग्रे अह्नाम् ।
व्यु प्रथते वितरं वरीयो देवेभ्यो अदितये स्योनम् ॥

29. O men, in this world, the Immortal God, All-pervading like space, beyond the light of day, early in the morning before dawn, grants to the learned and immortal soul happiness that removes miseries and is most excellent. Know and realise Him following the instructions of the vedas!

३०. व्यचस्वतीर्विया वि श्रयन्तां पतिभ्यो न जनयः शुम्भमानाः ।
देवीर्द्वारो बृहतीर्विश्वमिन्वा देवेभ्यो भवत सुप्रायणाः ॥

30. O men, learn all sciences, just as wives, highly cultured and virtuous, well experienced in all domestic dealings, dwellers in nice houses, decorated with ornaments, tall like doors, deck their beauty for their noble husbands, and serve them!

३१. आ सुष्वयन्ती यजते उपाके उपासानक्ता सदतां नि योनौ ।
दिव्ये योषणे बृहती सुरुक्मे अधि श्रियꣳ शुक्रपिशं दधाने ॥

31. O learned person, acquire prosperity by properly using day and night, that move continuously in the wheel of time, each close to each, seated at their stations, assuming light and darkness, lofty, fair and radiant beauty like two women!

---
[29]Those who say their prayer and remember God early in the morning before sunrise, attain to happiness and get freedom from misery.

CHAPTER XXIX

३२. दैव्या होतारा प्रथमा सुवाचा मिमाना यज्ञं मनुषो यजध्यै ।
प्रचोदयन्ता विदथेषु कारू प्राचीनं ज्योति: प्रदिशा दिशन्ता ॥

32. O men, learn fine arts from two skilled persons, who are competent amongst the learned, charitably disposed, well-known, sweet-voiced, executors of projects, inducers of men in scientific knowledge, and acts of sacrifice, preachers of the doctrines of the vedas, and expounders of mechanical knowledge!

३३. आ नो यज्ञं भारती तूयमेत्विडा मनुष्वदिह चेतयन्ती ।
तिस्रो देवीर्बर्हिरेदꣳ स्योनꣳ सरस्वती स्वपस: सदन्तु ॥

33. May Bharati, Ida, Saraswati, in this mechanical work, come unto us from all sides, speedily expounding the secrets of mechanical science, like a thoughtful person. May these three intellectual forces, guide us, the performers of nice enterprises, in this mighty project, the source of comfort.

३४. य इमे द्यावापृथिवी जनित्री रूपैरपिꣳशद्भुवनानि विश्वा ।
तमद्य होतरिषितो यजीयान् देवं त्वष्टारमिह यक्षि विद्वान् ॥

34. O seeker after knowledge, extremely fond of companionship, urged, receiving education from everywhere, thou deservest homage, as thou always rememberest that God, Who, in this world, creates different spheres, these Earth and Sun, the progenitors of various actions and brings about the creation and dissolution of the universe!

३५. उपावसृज त्मन्या समञ्जन् देवानां पाथ ऋतुथा हवींषि ।
वनस्पति: शमिता देवो अग्नि: स्वदन्तु हव्यं मधुना घृतेन ॥

35. O learned person, put into fire, at different seasons, with devotion, in the form of oblations, eatables mixed with honey and butter, fit to be taken by the learned. May the Sun, cloud and fire receive thy oblations!

३६. सद्यो जातो व्यमिमीत यज्ञमग्निर्देवानामभवत् पुरोगा: ।
अस्य होतु: प्रदिश्यृतस्य वाचि स्वाहाकृतꣳ हविरदन्तु देवा: ॥

36. The enlightened person, who speedily attains to fame, and manages different transactions, with truth-imbued of words of a learned fellow, and precedes scholars, and the remnants of whose properly performed Homa are eaten by the learned, deserves all round veneration.

[32] The word कारू in the verse means two persons, one of whom is skilled in teaching fine arts, and the other is expert in handicrafts.

[33] Bharati: The knowledge of fine arts.
Ida: Beautiful, trained, sweet voice.
Saraswati : Wisdom full of knowledge.

[35] Articles put into the fire in the performance of Havan, being rarefied reach the sun and cloud.

[36] Remnants: the शेष residue of the yajna.

३७. केतुं कृण्वन्नकेतवे पेशो मर्या अपेशसे ।
समुषद्भिरजायथाः ॥

37. O men, making the illiterate, literate, the poor, rich, shine, with the beams of knowledge.

३८. जीमूतस्येव भवति प्रतीकं यद्वर्मी याति समदामुपस्थे ।
अनाविद्धया तन्वा जय त्वꣳ स त्वा वर्मणो महिमा पिपर्तु ॥

38. The warrior's look is like the thunderous rain-cloud, when, armed with mail, he seeks the lap of battle. Be thou victorious with unwounded body, and let the strength of thy armour save thee.

३९. धन्वना गा धन्वनाऽऽजिं जयेम धन्वना तीव्राः समदो जयेम ।
धनुः शत्रोरपकामं कृणोति धन्वना सर्वाः प्रदिशो जयेम ॥

39. With military weapons let us win the Earth, with them the battle, with cannon let us win the ease-loving army of our foes. War-like weapons destroy the ambitions of the foeman. Armed with the bow may we subdue all regions.

४०. वक्ष्यन्तीवेदा गनीगन्ति कर्ण प्रियꣳ सखायं परिषस्वजाना ।
योषेव शिङ्क्ते वितताधि धन्वꣳज्या इयꣳ समने पारयन्ती ॥

40. This bow-string strained on the bow whispers like a woman, and preserves us in the combat, as a wife, fain to speak, offering advice, embraces her affectionate, praiseworthy husband.

४१. ते आचरन्ती समनेव योषा मातेव पुत्रं विभृतामुपस्थे ।
अप शत्रून् विध्यताꣳ संविदाने आर्त्नी इमे विष्फुरन्ती अमित्रान् ॥

41. Just as a learned wife behaves towards her husband, and a mother towards her child, so these two bow-strings, well procured, together beat the foes, and in unison scatter asunder, the foes who hate us.

४२. बह्वीनां पिता बहुरस्य पुत्रश्चिश्चा कृणोति समनावगत्य ।
इषुधिः सङ्काः पृतनाश्च सर्वाः पृष्ठे निनद्धो जयति प्रसूतः ॥

42. With many a son, father of many daughters, he clangs and clashes as he goes to battle, with the quiver slung on the back, the born hero, vanquishes all the scattered armies.

४३. रथे तिष्ठन्नयति वाजिनः पुरो यत्र-यत्र कामयते सुषारथिः ।
अभीशूनां महिमानं पनायत मनः पश्चादनु यच्छन्ति रश्मयः ॥

43. The skilful driver, sitting in the cor.veyance, guides his horses in the front, in whichever direction he likes. Just as mind keeps the organs under

---

[37] He is an Apta आप्त, who makes the poor, rich, and the ignorant, wise.
[42] Quivers, arrows and bow-strings are the sons and daughters of a warrior.

control, so reins from behind, control the horse. See and admire the strength of these controlling reins.

४४. तीव्रान् घोषान् कृण्वते वृषपाण्योऽश्वा रथेभिः सह वाजयन्तः ।
अवक्रामन्तः प्रपदैरमित्रान् क्षिणन्ति शत्रुं१ रनपव्ययन्तः ॥

44. Warriors with arms in hand, conveying soldiers swiftly along conveyances, trample upon the foes devoid of friendship, with their forefeet.
Fast running horses neigh loudly. Soldiers not burdening their master economically, destroy their foes.

४५. रथवाहणं हविरस्य नाम यत्रायुधं निहितमस्य वर्म ।
तत्रा रथमुप शग्मं सदेम विश्वाहा वयं सुमनस्यमानाः ॥

45. Let us honour that aeroplane, each day that passes, with hearts full of joy, in which are laid necessary ingredients for propelling it, and gun, cannon, shield, bow, arrow, armour and military equipment of this warrior.

४६. स्वादुषंसदः पितरो वयोधाः कृच्छ्रेश्रितः शक्तीवन्तो गभीराः ।
चित्रसेना इषुबला अमृध्राः सतोवीरा उरवो व्रातसाहाः ॥

46. Let our rulers, be pertakers of savoury food, long-lived, patient in adversity, powerful, deep-minded, armed with wondrous army, strong in arrows, robust, possessors of long legs and broad chests, invincible, and conquerors of numerous hosts.

४७. ब्राह्मणासः पितरः सोम्यासः शिवे नो द्यावापृथिवी अनेहसा ।
पूषा नः पातु दुरितादृतावृधो रक्षा माकिर्नो अघशंस ईशत ॥

47. May virtuous people, promoters of truth, protectors, knowers of God and the vedas, and the Heaven and Earth indestructible in nature, conduce to our welfare. May God, the Nourisher, save us from sinful conduct, guard us, and let not the evil-wisher master us.

४८. सुपर्णं वस्ते मृगो अस्या दन्तो गोभिः सन्नद्धा पतति प्रसूता ।
यत्रा नरः सं च वि च द्रवन्ति तत्रास्मभ्यमिषवः शर्म यंसन् ॥

48. O brave soldiers give us protection in the army, where there are commanders, adequate transport arrangements, where arrows and weapons are used swiftly like a deer, controlled with cow-leather strings, which pounces upon the enemy forcibly, duly persuaded, and its warriors run together or go hither and thither in different directions!

४९. ऋजीते परि वृङ्ग्धि नोऽश्मा भवतु नस्तनूः ।
सोमो अधि ब्रवीतु नोऽदितिः शर्म यच्छतु ॥

49. O learned person, drive straight away diseases from our body, so that it may be strong like stone. Give us instructions about efficacious medicine and Earth, and grant us happiness!

५०. आ जङ्घन्ति सान्वेषां जघनाँ२ उप जिघ्नते ।
अश्वाजनि प्रचेतसोऽश्वान्त्समत्सु चोदय ॥

50. O queen, who trainest horses, just as heroes, whip sharply the back of these horses, and lead young soldiers, so shouldst thou drive sagacious chargers in the battles!

५१. अहिरिव भोगैः पर्येति बाहुं ज्याया हेति परिबाधमानः ।
हस्तघ्नो विश्वा वयुनानि विद्वान् पुमान् पुमाँ॰ सं परि पातु विश्वतः ॥

51. May the energetic learned person, discharging arrow from the bow-string, and extirpating the opposing foe from all sides, protect the virile-person, in every way, and thundering like a cloud with his armies, acquire all sorts of worldly knowledge.

५२. वनस्पते वीड्वङ्गो हि भया अस्मत्सखा प्रतरणः सुवीरः ।
गोभिः सन्नद्धो असि वीडयस्वास्थाता ते जयतु जेत्वानि ॥

52. O king powerful like the Sun, be our friend, conqueror of foes, yoked with brave, victorious heroes, firm and strong in body!
Thou art the possessor of various parts of Earth, make us strong. May thy commander-in-chief win foes deserving defeat.

५३. दिवः पृथिव्याः पर्योज उद्भृतं वनस्पतिभ्यः पर्याभृतँ सहः ।
अपामोज्मानं परि गोभिरावृतमिन्द्रस्य वज्रँ हविषा रथं यज ॥

53. O learned person, give us the vitality possessed by the Sun and Earth, the strength of trees, the vitalising juice of waters. Fill thy car with warlike weapons shining like the sun's rays!

५४. इन्द्रस्य वज्रो मरुतामनीकं मित्रस्य गर्भो वरुणस्य नाभिः ।
सेमां नो हव्यदातिं जुषाणो देव रथ प्रति हव्या गृभाय ॥

54. O beautiful, highly educated person, accepting gifts we offer, know the significance of the fall of lightning, realise the force of the army of men, the inner feelings of friends, the promptings of the soul of the virtuous, and enjoy our company, and all acceptable objects!

५५. उप श्वासय पृथिवीमुत द्यां पुरुत्रा ते मनुतां विष्ठितं जगत् ।
स दुन्दुभे सजूरिन्द्रेण देवैर्दूराद्दवीयो अप सेध शत्रून् ॥

55. O commander, thundering aloud like the drum, being full of supremacy, with the help of the learned, drive thou afar, yea, very far, our foemen. Grant life to the denizens of the Earth, and persons exalted like Heaven. Regard the world as pervaded with space and lightning. May thy rule give thee pleasure!

CHAPTER XXIX

५६. आ क्रन्दय बलमोजो न आधा निष्टनिहि दुरिता बाधमानः ।
अप प्रोथ दुन्दुभे दुच्छुना इत इन्द्रस्य मुष्टिरसि वीडयस्व ॥

56. O commander, whose army thunders like the war drum, drive away all dangers, fill us full of vigour, gain supremacy, expand the army, make those weep, who behave like depraved dogs, let thy administration be well knit like the fist, make efficient arrangements for electricity in the army, and enjoy all comforts!

५७. आमूरज प्रत्यावर्तयेमाः केतुमद्दुन्दुभिर्वावदीति ।
समश्वपर्णाश्चरन्ति नो नरोऽस्माकमिन्द्र रथिनो जयन्तु ॥

57. O commander, drive thither away the troops of the enemy, and bring back ours safe after victory. Let our cavalry march forth, in accompaniment with the beating of war-drums. Let our car-warriors be triumphant!

५८. आग्नेयः कृष्णग्रीवः सारस्वती मेषी वभ्रः सौम्यः पौष्णः श्यामः शितिपृष्ठो बार्हस्पत्यः शिल्पो वैश्वदेव ऐन्द्रोऽरुणो मारुतः कलमाष ऐन्द्राग्नः सँहितोऽधोरामः सावित्रो वारुणः कृष्ण एकशितिपात्पेत्वः ॥

58. The black necked animal is ferocious like fire; the ewe is mild like speech; the brown animal is calm and pleasant like the Moon; the dusky animal is strong in body; the black-backed animal is fiery like the Sun; the dappled animal possesses various qualities; the red animal is full of heat like the Sun; the black and white coloured animal is fast like the air; the strong bodied animal possesses the qualities of the Sun and fire; the bird that flies low is furious like the Sun; the black coloured bird with one foot is calm and peaceful like water.

५९. अग्नयेऽनीकवते रोहिताञ्जिरनड्वानधोरामौ सावित्रौ पौष्णौ रजतनाभी वैश्वदेवौ पिशङ्गौ तूपरौ मारुतः कलमाष आग्नेयः कृष्णोऽजः सारस्वती मेषी वारुणः पेत्वः ॥

59. A red-marked ox is strong and strenuous like the learned commander of the army; animals with white spots below are active like the Sun; animals with silvery navel are full of force; yellow hornless animals are imbued with many qualities; black and white animal is swift like air; the black-faced he-goat is ferocious like fire; the ewe is sweet like speech; the fast running animal is fast like water.

६०. अग्नये गायत्राय त्रिवृते राथन्तरायाष्टाकपाल इन्द्राय त्रैष्टुभाय पञ्चदशाय बार्हतायैकादशकपालो विश्वेभ्यो देवेभ्यो जागतेभ्यः सप्तदशेभ्यो वैरूपेभ्यो द्वादशकपालो मित्रावरुणाभ्यामानुष्टुभाभ्यामेकविँशाभ्यां वैराजाभ्यां पयस्या बृहस्पतये पाङ्क्ताय त्रिणवाय शाक्वराय चरुः सवित्र औष्णिहाय त्रयस्त्रिँशाय रैवताय द्वादशकपालः प्राजापत्यश्चरुरदित्यै विष्णुपत्यै चरुरग्नये वैश्वानराय द्वादशकपालोऽनुमत्या अष्टाकपालः ॥

60. To the fiery soul possessing the qualities of Satva, Rajas and Tamas, the crosser of ocean by means of ships, expounded in Gayatri metre, should be offered the food cooked in eight pot-herds. To the highly strong soul, well-versed in fifteen kinds of Trishtup metre, be offered the food cooked in eleven pot-herds. To the divine persons, endowed with diverse qualities, as described in all the seventeenfold Jagati metre, should be offered the food cooked in twelve pot-herds. To Pran and Udan delineated in Anushtup and twentyone fold virat metres, should be offered a mess of curdled milk. To the protectors of the great, sublime in assemblies, renowned in action, contemplation and knowledge, celebrated for strength should be offered special food. To the man acquiring supremacy, coupled with thirty three kinds of wealth, mentioned in Ushnik metre, should be offered the food cooked in twelve pot-herds. To father and mother should be offered the food prepared in the cooking pot; the same be offered to the entire space protected by the All-pervading God. To the brilliant amongst all men, shining like lightning, be offered the food cooked in twelve pot-herds. For the follower, refined food should be prepared in eight pot-herds.

---

⁶⁰The significance of pot-herds and the food prepared therein is not clear to me. According to Pt. Jaidev Vidyalankar, the word कपाल (pot-herd) merely denotes division. अष्टकपाल means a mature thought well considered by eight learned persons. Similarly एकादशकपाल द्वादशकपाल mean an idea which is the result of the deliberations of eleven and twelve scholars. Food has been compared to the well thought out idea, resulting from the joint mental cooking of learned persons.

CHAPTER XXX

१. देव सवित: प्र सुव यज्ञं प्र सुव यज्ञपतिं भगाय ।
दिव्यो गन्धर्व: केतपू: केतं न: पुनातु वाचस्पतिर्वाचं न: स्वदतु ॥

1. O Divine God, create for wealth and supremacy, the king, who is glorious, the protector of the Earth, the purifier of knowledge, the cleanser of our wisdom, the master of speech, who renders our speech sweet, smooth, mild and lovely. Make his rule successful !

२. तत्सवितुर्वरेण्यं भर्गो देवस्य धीमहि ।
धियो यो न: प्रचोदयात् ॥

2. Let us adore the supremacy of that divine God, the Creator of the universe, Self-illumined, and Sublime. We invoke Him to direct our understanding aright.

३. विश्वानि देव सवितर्दुरितानि परा सुव ।
यद्भद्रं तन्न आ सुव ॥

3. O God, full of noble attributes, actions and nature, send far away all vices and calamities, and grant us virtues!

४. विभक्तारꣽ हवामहे वसोश्चित्रस्य राधस: ।
सवितारं नृचक्षसम् ॥

4. We praise God, the Procurer of comforts, the Distributor of wondrous wealth, the Creator, and the Seer of men.

५. ब्रह्मणे ब्राह्मणं क्षत्राय राजन्यं मरुद्भ्यो वैश्यं तपसे शूद्रं तमसे तस्करं नारकाय वीरहणं पाप्मने क्लीबमाक्रयाया अयोगूं कामाय पुंश्चलूमतिकृष्टाय मागधम् ॥

5. O God create a Brahmana, who knows the veda and God, for propagating the knowledge of God and the veda; a Kshatriya prince for the safety of kingdom; a vaisha for rearing the cattle; a Shudra for hard labour and service.

---

[1]Western scholars like Griffith, Colebrooke, Weber, Wilson, Muir, Oldenberg, and Max Muller consider this and the next chapter meant for human sacrifice. This is an erroneous idea.

Just as Ashvamedha does not mean Horse sacrifice, but the improvement of land for growing more food, so Purushmedha does not mean human sacrifice, but the perfection of man for spiritual and worldly advancement. This interpretation put upon these two words by Rishi Dayananda is highly logical and rational. 'Tis pity the western scholars, following Mahidhar and Sayana, have miserably failed to understand the true purport of these words.

[3]This verse occurs in 3—35, and 22—9. It is called Savitri or Gayatri Mantra.

[4]God being present in our soul, sees all our actions, good and bad,

Cast aside the thief, who steals in darkness; the destroyer of heroes, who passes his days in jail, the eunuch mentally disposed to licentiousness, the dacoit bent on looting and harming people; the harlot full of lust; and the bard disposed to abuse!

६. नृत्ताय सूतं गीताय शैलूषं धर्माय सभाचरं नरिष्ठायै भीमलं नर्माय रेभ॒ हसाय कारिमानन्दाय स्त्रीषखं प्रमदे कुमारीपुत्रं मेधायै रथकारं धैर्याय तक्षाणम् ।

6. O God, create for dance a bard; for song a public dancer; for duty one who administers justice; for sweetness a panegyrist; for pleasure a wife-lover husband; for dexterity a car-builder; for firmness a carpenter.

Cast aside, a debauchee who indulges in conversation with the dissolute; a ridiculer fond of derision; an illegitimate virgin's son, addicted to carelessness.

७. तपसे कौलालं मायायै कर्मारं॒ रूपाय मणिकारं॒ शुभे वप॒ शरव्याया इषुकारं॒ हेत्यै धनुष्कारं कर्मणे ज्याकारं दिष्टाय रज्जुसर्जं मृत्यवे मृगयुमन्तकाय श्वनिनम् ॥

7. O God, create for penance a potter's son; for sharpening intellect an artificer; for beauty a jeweller; for welfare a sower; for arrows a maker of shafts; for destructive weapons a bowyer; for victory a bowstring maker; for control a ropemaker. Cast aside a hunter bent on murder; and a dog-rearer the helper of the murderer!

८. नदीभ्य: पौञ्जिष्ठ॒मृक्षीकाभ्यो नैषादं पुरुषव्याघ्राय दुर्मदं गन्धर्वाप्सरोभ्यो व्रात्यं प्रयुग्भ्य उन्मत्त॒ सर्पदेवजनेभ्योऽप्रतिपद्मयेभ्य: कितवमीर्यतायाऽकितवं पिशाचेभ्यो विदलकारीं यातुधानेभ्य: कण्टकीकारीम् ॥

8. O God, cast aside the vile man who pollutes rivers; Nishada's son, hankering after libidinous women; a degraded arrogant man, friend of a person harmful like a tiger; an uneducated person attached to low dancing and singing women; the demented, given to the application of magical rites; an untrustworthy person who befriends the serpents and the fools; a gambler who acquires wealth by unlawful means; a non-gambler who creates unnecessary excitement; a woman who creates split amongst the Pishachas, the thorny woman who favours the freebooters!

[6]सूत: the son of a Kshatriya by a Brahmana woman, who generally does the business of dancing.

[8]पौञ्जिष्ठ: the son of a Nishad by a Shudra woman, a vile person. Nishada is the name of one of the wild aboriginal tribes in India, such as, hunters, fishermen etc. man of a degraded tribe in general an outcast, a chandala, the son of a Brahmana by a Shudra woman.

Pishachas: those whose aims and ambitions have been destroyed through immoral conduct, or those who are fond of eating raw meat mixed with blood.

९. सन्धये जारं गेहायोपपतिमार्यै परिवित्तं निर्‌कृत्यै परिविविदानमराध्या एदिधिषु: पतिं निष्कृत्यै पेशस्कारीं॒ संज्ञानाय स्मरकारीं प्रकामोद्यायोपसदं वर्णयानुरुधं बलायोपदाम् ॥

9. O God, cast aside a lover, who cohabits with another's wife; a paramour having illicit connection with a domestic woman; an unmarried elder brother suffering from the pangs of passion; younger brother who has married before his elder to inherit his father's property; the husband of a younger sister whose elder sister has not been married, for ulterior motives of greed; a licentious adorned woman who pretends for penance; a lustful go-between woman bent on arousing passions; a by-sitter for garrulity, an obstinate man who insists upon acceptance; and him who offers presents in the shape of bribe, to gain strength.

१०. उत्सादेभ्य: कुब्जं प्रमुदे वामनं द्वार्भ्य: स्रामं॒ स्वप्नायान्धमधर्माय बधिरं पवित्राय भिषजं प्रज्ञानाय नक्षत्रदर्शमाशिक्षायै प्रश्निनमुपशिक्षाया अभिप्रशिनं मर्यादायै प्रश्नविवाकम् ॥

10. O God, keep aside a hunch-back bent on destruction; a dwarf given to carnal pleasures; a blear-eyed man as a gate-keeper; a blind man for sleep; and a deaf man devoid of righteousness. O God create a physician for purifying our body with the eradication of disease; an astronomer for the advancement of knowledge; an inquisitive man full of craving for knowledge; an extra inquisitive man for desire of extra knowledge; and a question-solver for establishing moral law!

११. श्रमेभ्यो हस्तिपं जवायाश्वपं पुष्ट्यच्च गोपालं वीर्यायाविपालं तेजसेऽजपालमिरायै कीनाशं कीलालाय सुराकारं भद्राय गृहप॒ श्रेयसे वित्तधमाध्यक्ष्यायानुक्षत्तारम् ॥

11. O God, create an elephant-keeper for deep walking; a horse-keeper for speed; a cowherd for nourishment; a shepherd for manliness; a goatherd for enhancing keenness, a ploughman for growing more food; a preparer of Soma for obtaining essence of medicines and food; a house-guard for weal; a possessor of wealth for well-being; and an obedient attendant for supervision!

---

[9]Upapati: Second husband, a paramour who uses a woman as his wife in the presence of her legal husband.

Parivittam: an elder brother who is unmarried, while his younger brother is married. This means that elder brother should be married first. The State should enact a law, that no younger brother be married before his elder brother is married. The words convey condemnation of the elder brother, a prey to lust, who pleads for his marriage.

Parivividanam: younger brother who marries before his elder.

Edidhishu-pati: the husband of a younger sister; whose elder sister is unmarried. Such a marriage should ordinarily be prohibited by law.

[10]A man suffering from eye-disease should not be appointed as a gate-keeper.

A blind man should not be appointed as a watchman, otherwise you can't have a sound sleep, as he cannot protect you against thieves.

A deaf man cannot listen to religious preachings, and hence does not know what is truth and Dharma.

१२. भार्यै दार्वाहारं प्रभाया अग्न्येधं ब्रध्नस्य विष्टपायाभिषेक्तारं वर्षिष्ठाय नाकाय
परिवेष्टारं देवलोकाय पेशितारं मनुष्यलोकाय प्रकरितारꣳ सर्वेभ्यो लोकेभ्य उपसेक्तार-
मव ऋत्यै बधायोपमन्थितारं मेधायै वासः पल्पूलीं प्रकामाय रजयित्रीम् ॥

12. O God create a wood-bringer for Light; a fire-kindler for brightness; a besprinkler for horse's path; a high steward for highest happiness, a master of all sorts of knowledge, for the sight of the learned; a distributor of knowledge, for the benefit of humanity; a magnanimous person who contributes to the happiness of all, a washer-woman for cleanliness; an affectionate wife for domestic happiness. O God, cast aside a wicked person bent on teasing, murdering, and offering opposition!

१३. ऋतये स्तेनहृदयं वैरहत्याय पिशुनं विविक्त्यै क्षत्तारमौपद्रष्ट्वायानुक्षत्तारं बलायानुचरं
भूम्ने परिष्कन्दं प्रियाय प्रियवादिनमरिष्ट्या अश्वसादꣳ स्वर्गाय लोकाय भागदुघं
वर्षिष्ठाय नाकाय परिवेष्टारम् ॥

13. O God cast aside, a thievish hearted man bent on violence, a slanderer bent on homicide. O God create, a religious-minded man for discrimination; an ascetic as a wise counsellor; a servant for strength; an observer of celibacy for plenty of progeny; a sweet speaker for affection; a cavalier for safety; a collector of taxes for enjoying full happiness; a talented man spreading knowledge for highest happiness!

१४. मन्यवेऽस्तापं क्रोधाय निसरं योगाय योक्तारꣳ शोकायाभिसर्त्तारं क्षेमाय विमोक्ता-
रमुत्कूलनिकूलेभ्यस्त्रिष्ठिनं वपुषे मानस्कृतꣳ शीलायाऽञ्जनीकारीं निर्ऋत्यै कोशकारीं
यमायासूम् ॥

14. O God drive away, a mentally angry man, blazing like red hot iron; an invader full of ire; an assailant destined for grief; an embarrassed barren woman bent on violence!
O God create a yogi for the practice of yoga; an alleviator of sufferings for welfare; a mechanic skilled in running ships; car and aeroplanes for going to high and low places; a thoughtful person for welfare of the body; a well-behaved wife of noble deeds for a Brahmchari; a wealthy lady for acquiring land!

१५. यमाय यमसूमथर्वभ्योऽवतोकाꣳ संवत्सराय पर्यायिणीं परिवत्सरायाविजातामिदा-
वत्सरायातीत्वरीमिद्वत्सरायातिष्कद्वरीं वत्सराय विजर्जराꣳसंवत्सराय पलिक्नीमृभुभ्यो-
ऽजिनसन्धꣳ साध्येभ्यश्चर्मम्नम् ॥

15. O God, for administration create a woman who gives birth to rulers; for the harmless physicians a woman who has miscarried; for the Samvatsar,

---

[13]अनुक्षत्तारः is an ascetic who offers wise counsel to great men at the time of danger. This post was held by Sanjaya for Dhirtarashtra, Vidura for Duryodhan, and Sumanta for Dashratha.
[15]A woman suffering from miscarriage should be treated by learned, sympathetic physicians.

CHAPTER XXX

first year, a woman who gives birth to male and female child alternately; for the Parivatsar, second year, a celibate virgin; for the Idvatsar, 3rd year, one who is fond of roaming; for the Idvatsar, fifth year, one who is highly learned; for one year, an ailing woman; for four years, one with grey hair, for the wise, a friend of the invincible, and for executive projects, men of skill and proficiency!

१६. सरोभ्यो धैवरमुपस्थावराभ्यो दाशं वैशन्ताभ्यो बैन्दं नड्वलाभ्य: शौष्कलं पाराय मार्गा-रमवाराय केवर्त्तं तीर्थेभ्यो ब्रान्दं विषमेभ्यो मैनाल(ँ) स्वनेभ्य: पर्णकं गुहाभ्य: किरात(ँ) सानुभ्यो जम्भकं पर्वतेभ्य: किम्पूरुषम् ॥

16. O God, create the son of a fisherman for crossing ponds; a paid servant for menial service; the son of a Nishada for managing small tanks; a dry fish clearer for reed-beds, a celibate who controls passions for uneven impassable places; a boatsman for crossing watery places; an engineer for constructing bridges over rivers!
O God, drive away a hunter's son bent upon killing deer; a contemptible Bhil for sounds; a Kirata for caverns; a destructive savage for living on mountain-heights; a wild man for living in mountains!

१७. बीभत्सायै पौल्कसं वर्णाय हिरण्यकारं तुलायै वाणिजं पश्चादोषाय ग्लाविनं विश्वेभ्यो भूतेभ्य: सिध्मलं भूत्यै जागरणमभूत्यै स्वपनमार्त्यै जनवादिनं व्यृद्ध्या अपगल्भ(ँ) स(ँ)शराय प्रच्छिदम् ॥

17. O God drive away a sweeper's son bent on ferocity; a dissatisfied person given to back-biting; a slothful person destined for poverty; a shameless person bent on losing wealth; a destroyer and splitter bent on violence!
O God create a goldsmith for beautifying ornaments; a merchant for exact weighing; a bringer of happiness for all human beings with his assistants; a watchful man for prosperity; an eloquent debater for alleviation of suffering!

A woman who gives birth to a male and female child alternately should observe celibacy for one year, to be free from this defect. The question of the marriage of the virgin girls should be decided in the second year.
A girl fond of roaming should wait for marriage for three years.
A learned woman should not be married, but should wait for five years.
An ailing woman should observe celibacy for one year.
A husband should wait for four years for progeny in the case of a wife grown grey-haired before time.
Samvatsar, Parivatsar, Idavatsar, Anuvatsar, Idvatsar constitute a cycle of five years.
[16]Nishada: the son of a Brahmana by a Shudra woman, a fisherman, Bhil is a black man, who carries bows and arches in his hands, and shoots you in the direction from where he hears your sound.
Kirata: a savage who lives by hunting and resides in pits and caves.
A dry fish clearer: A person who clears the reed-beds of dry, dead fish in summer, and thus earns his living by labour, but does not eat them, or sell them, for his livelihood.

१८. अक्षराजाय कितवं कृतायादिनवदर्श त्रेतायें कल्पिनं द्वापरायाधिकल्पिनमास्कन्दाय सभास्थाणुं मृत्यवे गोव्यच्छमन्तकाय गोघातं क्षुधे यो गां विकृन्तन्तं भिक्षमाण उपतिष्ठति दुष्कृताय चरकाचार्यं पाप्मने संलगम् ॥

18. O God drive away a gambler, friend of the dice-king; a person with evil designs for murdering cows; a cow-killer for gallows; one who for hunger goes begging to a man who is cutting up a cow; a leader of meat eaters bent on misdeed; the son of a depraved person, befriending a sinner!

O God, create a wise person who soon realizes the shortcomings in the acts performed; a person who is fit in childhood, youth and old age; one endowed with capability for this world and the next; a leader of the Assembly for drying up the resources of the enemy!

१९. प्रतिश्रुत्कायाः अर्तनं घोषाय भषमन्ताय बहुवादिनंभनन्ताय मूकꣳ शब्दायाडम्बराघातं महसे वीणावादं क्रोशाय तूणवध्ममवरस्पराय शङ्ख्ध्मं वनाय वनपमन्यतोरण्याय दावपम् ॥

19. O God, create a man of iron determination for the implementation of vow; a loud-voiced man for proclamation; a comprehensive speaker for establishing propriety of conduct; a mute for unending lawless discussion; a lute-player for great festivals; a conch-blower, for calling neighbouring and distant people; a forest-guard, for the protection of forest; and drive away a creator of uproar bent on uttering frightening sounds; a flute-blower intending singing songs of lamentation; a forest burner contemplating the destruction of jungles!

२०. नर्माय पुंश्चलूꣳ हसाय कारिं यादसे शाबल्यां ग्रामण्यं गणकमभिक्रोशकं तान्महसे वीणावादं पाणिघ्नं तूणवध्मं तान्नृत्तायानन्दाय तलवम् ॥

20. O God, drive away a harlot fond of pastime; a strange mad man inclined to laughter; the daughter of a man with spotty skin bent on killing aquatic creatures; create for reverence, the following, a headman, a mathematician, a watchman. Create a lute-player, a player on musical instruments with hands, a flutist for dance; and a hand clapper for pleasure!

२१. अग्नये पीवानं पृथिव्यै पीठसर्पिणं वायवे चाण्डालमन्तरिक्षाय वꣳशनर्तिनं दिवे खलतिꣳ सूर्याय द्यर्यक्षं नक्षत्रेभ्य: किमिरं चन्द्रमसे किलासमह्ने शुक्लं पिङ्गाक्षꣳ रात्र्यै कृष्णं पिङ्गाक्षम् ॥

21. O God, create bulky substances for fire; serpents to crawl on earth; a pole-dancer for mid-air; a monkey-like green-eyed man for the Sun; a whitish person for giving pleasure like the Moon; a white yellow-eyed man for day, and drive away an impure person who emits foul air from his body; a bald prone to jest and joke; a spotty man who is bent upon opposing the rulers; a black man with yellow eyes who prefers darkness!

---

[19]Just as a mute remains silent to an unending discussion ungoverned by rules and regulations, so we should observe silence in a futile discussion.
[21]Fire burns the bulky substances.

CHAPTER XXX

२२. अर्थैतानष्टौ विरूपाना लभतेऽतिदीर्घं चातिह्रस्वं चातिस्थूलं चातिकृशं चातिशुक्लं चाति-
कृष्णं चातिकुल्वं चातिलोमशं च ।
अशूद्रा अब्राह्मणास्ते प्राजापत्याः ।
मागधः पुंश्चली कितवः क्लीबोऽशूद्रा अब्राह्मणास्ते प्राजापत्याः ॥

22. O kings, just as a learned man comes in contact with the eight following variform men, one too tall, one too short, one too stout, one too thin, one too white, one too black, one too bald, one too hairy, so should ye do!

Those connected with the kings, who are neither Shudras nor Brahmanas should also come in their contact.

A murderer, a harlot and eunuch, neither of Shudra nor Brahmana caste should be made to dwell at a distance. Loyal subjects and devotees of God should dwell near.

---

[22]People of low character should not be allowed to mix with others and spread the contagion of their vices.
They should be kept in prison or far away from the town.

CHAPTER XXXI

१. सहस्रशीर्षा पुरुषः सहस्राक्षः सहस्रपात् ।
स भूमिꣳ सर्वतः स्पृत्वाऽत्यतिष्ठद्दशाङ्गुलम् ॥

1. The Almighty God, hath the power of a thousand heads, a thousand eyes; a thousand feet.
Pervading the Earth on every side He transgresses the universe.

२. पुरुष एवेदꣳ सर्वं यद्भूतं यच्च भाव्यम् ।
उतामृतत्वस्येशानो यदन्नेनातिरोहति ॥

2. God, the Lord of final emancipation is in truth the Creator of all that hath been and what yet shall be; and what grows on earth.

३. एतावानस्य महिमातो ज्यायाꣳश्च पूरुषः ।
पादोऽस्य विश्वा भूतानि त्रिपादस्यामृतं दिवि ॥

3. The visible and invisible universe displays His grandeur. Yea, He is greater than this universe.
All worlds are but a part of Him, the rest lies in His Immortal, Resplendent Nature.

---

[1] Mr. Griffith translates दशाङ्गुलम् (Dashangulam) as a space of ten fingers, which is meaningless.
Thousand means innumerable. Dash Angulam (दशाङ्गुलम्) the world which is made up of ten parts, i.e., five gross and five subtle elements. Five gross elements are earth, water, air, fire and atmosphere. Five subtle elements are sight (रूप), smell (गंध), speech (शब्द), taste (रस), touch (स्पर्श).

[2] The word (अन्न) has been wrongly interpreted as food and nourishment.
Colebrooke translates the line: 'He is that, which grows by nourishment.' God is not a materiel object which requires nourishment for growth. He is Everlasting and Immaterial.
Muri renders it thus: 'He is also the Lord of immortality since by food He expands:'
Professors Ludwig and Wilson also give the same explanation.
Sayana interprets it thus: 'He is the Lord or Distributor of immortality because He becomes the visible world in order that living beings may obtain the fruits of their actions and gain moksha or final liberation from their bonds! This interpretation is highly irrational and illogical. God being immaterial cannot assume a visible form. He is spoken of in the vedas as अकायम् without a body. The interpretation of the western scholars is mostly based on that of Sayana.
Swami Dayananda interprets अन्न as Earth, out of which grow all trees, vegetables, and corns.

[3] God is indivisible. He can't be spoken of as having parts.
The words Pad a fourth and Tripad three-fourths are used figuratively to show His immensity and world's littleness.

CHAPTER XXXI

४. त्रिपादूर्ध्व उदैत्पुरुषः पादोऽस्येहाभवत् पुनः ।
ततो विष्वङ् व्यक्रामत्साशनानशने अभि ॥

4. God, with three-fourths of His grandeur rises higher than all, separate from the world, enjoying liberation. With one fourth of His grandeur He creates and dissolves the universe again and again. Then pervading the animate and inanimate creation He resides therein.

५. ततो विराडजायत विराजो अधि पूरुषः ।
स जातो अत्यरिच्यत पश्चाद्भूमिमथो पुरः ॥

5. God creates the universe, and lords over it.
He, then pre-existent, remains aloof from the world, and afterwards creates the Earth.

६. तस्माद्यज्ञात्सर्वहुतः सम्भृतं पृषदाज्यम् ।
पशूंस्तांश्चक्रे वायव्यानारण्या ग्राम्याश्च ये ॥

6. From that great God, adorable by all, were created curd and clarified butter.
He creates the wild and tame animals swift like air.

७. तस्माद्यज्ञात् सर्वहुत ऋचः सामानि जज्ञिरे ।
छन्दांसि जज्ञिरे तस्मादयजुस्तस्मादजायत ॥

7. From that Adorable God unto Whom people make every kind of sacrifice, were created the Rigveda, the Samaveda. From Him was created the Atharvaveda and also the Yajurveda.

८. तस्मादश्वा अजायन्त ये के चोभयादतः ।
गावो ह जज्ञिरे तस्मात्तस्माज्जाता अजावयः ॥

8. From God were born horses, and from Him were born all cattle with two rows of teeth.
From Him were generated kine, from Him were goats and sheep produced.

९. तं यज्ञं बर्हिषि प्रौक्षन् पुरुषं जातमग्रतः ।
तेन देवा अयजन्त साध्या ऋषयश्च ये ॥

9. O men know Him, the perfect God, existent before the creation of the

---

⁴What eats is the animate, and what eats not is the inanimate creation.
⁵The creation of the Earth is mentioned for distinction, through Earth is ordinarily included in the creation of the universe.
⁶Wild animals of the forest, like lion, and tame animals of the village like cow, which are quick in motion like the air have been created by God. The word वायव्यान has been translated by some as birds of air, but Rishi Dayananda translates it as fast like air.
अन्नं हि पृषदाज्यम् शत० 3-8-4-8.
According to Shatpath Brahmana पृषदाज्यम् may also mean food.
⁹Rishis: men who know the significance of vedic verses.

world, and highly adorable, Him the learned, the yogis and the Rishis realise in the innermost recesses of their hearts, and worship as directed by the vedas preached by Him!

१०. यत्पुरुषं व्यदधुः कतिधा व्यकल्पयन् ।
मुखं किमस्यासीत् किं बाहू किमरू पादा उच्येत ॥

10. O learned people, ye realise the perfect God in diverse ways; and describe Him in manifold manners! In this creation of God, who is exalted like the mouth? Who possesses the strength like arms? Who does the work of things? Who is low like the feet?

११. ब्राह्मणोऽस्य मुखमासीद्बाहू राजन्यः कृतः ।
ऊरू तदस्य यद्वैश्यः पद्भ्याꣳ शूद्रो अजायत ॥

11. In God's creation, the Brahmana in body-politic is like the head in the body, a Kshatriya is like arms, a Vaisha is like thighs, and a Shudra is considered as feet.

१२. चन्द्रमा मनसो जातश्चक्षोः सूर्यो अजायत ।
श्रोत्राद्वायुश्च प्राणश्च मुखादग्निरजायत ॥

12. The Moon was engendered from His strength of knowledge; the sun was born from His power of refulgence, the air and ten vital breaths were born from His power of space, fire was born from His power of destruction.

१३. नाभ्या आसीदन्तरिक्षꣳ शीर्ष्णो द्यौः समवर्तत ।
पद्भ्यां भूमिर्दिशः श्रोत्रात्तथा लोकाꣳ अकल्पयन् ॥

13. Mid-air was produced from His central power of space; from His excellent head-like strength was fashioned the sky. Earth came into being from primordial power; and the quarters from His power of space. Similarly were other regions created.

१४. यत्पुरुषेण हविषा देवा यज्ञमतन्वत ।
वसन्तोऽस्यासीदाज्यं ग्रीष्म इध्मः शरद्धविः ॥

[11]Brahmana: one who knows God and the veda, and is their devotee.
Kshatriya: He who is warlike in spirit, and defends the country like soldiers.
Vaisha: the agriculturist and tradesman, the chief supporter of the society.
Shudra: A labourer on whose toil and industry all prosperity ultimately depends.
This verse contains reply to the questions raised in the previous verse. The four castes in the society have been compared to the four parts of the body.
Commentators like Mahi Dhar and Ubbat translate this verse to mean that a Brahmana is born out of God's mouth, a Kshatriya out of His arms, a vaisha out of His thighs, and a Shudra out of His feet. This interpretation is wrong as God has got no body.

[12]Ten vital breaths: Pran air in the heart, Apan in the anus, Saman in the navel, Udan in the throat, Vyan in the whole body, and Nag, Kurma, Krikal, Dev Dutt, Dhananjaya.

14. When the learned perform, meditating upon the Adorable God, the sacrifice of mental worship, then morning is its butter, mid-day its fuel, and mid-night its oblation.

१५. सप्तास्यासन् परिधयस्त्रि: सप्त समिध: कृता: ।
देवा यद्यज्ञं तन्वाना अबध्नन् पुरुषं पशुम् ॥

15. The mental sacrifice, performing which, the learned concentrate upon the knowable God in their hearts, has seven coverings and twenty one kinds of kindling fuel.

१६. यज्ञेन यज्ञमयजन्त देवास्तानि धर्माणि प्रथमान्यासन् ।
ते ह नाकं महिमान: सचन्त यत्र पूर्वे साध्या: सन्ति देवा: ॥

16. The learned worship God through mental contemplation. Their holy ordinances for the worship of God are immemorial. Such noble souls in particular enjoy the happiness of final beatitude, in which dwell the ancient yogis and learned devotees.

१७. अद्भ्य: सम्भृत: पृथिव्यै रसाच्च विश्वकर्मण: समवर्तताग्रे ।
तस्य त्वष्टा विदधद्रूपमेति तन्मर्त्यस्य देवत्वमाजानमग्रे ॥

17. God creates in the beginning with His urge this world nourished by waters, earth and sun. Fixing its form, He assigns in the beginning the wisdom and duties of mankind.

१८. वेदाहमेतं पुरुषं महान्तमादित्यवर्णं तमस: परस्तात् ।
तमेव विदित्वाति मृत्युमेति नान्य: पन्था विद्यतेऽयनाय ॥

18. I know this Mighty, Perfect God, Who is Refulgent like the Sun and free from ignorance.
He only who knows Him feels not the pangs of death. For salvation there is no other path save this.

[14]Sacrifice: Yajna.
Its: of the Yajna.
In the absence of outward provisions a mental sacrifice is to be performed. Then morning, mid-day and mid-night should be imagined to serve the purpose of butter, fuel and oblation of the yajna.

[15]Seven coverings are the seven metres Chhandas in which the vedic verse encompass the yajna.
Twenty one kinds of fuel: Matter, Mahat, Tatva (Intellect), Ahankar (Egotism), five subtle elements (सूक्ष्मभूत), five gross elements (स्थूलभूत) five organs of cognition, (ज्ञानेन्द्रिय) satva, Rajas, Tamas, three qualities. These twenty one materials serve as fuel to the contemplative yajna, the learned perform. Griffith says 'This pantheistic hymn, which is generally called the Purushasukta, is of comparatively recent origin. Nothing can be farther from truth than this statement. The hymn is the part and parcel of the Yajurveda, and is hence as old and immemorial as the Veda itself.

[16]Holy ordinances: The teachings of the Vedas.

[18]Knowledge of God alone is the sure path for salvation.

१९. प्रजापतिश्चरति गर्भे अन्तरजायमानो बहुधा वि जायते ।
तस्य योनि परि पश्यन्ति धीरास्तस्मिन् ह तस्थुर्भुवनानि विश्वा ॥

19. God, the Protector of men, pervades the soul in the womb and the hearts of all. Being unborn, He manifests himself in various ways. Yogis alone realise His true nature. In Him stand all existing worlds.

२०. यो देवेभ्य आतपति यो देवानां पुरोहितः ।
पूर्वो यो देवेभ्यो जातो नमो रुचाय ब्राह्मये ॥

20. The sun gives light and heat to the useful objects like the Earth; stands first and foremost in the centre for the good of all heavenly bodies, is born ere the Earth etc. and being the creation of Gracious God gives us food.

२१. रुचं ब्राह्मं जनयन्तो देवा अग्रे तदब्रुवन् ।
यस्त्वैवं ब्राह्मणो विद्यात्तस्य देवा असन् वशे ॥

21. The learned persons in the beginning, making thee a lovable devotee of God, preach the eternity of God, Soul and Matter. The Brahmana who thus knows the nature of God, shall have learned persons in his control.

२२. श्रीश्च ते लक्ष्मीश्च पत्न्यावहोरात्रे पार्श्वे नक्षत्राणि रूपमश्विनौ व्यात्तम् ।
इष्णन्निषाणामुं म इषाण सर्वलोकं म इषाण ॥

22. Grandeur and Fortune are Thy two wives. Thy sides are Day and Night. Constellations are Thy form: the Aswins are Thy open Mouth. Imploring grant salvation unto me, grant me all sorts of knowledge and pleasures.

²¹Thee: A devotee of God.
²²Thy God's Aswins: The Sun and Moon.
Just as wives serve and protect their husbands, so God protects all through His grandeur and might.
Day and Night are two phases of the Sun. When it rises and shines it is day, when it sets it is night. So when God shines in our heart, it is day through His lustre and Knowledge. It is night when darkness (ignorance) prevails in the soul, and we forget God. All luminous objects exhibit the beauty and glory of God. In this Purushsukta the metamorphosic nature of God is spoken of figuratively.

CHAPTER XXXII

१. तदेवाग्निस्तदादित्यस्तद्वायुस्तदु चन्द्रमा: ।
तदेव शुक्रं तद्ब्रह्म ता श्रापः स प्रजापतिः ॥

1. God is Agni being Self-refulgent; He is Aditya as He engulfs all at the time of dissolution of the universe; He is Vayu as He is All-powerful; He is Chandrama as He is full of pleasure and is the giver of pleasure; He is Shukra as He is pure and quick in action; He is Brahma as He is great; He is Apa being All-pervading; He is Prajapati as He is the guardian of His creatures.

२. सर्वे निमेषा जज्ञिरे विद्युतः पुरुषादधि ।
नैनमूर्ध्वं न तिर्यञ्चं न मध्ये परि जग्रभत् ॥

2. All divisions of time sprang from the Resplendent, Perfect God. No one hath comprehended Him from above, across, or in the midst.

३. न तस्य प्रतिमा अस्ति यस्य नाम महद्यशः ।
हिरण्यगर्भ इत्येष मा मा हिꣳसीदित्येषा यस्मान्न जात इत्येषः ॥

3. There is no image of Him whose glory verily is great. He sustains within Himself all luminous objects like the Sun etc. May He not harm me, this is my prayer. As He is unborn, He deserves our worship.

४. एषो ह देवः प्रदिशोऽनु सर्वाः पूर्वो ह जातः स उ गर्भे अन्तः ।
स एव जातः स जनिष्यमाणः प्रत्यङ् जनास्तिष्ठति सर्वतोमुखः ॥

4. O learned persons, this very God pervadeth all regions. He was present in the minds of all in the last cycle of creation; He is present now, and will be present in future cycles. He exists, controlling everything, with His power of facing all directions!

५. यस्माज्जातं न पुरा किं चनैव य आबभूव भुवनानि विश्वा ।
प्रजापतिः प्रजया सꣳररानस्त्रीणि ज्योतीꣳषि सचते स षोडशी ॥

5. Before Whom, naught whatever sprang to being; Who with His presence aids all creatures. God, the Guardian of His subjects, rejoicing in His offspring, maintains the three great Lustres. He is Shodashi.

ᵃGod is indivisible, hath no physical organs, and is ubiquitous.
ᵇThis verse condemns idol-worship, and incarnation.
See Yajurveda Chapter 25, 'verses 10, 13, 12, and 8, 36, 37.
सर्वतोमुखः: He without possessing the physical organs, does their work.
ᵈThree great Lustres: Lightning, Sun and Moon.

६. येन द्यौरुग्रा पृथिवी च दृढा येन स्व स्तभितं येन नाकः ।
यो अन्तरिक्षे रजसो विमानः कस्मै देवाय हविषा विधेम ॥

6. May we realise with love and devotion, God, the Embodiment of happiness; Who has made the heavens strong, and the beautiful Earth firm, is full of pleasure, and being free from all miseries is all Bliss and is the Maker of all worlds in the space.

७. यं क्रन्दसी अवसा तस्तभाने अभ्यैक्षेतां मनसा रेजमाने ।
यत्राधि सूर उदितो विभाति कस्मै देवाय हविषा विधेम ।
आपो ह यद्बृहतीर्यश्चिदापः ॥

7. Whom, the Sun and Earth, the supporters of all, moving in their orbits, worthy of praise for their virtues, affording shelter to humanity, do acknowledge; in Whom the Sun shines in full; Who shines after manifesting great waters and vast space; Whom the teacher and preacher visualise through intellect; may we through concentration realise Him, who is full of lustre and happiness.

८. वेनस्तत्पश्यन्निहितं गुहा सद्यत्र विश्वं भवत्येकनीडम् ।
तस्मिन्निदᳪ सं च वि चैति सर्वᳪ स ओतः प्रोतश्च विभूः प्रजासु ॥

8. The sage beholdeth the eternal conscious God hidden in the inmost recesses of the heart; in Whom this world hath found a solitary abode. In Him is this universe dissolved and then created. He is ubiquitous, and pervades souls and matter like warp and woof.

९. प्र तद्वोचेदमृतं नु विद्वान् गन्धर्वो धाम विभृतं गुहा सत् ।
त्रीणि पदानि निहिता गुहास्य यस्तानि वेद स पितुः पिताऽसत् ॥

9. May the learned person, who knows the vedas, soon expatiate upon the Eternal and Conscious God, the Imperishable abode of salvation, and hidden in intellect. There are three steps of eternal God, placed in comprehension. He who knows them becomes the watchman of God through theism.

Shodashi: Possessing sixteen powers; as enumerated in the Prashna Upanishad, question sixth.
They are: 1. Vital breath, Pran 2. Faith, Shraddha. 3. Space, Akash. 4. Air 5. Fire 6. Water 7. Earth 8. Senseorgan, Indriya. 9. Mind 10. Grain (corn) 11. Semen, Virya. 12. Austerity, Tapsa, 13. Vedic hymns 14. Moral duty 15. Worlds 16. Name.
This universe possessing these 16 powers and attributes is created by God and resides in Him who is the master of this universe with sixteenfold attributes and powers.
⁹Three steps: Creation, Sustenance and Dissolution of the universe, or present, past and future.
The word soon enjoins upon all the knowers of the vedas to lose no time in preaching the vedic truths.

CHAPTER XXXII

१०. स नो बन्धुर्जनिता स विधाता धामानि वेद भुवनानि विश्वा ।
यत्र देवा अमृतमानशानास्तृतीये धामन्नध्यैरयन्त ॥

10. He is our Brother, our Father and Begetter. He knows all beings and all worlds. In Him, the third high stage, the learned obtaining the bliss of salvation, move at will.

११. परीत्य भूतानि परीत्य लोकान् परीत्य सर्वाः प्रदिशो दिशश्च ।
उपस्थाय प्रथमजामृतस्यात्मनाऽऽत्मानमभि सं विवेश ॥

11. God manifests Himself pervading the five elements, the worlds and all the Quarters and Mid-quarters.
The learned person having studied the four vedas created in the beginning, unites himself with God, the Embodiment of Truth.

१२. परि द्यावापृथिवी सद्य इत्वा परि लोकान् परि दिशः परि स्वः ।
ऋतस्य तन्तुं विततं विचृत्य तदपश्यत्तदभवत्तदासीत् ॥

12. God fully pervading the Heaven and Earth, the worlds, the Quarters, the eternal bliss; controlling the lengthened thread of Matter, views it, masters it, was its master and will remain so.

१३. सदसस्पतिमद्भुतं प्रियमिन्द्रस्य काम्यम् ।
सनि मेधामयासिषꣳ स्वाहा ॥

13. Having worshipped with truthful action and speech, God Wondrous, the lovely Friend of Soul, may I acquire wisdom which discriminates between truth and untruth.

१४. यां मेधां देवगणाः पितरश्चोपासते ।
तया मामद्य मेधयाऽग्ने मेधाविनं कुरु स्वाहा ॥

14. That wisdom which the sages and scholars long for; with that wisdom, O God, with Thy truthful speech, make me wise today.

१५ मेधां मे वरुणो ददातु मेधामग्निः प्रजापतिः ।
मेधामिन्द्रश्च वायुश्च मेधां धाता ददातु मे स्वाहा ॥

15. May the Supreme God grant me wisdom, in consonance with the performance of religious duty. May the Omniscient God and Protector of man

---

[10] The third high station: God is higher than matter and soul. Matter is the first, soul and the second God the third stage of man's evolution of knowledge.
[11] Five elements: Water, air, fire, earth, ether.
[14] Truthful speech: Knowledge of the vedas.
Today: Ever (Tomorrow never comes).

grant me wisdom. May the Omnipotent God grant me wisdom, May the Almighty Father grant me wisdom, May the Ruler of the universe grant me wisdom.

१६. इदं मे ब्रह्म च क्षत्रं चोभे श्रियमश्नुताम् ।
मयि देवा दधतु श्रियमुत्तमां तस्यै ते स्वाहा ॥

16. O God, through Thy grace, leading a life of truth, may these Brahmanas and Kshatriyas of my country enjoy the splendour and wealth of my government. Just as the learned persons bestow best splendour and wealth on me, so O seeker after truth may we try for that splendour and wealth for thee!

CHAPTER XXXIII

१. अस्याजरासो दमामरित्रा अर्चंद्धूमासो अग्नयः पावकाः ।
शिवतीचयः श्वात्रासो भुरण्यवो वनर्षदो वायवो न सोमाः ॥

1. In this God's creation, may the fires, ever active, protectors against foes, coupled with fragrant smoke, purifying, white wealth-producing, ever stirring, recipients of prosperity, seated in woods, rays and water, and potent like winds preserve our houses.

२. हरयो धूमकेतवो वातजूता उप द्यवि ।
यतन्ते वृथगग्नयः ॥

2. Various flames of fire, moving in nature, bannered with the smoke, fanned by the wind, rise, aloft to heaven.

३. यजा नो मित्रावरुणा यजा देवाँ२ ऋतं बृहत् ।
अग्ने यक्षि स्वं दमम् ॥

3. O learned person, honour our friends, revered persons, and scholars. Preach grand truth unto us, and manage thy domestic affairs!

४. युक्ष्वा हि देवहूतमाँ२ अश्वाँ२ अग्ने रथीरिव ।
नि होता पूर्व्यः सदः ॥

4. O learned person, just as a charioteer yokes fast horses highly praised by the experts, so shouldst thou arrange fast burning fires, and verily take thy seat as Hota instructed by the aged sages!

५. द्वे विरूपे चरतः स्वर्थें अन्याऽन्या वत्समुप धापयेते ।
हरिरन्यस्यां भवति स्वधावाञ्छुक्रो अन्यस्यां ददृशे सुवर्चाः ॥

5. Just as two women, with fair aim, unlike in semblance, feed themselves, and each in succession nourishes a child in embryo, and one bears a quiet, fascinating babe, and the other an active, fair, shining babe, so do dark and bright night and day exist, and work for uplift of the world as a child. In one of them is born the peaceful Moon, pleasing to the mind; and in the other is born the beautiful, purifying and lustrous Sun.

---

[1]Fires: Electricity and the sacrificial fire.
[2]Bannered with the smoke: Smoke acts like the flag of fire. Just as a flag from a distance gives us the impression of any army, so smoke seen from a distance gives us the idea of fire. We should utilise these fires for worldly purposes.
[3]See 13—37.

६. अयमिह प्रथमो धायि धातृभिर्होता यजिष्ठो अध्वरेष्वीड्यः ।
यमप्रवानो भृगवो विरुरुचुर्वनेषु चित्रं विभ्वं विशे-विशे ॥

6. The explorers, in this world, hold for the people, this fire, vastly expanded, comfort-giving, praiseworthy, investigable in all useful projects.

The learned, and the householders with their disciples and children, specially kindle in woods this fire, wondrous in its attributes, actions and nature, spreading to every place.

७. त्रीणि शता त्री सहस्राण्यग्निं त्रिँशच्च देवा नव चासपर्यन् ।
और्क्षन् घृतैरस्तृणन् बर्हिरस्मा आदिद्धोतारं न्यसादयन्त ॥

7. The skilled mechanics should utilise fire in making automobiles travel for 3339 miles. Fire and water should be employed in making them cover the atmosphere. For this fire, the sacrificer should constantly be seated, to perform Havan.

८. मूर्धानं दिवो अरतिं पृथिव्या वैश्वानरमृत आ जातमग्निम् ।
कविँ सम्राजमतिथिं जनानामासन्ना पात्रं जनयन्त देवाः ॥

8. The learned manifest fire, the head of heaven, resident of Earth, the benefactor of humanity, properly employed in the Yajna, surpassing in beauty, blazing with lustre, the guest of men, created by the mouth-like power of God for the sake of protection.

९. अग्निवृँ त्राणि जङ्घनद्द्रविणस्युर्विपन्यया ।
समिद्धः शुक्र आहुतः ॥

9. Just as the brilliant, active sun slays the clouds, so should a wise man, aspiring after wealth, remove his vices, having recourse to various devices.

१०. विश्वेभिः सोम्यं मध्वग्न इन्द्रेण वायुना ।
पिबा मित्रस्य धामभिः ॥

10. Just as the sun, with the aid of All-sustaining air, drinks the sweet essence of all medicinal herbs, so should a learned person enjoy the essence of the medicinal herbs of his friend.

[6] Fire means electricity.
[7] Distance of 3339 miles means, the automobiles can be made to travel in a non-stop flight thousands of miles, far and wide.
It is not clear why this number of 3339 has been selected to convey the idea of an aeroplane's flight.
[8] The head of heaven: the sun full of fire.
The guest of men: Respected by men like a guest.
Fire should be used by the learned in propelling automobiles.
Just as a powerful and oratorical speech from the mouth instructs men and protects them from dangers, so does electricity protect us.

११. आ यदिषे नृपतिं तेज आनट् शुचि रेतो निषिक्तं द्यौरमीके ।
अग्नि: शर्धमनवद्यं युवानꣳ स्वाध्यं जनयत् सूदयच्च ॥

11. When, for rain, the pure light, coming out of the fire of a yajna full of ghee oblations, reaches the Sun; he creates in the atmosphere and sends in the form of rain, water, invigorating, pure, youth-infusing, and drinkable.

१२. अग्ने शर्ध महते सौमगाय तव द्युम्नान्युत्तमानि सन्तु ।
सं जास्पत्यꣳ सुयममा कृणुष्व शत्रूयतामभि तिष्ठा महाꣳसि ॥

12. Show thyself strong for mighty bliss, O king most excellent be thy effulgent splendours. Strengthen through Brahmcharya the well-knit bond of wife and husband, and trample down the might of those who hate us!

१३. त्वाꣳहि मन्द्रतममर्कशोकैर्ववृमहे महि न: श्रोष्यग्ने ।
इन्द्रं न त्वा शवसा देवता वायुं पृणन्ति राधसा नृतमा: ॥

13. O learned teacher, as thou payest attention to the weighty words of ours, the Brahmcharis; so we, along with men resplendent like the sun, accept thee deserving of highest reverence!
The best men, with strength and wealth, please thee, godly in nature powerful like the sun and bounteous like the air.

१४. त्वे अग्ने स्वाहुत प्रियास: सन्तु सूरय: ।
यन्तारो ये मघवानो जनानामूर्वान् दयन्त गोनाम् ॥

14. O well read learned person, may the heroes amongst men, self-controllers, wealthy patrons, destroyers of the killers of kine, all these sages, be dear unto thee!

१५. शृधि श्रुत्कर्ण वह्निभिर्देवैरग्ने सयावभि: ।
आ सीदन्तु बर्हिषि मित्रो अर्यमा प्रातर्यावाणो अध्वरम् ॥

15. O supreme ruler, hearer of the grievances of the subjects, listen to the important state business in the company of thy ministers, administrators and learned officials. In this spacious Assembly Hall seat thyself, the impartial friend of all, the Lord—worthy of respect, along with officials who resort to their duty early in the morning!

१६. विश्वेषामदितिर्यज्ञियानां विश्वेषामतिथिमनुषाणाम् ।
अग्निर्देवानामव आवृणान: सुमृडीको भवतु जातवेदा: ॥

16. O head of the state thou art the wisest amongst all the honourable learned persons, most adorable amongst all men, responsible for protection, gracious to all, highly renowned for thy knowledge and concentration of mind through the practice of yoga!

[11]He: Sun.
[16]A person of these qualities should be elected as the head of the State.

१७. महो अग्ने: समिधानस्य शर्मंण्यनागा मित्रे वरुणे स्वस्तये ।
श्रेष्ठे स्याम सवितु: सवीमनि तद्देवानामवो व्रधा वृणीमहे ॥

17. May we the state officials, live free from sin, under the shelter of the highly brilliant head of the state, excellent, friendly and worthy of reverence.
We crave today for bliss, and gracious favour of the learned, who live under the command of God, as given in the vedas.

१८. आपश्चित्पिप्यु स्तर्यो न गावो नक्षन्नृतं जरितारस्त इन्द्र ।
याहि वायुर्न नियुतो नो अच्छा त्वँ हि धीभिर्दयसे वि वाजान् ॥

18. O highly learned person, thy panegyrists wax like waters, attain to true knowledge like expanding rays. May the persons possessing knowledge vast like mind come near us, may thou possess the qualities of swiftness and force like air!
Thou art worthy of reverence, as thou art highly kind to us through thy wisdom and deeds.

१९. गाव उपावतावतं मही यज्ञस्य रप्सुदा ।
उभा कर्णा हिरण्यया ॥

19. Just as the cows and sun's rays protect the beautifying Heaven and Earth, so should the learned protect both the ears coupled with golden ornaments, and parts of altar in a yajna.

२०. यदद्य सूर उदितेऽनागा मित्रो अर्यमा ।
सुवाति सविता भग: ॥

20. May the sinless, affectionate, just, and glorious king, the urger of the laws of administration, improve our health.

२१. आ सुते सिञ्चत श्रियँ रोदस्योरभिश्रियम् ।
रसा दधीत वृषभम् ।
तं प्रत्नथा अयं वेन: ॥

21. O happiness-giving people, elect him as your ruler, who is most mighty, lends lustre to heaven, and earth, is full of beauty and sustains you!

२२. आतिष्ठन्तं परि विश्वे अमूषञ्छ्रियो वसानश्चरति स्वरोचि: ।
महत्तद्वृष्णो असुरस्य नामा विश्वरूपो अमृतानि तस्थौ ॥

[17]Today: Ever.
[19]Griffith writes, the meaning of Rapsuda is uncertain. Rishi Dayananda translates the word as givers of beauty. There is no uncertainty in this meaning येरप्सु रूपं दत्तरते । (Rishi Dayananda's Commentary). Things which lend beauty.
[21]He alone is fit to be elected a king, who possesses the characteristics mentioned in the verse. For the translation of (तं प्रत्नथा । अयं वेन:) See Chapter 7, verses 12, 16.

22. O learned people ye all should use in your projects electricity, full of splendour, Self-effulgent, pervading all substances, ever active, present in all indestructible elements, well-established, bringer of rain, killer, and dignified in nature!

२३. प्र वो महे मन्दमानायान्धसोऽर्चा विश्वानराय विश्वाभुवे ।
इन्द्रस्य यस्य सुमखꣳ सहो महि श्रवो नृम्णं च रोदसी सपर्यतः ॥

23. Worship Him, Whose beautiful sacrifice, wealth, strength, and mighty glory are enjoyed by the Heaven and Earth, Who is the Creator of all beings, the Embodiment of great happiness, All-pervading and Supplier of food.

२४. बृहन्निदिध्म एषां भूरि शस्तं पृथुः स्वरुः ।
येषामिन्द्रो युवा सखा ॥

24. They alone perform laudable deeds, whose friend is God, Brilliant, Omnipresent, Majestic, ever young, Exalted, and Supreme.

२५. इन्द्रेहि मत्स्यन्धसो विश्वेभिः सोमपर्वभिः ।
महाꣳ अभिष्टिरोजसा ।

25. O learned person, fit for great veneration, due to thy strength, come and delight thyself with diverse juices of medicinal herbs and food!

२६. इन्द्रो वृत्रमवृणोच्छर्धनीतिः प्र मायिनामिनाद्वर्पणीतिः ।
अहन् व्यꣳसमुशधग्वनेष्वाविर्धेना अक्रुणोद्ब्राम्याणाम् ॥

26. He alone is fit to be elected the head of the State, who possesses power, knows how to arrange his army in different military arrays, is majestic like the sun; challenges for battle his impious foes, chastises the wily and deceitful persons, kills the dacoits hidden in forests, and makes apparent the words of preachers who diffuse happiness.

२७. कुतस्त्वमिन्द्र माहिनः सन्नेको यासि सत्पते किं त इत्था ।
सं पृच्छसे समराणः शुभानैर्वोचेस्तन्नो हरिवो यत्ते अस्मे ।
महाꣳ इन्द्रो य ओजसा
कदा चन स्तरीरसि
कदा चन प्र युच्छसि ॥

27. O King, the protector of the virtuous, highly venerable, why dost thou go alone? What is thy purpose in doing so? Lord of fascinating horses, we

---

²³Beautiful sacrifice: The great beautiful yajna in the shape of creation.
Enjoyed by the Heaven and Earth: Enjoyed by sentient beings and birds, animals and reptiles not developed in knowledge living on the earth and in the atmosphere.
²⁷A king should do nothing without consulting his ministers. He is a constitutional head. The responsibility of running the state does not devolve upon him alone. It is joint with his advisers and counsellors. See 7-40, 8-2, 3; for translation of the words from महाँ to प्रयुच्छसि ।

are thy well-wishers, consult us in thy true behaviour and tell us in blissful words, the reason of thy prefering solitude!

२८. आ तत्त इन्द्रायव: पनन्ताभि य ऊर्वं गोमन्तं तितृत्सान् ।
सकृत्स्वं ये पुरुपुत्रां महीꣳसहस्रधारां बृहतीं दुदुक्षन् ॥

28. O King, advance those persons who wish to utilise according to their desire, the Earth, which bears at one time many kinds of cereals, is the mother of many sons, the sustainer of numberless human beings, great, and lofty, who wish to kill the wicked, the voluptuous, and harmful persons in the front, and thus extol thy administration!

२९. इमां ते धियं प्र भरे महो महीमस्य स्तोत्रे धिषणा यत्त आनजे ।
तमुत्सवे च प्रसवे च सासहिमिन्द्रं देवास: शवसामदन्नु ॥

29. O King, I acknowledge this mighty wisdom of thine. My intellect manifests thee in praise. The learned on great festive occasions and childbirth bring joy unto thee, the master of intense endurance and the conqueror of foes with thy strength!

३०. विभ्राड् बृहत्पिबतु सोम्यं मध्वायुर्दधद्यज्ञपतावविह्रुतम् ।
वातजूतो यो अभिरक्षति त्मना प्रजा: पुपोष पुरुधा वि राजति ॥

30. The king, who shining like the wind-urged sun, grants full prolonged life to the sacrifice's lord, in person guards and nourishes the subjects, and variously sheds his lustre, should drink the glorious sweet juice of medicinal herbs.

३१. उदु त्यं जातवेदसं देवं वहन्ति केतव: ।
दृशे विश्वाय सूर्यम् ॥

31. O men know ye the illumined sun present in all created objects, whose rays shine wondrously for making the world visible!

३२. येना पावक चक्षसा भूरण्यन्तं जनाꣳ अनु ।
त्वं वरुण पश्यसि ॥

32. O pure king, with that same eye wherewith thou lookest as a guardian, look thou upon us, so that we may follow in thy wake!

३३. देव्यावध्वर्यू आ गतꣳ रथेन सूर्यत्वचा ।
मध्वा यज्ञꣳ समञ्जाथे ॥
तं प्रत्नथा ꣳयं वेनश्चित्रं देवानाम् ॥

²⁹I: Purohit, priest.
³¹See 7—41.
The verse may also mean, just as the rays of the sun exhibit Him, so do the learned display through their knowledge the grandeur of God, knower of all created objects.
³³See 7-12, 16, 42.

33. Ye two divine performers of harmless sacrifice, come hither upon a plane with sun-bright exterior, and clearly accomplish your journey, battle, and yajna with agreeable provisions.

३४. आ न इडाभिर्विदथे सुशस्ति विश्वानरः सविता देव एतु ।
अपि यथा युवानो मत्सथा नो विश्वं जगदभिपित्वे मनीषा ॥

34. O young preachers, having acquired knowledge through celibacy, just as a learned, person, the leader of all, endowed with noble qualities, brilliant like the sun, highly lauded for his speeches on knowable conduct, visits all our sons and cattle; so should ye approach and gladden us, and purify our intellect!

३५. यदद्य कच्च वृत्रहन्नुदगा अभि सूर्य ।
सर्वं तदिन्द्र ते वशे ॥

35. O slayer of foes like sun, the slayer of clouds, father of supremacy in knowledge, giver of food, noble man, all things are in thy power today, when wilt thou harness them!

३६. तरणिर्विश्वदर्शतो ज्योतिष्कृदसि सूर्य ।
विश्वमा भासि रोचनम् ॥

36. O king lustrous like the sun, that dispels darkness, is visible to all, produces light and illumines the whole universe, thou illuminest thy state with justice and humility, and art hence worthy of veneration!

३७. तत्सूर्यस्य देवत्वं तन्महित्वं मध्या कर्तोर्विततꣳ सं जभार ।
यदेदयुक्त हरितः सधस्थादादरात्री वासस्तनुते सिमस्मै ॥

37. O men, understand the divinity and greatness of God, the soul of the animate and inanimate creation; Who dissolves in Himself the quarters in the atmosphere, and this vast created universe, and spreads for all darkness like night; Who again creates the universe with His invisible, divine might!

३८. तन्मित्रस्य वरुणस्याभिचक्षे सूर्यो रूपं कृणुते द्योरुपस्थे ।
अनन्तमन्यद्रुशदस्य पाजः कृष्णमन्यद्धरितः सं भरन्ति ॥

38. God, away from darkness, creates that form of Apan and Udan, whereby the man beholds and perceives.
Immeasurable are His Immaculate Nature and power, different from soul, and different from Matter, full of ignorance and darkness, wherein reside the quarters.

[35]Slayer of foes: King.
[37]This verse describes the process of the creation and dissolution of the universe by God. Griffith remarks, the stanza is difficult and no thoroughly satisfactory explanation of it has yet been offered. The verse is clear and full of sense as interpreted by Maharshi Dayananda.

३९. बण्महाँ२ असि सूर्यं बडादित्य महाँ२ असि ।
महस्ते सतो महिमा पनस्यतेऽद्धा देव महाँ२ असि ॥

39. Verily, O God, Thou art great, truly Indestructible, Omniscient God, Thou art great!

As Thou art great indeed Thy greatness is admired. Yea, verily Thou, God, art great!

४०. बट् सूर्य श्रवसा महाँ२ असि सत्रा देव महाँ२ असि ।
महत्त्वा देवानामसूर्यः पुरोहितो विभु ज्योतिरदाभ्यम् ॥

40. Yea, God, Thou art great in fame. Thou, evermore, O God, art great. Thou by Thy greatness art the friend of the learned from the beginning, the Well-wisher of vital breaths, Unconquerable, Ubiquitous, and Refulgent!

४१. श्रायन्त इव सूर्यं विश्वेदिन्द्रस्य भक्षत ।
वसूनि जाते जनमान ओजसा प्रति भागं न दीधिम ॥

41. O people, just as we, manifest all substances depending upon God, Who shines in this world and the world to be, created through His might; and enjoy the portion allotted to us, so should ye enjoy your share of prosperity!

४२. श्रद्धा देवा उदिता सूर्यस्य निरँहसः पिपृता निरवद्यात् ।
तन्नो मित्रो वरुणो मामहन्तामदितिः सिन्धुः पृथिवी उत द्यौः ॥

42. O learned persons, save us today from sin and blamable affliction, when the sun hath ascended. May friends, noble persons, atmosphere, sea, Earth and light all honour our determination!

४३. आ कृष्णेन रजसा वर्तमानो निवेशयन्नमृतं मर्त्यं च ।
हिरण्येन सविता रथेना देवो याति भुवनानि पश्यन् ॥

43. The lustrous Sun, with its effulgent and moving nature, revolving repeatedly, bound with the solar system through gravitation, exhibiting all regions, fixing the immortal and mortal in their respective stations, comes and goes at the time of rising and setting.

४४. प्र वावृजे सुप्रया बर्हिरेषामा विश्पतीव वीरिट इयाते ।
विशामक्तोरुषसः पूर्वहूतौ वायुः पूषा स्वस्तये नियुत्वान् ॥

[41] The verse is considered by Griffith to be difficult and obscure. I don't understand why he holds this view. Its sense is clear and explicit.

[42] When the sun hath ascended may also mean, when the light of knowledge and wisdom hath dawned upon us. Mitra and Varuna have been translated by some commentators as day and night whereas Rishi Dayananda translates them as friends and noble persons.

Today means ever.

[43] Immortal: Matter.

Mortal: Men who are prone to death.

CHAPTER XXXIII

44. The air and Sun, extolled by forefathers, moving nicely, endowed with swiftness, move with intensity for the welfare of human beings.
Like the kings in the midst of their subjects, they come and go, and get water at night and morning.

४५. इन्द्रवायू बृहस्पतिं मित्राग्निं पूषणं भगम् ।
आदित्यान् मारुतं गणम् ॥

45. Electricity, air, Sun, breath, fire, invigorating wealth, twelve months, and the host of wind should be properly utilised.

४६. वरुण: प्राविता भुवन्मित्रो विश्वाभिरूतिभि: ।
करतां न: सुराधस: ॥

46. O learned teacher and preacher, just as a well-read person, like Udan and a friend dear like Pran guard us with all aids, so should ye both make us exceedingly rich!

४७. अधि न इन्द्रैषां विष्णो सजात्यानाम् । इता मरुतो अश्विना ।
तं प्रत्नथा ऽयं वेनो ये देवास
आ न इडाभिर्विश्वेभि: सोम्यं मध्वोमासश्चर्षणीधृत: ॥

47. O highly learned person, O Omnipresent God, noblemen, O teacher and preacher, may ye lord over us and our associates!

४८. अग्न इन्द्र वरुण मित्र देवा: शर्ध: प्र यन्त मारुतोत विष्णो ।
उभा नासत्या रुद्रो अध ग्ना: पूषा भग: सरस्वती जुषन्त ॥

48. O learned persons, the expositors of knowledge, the embodiments of supremacy, the masters of excellence, friendly, sociable and penetrating, grant us physical and spiritual strength!
May both the truthful teacher and preacher, the chastisers of the ignoble, well disciplined speech, and our protector, a wealthy person, and a highly educated wife serve us.

४६. इन्द्राग्नी मित्रावरुणादितिꣳ स्व: पृथिवीं द्यां मरुत: पर्वताꣳ्र अप: ।
हुवे विष्णुं पूषणं ब्रह्मणस्पतिं भगं नु शꣳसꣳ सवितारमूतये ॥

49. May I eagerly praise for help and happiness, conjoint electricity and fire, intermingled Pran and Udan, the sky, the Earth, the Sun, the thoughtful persons, the clouds, the waters, the All-pervading God, the invigorating cereals, God, the guardian of the world and the vedas, prosperity, and laudable king.

---
44 Water: Dew.
45 Aditya: The word may also mean beams of the Sun.
47 See 7-12, 16, 19, 33-35, 10, 7-33.

५०. अस्मे रुद्रा मेहना पर्वतासो वृत्रहत्ये भरहूतौ सजोषाः ।
यः शंसते स्तुवते धायि पज्र इन्द्रज्येष्ठा अस्मांर॒ अवन्तु देवाः ॥

50. May those learned persons, who in our midst are bounteous, chastisers of the ignoble, performers of festivals, accordant in call to battle for slaying the foe, acknowledging their ruler as their head, protect us and him who preaches virtue, praises God, and preserves the accumulated wealth.

५१. अर्वाञ्चो अद्या भवता यजत्रा आ वो हार्दि भयमानो व्ययेयम् ।
त्राध्वं नो देवा निजुरो वृकस्य त्राध्वं कर्तादवपदो यजत्राः ॥

51. Ye sociable, holy persons, turn yourselves hitherward this day, that fearing I may know your internal intentions. Protect us from the violent thief and dacoit. Save us ye admirer of the learned, from the pit in which we are liable to fall.

५२. विश्वे अद्य मरुतो विश्व ऊती विश्वे भवन्त्वग्नयः समिद्धाः ।
विश्वे नो देवा अवसा गमन्तु विश्वमस्तु द्रविणं वाजो अस्मे ॥

52. May this day all mortals, all officials, all enkindled fires, be our protectors with their act of protection. May all godly persons come hither with their protection. My we possess all riches and provisions.

५३. विश्वे देवाः शृणुतेमं हवं मे ये अन्तरिक्षे य उप द्यविष्ठ ।
ये अग्निजिह्वा उत वा यजत्रा आसद्यास्मिन्बर्हिषि मादयध्वम् ॥

53. All learned persons, may ye know all venerable objects that reside in heaven, and air's mid region, and are full of fire like the tongue. May ye listen to this mode of my studies, and seated in the Assembly be joyful.

५४. देवेभ्यो हि प्रथमं यज्ञियेभ्योऽमृतत्वं सुवसि भागमुत्तमम् ।
आदिद्दामानं सवितर्व्यूर्णुषेऽनूचीना जीविता मानुषेभ्यः ॥

54. O God, as Thou bestowest on the learned performers of sacrifice, the noblest and highest bliss of immortality, and preachest for the good of humanity, the light of knowledge that conduces to happiness, and actions worth knowing, Thou art hence worthy of worship!

५५. प्र वायुमच्छा बृहती मनीषा बृहद्रयिं विश्ववारं रथप्राम् ।
द्युतद्यामा नियुतः पत्यमानः कविः कविमियक्षसि प्रयज्यो ॥

55. O learned performer of sacrifice, approaching men of iron determination, with thy intense wisdom, thou promptly honourest the sage, and wishest to utilise the air, all-bounteous, encompasser of all substances, pervader of all aeroplanes, and fanner of fire!

⁶³May: Pupil's.

५६. इन्द्रवायू इमे सुता उप प्रयोभिरा गतम् ।
इन्दवो वामुशन्ति हि ॥

56. O masters of the sciences of electricity and air, for ye are all these substances prepared. The juices of medicinal herbs are yearning for ye both. Hence come with your excellent qualities, deeds and nature and enjoy them!

५७. मित्रं हुवे पूतदक्षं वरुणं च रिशादसम् ।
धियं घृताचीं साधन्ता ॥

57. I acknowledge a friend of holy strength and a foe-destroying virtuous man, who possess wisdom and peaceful silence of the night.

५८. दस्रा युवाकवः सुता नासत्या वृक्तबर्हिषः ।
आ यातं रुद्रवर्त्तनी ।
तं प्रत्नथा ॐ वेनः ॥

58. O lovers of truth, kingly extirpators of the impious, come, and enjoy the substances prepared for your meals; eagerly waiting for ye both!

५९. विदद्यदी सरमा रुग्णमद्रेर्महि पाथः पूर्व्यं सध्र्यक्कः ।
अग्रं नयत्सुपद्यक्षराणामच्छा रवं प्रथमा जानती गात् ॥

59. A wife, obedient to her husband, renowned, light-footed, eloquent in speech, sympathetic to the patients, attains to happiness when she lives peacefully with her husband, and nicely cooks the food highly efficacious, and grown through rain, conducive to our physical growth, brought daily in use, and relished by our ancestors.

६०. नहि स्पशमविदन्न्यमस्माद्वैश्वानरात्पुर एतारमग्ने ।
एमेनवृमधन्नमृता अमर्त्यं वैश्वानरं क्षेत्रजित्याय देवाः ॥

60. The divine immortal souls recognise none as their protector, but this loving and foremost God. For sovereignty of this land, they glorify with their praise, the Eternal God, the Friend of all.

६१. उग्रा विघनिना मृध इन्द्राग्नी हवामहे ।
ता नो मृडात ईदृशे ॥

61. We invoke the head of the State and the commander-in-chief, strong, and dispellers of foes. May they be kind to us in the battle-field.

६२. उपास्मै गायता नरः पवमानायेन्दवे ।
अभि देवाँ२ इयक्षते ॥

---

[56] See 7-8.
[58] Ye both: The king and Purohit (priest).
See 7-12, 16.

62. O teacher instruct in religious lore this student, anxious for maintaining good character, and willing to honour the learned!

६३. ये त्वाऽहिहत्ये मघवन्नवर्धन्ये शाम्बरे हरिवो ये गविष्टौ ।
ये त्वा नूनमनुमदन्ति विप्रा: पिबेन्द्र सोमꣳ सगणो मरुद्भि: ॥

63. O venerable wealthy commander of the army, just as in the conflict between the sun and the cloud, rays make the sun victorious, so learned persons encourage thee. O heroic person, possessing horses shining like the praiseworthy rays, the learned advance thee like lightning in the fight between the sun and the cloud. Verily do these persons rejoice following in thy wake and affording thee protection. O valorous person, just as the sun with its host of winds imbibes water, so do thou drink with thy man the juice of medicinal herbs!

६४. जनिष्ठा उग्र: सहसे तुराय मन्द्र ओजिष्ठो बहुलाभिमान: ।
अवर्धन्निन्द्रं मरुतश्चिदत्र माता यद्वीरं दधनद्धनिष्ठा ॥

64. O King, thy most wealthy mother has been nourishing thee a hero, just as air strengthens the Sun, so learned persons strengthen thee. Create pleasure, being mighty for victorious valour, exulting, strongest, full of pride and courage!

६५. आ तू न इन्द्र वृत्रहन्नस्माकमर्धमा गहि ।
महान्महीभिरूतिभि: ॥

65. O King, the slayer of foes, work hard for our advancement. Mighty one, protect us with thy mighty aids!

६६. त्वमिन्द्र प्रतूर्तिष्वभि विश्वा असि स्पृध: ।
अशस्तिहा जनिता विश्वतूरसि त्वं तूर्य तरुष्यत: ॥

66. Thou in thy battles, King, art subduer of all hostile bands. Thou art the destroyer of the depraved, the genitor of happiness, the slayer of foes, the conqueror, vanquish the foes who wish to kill us!

६७. अनु ते शुष्मं तुरयन्तमीयतु: क्षोणी शिशुं न मातरा ।
विश्वास्ते स्पृध: स्नथयन्त मन्यवे वृत्रं यदिन्द्र तूर्वसि ॥

67. O King, just as sire and mother walk after the child, so do thy enemies and their territories fall into thy hands. When thou killest thy unjust foe, all his forces are weakened before thy indignation!

६८. यज्ञो देवानां प्रत्येति सुम्नमादित्यासो भवता मृडयन्त: ।
आ वोऽर्वाची सुमतिर्ववृत्यादꣳहोश्चिद्या वरिवोवित्तरासत् ॥

68. Struggle is a source of happiness for the learned. O well-read scholars

---

[68]See 8-4.

remain firm in happiness. Let your favour be directed towards us; which may bring us riches even from the sinful foe!

६९. अदब्धेभिः सवितः पायुभिष्ट्वꣳ शिवेभिरद्य परि पाहि नो गयम् ।
हिरण्यजिह्वः सुविताय नव्यसे रक्षा माकिर्नो अघशꣳस ईशत ॥

69. O King with non-violent, propitious aids, protect this day, on all sides, our progeny, riches and home. Master of speech conducive to the welfare of all, keep us for newest bliss; let not the evil-wisher lord over us!

७०. प्र वीरया शुचयो दद्रिरे वामध्वर्युभिर्मधुमन्तः सुतासः ।
वह वायो नियुतो याह्यच्छा पिबा सुतस्यान्धसो मदाय ॥

70. O officials and people, your noble persons full of praiseworthy knowledge, education and nice instructions, with the help of the non-violent and just, rend asunder the foes with an army of brave soldiers!
O King, strong like the wind, possess the qualities of joining and separating like the air, invade courageously thy enemies, and drink for thy rapture the sap of well-prepared food!

७१. गाव उपावतावतं मही यज्ञस्य रप्सुदा ।
उभा कर्णा हिरण्यया ॥

71. O men, just as both immense Sun and Earth, full of brilliance, the fulfillers of all transactions, the bestowers of beauty, guard this organised world like a well, and rays also guard it, so should ye guard them!

७२. काव्ययोराजानेषु ऋत्वा दक्षस्य दुरोणे ।
रिशादसा सधस्थ आ ॥

72. O teacher and preacher, the dispellers of the sins of nescience, come ye with force of intellect to the study circles where are studied the works of poets on worldly and spiritual topics, to the meeting place and the dwelling of a scholarly person!

७३. दैव्याबध्वर्यू आ गतꣳ रथेन सूर्यत्वचा ।
मध्वा यज्ञꣳ समञ्जाथे ।
तं प्रत्नथा ꣳयं वेनः ॥

73. Ye two learned persons, believers in non-violence, come hither in a sun-bright plane, and explain fully to us the conduct of life!

[71] This verse is the same as 33-19, but with a quite different significance.
Like a well: Just as peasants guard their fields and garden with water from a well, so do the Sun and Earth guard this world. Them: The Sun and Earth.
[72] Mr. Griffith says "The verse is difficult and obscure."
To me these remarks seem to be unreasonable.
[73] रथेन may mean a plane, a motor car or a motor-boat as it is used in air, on land or water.
Two: The teacher and preacher.
For two pratikas see 7-12, 16.

७४. तिरश्चीनो विततो रश्मिरेषामधः स्विदासी३ दुपरि स्विदासी३त् ।
रेतोधा आसन्महिमान आसन्त्स्वधा अवस्तात्प्रयतिः परस्तात् ॥

74. The transverse and extended light of the sun and lightning is found above and below. It is struggling from hither and thither. With its knowledge men should gain strength, and become venerable and philanthropic with their wealth.

७५. आ रोदसी अपृणदा स्वर्मंहज्जातं यदेनमपसो अधारयन् ।
सो अध्वराय परि णीयते कविरत्यो न वाजसातये चनोहितः ॥

75. Electricity hath filled the Heaven and Earth and the great apparent realm of light. This fire is utilised through application; being the cause of sound, it is used for non-violent industrial concerns. For fastness in battle it is used as a horse that covers distances quickly. It is helpful for the growth of food grains from the Earth.

७६. उक्थेभिर्वृहन्तमा या मन्दाना चिदा गिरा ।
आजूर्वैराविवासतः ॥

76. The teacher and preacher are deserving of praise, who like the King and Commander of the army, the bestowers of happiness and chastisers of the irreligious sinners, spread technical knowledge through vedic verses, speech and proclamations.

७७. उप नः सूनवो गिरः शृण्वन्त्वमृतस्य ये ।
सुमृडीका भवन्तु नः ॥

77. May our sons listen about the Immortal God, to the eternal preachings of the vedas from their teachers, and bring us joy.

७८. ब्रह्माणि मे मतयः शं सुतासः शुष्म इयर्ति प्रभृतो मे अद्रिः ।
आ शासते प्रति हर्यन्त्युक्थेमा हरी वहतस्ता नो अच्छ ॥

78. Endowed with knowledge and good education, the prosperous, wise persons, expect riches, and desire for vedic instructions from me. Just as the strong cloud well fed through Homa, brings me joy, so should the teacher and the taught teach us different sorts of vedic knowledge.

७९. अनुत्तमा ते मघवन्नकिर्नु न त्वावाँर् अस्ति देवता विदानः ।
न जायमानो नशते न जातो यानि करिष्या कृणुहि प्रवृद्ध ॥

79. O Mighty God, The nature is matchless. Among the learned sages not one is found Thy equal!

[78]The teacher, Acharya. The verse means, there should be mutual exchange of knowledge. The pupils should learn from the teachers, from those who are more learned than themselves.
Me: A learned person.

Thou wast never born, nor is born. None can comprehend what Thou hast done or shalt do.

८०. तदिदास भुवनेषु ज्येष्ठं यतो जज्ञ उग्रस्त्वेषनृम्णः ।
सद्यो जज्ञानो नि रिणाति शत्रूननु यं विश्वे मदन्त्यूमाः ॥

80. In all the worlds God is the Best and Highest whence sprang the valiant, wealthy hero. Quickly when born he overcomes his foemen. All benefactors of humanity who follow God derive joy.

८१. इमा उ त्वा पुरूवसो गिरो वर्धन्तु या मम ।
पावकवर्णाः शुचयो विपश्चितोऽभि स्तोमैरनूषत ॥

81. May these my songs of praise verily exalt Thee, God, Who is omnipresent.
Men, radiant like fire, pure, full of knowledge, sing Thy praises admiring material objects.

८२. यस्यायं विश्व आर्यो दासः शेवधिपा अरिः ।
तिरश्चिदर्ये रुशमे पवीरवि तुभ्येत्सो अज्यते रयिः ॥

82. O King, this man of high character is obedient to thee. The miser who hides his treasure is thy enemy. The hidden wealth of a wealthy trader, protected against arms and violence, is meant for thee!

८३. अयꣳ सहस्रमृषिभिः सहस्कृतः समुद्र इव पप्रथे ।
सत्यः सो अस्य महिमा गृणे शवो यज्ञेषु विप्रराज्ये ॥

83. The King is endowed with innumerable branches of knowledge through sages, the knowers of the vedas, possesses vast strength, and is famous for his noble actions, His greatness is spread vast like the ocean. I praise firmness in the administration of the wise and well-organised government functions.

८४. अदब्धेभिः सवितः पायुभिष्ट्वꣳ शिवेभिरद्य परि पाहि नो गयम् ।
हिरण्यजिह्वः सुविताय नव्यसे रक्षा माकिर्नो अघशꣳस ईशत ॥

84. O supreme King, protect this day our dependants from all sides with different kinds of harmless, lucky aids. Endowed with speech contributing to the welfare of all, protect us for newest prosperity, whereby no evil-minded thief may have his sway over us!

---

[80] When born: It does not refer to physical birth. It refers to intellectual and spiritual birth, after he has received military training from his teacher, and become twice born.
[81] Material objects, created by God, sing His glory. The learned seeing the wonderful, beautiful world created by God, sing the praise of God expressing their admiration for all material objects.
[83] I: A member of the subjects.
[84] This verse is the same as 33—69. The meanings of both are different. Hence there is no repetition. In the verse 69 गयम् means, riches and house, whereas here it means the dependants, which altogether changes the significance.

८५. आ नो यज्ञं दिविस्पृशं वायो याहि सुमन्मभिः ।
अन्तः पवित्र उपरि श्रीणानोऽय॒ शुक्रो अ्यामि ते ॥

85. O king, quick like air, just as I, internally pure, believing in progress, active and valorous, with nice store of knowledge, attend thy literary conclaves, so shouldst thou ours!

८६. इन्द्रवायू सुसन्दृशा सुहवेह हवामहे ।
यथा नः सर्वं इज्जनोऽनमीवः सङ्गमे सुमना असत् ॥

86. We accept as our masters in this world, the king and the Commander-in-chief, fair to see and fit to be invoked, so that in the Assembly and battle, all our men be happy and free from disease.

८७. ऋधगित्था स मर्त्यः शशमे देवतातये ।
यो नूनं मित्रावरुणावभिष्टय आचक्रे हव्यदातये ॥

87. The prosperous person, who for the acquisition of noble traits, the acquirement of desired happiness, obtaining things worthy of possession, verily serves the king and public leaders, becomes thereby peaceful in mind and free from trouble.

८८. आ यातमुप भूषतं मध्वः पिबतमश्विना ।
दुग्धं पयो वृषणा जेन्यावसू मा नो मर्धिष्टमा गतम् ॥

88. O king and public leaders, valiant, conquerors of riches, immersed in knowledge, attain to happiness, adorn the subjects, drink the medically prepared juice, arrange for the supply of water, injure us not, and gain victory through righteousness!

८९. प्रेतु ब्रह्मणस्पतिः प्र देव्येतु सूनृता ।
अच्छा वीरं नर्यं पङ्क्तिराधसं देवा यज्ञं नयन्तु नः ॥

89. May the master of wealth and vedic lore come nigh unto us, may we cultivate truthful speech. May the learned associate with an exalted and brave person, the lover of humanity and follower of the path of rectitude.

९०. चन्द्रमा अप्स्वन्तरा सुपर्णो धावते दिवि ।
रयिं पिशङ्गं बहुलं पुरुस्पृह॒ हरिरेति कनिक्रदत् ॥

90. The moon with beautiful gaits, like a loud-neighing horse, runs in the atmosphere, receiving light from the sun. Object of many a man's desire, abundantly golden-hued, she acquires beauty, lustre and grandeur.

९१. देव-देवं वोऽवसे देव-देवमभिष्टये ।
देव-देव॒ हुवेम वाजसातये गृणन्तो देव्या धिया ॥

91. Singing their praises with godlike wisdom, let us invoke each learned person for your protection; each scholar for the acquisition of desired happiness, and each sage for enjoying progress.

९२. दिवि पृष्टो अरोचतानिर्वैश्वानरो बृहन् ।
क्षमया वृधान ओजसा चनोहितो ज्योतिषा बाधते तमः ॥

92. O learned persons, just as the Sun, set in heaven, the benefactor of humanity, increasing in his power on Earth, ripens medicines and grows food, removes darkness of the night with his lustre, and shines forth, so should ye dispel ignorance and gain glory!

९३. इन्द्राग्नी अपादियं पूर्वागत् पद्वतीभ्यः ।
हित्वी शिरो जिह्वया वावदच्चरत्रि॒ शतपदा न्यक्रमीत् ॥

93. O teacher and preacher; this footless Dawn, first comes to those with feet. Being headless, speaking loudly with the tongue of birds, she goes down for twenty four hours!

९४. देवासो हि ष्मा मनवे समन्यवो विश्वे साक॒ सरातयः ।
ते नो अद्य ते अपरं तुचे तु नो भवन्तु वरिवोविदः ॥

94. May all learned persons, equally charitably disposed, and equally full of righteous indignation, in unison, be the bringers of riches, today and hereafter, for a thoughtful person, for us and our progeny.

९५. अपाधमदभिशस्तीरशस्तिहाथेन्द्रो द्युम्न्याभवत् ।
देवास्त इन्द्र सख्याय येमिरे बृहद्भ्वानो मरुद्गण ॥

95. O King refulgent with fame, lord of the hosts of men, the learned strive to win thy love. O supreme King, suppressor of violence from all sides, chastiser of the ignoble, be thou the master of riches!

९६. प्र व इन्द्राय बृहते मरुतो ब्रह्मार्चत ।
वृत्र॒ हनति वृत्रहा शतक्रतुर्वज्रेण शतपर्वणा ॥

96. O men, the Commander of the army with manifold acts, affording protection to the millions, with warlike weapons, like sun the slayer of clouds, slays the foes for mighty prestige, and secures wealth and food for ye, so should ye show him respect!

⁹¹Their: the Vishvedevas, the learned sages and saints.
 Your: the common people, the subjects.
⁹³This verse is applicable to Dawn and Tongue. Rishi Dayananda, Sayana, and Mahidhar have interpreted it differently. I have given the interpretation of Maharshi Dayananda. Dawn, without foot moving in the sky, appears when men with feet are sleeping. Birds like cock announce with their tongue its arrival. It leaves its head, the sun. It reappears after passing through thirty divisions of day and night, i.e., 24 hours.

९७. अस्येदिन्द्रो वावृधे वृष्ण्यꣳ शवो मदे सुतस्य विष्णवि ।
अद्या तमस्य महिमानमायवोऽनु ष्टुवन्ति पूर्वथा ॥
इमा उ त्वा यस्यायमयꣳ सहस्रमूर्ध्व ऊ षु ण: ॥

97. O men, the mighty king, always enhances his power and valour, and arranges for the supply of water, for the happiness of the world created by God. Human beings anxious for the fruit of their actions sing the glory of God like their forefathers. Praise ye also Him!

⁹⁷For four Pratikas (limbs) see 33—81, 82, 83 and 11—42.

CHAPTER XXXIV

१. यज्जाग्रतो दूरमुदैति दैवं तदु सुप्तस्य तथैवैति ।
दूरङ्गमं ज्योतिषां ज्योतिरेकं तन्मे मन: शिवसङ्कल्पमस्तु ॥

1. That which, divine, mounts far when man is waking, that which returns to him when he is sleeping.
The lights' one light that goeth to a distance, may that, my mind, be moved by auspicious resolve.

२. येन कर्माण्यपसो मनीषिणो यज्ञे कृण्वन्ति विदथेषु धीरा: ।
यदपूर्वं यक्षमन्त: प्रजानां तन्मे मन: शिवसङ्कल्पमस्तु ॥

2. Whereby the virtuous, thoughtful and wise persons, in religious performances, learned assemblies and battles, perform their duties. The peerless spirit stored in living creatures, may that, my mind be moved by auspicious resolve.

३. यत्प्रज्ञानमुत चेतो धृतिश्च यज्ज्योतिरन्तरमृतं प्रजासु ।
यस्मान्न ऋते किं चन कर्म क्रियते तन्मे मन: शिवसङ्कल्पमस्तु ॥

3. That which is wisdom, intellect, and firmness, immortal light which creatures have within them. That without which men can do no single action, may that, my mind, hanker after God and be moved by noble resolve.

४. येनेदं भूतं भुवनं भविष्यत् परिगृहीतममृतेन सर्वम् ।
येन यज्ञस्तायते सप्तहोता तन्मे मन: शिवसङ्कल्पमस्तु ॥

4. Whereby, coupled with immortal God, the past, present and future all are comprehended, whereby spreads sacrifice by Seven Hotas, may that, my mind, aim at salvation.

५. यस्मिन्नृच: साम यजूंषि यस्मिन् प्रतिष्ठिता रथनाभाविवारा: ।
यस्मिंश्चित्तं सर्वमोतं प्रजानां तन्मे मन: शिवसङ्कल्पमस्तु ॥

5. Wherein the Richas, Samans, Yajur-verses and the Atharvaveda, like spokes within a cart's nave, are included, and all the knowledge of human beings is inwoven, may that, my mind, be actuated with the noble resolve of propagating the Vedas.

¹The lights' one light: The sole illuminator of all perceptive senses.
⁴Seven Hotas: The seven organs in the head, two eyes, two ears, two nostrils and mouth. They play an important part in performing the functions of this bodily sacrifice.
Seven Hotas may also mean, five breaths, Soul and primary Matter.

६. सुषारथिरश्वानिव यन्मनुष्यान्नेनीयतेऽभीशुभिर्वाजिन इव ।
हृत्प्रतिष्ठं यदजिरं जविष्ठं तन्मे मनः शिवसङ्कल्पमस्तु ॥

6. As a skilful charioteer drives with reins the fleet-foot horses, so does the mind control men. It dwells within the heart, is free from old age, drives men into sensuality, and is most rapid. May that, my mind, be moved by right intention.

७. पितुं नु स्तोषं महो धर्माणं तविषीम् ।
यस्य त्रितो व्योजसा वृत्रं विपर्वमदर्यत् ॥

7. I glorify eagerly the king who possesses food, justice and a strong army. He conquers the foes, just as the sun rends limb by limb the cloud filled with water.

८. अग्निदनुमते त्वं मन्यासै शं च नस्कृधि ।
क्रत्वे दक्षाय नो हिनु प्रण आयूँषि तारिषः ॥

8. O learned king of favourable disposition, grant us happiness, which thou dost consider conducive. Urge us to wisdom, and strength; and prolong the days of our life!

९. अनु नोऽद्यानुमतिर्यज्ञं देवेषु मन्यताम् ।
अग्निश्च हव्यवाहनो भवतं दाशुषे मयः ॥

9. May the man of favourable knowledge approve friendly this day our sacrifice among the learned. May he and master of the science of oblation-bearing fire, bring bliss to the charitably disposed person.

१०. सिनीवालि पृथुष्टुके या देवानामसि स्वसा ।
जुषस्व हव्यमाहुतं प्रजां देवि दिदिड्ढि नः ॥

10. O lovely, strong, broad-tressed, famous, beautiful, educated virgin, sister of the learned, accept the desired husband, and grant us progeny!

११. पञ्च नद्यः सरस्वतीमपि यन्ति सस्रोतसः ।
सरस्वती तु पञ्चधा सो देशेऽभवत्सरित् ॥

11. Five organs of cognition, emanating from their common source, the mind, like five rivers speed onward to speech. The flowing speech, in its dwelling place, the mouth, becomes fivefold.

१२. त्वमग्ने प्रथमो अङ्गिरा ऋषिर्देवो देवानामभवः शिवः सखा ।
तव व्रते कवयो विद्मनापसोऽजायन्त मरुतो भ्राजदृष्टयः ॥

12. O God, may Thou the Most-renowned, the Assuager of souls, Master of knowledge, the Scholar of scholars, be our Well-wisher and Friend !

[9]Sacrifice: Yajna.
[11]Saraswati: The speech.
Fivefold: Speech describes the five organs of cognition, the Gyan-Indriyas.

After Thy holy Law, sages and ordinary mortals, wise and prudent in actions with their splendid weapons, are born.

१३. त्वं नो अग्ने तव देव पायुभिर्मघोनो रक्ष तन्वश्च वन्द्य ।
त्राता तोकस्य तनये गवामस्यनिमेष रक्षमाणस्तव व्रते ॥

13. O God, noble in qualities, actions and nature, preserve our wealthy patrons and our bodies with Thy succours. O Venerable God, Guard art thou of our sons, grandsons and cows, incessantly protecting in Thy holy law!

१४. उत्तानायामव भरा चिकित्वान्त्सद्यः प्रवीता वृषणं जजान ।
अरुषस्तूपो रुशदस्य पाज इडायास्पुत्रो वयुनेऽजनिष्ट ॥

14. O learned person, just as a well-versed, aspiring scholar performs sacrifice (yajna) for the sake of rain in this vast Earth and atmosphere, and the son of a praiseworthy woman, acting as the promoter of non-violent persons, becomes famous for his knowledge and establishes his beautiful strength, so shouldst thou nourish thyself!

१५. इडायास्त्वा पदे वयं नाभा पृथिव्या अधि ।
जातवेदो निधीमह्याग्ने हव्याय वोढवे ॥

15. O sagacious king, we establish thee on the Earth in its centre in the post of a ruler, for granting us valuable substances!

१६. प्र मन्महे शवसानाय शूषमाङ्गूषं गिर्वणसे अङ्गिरस्वत् ।
सुवृक्तिभिः स्तुवत ऋग्मियायार्चामार्कं नरे विश्रुताय ॥

16. O men, just as we, with sinless acts, for the sake of knowledge, the reciters in well-trained utterances of vedic verses, replete with instructions, expatiate on religious lore, and long for the hero, the force of knowledge, and scriptures, dear like vital breath, and honour this venerable person, so should ye!

१७. प्र वो महे महि नमो भरध्वमाङ्गूष्यं शवसानाय साम ।
येना नः पूर्वे पितरः पदज्ञा अर्चन्तो अङ्गिरसो गा अविन्दन् ॥

17. O men, just as the knowers of the true nature o soul, showing respect unto us, knowing all the branches of the science of creation, and learned ancestors, for the great man imbued with physical and spiritual force, and for you, grant us disciplined speech and the knowledge of the Samaveda, highly useful for the attainment of strength, unto them should ye show respect and offer food!

१८. इच्छन्ति त्वा सोम्यासः सखायः सुन्वन्ति सोमं दधति प्रयांसि ।
तितिक्षन्ते अभिशस्तिं जनानामिन्द्र त्वदा कश्चन हि प्रकेतः ॥

---

[15] We: Preacher and teacher.

18. O king, honour those, who are affluent, friendly, gleaners of might, masters of knowledge, silent endurers of the abuses of the people. None is wiser than thee, hence all long for thee!

१९. न ते दूरे परमा चिद्रजाꣳ स्या तु प्र याहि हरिवो हरिभ्याम् ।
स्थिराय वृष्णे सवना कृतेमा युक्ता ग्रावाण: समिधाने अग्नौ ॥

19. O king, just as in the kindled fire these morning yajnas are performed, whereby the clouds come together, so come thou hither in conveyances moved by water and fire for acquiring permanent happiness. In this way even the distant places are not far for thee!

२०. आषाढं युत्सु पृतनासु पप्रिꣳ स्वर्षामप्सां वृजनस्य गोपाम् ।
भरेषुजाꣳ सुक्षितिꣳ सुश्रवसं जयन्तं त्वामनु मदेम सोम ॥

20. Invincible in fight, saviour of armies, giver of happiness, giver of life, protector of might, winner of battles, sovereign lord of the Earth, exceeding famous, victor, in thee may we rejoice, O King!

२१. सोमो धेनुꣳ सोमो अर्वन्तमाशुꣳ सोमो वीरं कर्मण्यं ददाति ।
सादन्यं विदथ्यꣳ सभेयं पितृश्रवणं यो ददाशदस्मै ॥

21. To him who reveres the king, teacher or preacher, he gives speech, full of learning, wealth, conducive to truthful conduct, a fleet steed, a brave son, active in duties, well-mannered, skilled in the performance of sacrifice (yajna), recipient of knowledge from his father, and competent in council.

२२. त्वमिमा ओषधी: सोम विश्वास्त्वमपो अजनयस्त्वं गा: ।
त्वमा ततन्थोर्वन्तरिक्षं त्वं ज्योतिषा वि तमो ववर्थ ॥

22. These herbs, these milch-kine, and these running waters, all these, O Soma, Thou hast generated. The spacious firmament hast Thou expanded, and with light hast Thou dispelled darkness!

२३. देवेन नो मनसा देव सोम रायो भागꣳ सहसावन्नभि युध्य ।
मा त्वा तनदीशिषे वीर्यस्योभयेभ्य: प्रचिकित्सा गविष्टौ ॥

23. O King, possessing a strong army, might, and fine attributes, with thy godly spirit, win for us a share of riches!
Thou art the lord of valour, let none subdue thee. With a desire for extreme happiness, in this world and the next, remove our impediments just as a disease is removed.

[18]In this verse are mentioned the attributes of an (Apta), an ideal sage.
[19]The word हरिव: has been translated by Swami Dayananda as king, the possessor of horses.
[21]The word Soma may mean God as well. He means a learned person.
[22]Soma means God.

२४. अष्टौ व्यख्यत् ककुभः पृथिव्यास्त्री धन्व योजना सप्त सिन्धून् ।
हिरण्याक्षः सविता देव आगाद्दधद्रत्ना दाशुषे वार्याणि ॥

24. The radiant, urging sun, comes giving choice treasures to the charitably disposed person. His brightness illumines the earth's eight directions, the three regions, and the seven rivers upto twelve miles.

२५. हिरण्यपाणिः सविता विचर्षणिरुभे द्यावापृथिवी अन्तरीयते ।
अपामीवां बाधते वेति सूर्यमभि कृष्णेन रजसा द्यामृणोति ॥

25. The sun, the recipient of water with his hands, the radiant rays, the exhibitor of all substances, the creator of all edibles, rises and moves between the Heaven and Earth, and removes the disease of darkness. At the time of setting it fills the atmosphere on all sides with dark night.

२६. हिरण्यहस्तो असुरः सुनीथः सुमृडीकः स्ववाँ यात्ववर्ड् ।
अपसेधन् रक्षसो यातुधानानस्थाद्देवः प्रतिदोषं गृणानः ॥

26. The Sun, with its hands of gleaming rays, kind benefactor, the bringer of rain, the giver of happiness, self refulgent, driving off demons and thieves, rises, removing human physical weaknesses. May he bring us happiness, illuminating all substances.

२७. ये ते पन्थाः सवितः पूर्व्यासोऽरेणवः सुकृता अन्तरिक्षे ।
तेभिर्नो अद्य पथिभिः सुगेभी रक्षा च नो अधि च ब्रूहि देव ॥

27. O highly learned fellow, brilliant like the Sun, thy dustless pathways, followed by the ancient scholars, are well established in the air's mid region, like those of the Sun. Come by those paths so fair to travel: make us ever tread upon them, preserve us and instruct us!

२८. उभा पिबतमश्विनोभा नः शर्म यच्छतम् ।
अविद्रियाभिरूतिभिः ॥

28. O teacher and preacher, lustrous like the Sun and Moon, grant us well protected, faultless, comfortable houses where ye may drink nice juices!

२९. अग्नस्वतीमश्विना वाचमस्मे कृतं नो दस्रा वृषणा मनीषाम् ।
अद्यूत्येऽवसे नि ह्वये वां बृधे च नो भवतं वाजसातौ ॥

29. O learned teacher and preacher, the dispellers of afflictions, and givers of joys, make ye our speech and wisdom effectual. Protect us against gambling, strive for your prosperity in battle. I praise ye both; work for my advancement!

---

[24]Eight directions: Four main directions: North, East South, West, and the four minor directions.
    Three regions: Heaven, firmament and earth.
    Seven rivers: Seven oceans or strata of vapour extending high up from the earth for twelve miles, upto the upper portion of the clouds.

३०. द्युभिरक्तुभि: परि पातमस्मानरिष्टेभिरश्विना सौभगेभि: ।
तन्नो मित्रो वरुणो मामहन्तामदिति: सिन्धु: पृथिवी उत द्यौ: ॥

30. O King and Commander of the army, just as the Earth, Ocean, atmosphere and heaven protect us, so ye both, friendly and chastisers of the wicked, through day and night, protect us on every side, with harmless riches!

३१. आ कृष्णेन रजसा वर्तमानो निवेशयन्नमृतं मर्त्यं च ।
हिरण्ययेन सविता रथेना देवो याति भुवनानि पश्यन् ॥

31. O learned persons, with full observation, use full well the lustrous electricity, which resides in the solar system, standing through attraction, fixes in its respective sphere the immortal cause and the mortal effect, and with its blazing, beautiful nature, grants prosperity, and pervades material objects!

३२. आ रात्रिं पार्थिवं रज: पितुरप्रायि धामभि: ।
दिव: सदांसि बृहती वि तिष्ठस आ त्वेषं वर्तते तम: ॥

32. O men, use properly the great Night, which covers the places of light, which hath filled the planet Earth and Sun's mid regions, whose terrific darkness comes and goes!

३३. उषस्तच्चित्रमा भरास्मभ्यं वाजिनीवति ।
येन तोकं च तनयं च धामहे ॥

33. O Dawn enriched with ample wealth, bestow on us that wondrous light wherewith we may support the babies and young sons, as does an accomplished wife!

३४. प्रातरग्निं प्रातरिन्द्रं हवामहे प्रातर्मित्रावरुणा प्रातरश्विना ।
प्रातर्भगं पूषणं ब्रह्मणस्पतिं प्रात: सोममुत रुद्रं हुवेम ॥

34. We invoke God at dawn, we pray for progress at dawn, we practice breath control at dawn, we respect father and mother, at dawn. At dawn we invoke God, the Lord of the vedas, the Sustainer of all, and Adorable by all. We use medicinal herbs in the morning, and at dawn we try to realise the true nature of soul.

३५. प्रातर्जितं भगमुग्रं हुवेम वयं पुत्रमदितेर्यो विधर्ता ।
आध्रश्चिद्यं मन्यमानस्तुरश्चिद्राजा चिद्यं भगं भक्षीत्याह ॥

35. God is the Master of infinite power, the Sustainer of manifold worlds, the Conqueror of all the Object of adoration by all, the aweinspiring Chastiser of the wicked, may, we worship Him in morning. Thinking of Whom the

---

[31] This verse is the same as 33-43 with a different significance. In 33-43 there is a mention of sun, but here electricity is the subject matter. There is no fault of repetition.

३६. भग प्रणेतर्भग सत्यराधो भगेमां धियमुदवा ददन्न: ।
भग प्र नो जनय गोभिरश्वैर्भग प्र नृभिनृ॑वन्त: स्याम ॥

36. O Glorious God, Goader of men to action, Giver of wealth, Master of riches, fit for adoration, grant us wisdom and afford us protection!

O God, the Giver of knowledge, increase our store of kine and horses. O God, may we be rich in men and heroes!

३७. उतेदानीं भगवन्त: स्यामोत प्रपित्व उत मध्ये अह्नाम् ।
उतोदिता मघवन्त्सूर्यस्य वयं देवानाᳪं सुमतौ स्याम ॥

37. O noble, pure God, may prosperity be ours at present, in future, and during the day-time!

May we, O Bounteous Lord, at the rising of the Sun, be happy, in the wake of the excellent wisdom of the learned!

३८. भग एव भगवाᳪं अस्तु देवास्तेन वयं भगवन्त: स्याम ।
तं त्वा भग सर्व इज्जोहवीति स नो भग पुर एता भवेह ॥

38. O learned persons, God verily is Supreme. May we become supreme through Him. O God, all invoke Thee. O Supreme God, be Thou our leader in this world!

३९. समध्वरायोषसो नमन्त दधिक्रावेव शुचये पदाय ।
अर्वाचीनं वसुविदं भगं नो रथमिवाश्वा वाजिन आ वहन्तु ॥

39. O men, Dawns like a disciplined horse, incline us to acquire a pure, desirable, non-violent conduct!

As strong steeds draw a chariot, may they remind us of the presence of the Mighty God, the Lord of riches.

४०. अश्वावतीर्गोमतीर्न उषासो वीरवती: सदमुच्छन्तु भद्रा: ।
घृतं दुहाना विश्वत: प्रपीता यूयं पात स्वस्तिभि: सदा न: ॥

40. O learned ladies, just as Dawns, full of nice cold water, and manifold beams, awakeners of heroic persons; auspicious; bestowers of pure water, advancing magnificently from all sides, dawn on our assembly, so should ye adorn our assembly and preserve us evermore with your health giving joys!

४१. पूषन् तव व्रते वयं न रिष्येम कदा चन ।
स्तोतारस्त इह स्मसि ॥

[39]They : Dawns.

At dawn man's mind is reflective, inclined to the worship of God, and contemplation of noble righteous deeds.

41. O nourishing God, may we following Thy Law, never suffer pain. We, in this world, are singers of Thy praise!

४२. पथस्पथः परिपतिं वचस्या कामेन कृतो अभ्यानडर्कम् ।
स नो रासच्छुरुधश्चन्द्राग्रा धियं-धियं सीषधाति प्र पूषा ॥

42. O men, Mighty God, with His vedic speech, noble intention, saintly Nature, gives us from time immemorial sources of happiness which keep afflictions away. He excellently establishes our wisdom and actions. He ever possesses good qualities, acts and nature. May we praise the Adorable God, Who guards all pathways!

४३. त्रीणि पदा वि चक्रमे विष्णुर्गोपा अदाभ्यः ।
अतो धर्माणि धारयन् ॥

43. The Merciful, Protecting, All-Pervading God, establishing His sacred laws, is thenceforth the Creator of the three steps of the causal, subtle and gross forms.

४४. तद्विप्रासो विपन्यवो जागृवाꣳसः समिन्धते ।
विष्णोर्यत्परमं पदम् ॥

44. The ever vigilant, the singers of the praise of God, and the learned yogis, realise His most sublime Nature.

४५. घृतवती भुवनानामभिश्रियोर्वी पृथ्वी मधुदुघे सुपेशसा ।
द्यावापृथिवी वरुणस्य धर्मणा विष्कभिते अजरे भूरिरेतसा ॥

45. By God's decree, the Sun and the Earth, full of light and water, ornamentors of the world created, vast, full of diverse objects, filled with sweet water, beautiful in their form, imperishable, rich in seed, stand apart firmly established.

४६. ये नः सपत्ना अप ते भवन्त्विन्द्राग्निभ्यामव बाधामहे तान् ।
वसवो रुद्रा आदित्या उपरिस्पृशं मोग्रं चेत्तारमधिराजमक्रन् ॥

46. Let those who are our foemen stand apart from us. With airy and fiery weapons we will drive them off. The Vasus, Rudras, and Adityas have exalted me, made me pre-eminent, mighty, thinker, and sovereign lord.

४७. आ नासत्या त्रिभिरेकादशैरिह देवेभिर्यातं मधुपेयमश्विना ।
प्रायुस्तारिष्टं नी रपाꣳसि मृक्षतꣳ सेधतं द्वेषो भवतꣳ सचाभुवा ॥

⁴²The word Pusha means God as well as an Apta person. The verse is applicable to an Apta person also.
⁴³Three steps may also mean Earth, atmosphere and Sun, or the three conditions of the soul, waking (Jagrit), sleeping (Swapna), profound sleeping (Sushupti). These words may also mean, creation, sustenance and dissolution of the universe.
⁴⁶Thinker : Distinguisher between truth and untruth.
Vasus, Rudras, Adityas : Those who observe celibacy for 24, 36 and 48 years ; or eight vasus, eleven Rudras, ten pranas and soul, twelve Adityas, the months of the year.

47. O devotees of truth, ye learned persons amongst the officials and the subjects, knowing the thirty three gods, come for enjoying medicinal juices. Wipe out sins, ward off enemies, perform noble deeds with zeal and energy; and prolong the days of life!

४८. एष व स्तोमो मरुत इयं गीर्मान्दार्यस्य मान्यस्य कारोः ।
एषा यासीष्ट तन्वे वयां विद्यामेष वृजनं जीरदानुम् ॥

48. O mortals, may this praise and speech of the magnanimous, laudable and energetic artisan be conducive to your benefit. Protect well with food the body of the aged. For long life may we acquire strength, knowledge and food!

४९. सहस्तोमाः सहच्छन्दस आवृतः सहप्रमा ऋषयः सप्त दैव्या । पूर्वेषां पन्थामनुदृश्य धीरा अन्वालेभिरे रथ्यो न रश्मीन् ॥

49. Those who study together the religious lore, who read together the vedas and enjoy happiness, who return home from the Gurukula after observing Brahmcharya and completing their studies, who are together advanced in knowledge, who are masters of seven divine forces, are veritable Rishis, the knowers of the vedas. Such calm, wise persons viewing the path of ancient sages take up the reins of noble deeds like a chariot-driver.

५०. आयुष्यं वर्चस्यॐ रायस्पोषमौद्भिदम् ।
इदॐ हिरण्यं वर्चस्वज्जैत्रायाविशताद् माम् ॥

50. Bestowing length of life, splendour, increase of wealth, and conquering power, may this brightly shining gold and food be attached to me for victory.

५१. न तद्रक्षाॐसि न पिशाचास्तरन्ति देवानामोजः प्रथमजॐ ह्येतत् ।
यो बिभर्ति दाक्षायणॐ हिरण्यॐ स देवेषु कृणुते दीर्घमायुः
स मनुष्येषु कृणुते दीर्घमायुः ॥

51. The strength acquired by the learned in the Brahmcharya Ashrama, can be destroyed neither by demons nor by fiends. Whoever possesses the strength of celibacy, lives a long life among the sages, and also lives a long life among thoughtful persons.

५२. यदाबध्नन् दाक्षायणा हिरण्यॐ शतानीकाय सुमनस्यमानाः ।
तन्म आ बध्नामि शतशारदायायुष्माञ्जरदष्टिर्यथासम् ॥

⁴⁷Thirtythree gods : Eight Vasus, Eleven Rudras, Twelve Adityas, Lightning and Yajna. The verse indicates how philanthropists and benefactors of humanity should lead their life.

⁴⁹Seven divine forces : Five senses of cognition, Gyan-Indriyas, the mind, and soul. Griffith mentions these forces according to Ludwig, as seven godlike Rishis, i.e., Bhardwaja, Kashyapa, Gotama, Atri, Vasishtha, Vishwamitra, and Jamadagni. This interpretation is incorrect, as there is no historical reference in the vedas.

52. Noble persons with benevolent thoughts, full of sagacity and learning, lords of hundreds of soldiers, bind me in knowledge which distinguishes between truth and untruth. I possess that in me for life through hundred autumns, that I may live till ripe old age overtakes me.

५३. उत नोऽहिर्बुध्न्यः शृणोत्वज एकपात्पृथिवी समुद्रः ।
विश्वे देवा ऋतावृधो हुवानाः स्तुता मन्त्राः कविशस्ता अवन्तु ॥

53. May the unborn God, the Support of all like the atmosphere, Indestructible, the Expander of the world, the Creator of all regions, the Master of permanent knowledge, hear our words. May all the learned persons, the protagonists of truth, vying with each other for advancement, and texts recited by the sages protect us.

५४. इमा गिर आदित्येभ्यो घृतस्नूः सनाद्राजभ्यो जुह्वा जुहोमि ।
शृणोतु मित्रो अर्यमा भगो नस्तुविजातो वरुणो दक्षो अंशः ॥

54. I listen with rapt attention to these eternal true sayings of the vedas preached by majestic kings.
May associates, intelligentsia, distributors, and noble persons hear our words purifying the conduct like water.

५५. सप्त ऋषयः प्रतिहिताः शरीरे सप्त रक्षन्ति सदमप्रमादम् ।
सप्ताप: स्वपतो लोकमीयुस्तत्र जागृतो अस्वप्नजौ सत्रसदौ च देवौ ॥

55. Seven Rishis are established in the body; these seven guard it with unceasing care.
These seven enter the soul in the body of him who lies asleep. At that time two sleepless gods, the protectors of soul, keep waking.

५६. उत्तिष्ठ ब्रह्मणस्पते देवयन्तस्त्वेमहे ।
उप प्र यन्तु मरुतः सुदानव इन्द्र प्राशूर्भवा सचा ॥

56. Arise, O learned persons, the guardian of vedic wealth, we longing for learned teachers pray to thee. May those persons who give good gifts, approach thee, and enjoy thou in a righteous manner the gifts offered!

⁵²Dakshayana दाक्षायणा According to Macdonell Daksha is in the Veda a creative Power associated with Aditi (Infinity or Eternity), the mother of the Adityas. In past Vedic literature he is generally regarded as the son of Brahma, and placed at the head of Prajapatis or Lords of Created Beings.

Rishi Dayananda translates the word as men possessing sagacity and learning. Failure on the part of Western scholars to understand the yaugic, derivative meaning of words leads them to concoct imaginary theories which have no hearing on the context and simply confuse the meaning.

⁵⁵Seven Rishis: Touch, Sight, Hearing, Taste, Smell, Mind and Intellect.
Two sleepless gods: Inbreath and outbreath Pran and Apana.
⁵⁶Pray to thee: Request thee to impart knowledge to us.

५७. प्र नूनं ब्रह्मणस्पतिमंन्त्रं वदत्युक्थ्यम् ।
यस्मिन्निन्द्रो वरुणो मित्रो अर्यमा देवा ओकाꣳसि चक्रिरे ॥

57. God, in Whom the Sun, Moon, breaths, air and all good attributes, seek their dwelling-place, is verily the Guardian of the vedic lore. He preaches the solemn hymn of praise.

५८. ब्रह्मणस्पते त्वमस्य यन्ता सूक्तस्य बोधि तनयं च जिन्व ।
विश्वं तद्भद्रं यदवन्ति देवा बृहद्वदेम विदथे सुवीराः ॥
य इमा विश्वा ।
विश्वकर्मा ।
यो नः पिता ।
ब्रह्मणपतेऽस्नस्य नो देहि ॥

58. O God, Protector of the universe, the learned sing Thy praise in the yajna, and we brave people accept Thee as Mighty, be Thou the Regulator of this our hymn, instruct the lover of knowledge, and satisfy all virtuous souls.

---

⁵⁷Dwelling-place : God is the shelter of all material objects in their nascent and gross condition. All material substances reside in His protection and care.
⁵⁸The four Pratikas that follow are taken respectively from 17-17, 17-26, 17-27, 11-83; for certain Karma Kandas.

CHAPTER XXXV

१. अपेतो यन्तु पणयोऽसुम्ना देवपीयव: ।
अस्य लोक: सुतावत: ।
द्युभिरक्तुभिरक्तुभिर्व्यक्तं यमो ददात्ववसानमस्मै ॥

1. Businessmen who torment others, and are inimical to the learned, should get away from here. May the Beautiful God, grant this soul, the singer of vedic hymns, full opportunity for work with the lustre of knowledge during all the days and nights of life.

२. सविताते शरीरेभ्य: पृथिव्यांल्लोकमिच्छतु ।
तस्मै युज्यन्तामुस्रिया: ॥

2. O soul, God grants for thy bodies in different births, according to thy deeds a happy or unhappy place on this earth. May radiant beams prove helpful to thee!

३. वायु: पुनातु सविता पुनात्वग्नेर्भ्राजसा सूर्यस्य वर्चसा ।
वि मुच्यन्तामुस्रिया: ॥

3. O soul, let air purify thee, let God purify thee with lightning's glitter and sun's lustre. Let beams release thee!

४. अश्वत्थे वो निषदनं पर्णे वो वसतिष्कृता ।
गोभाज इत्किलासथ यत्सनवथ पूरुषम् ॥

4. O souls, God has placed ye in this ephemeral world, and made your mansion in this life, ever changing like a leaf Worship the Perfect God alone. Through His grace, establish yourselves laboriously in religion, and acquire worldly possessions, vedic lore and control over passions!

५. सविता ते शरीराणि मातुरुपस्थ आ वपतु ।
तस्मै पृथिवि शं भव ॥

[2] After death the subtle soul is carried to different worlds through beams, before it is reborn. On this earth, soul derives happiness or suffering according to his good and bad deeds through the dispensation of God.

[3] When souls go out after death leaving the bodies, and attain to lightning, sun's lustre and air, and re-enter the womb, at that time the sun's beams, with whose aid the souls roam in the solar system, leave them.

[4] Ashwatha: The unstable world, which may or may not exist tomorrow, there is no certainty of life. Hence man should worship God, and alienating himself from the unsteady world yoke himself with God for acquiring real happiness.

The word अश्वत्थे has been translated by Griffith as Fig Tree, which is meaningless, See 12—79.

5. O girl, forbearing like the earth, the father establishes thy asylum on the Earth, kind like a mother, Be pleasant unto him!

६. प्रजापतौ त्वा देवतायामुपोदके लोके नि दधाम्यसौ । अप नः शोशुचदघम् ॥

6. O soul, May God soon drive away our sin. I establish thee in Him, the Protector of men and Worthy of worship, near a beautiful place full of water!

७. परं मृत्यो अनु परेहि पन्थां यस्ते अन्य इतरो देवयानात् ।
चक्षुष्मते शृण्वते ते ब्रवीमि मा नः प्रजाँ रीरिषो मोत वीरान् ॥

7. Go hence, O Death, pursue thy special pathway apart from that which the virtuous are won't to tread. To thee that sees and hears, I say, 'Kill not our offspring, injure not our heroes!

८. शं वातः शँ हि ते घृणिः शं ते भवन्त्विष्टकाः ।
शं ते भवन्त्वग्नयः पार्थिवासो मा त्वाऽभि शूशुचन् ॥

8. Pleasant to thee be wind and Sun, and pleasant be the bricks to thee. Pleasant to thee be the terrestrial fires; let not these things put thee to grief.

९. कल्पन्तां ते दिशस्तुभ्यमापः शिवतमास्तुभ्यं भवन्तु सिन्धवः ।
अन्तरिक्षँ शिवं तुभ्यं कल्पन्तां ते दिशः सर्वाः ॥

9. O soul, let the regions, the waters, and the seas be most propitious for thee. Auspicious unto thee be the atmosphere. Prosper all sub-quarters well for thee!

१०. अश्मन्वती रीयते सँ रभध्वमुत्तिष्ठत प्र तरता सखायः ।
अत्रा जहीमोऽशिवा ये असञ्छिवान्वयमुत्तरेमाभि वाजान् ॥

10. On flows this stormy, sensual river-like world, work cautiously, my friends, arise and overcome all obstacles.
Let us abandon what is profitless in this world, and enjoy excellent foods.

११. अपाघमप किल्बिषमप कृत्यामपो रपः ।
अपामार्ग त्वमस्मदप दुःस्वप्न्यँ सुव ॥

11. O God, the Remover of sins, drive away from us sin, the impurity of soul, evil deeds, the offence committed by our unsteady external organs, and evil thoughts!

---

[5] A daughter should be devoted to her parents even after marriage and should not sever her connection with them.
    Asylum: Relation, shelter, resort.

[8] Bricks: house or altar made of bricks. The word Ishtika may also mean day and night, vide Shatapath Brahmana.

अहोरात्राणि वै इष्टकाः शत 9—1—2—18.

[11] Just as the medicine Apamarga cures our physical ills, so does God purify our soul and free it from all shortcomings.

१२. सुमित्रिया न आप ओषधय: सन्तु दुर्मित्रियास्तस्मै सन्तु योऽस्मान्द्वेष्टि यं च वयं द्विष्म: ॥

12. To us let waters, and the medicinal plants be friendly, to him who hates us, whom we hate, unfriendly.

१३. अनड्वाहमन्वारभामहे सौरभेयँ स्वस्तये ।
स न इन्द्र इव देवेभ्यो वह्नि: सन्तरणो भव ॥

13. Electricity carries us the learned to distant places. Just as an ox carries the cart, so we use this electricity for prosperity in preparing planes and seating people therein. May that serve as lightning for you.

१४. उद्वयं तमसस्परि स्व: पश्यन्त उत्तरम् ।
देवं देवत्रा सूर्यमगन्म ज्योतिरुत्तमम् ॥

14. May we always keeping in view, eagerly know and realize God, free from the darkness of ignorance, Self-Effulgent, Releaser from afflictions, the most Learned to the learned, the Light that is most Excellent.

१५. इमं जीवेभ्य: परिधिं दधामि मैषां नु गादपरो अर्थमेतम् ।
शतं जीवन्तु शरद: पुरूचीरन्तर्मृत्युं दधतां पर्वतेन ॥

15. So that none may confiscate speedily the wealth amassed through exertion by these souls, I establish a law of morality, following which you can live for a hundred lengthened autumns, and keep death away through celibacy and knowledge.

१६. अग्न आयूँषि पवस आ सुवोर्जमिषं च न: ।
आरे बाधस्व दुच्छुनाम् ॥

16. O God, Thou purifiest our lives. Grant us vigorous strength and knowledge. Punish adequately the violent far or near!

१७. आयुष्मानग्ने हविषा वृधानो घृतप्रतीको घृतयोनिरेधि ।
घृतं पीत्वा मधु चारु गव्यं पितेव पुत्रमभि रक्षतादिमान्त्स्वाहा ॥

17. O King brilliant like fire, just as fire fanned by butter, with source of lustre, waxes with oblations, so shouldst thou live long!

[12]Hate the sin and not the sinner. We should work for the amelioration and betterment of even the sinner. We should hate the sin of others, who in turn should hate our sin and not us.
[13]That: Electricity.
As lightning: Just as lightning is highly fast in motion, so is electricity.
[14]See 20—21.
[15]I: God.
God has laid down for men the rule of conduct that they should follow religion and shun irreligiousness, and not snatch the wealth of others.
[16]See 19-38.

When thou hast assimilated the cow's fair savoury ghee, guard nicely, as a father guards his son, thy subjects.

१८. परीमे गामनेषत पर्यंग्निमहृषत ।
देवेष्वक्रत श्रव: क इमाँर आ दधर्षति ॥

18. If all study the vedas, enter domestic life after due ceremony listen to the spiritual teachings of the learned; who will then attack them with success?

१९. क्रव्यादमग्निं प्र हिणोमि दूरं यमराज्यं गच्छतु रिप्रवाह: ।
इहैवायमितरो जातवेदा देवेभ्यो हव्यं वहतु प्रजानन् ॥

19. I, the knower, drive away the eater of raw meat, and the tormentor of men like fire, and cast aside the sinners.
Let all criminals be brought before the Court of Justice. Let a noble soul, in this world, derive useful knowledge from the learned.

२०. वह वपां जातवेद: पितृभ्यो यत्रैनान्वेत्थ निहितान् पराके ।
मेदस: कुल्या उप तान्त्स्त्रवन्तु सत्या एषामाशिष: सं नमन्तां स्वाहा ॥

20. O intelligent person, thou knowest thy parents established far away, for them cultivate the land. Let rivulets full of water flow to meet them, and let their truthful wishes be accomplished in a decent manner!

२१. स्योना पृथिवि नो भवानृक्षरा निवेशनी ।
यच्छा न: शर्म सप्रथा: ।
अप न: शोशुचदघम् ॥

21. O wife calm like the Earth, give us far reaching pleasure, as does the Earth, free from thorn, our resting-place. Just as a just ruler drives away our sin, so shouldst thou eradicate our evil!

२२. अस्मात्त्वमधि जातोऽसि त्वदयं जायतां पुन: ।
असौ स्वर्गाय लोकाय स्वाहा ॥

22. O learned person, thou art foremost amongst men. May this son born anew from thee, be fair to look at, and enjoy fair reputation and happiness!

---

[19]I: The King.
[20]वपां has been translated by Griffith as fat, and land by Maharshi Dayananda, which yields corn, fruits and vegetable. We should serve and revere our parents and carry out their wishes.

CHAPTER XXXVI

१. ऋचं वाचं प्र पद्ये मनो यजुः प्र पद्ये साम प्राणं प्र पद्ये चक्षुः श्रोत्रं प्र पद्ये ।
वागोजः सहौजो मयि प्राणापानौ ॥

1. May inbreath and outbreath be strengthened in my soul. May my speech acquire mental strength, whereby I may gain physical strength.

May my speech be commendable like the Rigveda, my mind reflective like the Yajurveda. May I master the Samaveda, the expositor of the science of yoga. May I possess good eyes and ears.

२. यन्मे छिद्रं चक्षुषो हृदयस्य मनसो वातितृणं बृहस्पतिर्मे तद्दधातु ।
शं नो भवतु भुवनस्य यस्पतिः ॥

2. Whatever defect I have of eye or heart, or perplexity of mind, that may God amend. Gracious to us be He, Protector of the world.

३. भूर्भुवः स्वः ।
तत्सवितुर्वरेण्यं भर्गो देवस्य धीमहि ।
धियो यो नः प्रचोदयात् ॥

3. Oh men, just as we having studied the science of moral duty, the science of contemplation, and the science of sacred knowledge, meditate upon God, the Reliever of afflictions, Inaccessible through physical organs, the Giver of affluence, the Object of desire, the Impeller of our intellects, so should ye do!

४. कया नश्चित्र आ भुवदूती सदावृधः सखा ।
कया शचिष्ठया वृता ॥

4. With what help does the ever-prospering, wonderful God become our Friend? With what constant, most mighty wisdom does He impel us to noble attributes, actions and natures?

५. कस्त्वा सत्यो मदानां मँहिष्ठो मत्सदन्धसः ।
दृढा चिदारुजे वसु ॥

---

[1] चक्षुः श्रोत्रम These words have been interpreted by Pt. Jaidev Vidyalankar, as studying the Atharvaveda with attention as one listens with one's ears. This interpretation is plausible as it refers to the four instead of the three vedas.

[3] See 3-35, 22-9, 30-2.

This is Gayatri Mantra. This Mantra occurs four times in the Yajurveda. Swami Dayananda has interpreted it differently each time. In all the vedas this verse occurs six times.

[4] See 27-39.

5. O man, God, the Most advanced in happiness, the Embodiment of joy grants thee happiness through food; and gives thy soul, the eradicator of misery, durable wealth!

६. अभी षु णः सखीनामविता जरितृणाम् ।
शतं भवास्यूतिभि: ॥

6. O God, Thou granting us manifold glories, and protecting us from all sides, dost fairly guard us, Thy friends, who praise Thee!

७. कया त्वं न ऊत्याभि प्र मन्दसे वृषन् ।
कया स्तोतृभ्य आ भर ॥

7. O God, the Showerer of joys from all sides, with what aid dost Thou delight us, in what way dost Thou bestow happiness on thy worshippers!

८. इन्द्रो विश्वस्य राजति ।
शं नो अस्तु द्विपदे शं चतुष्पदे ॥

8. O God, like lightning Thou shinest in the universe, may weal attend our bipeds and our quadrupeds!

९. शं नो मित्र: शं वरुण: शं नो भवत्वर्यमा ।
शं न इन्द्रो बृहस्पति: शं नो विष्णुरुरुक्रम: ॥

9. May God, friendly like breath, be gracious unto us; may God, Tranquiliser like water be king to us; may God the Just be benevolent to us; may God the Mighty, and Guardian of the vedic speech be comfort-giving to us, may the All-pervading God, the Vigilant Creator of the universe be pleasant to us.

१०. शं नो वात: पवतां शं नस्तपतु सूर्य: ।
शं न: कनिक्रदद्देव: पर्जन्यो अभि वर्षतु ॥

10. May the wind blow pleasantly for us, May the Sun warm us pleasantly. May lightning roar for us. May cloud send the rain on us pleasantly.

११. अहानि शं भवन्तु न: शं रात्री: प्रति धीयताम् ।
शं न इन्द्राग्नी भवतामवोभि: शं न इन्द्रावरुणा रातहव्या ।
शं न इन्द्रापूषणा वाजसातौ शमिन्द्रासोमा सुविताय शं यो: ॥

11. May days pass pleasantly for us. May nights draw near delightfully. May lightning and fire, with their aids, bring us happiness. May the Sun and rain, givers of joy, comfort us.

१२. शं नो देवीरभिष्टय आपो भवन्तु पीतये ।
शं योरभि स्रवन्तु न: ॥

⁵See 27-40.

12. May beautiful waters be pleasant to us to drink and acquire happiness, and flow with health and strength to us.

१३. स्योना पृथिवि नो भवानृक्षरा निवेशनी ।
यच्छा न: शर्म सप्रथा: ॥

13. O wife, calm like the Earth, just as the Earth free from thorns and pits, the resting place for all durable substances, is comfortable for us, so shouldst thou be. Just as wide Earth gives us place for dwelling, so shouldst thou delight-affording, give us domestic happiness!

१४. आपो हि ष्ठा मयोभुवस्ता न ऊर्जे दधातन ।
महे रणाय चक्षसे ॥

14. O peaceful, learned, noble wives, just as beneficent waters sustain us for a big famous fight and energy, so should ye endear yourselves to us!

१५. यो व: शिवतमो रसस्तस्य भाजयतेह न: ।
उशतीरिव मातर: ॥

15. O noble wives, give us your most propitious affection in this world, like mothers longing for progeny!

१६. तस्मा अरं गमाम वो यस्य क्षयाय जिन्वथ ।
आपो जनयथा च न: ॥

16. O wives, just as ye make us calm like water, so should we make ye peaceful. As each of ye satisfies her husband for decent living for him, so may we acquire power and wealth for him.

१७. द्यौ: शान्तिरन्तरिक्षꣳ शान्ति: पृथिवी शान्तिराप: शान्तिरोषधय: शान्ति: ।
वनस्पतय: शान्तिर्विश्वे देवा: शान्तिर्ब्रह्म शान्ति: सर्वꣳ शान्ति: शान्तिरेव शान्ति सा मा शान्तिरेधि ॥

17. May sky be peaceful.
May atmosphere be peaceful.
May Earth be peaceful.
May waters be peaceful.
May medicinal herbs be peaceful.
May plants be peaceful.

[12]The verse may also mean, as interpreted by Maharshi Dayananda in Panch Maha Yajna Vidhi, May God, the Illuminator of all, Pleasure-giver to all, and All-pervading, for desired happiness and the acquisition of complete joy, be blissful to us. May He shower felicity on us from all sides. This is the first mantra of Sandhya (vedic prayer).
[13]See 35-21.
[14]See 11-50.
[15]See 11-51.
[16]See 11-52.

May all the learned persons be peaceful. May God and the vedas be peaceful. May all the objects be peaceful; May peace itself be peaceful. May that peace come unto me.

१८. दृते दृꣳह मा मित्रस्य मा चक्षुषा सर्वाणि भूतानि समीक्षन्ताम् ।
मित्रस्याहं चक्षुषा सर्वाणि भूतानि समीक्षे ।
मित्रस्य चक्षुषा समीक्षामहे ॥

18. O God, the Dispeller of ignorance and darkness, strengthen me, May all beings regard me with the eye of a friend. May I regard all beings with the eye of a friend. With the eye of a friend do we regard one another!

१९. दृते दृꣳह मा । ज्योक्ते सन्दृशि जीव्यासं ज्योक्ते
सन्दृशि जीव्यासम् ॥

19. Do, O God, the Preventer of mental delusion, strengthen me. Long may I live to look on Thee. Long may I live to look on Thee!

२०. नमस्ते हरसे शोचिषे नमस्ते अस्त्वर्चिषे ।
अन्याँस्ते अस्मत्तपन्तु हेतयः पावको अस्मभ्यꣳ शिवो भव ॥

20. Obeisance to God, the Queller of sins, the Source of light. Obeisance to God Worthy of adoration. May Thy punishments torment others. Be Thou Purifier, and Propitious unto us!

२१. नमस्ते अस्तु विद्युते नमस्ते स्तनयित्नवे ।
नमस्ते भगवन्नस्तु यतः स्वः समीहसे ॥

21. Homage to Thee God pervading like lightning, Homage to Thee God, the Inspirer of awe for the sinners. Homage, O Bounteous Lord to Thee, as Thou desirest to give us happiness.

२२. यतो यतः समीहसे ततो नो अभयं कुरु ।
शं नः कुरु प्रजाभ्योऽभयं नः पशुभ्यः ॥

22. O God, from whatsoever place, Thou desirest, give us freedom from fear thence. Give to our people and our beasts happiness and fearlessness!

२३. सुमित्रिया न आप ओषधयः सन्तु दुर्मित्रियास्तस्मै सन्तु
योऽस्मान् द्वेष्टि यं च वयं द्विष्मः ॥

23. O God, let waters and plants be friendly to us; unfriendly to him who hates us, and whom we hate!

---

[19] 'Long may I live to look on thee': Those words have been used twice for the sake of emphasis.
[20] See 6-22.

२४. तच्चक्षुर्देवहितं पुरस्ताच्छुक्रमुच्चरत् ।
पश्येम शरद: शतं जीवेम शरद: शतं ॐ श्रृणुयाम शरद: शतं प्र ब्रवाम शरद: शतमदीना:
स्याम शरद: शतं भूयश्च शरद: शतात् ॥

24. O God, Thou art the Well-wisher of the learned. Immaculate, the Exhibitor of every thing like the eye, the Eternal knower of every thing. Through Thy kindness may we see for a hundred years; may we live for a hundred years; may we listen for a hundred years to vedic lore; may we preach the vedas for a hundred years; may we live content independently for a hundred years; yea, even beyond a hundred years, see, live, hear, preach and be not dependent.

CHAPTER XXXVII

१. देवस्य त्वा सवितुः प्रसवेऽश्विनोर्बाहुभ्यां पूष्णो हस्ताभ्याम् ।
आ दटे नारिरसि ॥

1. O learned person, as thou art a leader, so in this world created by God, the Giver of all happiness, with the strength and valour of the teacher and preacher, and with the assistance of a nourisher, I accept thee!

२. युञ्जते मन उत युञ्जते धियो विप्रा विप्रस्य बृहतो विपश्चितः ।
वि होत्रा दधे वयुनाविदेक इन्मही देवस्य सवितुः परिष्टुतिः ॥

2. The Unequalled God, the Embodiment of knowledge, creates all beings. This is the great praise of Him, Who is Ubiquitous, and the Creator of the Universe. The noble and wise yogis concentrate their mind on and dedicate their action to, the Omnipresent God, the Highest knower. All should worship Him.

३. देवी द्यावापृथिवी मखस्य वामद्य शिरो राध्यासं देवयजने पृथिव्याः ।
मखाय त्वा मखस्य त्वा शीर्ष्णे ॥

3. O mistress and preachress, highly qualified like the Sun and Earth, may I nicely accomplish, this day, on the Earth, in the sacrificial abode of the learned, the excellent final stage of the sacrifice (yajna) conducted by ye both. O priest I accept thee for the yajna and the successful termination of the yajna!

४. देव्यो वम्रयो भूतस्य प्रथमजा मखस्य वोऽद्य शिरो राध्यासं देवयजने पृथिव्याः ।
मखाय त्वा मखस्य त्वा शीर्ष्णे ॥

4. O early born, young, brilliant, learned women, I accept ye, this day in a place where the learned assemble, as head of the contemplated sacrifice, connected with the Earth. O lady, the performer of the yajna, I acknowledge thee as head of the yajna!

५. इयत्यग्र आसीन्मखस्य तेऽद्य शिरो राध्यासं देवयजने पृथिव्याः ।
मखाय त्वा मखस्य त्वा शीर्ष्णे ॥

5. O learned person, at first I accept thee for due reverence, for the excellence of association. Thy sacrifice is well-merited. This day, on the Earth, I make thee duly prosper by honouring so many scholars!

*Yajna is connected with the Earth, as it is performed on it and for its betterment. Early born: Born before the birth of their sons.

६. इन्द्रस्यौज: स्थ मखस्य वोऽद्य शिरो राध्यासां देवयजने पृथिव्या: ।
मखाय त्वा मखस्य त्वा शीर्ष्णे ।
मखाय त्वा मखस्य त्वा शीर्ष्णे ।
मखाय त्वा मखस्य त्वा शीर्ष्णे ॥

6. O men, just as I acquire the vitality of a glorious person, so may I, this day, on that part of the earth where the learned are worshipped, like head, the chief organ, make ye prosperous!

May I perfect thee in the use of intellectual words of honour for the sages, and usage of loving conduct. May I perfect thee, the preacher of good qualities, in the art of artizanship, and usage of loving conduct. May I perfect thee in the dissemination of excellent science, and acquisition of knowledge. So should ye become valorous.

७. प्रैतु ब्रह्मणस्पति: प्र देव्येतु सूनृता ।
अच्छा वीरं नर्यं पङ्क्तिराधसं देवा यज्ञं नयन्तु न: ।
मखाय त्वा मखस्य त्वा शीर्ष्णे ।
मखाय त्वा मखस्य त्वा शीर्ष्णे ।
मखाय त्वा मखस्य त्वा शीर्ष्णे ॥

7. May the learned bring us in contact with a person, the dispeller of miseries, the leader of men, the controller of vast numbers in war, and the bestower of happiness. May we associate with a lord of wealth. May we acquire a truthful, good mannered, and well-read wife.

We seek thy shelter for the advancement of knowledge, and as an excellent means of happiness. We seek thy shelter for performing religious duties, and as a nice instrument for protecting religion. We seek thy shelter as a harbinger of happiness, as an advancer and giver of happiness.

८. मखस्य शिरोऽसि । मखाय त्वा मखस्य त्वा शीर्ष्णे ।
मखस्य शिरोऽसि । मखाय त्वा मखस्य त्वा शीर्ष्णे ।
मखस्य शिरोऽसि । मखाय त्वा मखस्य त्वा शीर्ष्णे ।
मखाय त्वा मखस्य त्वा शीर्ष्णे ।
मखाय त्वा मखस्य त्वा शीर्ष्णे ।
मखाय त्वा मखस्य त्वा शीर्ष्णे ॥

8. O learned person, as thou art the ornament of Brahmcharya Ashram, so we serve thee for acquiring knowledge, and for its right use. As thou art the master of deep thinking, so we serve thee for knowing the duties of domestic life, and nice execution of sacrifice. As thou art the grace of domestic

⁶Thee: The yajman, the performer of sacrifice.
I : The priest.
Ye : Men.
⁷Thy : A learned person.

life, so we serve thee for directing the domestic people in their actions, and excellent execution of sacrifice. We serve thee for success in noble enterprises, and leading righteous dealings!

We serve thee for learning yoga, and mastering all the intricacies of the science of yoga. We serve thee as giver of glory, and for performing all deeds of supremacy.

९. अश्वस्य त्वा वृष्ण: शक्ना धूपयामि देवयजने पृथिव्या: ।
मखाय त्वा मखस्य त्वा शीष्णे ।
अश्वस्य त्वा वृष्ण: शक्ना धूपयामि देवयजने पृथिव्या: ।
मखाय त्वा मखस्य त्वा शीष्णे ।
अश्वस्य त्वा वृष्ण: शक्ना धूपयामि देवयजने पृथिव्या: ।
मखाय त्वा मखस्य त्वा शीष्णे ।
मखाय त्वा मखस्य त्वा शीष्णे ।
मखाय त्वा मखस्य त्वा शीष्णे ।
मखाय त्वा मखस्य त्वा शीष्णे ॥

9. O sacrificer, on this Earth in a place where the learned perform yajna, with the powerful fire's strength of warding off bad smell, I fumigate thee for purifying the air, and for alleviating the brain disease of a purifier. On the Earth, in a place where the learned perform the yajna, with the strength of a powerful man, I fumigate thee for acquiring knowledge of the Earth, and knowing the principal part of the essential nature of learning. On this earth, in a place where the learned are worshipped, with the lustre of powerful, fast fire I urge thee for its application, and for doing noble deeds. I prepare thee for the completion of the yajna, for the completion of the best part of the yajna. I goad thee for fame, and the most important part of the yajna, I stimulate thee for performing the yajna, and the most important part of the yajna!

१०. ऋजवे त्वा साधवे त्वा सुक्षित्यै त्वा ।
मखाय त्वा मखस्य त्वा शीष्णे ।
मखाय त्वा मखस्य त्वा शीष्णे ।
मखाय त्वा मखस्य त्वा शीष्णे ।

10. O learned person we establish thee for sincerity, for honouring the learned, and for performing the yajna. We establish thee for philanthropy, for performing the yajna, and for finishing it to the end. We establish thee for land, for the yajna, and the best part of the yajna!

ºSacrificer : One who performs the yajna, yajman.
I : The priest.
Repetition in the verse is meant for the sake of emphasis.
Fumigate : Sitting in the yajnashala, the sacrificer is incited by the priest for various noble deeds.

११. यमाय त्वा मखाय त्वा सूर्यस्य त्वा तपसे ।
देवस्त्वा सविता मध्वानक्तु पृथिव्या: स॒ स्पृशस्पाहि ।
अर्चिरसि शोचिरसि तपोऽसि ॥

11. O learned person, a glorious, charitable man, receives thee for the administration of justice, for the observance of religious obligations, and for the performance of religious practices as ordained by God. May he unite thee with the sweetness of worldly objects, but protect thyself from their evil attachment!

As thou art noble, pure like the flame of fire, and embedded in religious austerity, hence we pay thee homage.

१२. अनाधृष्टा पुरस्तादग्नेराधिपत्य आयुर्मे दा: ।
पुत्रवती दक्षिणत इन्द्रस्याधिपत्ये प्रजां मे दा: ।
सुषदा पश्चाद्देवस्य सवितुराधिपत्ये चक्षुर्मे दा: ।
आश्रुतिरुत्तरतो धातुराधिपत्ये रायस्पोषं मे दा: ।
विधृतिरुपरिष्टाद्बृहस्पतेराधिपत्य ओजो मे दा: ।
विश्वाभ्यो मा नाष्ट्राभ्यस्पाहि मनोरश्वासि ॥

12. O woman, unconquerable in the East, in Agni's overlordship, give me life. Rich in sons, in the South, in Sun's overlordship give me offspring.

Fair-seated in the West, in God Creator's overlordship, give me spiritual sight. Excellent in hearing, in the North, in air's overlordship, give me increase of wealth.

Strong in convictions in the upper direction, in the overlordship of a learned master of the vedas, give me energy.

Being filled with a reflective mind, protect me from women given to adultery!

१३. स्वाहा मरुद्भि: परि श्रीयस्व
दिव: स॒ स्पृशस्पाहि । मधु मधु मधु ॥

13. O learned person, in the company of other men, act thou nobly, protect us from the lightning-fall!

Practice action, contemplation and knowledge.

१४. गर्भो देवानां पिता मतीनां पति: प्रजानाम् ।
सं देवो देवेन सवित्रा गत स॒ सूर्येण रोचते ॥

14. God pervades all the objects of Nature. He is Father of the wise, and Guardian of all living creatures.

He is Self Effulgent, and being Creator, shines like the shining man of knowledge. Let all attain to Him.

१५. समग्निरग्निना गत सं दैवेन सवित्रा स॒ सूर्येणारोचिष्ट ।
स्वाहा समग्निस्तपसा गत सं देव्येन सवित्रा स॒ सूर्येणारूरुचत ॥

15. Fire duly receives light from the Self-Effulgent God, and from the impelling sun created by God.
Know Him truly through righteous conduct.
Through religious practices, attain to God, the Self-Illuminator, the Stimulator, and the Glorifier of all material objects.

१६. धर्ता दिवो वि भाति तपसस्पृथिव्यां धर्ता देवो देवानाममर्त्यस्तपोजाः ।
वाचमस्मे नि यच्छ देवायुवम् ॥

16. God is the Sustainer of the Sun, who imparts heat to all objects in the atmosphere. He is Immortal and realisable through austerity. Effulgent God is the Sustainer of all the forces of Nature. He shines lustrously. May He grant us Vedic speech, full of excellent teachings and companion of the learned.

१७. अपश्यं गोपामनिपद्यमानमा च परा च पथिभिश्चरन्तम् ।
स सध्रीचीः स विषूचीर्वसान आ वरीवर्ति भुवनेष्वन्तः ॥

17. May I see God, the Protector, the Immovable, knowable through paths of virtue, here and hereafter. He encompassing the Quarters and subquarters, permeates all the worlds.

१८. विश्वासां भुवां पते विश्वस्य मनसस्पते विश्वस्य वचसस्पते सर्वस्य वचसस्पते । देवश्रुत्वं देव धर्म देवो देवान् पाह्यत्र प्रावीरनु वां देववीतये ।
मधु माध्वीभ्यां मधु माधूचीभ्याम् ॥

18. Lord of all earths, Lord of all minds, Lord of all vedic speech, thou Lord of speech entire; Brilliant, happiness bestowing God, Listener to the supplications of the learned, Guardian, protect in this world the righteous learned persons. Give us the pleasant knowledge of useful instructions and excellent teachings. Protect favourably the learned for acquiring divine virtues, with the help of the teacher and preacher who know the science of honey, antidote to poison!

१६. हृदे त्वा मनसे त्वा दिवे त्वा सूर्याय त्वा ।
ऊर्ध्वो अध्वरं दिवि देवेषु धेहि ॥

19. O God, we meditate on Thee, for the purity of heart, for the steadfastness of mind, for the manifestation of knowledge, and for learning the science of heavens. Foremost Thou. Preach Thou the sacrifice[19] free from violence, in noble dealings and amongst learned persons!

२०. पिता नोऽसि पिता नो बोधि नमस्ते अस्तु मा मा हिꣳसीः ।
त्वष्टृमन्तस्त्वा सपेम पुत्रान्पशून्मयि धेहि प्रजामस्मासु धेह्यरिष्टाऽ सह पत्या भूयासम् ॥

[19]Sacrifice : Yajna.

20. O God Thou art our Father, King-like instruct us fatherly. Obeisance be to Thee. Do not Thou harm me!

May we, the masters of material objects win Thee. Vouchsafe me sons and cattle. Grant us offspring. Safe may I remain together with my husband.

२१. अह: केतुना जुषताꣳ सुज्योतिर्ज्योतिषा स्वाहा ।
रात्रि: केतुना जुषताꣳ सुज्योतिर्ज्योतिषा स्वाहा ॥

21. O learned person or woman, enjoy nicely day and knowledge, in a wide awake manner, in the light of the Sun and Dharma.

May night full of brightness, with her lustre, intelligence and action serve us excellently.

CHAPTER XXXVIII

१. देवस्य त्वा सवितुः प्रसवेऽश्विनोर्बाहुभ्यां पूष्णो हस्ताभ्याम् ।
आ ददेऽदित्यै रास्नासि ॥

1. O learned woman, thou art charitable in thy definite behaviour. In this world created by the Agreeable God, with arms powerful like the sun and moon and with hands strong, protective and retentive like the air, I take thee!

२. इड एह्यदित एहि सरस्वत्येहि ।
असावेह्यसावेह्यसावेहि ॥

2. O woman, well-instructed like speech, come unto me. Thou comest unto me, I go unto thee. O giver of entire happiness, may thou get full happiness. May thy husband give thee happiness; so acquire him!

O highly learned woman, select a learned husband. Go to him who is advanced in knowledge!

३. अदित्यै रास्नाऽसीन्द्राण्या उष्णीषः ।
पूषाऽसि घर्माय दीष्व ॥

3. O woman, thou art constant bestower of knowledge, a turban for supreme state politics, a protector like the Earth, dedicate thyself to pleasant domestic life!

४. अश्विभ्यां पिन्वस्व सरस्वत्यै पिन्वस्वेन्द्राय पिन्वस्व ।
स्वाहेन्द्रवत् स्वाहेन्द्रवत् स्वाहेन्द्रवत् ॥

4. O learned woman, acquire excellence, satisfy well thy parents. Possessing body endowed with consciousness, please thy teachers with truthful speech!

Knowing the science of electricity rightly acquire supremacy.

५. यस्ते स्तनः शशयो यो मयोभूर्यो रत्नधा वसुविद्यः सुदत्रः ।
येन विश्वा पुष्यसि वार्याणि सरस्वति तमिह धातवेऽकः ।
उर्वन्तरिक्षमन्वेमि ॥

²This verse relates to marriage. Husband and wife are free in the choice of their life companion.

This verse may also mean O Rigveda may we master thee, O Samaveda may we master thee, O Yajurveda may we master thee.

May we master thee, master thee, master thee.

इडा वाङ् नाम । निघ० 1-11
अदितिर्वाङ् नाम । निघ० 1-11
सरस्वती वाङ् नाम । निघ० 1-11

³Just as the turban protects the head, so does a learned woman protect her country with her political sagacity.

5. O highly learned woman, thy breast milks the child and makes it sleep. Thy husband is bringer of happiness, possessor of noble qualities, master of riches, and charitable in nature. With his aid thou acquirest all desirable objects. Establish him in this house for acceptance. May I, through him rise to the vast summit of prosperity!

६. गायत्रं छन्दोऽसि त्रैष्टुभं छन्दोऽसि द्यावापृथिवीभ्यां त्वा परि गृह्णाम्यन्तरिक्षेणोप यच्छामि ।
इन्द्राश्विना मधुनः सारघस्य घर्मं पात वसवो यजत वाट् ।
स्वाहा सूर्यस्य रश्मये वृष्टिवनये ॥

6. O strong man, like the twentyfour syllables of the Gayatri metre, observe thou celibacy for twentyfour years; like fortyfour syllables of Trishtup metre, observe thou celibacy for fortyfour years!

I grasp thee dear wife beautified by the Sun and Earth, and accept thee who takes vow with water in hand. O husband and wife behave mutually like Pran and Apan to accomplish your tasks.

O Vasus, protect nicely the sacrifice and the sweet honey prepared by the bees. Work together well and nobly to make sun's beams bring rain!

७. समुद्राय त्वा वाताय स्वाहा ।
सरिराय त्वा वाताय स्वाहा ।
अनाधृष्याय त्वा वाताय स्वाहा ।
अप्रतिधृष्याय त्वा वाताय स्वाहा ।
अवस्यवे त्वा वाताय स्वाहा ।
अशिमिदाय त्वा वाताय स्वाहा ॥

7. O husband or wife, truly do I accept thee for purifying the air that moves in the atmosphere. Nicely do I accept thee for purifying the air in the water and the house. I enjoin thee to be fearless and unconquerable, and to know the air in medicinal herbs. Verily do I ask thee to be irresistible, and know the velocity of air. Nobly do I accept thee as protection-seeker, for knowing specially the force of breath. In a noble way do I accept thee for the juice in which eatable food creates viscosity, and for Udan breath!

[5]I : Preceptor, priest or teachress.
[6]Who takes vow : At the time of marriage, with water in hand, husband and wife take some vows.
Pran and Apan : Just as in-going and out-going breaths are inseparable from each other, so should the husband and wife work mutually to accomplish their domestic tasks.
Vasus : Those who have observed celibacy for 24 years, at the time they taste Madhuparka.
Sun's beams : They should perform Agnihotra daily, which brings timely rain.
[7]In this verse I refer to the husband or wife. The various duties of a married couple are enumerated in the verse.
Udan : One of the five vital airs or life wind, which rises up the throat and enters into the head, the other four being Pran, Apan, Saman and Vyan.
Udan breath serves as an aid to digestion.

८. इन्द्राय त्वा वसुमते रुद्रवते स्वाहेन्द्राय त्वाऽऽदित्यवते स्वाहेन्द्राय त्वाऽभिमातिघ्ने स्वाहा ।
सवित्रे त्व ऋभुमते विभुमते वाजवते स्वाहा बृहस्पतये त्वा विश्वदेव्यावते स्वाहा ॥

8. O husband or wife, in true words, do I accept thee for the wealthy and powerful offspring. Truly do I accept thee for the erudite, self-controlled, misery-killing offspring. In truthful words, do I accept thee for the foe-killing, and affluent offspring. Truly do I accept thee for the offspring knowing the science of Sun, and befriending the wise, understanding the mighty atmosphere, and possessing stores of provisions. In true words do I accept thee for the offspring, the guardian of the vedas, and the embodiment of noble virtues!

९. यमाय त्वाऽङ्गिरस्वते पितृमते स्वाहा ।
स्वाहा घर्माय
स्वाहा घर्मः पित्रे ॥

9. O husband or wife, I, resplendent like sacrifice, in true words do accept thee for the offspring, knowing the science of electricity, lover of justice, and friend of the learned. Verily do I accept thee for sacrifice. Truly do I accept thee as a protector!

१०. विश्वा आशा दक्षिणसद्भिश्वान् देवानयाडिह ।
स्वाहाकृतस्य घर्मस्य मधोः पिबतमश्विना ॥

10. O teacher and preacher, in this world, taste ye the remnants of this pleasant well-arranged sacrifice. Let the priest seated in the south of the altar, accompany and worship the learned in all quarters!

११. दिवि धा इमं यज्ञमिमं यज्ञं दिवि धाः ।
स्वाहाऽग्नये यज्ञियाय शं यजुभ्यः ॥

11. O husband or wife, with the verses of the Yajurveda, in a nice way, in the light of the Sun, in the fire fit for yajna, perform with pleasure, the duty of domestic life. In the light of knowledge, perform with pleasure in the company of the learned, the Sanyas yajna; the giver of true spiritual knowledge![11]

१२. अश्विना घर्मं पातꣳ हार्दिनमहर्दिवाभिरूतिभिः ।
तन्त्रायिणे नमो द्यावापृथिवीभ्याम् ॥

12. O well educated husband and wife, protect daily the yajna, which broadens our mental vision, gives us scientific and technical knowledge, and is worth preservation day and night, in various ways. Give food and show respect to the technician who brings the Sun and atmosphere in service!

---

[11] Husband and wife are allowed to become a Sanyasi (recluse) if developed spiritually.

१३. अपातामश्विना धर्ममनु धावापृथिवी अम॒ँसाताम् ।
इहैव रातय: सन्तु ॥

13. O husband and wife, protect together the domestic life like air and lightning. Like the Sun and Earth judge together the responsibilities of the married life, whereby in this domestic life let your boons of knowledge and pleasure be bestowed on all !

१४. इषे पिन्वस्वोर्जे पिन्वस्व ब्रह्मणे पिन्वस्व क्षत्राय पिन्वस्व द्यावापृथिवीभ्यां पिन्वस्व ।
धर्मासि सुधर्मेन्यस्मे नृम्णानि धारय ब्रह्म धारय क्षत्रं धारय विशं धारय ॥

14. O husband or wife, the recipient of truth, religious minded, thou art free from violence, hence establish wealth for us, learn the Veda, acquire sovereignty, and preserve the subjects. Hence enjoy overflow for food, enjoy overflow for vedic knowledge and God, enjoy overflow for energy, enjoy overflow for vedic knowledge and God, enjoy overflow for political power, enjoy overflow for Heaven and Earth!

१५. स्वाहा पूष्णे शरसे स्वाहा ग्रावभ्य: स्वाहा प्रतिरवेभ्य: ।
स्वाहा पितृभ्य ऊर्ध्वबर्हिभ्यो धर्मपावभ्य: स्वाहा द्यावापृथिवीभ्याँ स्वाहा विश्वेभ्यो देवेभ्य: ॥

15. Husband and wife should try to save powerful, violent persons from irreligious acts. They should respect the pupils who repeat the utterances of their preceptor. They should receive gladly the thundering clouds. They should respect the highly cultured people, who purify the world with sacrifice, and like seasons protect us. They should use respectful words for ladies and gentlemen dignified like the Sun and Earth. They should always speak the truth to all the learned people.

१६. स्वाहा रुद्राय रुद्रहूतये स्वाहा सं ज्योतिषा ज्योति: ।
अह: केतुना जुषता॒ँ सुज्योतिर्ज्योतिषा स्वाहा ।
रात्रि: केतुना जुषता॒ँ सुज्योतिर्ज्योतिषा स्वाहा ।
मधु हुतमिन्द्रतमे अग्नावश्याम् ते देव धर्म नमस्ते अस्तु मा मा हि॒ँसी: ॥

16. O husband or wife, for the soul that wisely extols the life breaths, let light combine with light in a righteous manner. Spend the day rightly combining the light of knowledge with the light of noble qualities!
Wisely spend the night, rightly combining the light of contemplation with the light of noble religious qualities. May we enjoy through smell the sweet butter oblations put in the highly blazing fire. O Supreme God, I bow unto Thee. Let not Thou injure me!

---

[13] Just as air and lightning, the Sun and Earth work together for the good of others, so should married couple live together peacefully realizing their responsibilities.

१७. अभीमं महिमा दिवं विप्रो बभूव सप्रथाः ।
उत श्रवसा पृथिवीᳪ᳭ सᳪ᳭ सीदस्व महाँ२ असि रोचस्व देववीतमः ।
वि धूममग्ने अरुषं मियेध्यच सृज प्रशस्त दर्शतम् ॥

17. O learned person, famous, chastiser of the wicked, majestic, possessing far-spread glory, and wise, thou condemnest the spread of ignorance. Seat thee well on earth with plenty to eat. Thou art mighty. Be happy, thou best entertainer of the learned. Loosen through Homa the smoke ruddy and beautiful to see!

१८. या ते घर्म दिव्या शुग्या गायत्र्याᳪ᳭ हविर्धाने ।
सा त आ प्यायतां निष्टचायतां तस्यै ते स्वाहा ।
या ते घर्मन्तरिक्षे शुग्या त्रिष्टुब्भ्याग्नीध्रे ।
सा त आ प्यायतां निष्टचायतां तस्यै ते स्वाहा ।
या ते घर्म पृथिव्याᳪ᳭ शुग्या जगत्याᳪ᳭ सदस्या ।
सा त आ प्यायतां निष्टचायतां तस्यै ते स्वाहा ॥

18. O learned husband or wife, may thy meditation and divine contemplation for preserving the knowledge of the pupils, and the provisions of the yajna increase and be ever accomplished. True speech for that act and thee!
O husband or wife bright like the day, that flight of thine in the air, with the help of electricity as expounded in Trishtup, may increase and be accomplished. True speech for that act and thee!
O husband or wife, lustrous like electricity, that shining performance of thine on the Earth, in the Assembly, or amongst the people, may increase and be accomplished. True speech for that performance and thee!

१९. क्षत्रस्य त्वा परस्पाय ब्रह्मणस्तन्वं पाहि ।
विशस्त्वा धर्मणा वयमनु क्रामाम सुविताय नव्यसे ॥

19. O king, guard the body of the Kshatriya and Brahmana for affording protection to others. Just as we follow thee for acquiring new supremacy, so let thy subjects follow thee in a spirit of devotion!

२०. चतुः स्त्रक्तिर्नाभिरृतस्य सप्रथाः स नो विश्वायुः सप्रथाः स नः सर्वायुः सप्रथाः ।
अप द्वेषो अप ह्वरोऽन्यव्रतस्य सश्चिम ॥

20. A godly person, like the four-cornered navel, serves in abundance, God, the Protector of the world and True in nature. May he, full of age and engagements teach us. May he, advanced in age and happiness instruct us in the knowledge of God, so that we may shun the hateful enemies, and cast aside the crooked persons.

२१. घर्मेतत्ते पुरीषं तेन वर्द्धस्व चा च प्यायस्व ।
वर्द्धिषीमहि च वयमा च प्यासिषीमहि ॥

21. O most Adorable God, this is Thy nourishing power. Be great thereby and make others also great. Be strong, make others strong!
Through your compassion, just as we advance, let us make others advance. Just as we grow great, let us make others great.

२२. अचिक्रदद्वृषा हरिर्महान्मित्रो न दर्शत: ।
सꣳ सूर्येण दिद्युतदृद्धिर्निधि: ॥

22. All should understand lightning-fire, the cause for rain, fast in motion, mighty, roaring, like friend fair to see, shining with the Sun in the atmosphere, the ocean of water.

२३. सुमित्रिया न आप ओषधय: सन्तु दुर्मित्रियास्तस्मै सन्तु योऽस्मान्द्वेष्टि यं च वयं द्विष्म: ॥

23. To us let waters and plants be friendly, to him who hates us, whom we hate, unfriendly.

२४. उद्वयं तमसस्परि स्व: पश्यन्त उत्तरम् ।
देवं देवत्रा सूर्यमगन्म ज्योतिरुत्तमम् ॥

24. May we, looking mentally upon God, free from darkness, highest of all, noblest amongst the noble, the light that is most excellent, nicely attain to happiness on all sides.

२५. एघोऽस्येधिषीमहि समिदसि तेजोऽसि तेजो मयि धेहि ॥

25. O God, Thou shinest in our souls, Thou art brilliant like the burning fuel, Thou art the Illuminator of knowledge like electricity, give me light. May we progress in full, having acquired Thee!

२६. यावती द्यावापृथिवी यावच्च सप्त सिन्धवो वितस्थिरे ।
तावन्तमिन्द्र ते ग्रहमूर्जां गृह्लाम्यक्षितं मयि गृह्लाम्यक्षितम् ॥

26. O God, far as the Heaven and Earth are spread in compass, far as the seven oceans are extended, so vast do I take with strength Thy indestructible power of perseverance. I imbibe in me Thy imperishable power!

२७. मयि त्यदिन्द्रियं बृहन्मयि दक्षो मयि क्रतु: ।
घर्मस्त्रिशुग्वि राजति विराजा ज्योतिषा सह ब्रह्मणा तेजसा सह ॥

27. With lustrous fulgency, with readily serviceable riches, the yajna shines with triple light. In my soul be that great mental force, in my soul be strength, wisdom and action.

[23]See 6-22.
[24]See 20-21, 27-10, 35-14.
[25]See 20-23.
[27]Triple light : the light of fire, lightning and Sun, or soft, medium and excessive light.

२८. पयसो रेत आभृतं तस्य दोहमशीमह्य॒त्तरामुत्तरा॒ँ समाम् ।
विष: संवृक् कृत्वे दक्षस्य ते सुषुम्णस्य ते सुषुम्णाग्निहुत: ।
इन्द्रपीतस्य प्रजापतिभक्षितस्य मधुमत उपहूत उपहूतस्य भक्षयामि ॥

28. O virtuous happy person, the strength through milk thou hast gained, may we through each succeeding year enjoy the bliss of drinking it. May we thereby for wisdom attain to thy wisdom and manifest strength. May I, the remover of the defects of milk brought near, invited, the performer of Homa, enjoy a share of the invigorating and savoury milk, drunk and tasted by the soul!

CHAPTER XXXIX

१. स्वाहा प्राणेभ्य: साधिपतिकेभ्य: ।
पृथिव्यै स्वाहा अग्नये स्वाहा ऽन्तरिक्षाय स्वाहा वायवे स्वाहा । दिवे स्वाहा सूर्याय स्वाहा ॥

1. Swaha to the vital breathings with their controlling lord, the soul.
To earth Swaha! To Agni Swaha!
To Firmament Swaha!
To Vayu Swaha! To Sky Swaha! To Surya Swaha!

२. दिग्भ्य: स्वाहा चन्द्राय स्वाहा नक्षत्रेभ्य: स्वाहा ऽद्भ्य: स्वाहा वरुणाय स्वाहा । नाभ्यै स्वाहा पूताय स्वाहा ॥

2. To the Quarters Swaha! To the Moon Swaha! To the Stars Swaha! To the Waters Swaha! To the Ocean Swaha! To the Navel Swaha! To the Purifying light Swaha!

३. वाचे स्वाहा प्राणाय स्वाहा प्राणाय स्वाहा ।
चक्षुषे स्वाहा चक्षुषे स्वाहा ।
श्रोत्राय स्वाहा श्रोत्राय स्वाहा ॥

3. To Speech Swaha! To Breath Swaha! To Dhananjaya Vayu Swaha! To the right eye Swaha! To the left eye Swaha ! To the right ear Swaha! To the left ear Swaha!

४. मनस: काममाकूतिं वाच: सत्यमशीय ।
पशुनाँ रूपमन्नस्य रसो यश: श्री: श्रयतां मयि स्वाहा ॥

4. The wish and purpose of the mind and truth of speech may I obtain. Bestowed on me be cattle's beauty, sweet taste of food, fame and grace, through truthful speech and virtuous conduct.

[1]Swaha : The sacrificial exclamation on making an offering.
It means, uttered in truthful speech. It denotes righteous action.
All the thirteen verses in this chapter relate to cremation; They are recited at the time of cremating the dead body. The dead body should never be interred in the ground, thrown in the jungle, or a river. Cremation is the only remedy against its pollution and spread of diseases from its offensive odour, Swami Dayananda has condemned in strong words the disposal of the corpse in ways other than cremation.
[2]People should send in all directions, by burning the body, its parts through fire.
[3]All parts of the body should be thoroughly burnt. Those who burn the dead body with odorous butter and sweet-scented provisions do a virtuous act.
Dhananjaya: A kind of vital air nourishing the body.
The different organs of the body are named to be burnt completely.
[4]Those who cremate the dead bodies properly attain to grace, fame, etc.

५. प्रजापतिः सम्प्रियमाणः सम्राट् सम्भृतो वैश्वदेवः सँसन्नो धर्मः प्रवृक्तस्तेज उद्यत
श्राशिवन: पयस्यानीयमाने पौष्णो विष्पन्दमाने मारुत: क्लथन् ।
मैंत्र: शरसि सन्ताय्यमाने वायव्यो ह्रियमाण आग्नेयो हूयमानो वाग्घुत: ॥

5. Worship Him alone Who retains the soul called Prajapati, (the nourisher of men); the well protected soul called Samrat, (filled with lustre); the well received soul called Vaishvadeva (Connected with all material objects), the soul separated from the body, called Dharma (full of brilliance); the soul progressing called Teja (light); the soul well received in water called Ashwin (connected with Pran and Apan); timely received soul called Paushan (the light connected with the Earth); the violent soul called Maruta (the light connected with man's body); the soul reared in water called Maitra (connected with friendly Pran); the attacking soul called vayavya (full of velocity like air); the soul invoked called Agneya (burning lustrous like fire), the soul recognised as head called vak (one that commands and gives orders).

६. सविता प्रथमेऽह्नग्निर्द्वितीये वायुस्तृतीय आदित्यश्चतुर्थे चन्द्रमा: पञ्चम ऋतु: षष्ठे
मरुत: सप्तमे बृहस्पतिरष्टमे ।
मित्रो नवमे वरुणो दशम इन्द्र एकादशे विश्वे देवा द्वादशे ॥

6. After death, the soul goes to the Sun on the first day; to Agni on the second; to Vayu on the third; to Aditya on the fourth; to Chandrama (the moon) on the fifth; to Ritu on the sixth; to Maruts on the seventh; to Brihaspati on the eighth; to Mitra on the ninth; to Varuna on the tenth; to Indra on the eleventh; to all divine, noble traits on the twelfth.

७. उग्रश्च भीमश्च ध्वान्तश्च धुनिश्च ।
सासह्वाँश्चाभियुग्वा च विक्षिप: स्वाहा ॥

7. The soul after death, according to its actions becomes fierce and calm; terrible and fearless; ignorant and enlightened; trembling and steadfast; forbearing and unforbearing; passionate and ascetic; and a prey to bewilderment.

८. अग्निँ हृदयेनाशनिँ हृदयाग्रेण पशुपतिं कृत्स्नहृदयेन भवं यक्ना ।
शर्वं मतस्नाभ्यामीशानं मन्युना महादेवमन्त: पर्शव्येनोग्रं देवं वनिष्ठुना वसिष्ठहनु: शिङ्गीनि कोश्याभ्याम् ॥

⁵Soul enters the body through water or semen. Twelve names for the soul have been enumerated in the verse, depicting its twelve qualities.
⁶Aditya : rays of the sun.
Ritu : Season, personified.
Maruts : Human beings.
Brihaspati : The Sutra Atma Vayu.
Mitra : Pran.
Varuna : Udan.
Indra : Lightning.
The soul roams after death, through different regions, for twelve days, before it takes its birth, being washed of its impurities.

8. The souls after death attain to fire with the heart; to lightning with the upper part of the heart; to Pashupati with the whole heart; to Bhava with the liver.

To Sharva with the two cardinal bones; to Ishana with righteous indignation; to Mahadeva with the intercostal flesh; to the Fierce God with the rectum; to handsome chinned person, to knowable and procurable powers with two lumps of flesh near the heart.

८. उग्रॅल्लोहितेन मित्रॅ सौव्रत्येन रुद्रं दौर्व्रेत्येनेन्द्रं प्रक्रीडेन मरुतो बलेन साध्यान् प्रमुदा । भवस्य कण्ठघॅ रुद्रस्यान्त: पार्श्व्यं महादेवस्य यक्नच्छव्रेस्य वनिष्ठु: पशुपते पुरीतत् ॥

9. Souls inside or outside the womb become virile through pure blood; lovely through virtuous deeds; chastisable through ignoble deeds; supreme through pastime; noble through spiritual force; achievers of aims through enjoyment. Suitable place for fire is between the ribs; for bile the liver; for waters the rectum; for soul the protector of bodily organs the pericardium.

१०. लोमभ्य: स्वाहा लोमभ्य: स्वाहा त्वचे स्वाहा त्वचे स्वाहा लोहिताय स्वाहा लोहिताय स्वाहा मेदोभ्य: स्वाहा मेदोभ्य: स्वाहा । माॅ सेभ्य: स्वाहा माॅ सेभ्य: स्वाहा स्नावभ्य: स्वाहा स्नावभ्य: स्वाहा ऽस्थभ्य: स्वाहा ऽस्थभ्य: स्वाहा मज्जभ्य: स्वाहा मज्जभ्य: स्वाहा । रेतसे स्वाहा पायवे स्वाहा ॥

10. To the hair Swaha! To the nails Swaha! Swaha for burning the external skin! Swaha for burning the internal skin! Swaha for burning the blood! Swaha for burning the heart's blood! Swaha for burning the fats! Swaha for burning all the wet parts of the body! Swaha for burning the external fleshy parts! Swaha for burning the internal fleshy parts! Swaha for burning the gross sinews! Swaha for burning the subtle sinews! Swaha for burning the tough bones! Swaha for burning the soft bones! Swaha for burning the marrows! Swaha for burning the internal part of the marrows! Swaha for burning the semen! Swaha for burning the anus!

११. आयासाय स्वाहा प्रायासाय स्वाहा संयासाय स्वाहा वियासाय स्वाहोद्यासाय स्वाहा । शुचे स्वाहा शोचते स्वाहा शोचमानाय स्वाहा शोकाय स्वाहा ॥

11. Take nourishing diet for physical exertion, for lofty adventure, for concerted effort, for endeavour by different organs, for enterprise, for physical and mental purity, for contemplative soul, for expounding nice ideas, and for spiritual power.

[8]Pashupati : God the protector of the cattle, the sustainer of the universe.
Bhava : The Omnipresent God.
Sharva : The Omniscient God.
Ishana : God the Lord of the universe.
Mahadeva : Great God.
[10]All parts of the body should completely be burnt to ashes.
Swaha : I put into the fire an oblation of butter and sacrificial provisions.

CHAPTER XXXIX

१२. तपसे स्वाहा तप्यते स्वाहा तप्यमानाय स्वाहा तप्ताय स्वाहा घर्माय स्वाहा ।
निष्कृत्यै स्वाहा प्रायश्चित्त्यै स्वाहा भेषजाय स्वाहा ॥

12. Exert for the performance of religious duty, the advancement of the man of penance, the Brahmchari devoted to study, the recluse, the people lustrous like the Sun. Try hard to avoid sins, expiate for them, and ward off physical ailments through medicine.

१३. यमाय स्वाहा ऽन्तकाय स्वाहा मृत्यवे स्वाहा ।
ब्रह्मणे स्वाहा ब्रह्महत्यायै स्वाहा विश्वेभ्यो देवेभ्यः स्वाहा द्यावापृथिवीभ्याꣳ स्वाहा ॥

13. Honour the just ruler. Keep away Death, the great Finisher. Worship God, the Destroyer of the wicked. Contemplate on God, the Great. Try for the preservation of vedic knowledge. Revere all learned persons, utilise all the forces of nature. Acquire the knowledge of Heaven and Earth.

CHAPTER XL

१. ईशा वास्यमिद ँ सर्वं यत्किं च जगत्यां जगत् ।
तेन त्यक्तेन भुञ्जीथा मा गृधः कस्य स्विद्धनम् ॥

1. O man, all moving beings in the universe are enveloped by the Omnipotent God. Enjoy what God hath granted thee. Covet not the wealth of any man!

२. कुर्वन्नेवेह कर्माणि जिजीविषेच्छत ँ समाः ।
एवं त्वयि नान्यथेतोऽस्ति न कर्म लिप्यते नरे ॥

2. Man, only doing unselfish, religious deeds in this world, should wish to live for a hundred years. So Karma cleaveth not to man. No way is there for thee but this for emancipation.

३. असुर्या नाम ते लोका अन्धेन तमसावृताः ।
ताँस्ते प्रेत्यापि गच्छन्ति ये के चात्महनो जनाः ॥

3. Verily, the men engulfed in the darkness of ignorance, and those who disobey the dictates of conscience, are sinners given to carnal pleasures. They, in this life, and after death, attain to those sexual enjoyments enwrapt in affliction and ignorance.

४. अनेजदेकं मनसो जवीयो नैनद्देवा आप्नुवन् पूर्वमर्षत् ।
तद्धावतोऽन्यानत्येति तिष्ठत्तस्मिन्नपो मातरिश्वा दधाति ॥

4. God is permanent, One, swifter than mind, beyond the reach of physical organs, speeding on before them. He through His Omnipresence, outstrips the physical organs running after passions.
Residing in Him doth soul perform action.

५. तदेजति तन्नैजति तद्दूरे तद्वन्तिके ।
तदन्तरस्य सर्वस्य तदु सर्वस्यास्य बाह्यतः ॥

---

¹It may also mean enjoy the universe in a spirit of renunciation. One should shun worldly enjoyments to enjoy real spiritual happiness.
तेन त्यक्तेन may also mean given to thee by God. Content thyself with what God has given thee.
Don't be greedy To whom do the riches belong? To none, then why run after money.
²So : Doing noble, religious deeds.
No way : For salvation there is no other way, but the performance of good deeds.
³The word Loka has been translated by some commentators as worlds, regions. Swami Dayananda translates it as men who see. There are no regions where pain and ignorance predominate.

5. God moves in the eyes of fools. He is motionless. He is far distant from the irreligious and ignorant, and near the yogis. He is within this entire universe, and surrounds it externally.

६. यस्तु सर्वाणि भूतान्यात्मन्नेवानुपश्यति ।
सर्वभूतेषु चात्मानं ततो न वि चिकित्सति ॥

6. The man, who sees all animate and inanimate creation in God, and God pervading all material objects, falls not a prey to doubt.

७. यस्मिन्त्सर्वाणि भूतान्यात्मेवाभूद्विजानतः ।
तत्र को मोहः कः शोक एकत्वमनुपश्यतः ॥

7. A man contemplating upon God, feels in Him all beings like unto himself. Such a yogi looking upon God as an unequalled One, becomes free from delusion and grief.

८. स पर्यगाच्छुक्रमकायमव्रणमस्नाविर शुद्धमपापविद्धम् ।
कविर्मनीषी परिभूः स्वयम्भूर्याथातथ्यतोऽर्थान् व्यदधाच्छाश्वतीभ्यः समाभ्यः ॥

8. God is All-pervading, Lustrous, Bodiless, Flawless, Sinewless, Pure, Unpierced by evil. He is Omniscient, Knower of the hearts of all, Censurer of the sinful, and self-existent. He truly reveals through the vedas all things for His subjects from His immemorial attributes, free from birth and death.

९. अन्धं तमः प्रविशन्ति येऽसंभूतिमुपासते ।
ततो भूय इव ते तमो य उ सम्भूत्या रताः ॥

9. Abandoning God, deep into the shade of blinding gloom fall the worshippers of eternal, unborn Matter. They sink to darkness deeper yet who are engaged in the material pleasures of the world.

१०. अन्यदेवाहुः सम्भवादन्यदाहुरसम्भवात् ।
इति शुश्रुम धीराणां ये नस्तद्विचचक्षिरे ॥

10. One fruit, they say, results from the knowledge of this created world, the Effect, another from the knowledge of eternal Matter, the Cause. That from the sages have we heard who have declared this lore to us.

⁶The man : he who has renounced the world and wishes for final emancipation. The reading of the Kanva recension is 'na vijugupsate' does not shrink away from them as alien and inferior to his ownself.

⁹They who worship the eternal uncreated matter are spiritually degraded, and are put to suffering. Those who worship and enjoy the material objects of the world are more degraded. God alone is worthy of worship. Asambhuti is undeveloped Prakriti. Nature in its causal or germinal state when it has not been evolved as the universe which is the effect. It is also called tamas, darkness or chaos. This worship is mere blindness, and ignorance.

¹⁰Each fruit from the worship of Cause and Effect fails to achieve the desired object, regarding the integration of soul with the Supreme Self.

११. सम्भूतिं च विनाशां च यस्तद्वेदोभयꣳ सह ।
विनाशेन मृत्युं तीर्त्वा सम्भूत्यामृतमश्नुते ॥

11. The man who knows simultaneously the effect and the cause, overcoming death through the knowledge of the cause, attains to salvation through the knowledge of the effect, the created world.

१२. अन्धं तम: प्र विशन्ति येऽविद्यामुपासते ।
ततो भूय इव ते तमो य उ विद्यायाꣳ रता: ॥

12. To blinding darkness go the men who worship Nescience. Those proud of little knowledge enter darkness that is darker still.

१३. अन्यदेवाहुर्विद्यया अन्यदाहुरविद्यया: ।
इति शुश्रुम धीराणां ये नस्तद्विचचक्षिरे ॥

13. Different is the fruit, they say, of knowledge and Nescience. Thus from the sages have we heard who have declared this lore to us.

१४. विद्यां चाविद्यां च यस्तद्वेदोभयꣳ सह ।
अविद्यया मृत्युं तीर्त्वा विद्ययाऽमृतमश्नुते ॥

14. He who simultaneously knoweth well these two, knowledge and Action, overcoming death by Action, by knowledge gaineth salvation.

१५. वायुरनिलममृतमथेदं भस्मान्तꣳ शरीरम् ।
ओ३म् क्रतो स्मर । क्लिबे स्मर । कृतꣳ स्मर ॥

15. O active soul, at the time of death, remember Om, remember God for thy vitality and thy eternity, remember thy deeds. Know that soul is immaterial and immortal but the body is finally reduced to ashes!

१६. अग्ने नय सुपथा राये अस्मान्विश्वानि देव वयुनानि विद्वान् ।
युयोध्यस्मज्जुहुराणमेनो भूयष्ठां ते नम उक्तिं विधेम ॥

16. O Divine, Lustrous, Benevolent God, most ample, respectful adoration do we bring Thee. Thou art All-Knowing. Remove from us the sin that leads

---

[11] One should know simultaneously the eternal Matter, the cause कारण of the universe, and the effect, कार्यं, the created world.
   Sambhuti : The world in which all substances are created.
   Vinasha : The eternal matter in which all substances are resolved at the time of dissolution.
   Knowledge of Matter frees one from the fear of death and the knowledge and practice of noble virtuous and religious deeds leads one to final beatitude. Ubbat translates Sambhuti as God the Great.
[12] Nescience : Worship of Matter, not God. Those who with a smattering of knowledge style themselves as highly learned fall into greater darkness.

us astray. Lead us through virtuous path to riches, happiness and all sorts of wisdom!

१७. हिरण्मयेन पात्रेण सत्यस्यापिहितं मुखम् ।
योऽसावादित्ये पुरुष: सोऽसावहम् ।
ओ३म् खं ब्रह्म ॥

17. O men, by Me, the Resplendent Protector, is covered the face of Eternal Cause, the Matter. The Spirit yonder in the Sun, that spirit dwelling there am I. I am vast like the atmosphere, Greatest of all in merit, action, and nature am I. Om is My name!

---

[17]Om is the best name of God. Om comes from the root श्रव (to protect). God is Om as He protects the universe and us all,

GLOSSARY AND INDEX

Adhi-Atmika, 171fn.
Adhi-Bhautika, 171fn.
Adhi-Daivika, 171fn.
Adhvaryu(s), the priest(s) who do the practical part of the scrifice, 9fn., 11fn., 65fn., 68, 131fn., 210, 254fn., 259, 272fn., 322fn.
Aditi, Infinity, Infinite nature, the mother of the Gods, 24fn., 25fn., 85fn., 308, 408fu.
Aditya, a son of Aditi, especially varuna and the sun, 7fn., 10fn., 377, 433
Adityas, Twelve months of the year or Varuna, Mitra, Aryaman, Bhaga, Daksha, Amsha and one or two others, 10, 13, 98, 105fn., 135, 162fn., 166, 170, 173, 256, 292, 296, 307, 315, 341, 354, 389, 406, 408fn.
aeroplane, 39, 106, 112, 174, 198, 211, 356, 361, 368, 390, 412
Aghanya, a wife worthy of veneration, 85fn.
Agni, the God of Fire and Light, 9fn., 10fn., 11fn., 19, 33, 34fn., 308, 310, 433; oblation bearer, 33; as soma, 106fn., 314fn; identified with the Sun, 178; identified with other Gods, 377; worlds messenger, 180fn.
Agni Hotra, oblation to Agni, 210; daily oblation to Agni and Gods, 20fn., 50fn., 59fn.
agriculture, 3, 45, 95, 139, 173, 237
Ahankar, egotism, 375fn.
Ahuti, oblation, 13
Air, 4, 5, 6, 11, 14, 24, 66fn., 89fn., 91fn., 303, 321fn., 372fn., 389, 391
altar, 8, 9, 200, 233
Ambika, sister of God Rudra, 29fn.
Angas, six constituent parts of the vedas, 57fn.
Angira, a member of the family of Angiras, 42
Animals, antilope, 313, 314, 315; ass, 315; bear, 314; black buck, 312, 314; black deer, 313; boar, 315; buck, 314; buffalo, 312, 314; camel, 315; cat, 313; cow, 1, 29, 58, 307, 370; deer, 312; elephant, 312; ghrinwan, 315; goat, 373; golattika, 314; goyal, 313; hare, 315; horse, 315, 373, 405; hyena, 315; ichneumon, 312; jackal, 313, 314; kundrirachi, 314; mongoose, 312; monkey, 313; nilgaya, 315; ox, 412; porcupine, 313; rat, 312; reddoe, 313; sheep, 373; tiger, 313, 366; tortoise, 314; wild goat, 313; wild ram, 313, 315; wolf, 313
Anna, food, 82fn.
Antriksha, the intermediate space between heaven and earth; the middle of the three spheres or regions of life, 10fn., 11fn., 20fn., 59fn.
Anushtup metre, a kind of metre consisting of four Padas or quarter verses of eight syllables each, 86fn., 128, 158, 272, 301, 309, 350, 364
Anushtup verses, 121, 123
Anuvatsar, the fourth year in the vedic cycle of five years, 369fn.
Apa, water, 82fn., 377
Apan, one of the vital airs which moves downwards and out through the anus, 7fn., 9fn., 10fn., 12fn., 20fn., 25, 66fn., 89fn., 91fn., 105fn., 162, 165, 174fn., 185, 204fn., 214fn., 219, 229fn., 316, 325, 374fn., 387, 408fn., 426, 433
Apnawana, an ancient Rishi, belonging to the Bhrigu family, 21fn.
Apratirath, the name of a hymn (RV. x.103) composed by Rishi Apratiratha, son of Indra, 210fn.
Apsaras, two airs that course through the veins and not female divinities, 176, 177
Apta, an ideal sage, 402, 406fn.
archery, 188
architect, 270, 287
Arithmetic, 105fn., 172, 200, 233
Arithmetical operations, 225
arrows, 361, 366
art of Government, 80
arteries, 318
Artha, utility, or worldly prosperity, 81fn., 105fn., 298fn., 299
Arthaveda, science of wealth subordinate to Atharvaveda, 98fn., 144fn.
Aryama, one of the Adityas commonly invoked with Mitra and Varuna, 25fn.
Asamaratha, matchless air, 177
Asanas, 9fn.

GLOSSARY AND INDEX

Ashada (Asarh), summer, 70, 161, 293
Ashvamedha, improvement of land for growing more crops and not horse sacrifice, 365fn.
Ashwatha, the unstable world, 410fn.
assembly, 46fn., 70, 191, 204, 261fn., 266, 268, 277, 279, 341, 370, 383, 390, 396, 429
astronomy, 43, 57, 103
Asuri Anushṭup Chhand, metre of thirteen syllables, 98fn.
Asuri Gayatri Chhand, metre of fifteen syllables, 98fn.
Asuri Pankti, metre of eleven syllables, 97fn.
Asvin (Aswin), mid September to mid October, 70, 165, 177, 293, 314, 433
Atharvaveda, 57, 227, 256, 339fn., 373, 399
Ati Ashti, metre with sixty eight syllables, 273fn., 349fn.
Ati Dhriti, metre with seventy six syllables, 273fn., 349fn.
Ati Jagati, metre with forty eight syllables, 273fn., 349fn.
Ati Shakwari, metre with sixty syllables, 273fn., 349fn.
Atichhand, name of a metre, 310
Atichhandas, Ati Dhriti, Ati Ashti, Ati Shakvari and Ati Jagati are known as Atichhandas, 349
atmosphere, 3, 73, 167, 298, 318, 372fn., 382, 388, 401, 408, 423
Atom, 4, 103
automobile, 382
Autumn, 309
Avayava, syllogism, 98fn.
Avbrith, expiatory bath for purification, 241fn.
Ayu, man, living being, 42
Ayurveda, science of medicine, 98fn., 99, 144fn., 238fn.

Baisakh, mid April to mid May, 293
bard, 366
besprinkler, 368
Bhadra, mid August to mid September, 70, 293
Bhadrapada, mid August to mid September, 164
Bharati, speech filled with vedic lore; a Goddess of speech, 336, 342, 345, 348, 354, 359
Bhardwaj Rishi, here it is not the name of a Rishi but means ear

Bhava, the omnipresent God, 434
Bhoomi, earth, 138
Bhrigu, one who can perform yagna, 21fn.
Bhutanampati, lord of spirits, 9fn.
Bhuvanpati, lord of the earth, 9fn.
Bhuvpati, lord of the atmosphere, 9fn.
Birds—alaja, 314; bat, 312, 314; black-bee, 312; bluejay, 311; chakravaka, 313; cormorant, 314; sushilika, 314; swan, 314
boatsman, 369
botanist, 50
bow, 193, 360
Brahma, 11fn., 12, 68, 131fn., 135, 210fn., 259, 272fn., 408fn.
Brahmchari, an unmarried religious student, 59, 76, 103, 197, 272, 273, 324fn., 368, 383, 435
Brahmchari—aditya, one who observes celibacy for fortyeight years, 7fn., 42, 60, 120, 121, 123, 168, 274fn., 316; rudra, one who observes celibacy for fortyfour years, 7fn., 42, 60, 120, 121, 123, 274; vasu, one who observes celibacy for twentyfour years, 7fn., 42, 60, 120, 121, 123, 168, 232, 274fn.
Brahmacharya ashram, the state of an unmarried religious student, 30fn., 54, 74, 98fn., 130fn., 146, 162, 184, 347, 407, 420
Brahmana, 7fn., 19fn., 36fn., 58, 73fn., 98fn., 100, 131, 162, 167, 179fn., 193, 290, 321, 327, 329fn., 365fn., 371, 374, 380, 429; crane, 311; cuckoo, 314; curlew, 313; dhanuksha, 313; duck, 311; eagle, 314; falcon, 313; gallinule, 312; goshadi, 312; goose, 31; heron, 313; kaalka, 314; kapinjala, 315; kaulika, 311; kulika, 312; owl, 31; paingraja, 314; parushna, 314; peacock, 311, 314; pelican, 314; pigeon, 311; pippaka, 315; sarga, 313; śayandaka, 313; sichapus, 312; sparrow, 313; srijaya, 313
bricks, 200, 411fn.
bridge, 369
Brihaspati, the chief offerer of prayers and sacrifices and therefore represented as the type of priestly order and the Purohita of the Gods with whom he intercedes for men, 12, 307, 314, 433
Brihat, one of the important hymns (of the Samaveda) composed in Brihati meter, 104, 127, 227, 310, 348
Brihati metre, a metre of thirtysix syllables, 272, 301, 347, 350

Colebrooke, 365fn., 372fn.

Commander, 67, 201, 206, 207, 235, 261, 262, 263, 310, 361, 394, 404
Conch-blower, 370
Constellations, 376
Consumption, 1
Corn, 7, 11
Couch-maker, 195
Cow, 1, 29, 58, 307, 370
Cowherd, 367
Cow-killer, 370
Creator, 1, 5, 317, 385, 419
Cuirass, 193

Dacoit, 390
Dakshinayan, the sun's progress south of the Equator, winter solstice, 224fn.
dancer, 366
Darbha-grass, a bunch of grass (Saccharum cylindricum) used during sacrificial rites, 233
Dashratha, 368fn.
Dasyus, savages, slaves, 72fn.
Daivi Anushtup Chhand, tri syllabic metre, 96fn.
Daivi Brihati Chhand, quadri syllabic metre, 96fn.
Daivi Gayatri Chhand, monosyllabic metre, 96fn.
Daivi Jagati Chhand, heptasyllabic metre, 97fn.
Daivi Pankti Chhand, pentasyllabic metre, 97fn.
Daivi Trishtup Chhand, six syllabic metre, 97fn.
Daivi Ushnik Chhand, disyllabic metre, 96fn.
Death, 435
demoniacal beings, 17
Devadutta, one of the vital airs exhaled while yawning, 10fn., 66fn., 89fn., 91fn., 169, 214fn., 374fn.
Dhananjay, vital air supposed to nourish the body, 10fn., 66fn., 87fn., 89fn., 91fn., 169, 176, 204fn., 214fn., 219, 374fn., 432
Dhanur Veda, the science of archery, a treatise considered as an upa-veda connected with the Yajurveda and derived from Visvamitra and Bhrigu, 68fn., 98fn., 144, 229
Dharma, prescribed conduct, duty, morality, 32, 81fn., 99, 105, 138, 298fn., 299, 367fn., 424, 433
Dharma Sabha, assembly for administration of the moral and spiritual needs of the people, 74fn.
Dhirtarashtra, the eldest son of Vyasa by the widow of Vichitra-virya, born blind, brother of Pandu and Vidura, husband of Gandhari, father of one hundred sons of whom the eldest was Duryodhana, 368fn.
Dhruva, the largest of three sacrificial ladles, 11fn.
Dhruva, the polar-star (personified as son of Uttanapada and grandson of Manu), 223
Dirghatama(s), father of Kakshivat rishi; he was born blind due to Brihaspati's curse, 24fn.
diseases, 143, 144
dissolution, 53, 378fn.
dog-rearer, 366
Drishtanta, illustration, 98fn.
Drona, a wooden vessel, bucket, trough; a soma vessel, 241
drummer, 193
dry fish clearer, 369
Duryodhan, eldest son of Dhritarastra, leader of the Kauravas in their war with Pandavas, 368fn.
Duties of the king, 99
Dwarf, 367
Dwipada, metre consisting of two padas, 351
Dyau, heaven, 10fn., 11fn.

Ear, 66fn.
Earth, 3, 6, 7, 9, 12, 20fn., 37, 44, 56, 66fn., 73, 89fn., 91fn., 95, 113, 145, 155, 169, 170, 177, 292, 295, 296, 303, 305, 306, 316, 317, 321, 325, 327, 337, 345, 347, 355, 356, 359, 361, 362, 372, 389, 406, 419, 425, 428, 430, 433
Edidhishu-pati, the husband of a younger sister whose elder sister is unmarried, 367fn.
Eggeling (Professor), 210fn.
Ego, 66fn.
Eight directions, 403fn.
eight Vasus, a class of Gods (who usually number eight); they were originally personifications of natural phenomena; their names are given differently by various texts, 10fn., 15, 89fn., 274, 275fn.
election of a ruler, 85, 90, 100, 131
electricity, 21, 68, 87, 88, 103, 104, 112,

GLOSSARY AND INDEX 443

113, 114, 115, 128, 155, 180fn., 183fn., 202, 212, 223, 234, 239, 280, 284, 296, 329, 340, 353, 355, 381fn., 385, 389, 391, 394, 404, 412, 425
elephant, 312
eleven names of a wife, 85
eleven Rudras, the sons of Rudra who is supposed to have sprung from Brahma's head and to have separated himself afterwards as half male and half female; the former half again separating itself into eleven Rudras, 89fn., 275
eleven substances, 66
Emancipator, 5
engineer, 284, 369
engineering works, 67
entrails, 318
Essence of waters, 90, 231
Ether, 19, 296
etymology, 57fn.
eugenics, 184
eunuch, 366, 371
ewe, 29
Eye, 66fn.

fiends, 15, 17
fifteenfold praise-songs, 104
fifteenfold objects, 98
fire, 4, 8, 9, 11, 14, 19, 20, 21, 22, 66fn., 70, 89fn., 91fn., 136, 166, 296, 297, 321fn., 327, 372fn., 381fn., 389
fire-kindler, 368
Five Bhutas, five elements, 105fn.
five castes, 329
Five classes of subjects, 72fn.
five elements, 91fn., 304fn.
Five Karma Indriyas, 105fn.
five Pranas, five vital airs, 131, 148fn.
Five regions, 97fn.
Five senses, 329
flutist, 370
forests, 4
forest-guard, 370
four Ashrams, 81fn.
Four horns, 216
Four-kinds of warriors, 73
Four Up-Vedas, a class of writing appended to the Vedas in a subordinate position; Ayurveda, the science of medicine to the Rigveda; the Dhanurveda, the science of archery, to the Yajurveda; the Ghandharva Veda, the science of music, to the Samaveda; the Shastra shāstra or science of arms, to the Atharvaveda, 98fn.
Four Varunas, four classes of people, tribe, order, caste (probably in contrast to the dark colour of the original inhabitants); refers to the four principal classes described in Manu's code viz., Brahmans, Kshatriyas, Vaisyas and Sudras, 81fn.
Fourteenfold objects, 98
Fuel, twentyone kinds, 375

gallows, 370
gambler, 366, 370
Gandharva, a heavenly being, also called Visva-vasu and Vayu-kesa, his duty is to keep watch over the heavenly Soma, 9fn.
Gandharva Veda, the science of music, considered as a branch of Samaveda, 98fn., 144
gastric juice, 12, 38, 318
gate-keeper, 367
Gayatri Mantra, prayer connected with the Gayatri, 25, 288, 365, 414
Gayatri metre, an ancient metre of twenty-four syllables, usually arranged in a triplet of eight syllables each, 7, 16, 36, 40, 86, 111, 158, 239, 272, 296, 301, 309, 349, 364, 426
Gayatri verses, sacred verses addressed to Savitri or the Sun as generator by every Brahman during the morning, noon and evening devotions; the Gayatri verse is personified as a Goddess, the wife of Brahma and mother of the four Vedas, 13, 104, 120, 121, 123, 127, 128, 158, 161, 346
geography, 57
geologist, 45, 113, 114
geology, 45, 46, 57, 95, 113, 173
goat, 307
goatherd, 367
gold, 42, 332
goldsmith, 369
grammar, 57fn.
Grassman (Professor), 246fn.
gravitation, 7
Griffith, 9fn., 14fn., 17fn., 65fn., 71fn., 79fn., 190fn., 222fn., 246fn., 264fn., 298fn., 347fn., 365fn., 372fn., 375fn., 384fn., 387, 388fn., 393fn., 413fn.
Grihastha, a house-holder in the second period of his religious life, performing the duties of the master of a house and father of a family after having finished

his studies, 82fn., 83fn.
Grihastha Ashram, the order of a house holder, 30fn., 98fn., 130fn., 160
Gurukula, the house of a teacher, 407
Gyan, higher knowledge, 163
Gyan Indriyas, organs of perception, 91fn.

harlot, 370, 371
Havan, oblation, burnt offering, 9, 22fn., 31fn., 40fn., 66, 182, 200fn., 277, 278, 346, 348, 349, 350, 382
Havya, anything to be offered as an oblation, sacrificial gift or food, 85fn.
headman, 370
head of the State, 67, 72, 74, 268, 383, 384, 385
Heaven, 19, 296, 303, 305, 306, 362
Heaven and Earth, 11, 170, 177, 203, 204, 205, 237, 264, 292, 304, 310, 314, 361, 379, 385, 394, 428
Heaven's head, 231, 382
helmet, 193
herbs, 4
Hetvabhasa, fallacy, 98fn.
Hinsa, violence, 6
Homa, the act of making an oblation to the devas or Gods by casting clarified butter into the fire, 3, 27fn., 167, 210, 224, 232, 236, 278, 343, 346, 347, 348, 349, 352, 429, 431
horse, 29, 307, 324, 356, 357, 361
horse-keeper, 367
house, 3, 14, 16, 23, 171, 194, 195
House of the people, 66, 74
humours, 60fn., 342
hunter, 366
hydrostatics, 57

Ichha, ambition, 82fn.
ichneumon, 309
Ida, praiseworthy speech, 85nf., 336, 342, 345, 354, 359
Idvatsar, last year of the cycle of five years, 369
Iguana, 314
Indra, in Vedic mythology, he rules over the deities of the intermediate region; he is addressed in prayers and hymns, more than any other deity as the lord of the Gods, 9fn., 45fn., 106fn., 308, 310, 433
Indrapatni, the wife of Indra, 342
Indriya, organ of sense, 82fn.
industrial works, 68

Ishana, one of the old names of Siva; also name of Vishnu; the lord of the ueiverse, 434

Jaati, a self-cantradictory answer based on mere similarity or dissimiliarity, 98fn.
Jagati metre a metre of fortyeight syllables, 7, 16, 36, 40, 86fn., 158, 273, 296, 301, 309, 348
Jagati verses, 121, 123, 158, 350, 351
Jagrit, waking, 322fn.
Jalpa, Discourse, 98fn.
Jamadagni Rishi, son of Bhargava Riciks and father of Parasurama; of ten named with Visvamitra as an adversary of Vasistha, 159
Jayestha, mid May to mid June, 161, 293
Jeeva, soul, 10fn.
jeweller, 366
Jnana higher knowledge derived from meditation on the Universal Spirit, 78fn., 158
Jnan Kand, portion of the Vedas which relate to the knowledge of the universal Spirit, 33fn.
Juhu, a curved wooden handle for pouring sacrificial butter into fire 11fn.
Jyoti, brilliance, 82fn., 85fn.
Jyotish, science of the movement of the Heavenly bodies, 98fn.

Kakshivant, (Kakshivat), a rishi famous as the author of several hymns of the Rigveda; he is the son of Usij and Dirghatamas, 24fn.
Kakup metre, metre of twentyeight syllables, 273, 301, 310
Kakup verses, 351
Kalash, a water-pot, pitcher or jar, 241
Kali, the worst of a class or number of objects, 214fn.
Kalpa, a period of time equal to one day of Brahma; it consists of one thousand yugas or four thousand, three hundred and twenty millions of human years' 34fn., 224
Kalpa, the most complete of the six vedangas which prescribes the ritual and lays down the rules for the performance of sacrifices, 98fn.
Kama, desire or longing for love, pleasure, enjayment especially of sexual love, 81fn., 105fn., 298fn., 229

Kamya, desirable, beautiful, amiable, agreeable, 85fn.

Karali (Karala), formidable, terrible, one of the seven tongues and nine Samidhis of Agni, 214fn.

Karma, act, action, performance, 78fn., 158, 163fn., 436

Karmakanda, that part of the Sruti which relates to ceremonial acts and sacrificial rites, 33fn.

Kartika, month i.e., mid-October to mid-November, 70, 165, 177, 293

Kidneys, 318

Kirata, a degraded mountain tribe residing in woods and mountains and living by hunting; for having neglected the prescribed religious rites, they came to be regarded as Mlecchas, 369

Knowledge of the Vedas—one-footed, 81; two-footed, 81; three-footed, 81; four-footed, 81; eight-footed, 81

Krikala, one of the five vital airs, 10fn., 66fn., 89fn., 91fn., 169, 374fn.

Kshatriya, member of the military or ruling class which later on became the second among the four castes, 7fn., 19fn., 36fn., 72fn., 98fn., 100, 131, 162, 167, 169, 179fn., 190fn., 199, 229, 321, 327, 329fn., 365, 374fn., 380, 429

Kumara, boy, youth, son, 209fn.

Kurma, one of the vital airs of the body causing the closing of the eyes, 10fn., 66fn., 89fn., 91fn., 169, 374fn.

Lake, 318
Lanman (Professor), 248fn.
laws of gravitation, 80
light, 8
lights' one light, 399
Ludwig (Professor), 216, 246fn., 372fn.
lute-player, 370

Macdonell, 408fn.
Magha, month i.e., mid January to mid February, 70, 184, 185, 293
Mahadeva, the great God, 434
Mahakalpa, great cycle of time, 224
Mahanamni, nine verses of the Samaveda beginning with the words vida maghavan, 301
Maha-Padma, a great number, 200
Mahat, intellect or the intellectual principle, 375fn.

Mahatattva, the great principle, 317
Mahendra, a great chief or leader, 310
Mahi, greatly, exceedingly, 85fn., 348
Mahidhar, 9fn., 13fn., 15fn., 17fn., 19fn., 20fn., 22fn., 24fn., 26fn., 27fn., 29fn., 38fn., 45fn., 71fn., 196fn., 208fn., 216fn., 246fn., 298fn., 339fn., 347fn., 365fn., 374fn., 397fn.
mail, 193
Maitra, friendly, amiable, 433
Manan, reflection, understanding intrinsic knowledge as one of the faculties connected with the senses, 98fn.
Manas, mind, 82fn.
Manojava, the speed or swiftness of thought; one of the seven tongues of Agni, 214fn.
Manu, father of the human race; identified with Praja-pati; but the name Manu is especially applied to fourteen successive mythical progenitors and sovereigns of the earth; among them the first Manu, Svayambhuva is said to be the famous 'code of Manu' and Kalpa and Grihya sutras; the seventh Manu, known as Vaivasvata is regarded as the ancestor of the present race of humans; he is also, like Noah of Old Testament, said to have been preserved from a great flood by Vishnu who assumed the form of a fish for this purpose, 71fn.
Margashirsha, month i.e., mid November to mid December, 70, 177, 293
Marutas, friends and companions of Indra; their names and number are variously given in the different texts; in the vedas, they are said to be the sons of Rudra and Prsni; they are the Gods of the middle sphere, 308, 333
Matrishwa (Matarisvan), developing within his mother i.e., within the fire stick; either Agni or of a divine being closely associated with him, 89fn.
matter, 321, 437
Max Muller, 365fn.
mechanic, 368
medicines, 3, 5
merchant, 369
meteors, 292
military machines, 57
military science, 43
Mitra, friend, companion; name of an Aditya, often invoked together with Va-

runa, 9fn., 25fn., 35fn., 64fn., 388fn., 433

Moksha, salvation, liberation from the cycle of births and deaths, 81fn., 105fn., 158, 298fn., 299

Moon, 7, 66, 89fn., 166, 296, 303, 305, 306, 363, 370, 381, 409

mortar, 8, 224

mosquito, 312

motions—One, 338; two, 338; ten, 338; twentythree, 338; thirty, 338

mrigshala, seat made of deer's skin, 315

Muir, 365fn., 372fn.

Mukti, final liberation or emancipation, 95fn.

murderer, 371

Musical instruments, 193, 207

Nag, One of the five airs of the human body which is expelled by eructation, 10fn., 66fn., 89fn., 91fn., 169, 219, 374fn.

Nakskatra, an asterism or constellation through which the moon passes, a lunar mansion; abode of the Gods or of pious persons after death, 10fn.

Nam, to yield or give away; keep quiet or be silent, 82fn.

Nichrid-Arshi Gayatri Chhand, metre of seventeen syllables, 98fn.

Nidhidhyasan, meditation, 99fn.

Nigrhasthan, a weak point in an argument or fault in syllogism, 98fn.

Nine gates of the body, 282

Nirnaya, complete ascertainment, decision, application of a complete argument, 98fn.

Nirukta, explanation or etymological interpretation of a word, 98fn.

Nishad !(Nishada), a wild non-aryan tribe in India, described as hunters, fishermen, robbers etc.; a man of any degraded tribe, an out-caste, especially the son of a Brahman by a Sudra woman, 131fn., 321fn., 329fn., 366fn.

niyama(s), restraint of the mind; the second of the eight steps of meditation mentioned in Yoga, 62, 63, 237, 328

Nobility, 228, 229

Objects—thirteen, 98; sixteen, 98; seventeen, 169; nineteen, 170; twentyone, 170; twentyfive, 170; twentyseven, 170; twentynine, 170; thirtyone, 170; thirtythree, 170

ocean, 3

Oldenburg, 365fn.

Om, every Hindu prayer begins and ends with this sacred monosyllable; it is considered as the highest object of profound religious meditation, the highest spiritual efficacy being attributed not only to the whole word but also to the three sounds A, U, M of which it consists; it is a symbol of the union of three gods, A representing Brahma, U representing Vishnu and M representing Siva; it also represents the three gunas, A rajas, U sattva and M tamas; 12fn.

One hundred and seven vital parts of the body, 141

Ox, 363

Panchdash stoma, a collection of verses occuring in the Atharvaveda, 274

Pankti metre, a sort of fivefold metre consisting of five Padas of eight syllables, 158, 272, 301, 310, 347

Pankti Shakvari, name of particular verses or hymns in Pankti metre, 105

Pankti verses, verses having stanzas of forty syllables, 350

Parivittam, an unmarried elder brother whose younger brother is married, 367fn.

Parivividanam, a younger brother who marries before his elder, 367fn.

Parliament, 46fn., 70

Pashupati, lord of animals; the elemental fire, the embodiment of the ritual sacrifice, the giver of life, 434

Patanjali, name of a celebrated grammarian and author of mahabhasya, 217fn.

Pausha, month i.e., mid December to mid January, 70, 177, 293

Pericardium, 318

pestle, 224

Phalguna, month i.e., mid February to mid March, 70, 184, 185, 293

Physician, 367

Pishacha, a class of demons, possibly so called either from their fondness for flesh, or from their yellowish appearance; in the Vedas, they are mentioned along with Asuras and Rakshasas, 366

ploughman, 367

Potter, 366

Powers of attraction and retention, 113

Praiser—fifteenfold, 167; seventeenfold, 167; twentyonefold, 167; tweentyfourfold, 167

GLOSSARY AND INDEX

Prajapati, lord of creatures; a supreme god above or among the Vedic deities, but also applied to Vishnu and Shiva later on, 98fn., 310, 377, 408fn., 433

Pramana, right measure, standard, authority, 98fn.

Pramey, basis, foundation, correct notion, 98fn.

Pran, the breath of life, respiration, spirit, vitality, 7fn., 9fn., 10fn., 13, 20fn., 25, 34fn., 64, 82fn., 89fn., 91fn., 105fn., 156, 158, 162, 164, 165, 167, 168, 169, 174fn., 176, 177, 185, 204fn., 214fn., 219, 223, 229fn., 271, 307, 309, 316, 318, 323, 325, 335fn., 354, 364, 389, 408fn., 426, 433

Pranayam, breathing exercises (three) performed during samdhya, 143, 252fn.

Prardh, a number beyond measure, 200

Prashnopanishad, 82fn., 83fn.

Prayojan, object, cause, motive, 98fn.

preservation, 53

President of the Republic, 70

President of the State, 74

Priesthood, 228, 229

Prishni, ray of light; the cow (wife of the bull-shaped Rudra, and mother of the Maruts) which represents the ocean or the earth, 13fn.

Prithvi, the earth, 10fn., 11fn., 12fn., 82fn.

pronounciation, 57fn.

prosody, 57fn., 98fn.

Purushmedha, the sacrifice of a man, 365fn.

Pushan, a vedic deity, 12fn.

qualities of a king, 130
qualities of a son, 117
Quiver, 193, 360

rain, 6, 309
Raivati metre, 176
Rajas, the second of the three Gunas or qualities (the other two being *sattva*, goodness, and *Tamas*, darkness; the darkening qualities like passion, emotion etc., 43fn., 170, 173fn., 233fn., 277fn., 364, 375fn.

Raj Sabha, assembly for conducting political affairs, 74fn.

Rakhshasas, demons, 15fn., 45fn.

ram, 29

Rathantra (Rathamtara), important hymns of the Samaveda, 104, 127, 227

Rathaprota, fixed in a car, a particular personification, 177

Ratna, jewel, gem, precious stone, 85fn.

Region— downward, 291, 292; eastern, 291; hitherward, 291; northern, 291; southern, 291; upward, 291, 292; western, 291

Revati, name of the verse in Rigveda. (I, 30, 13) beginning with Revati, 23, 105, 301

Rigveda, 19fn., 31, 33, 57, 65fn., 78, 81fn., 104fn., 127, 136, 210fn., 227, 229, 233, 234, 256, 339fn., 373, 399, 414, 425

Ritu, season, 433

rituals, 57fn.

Ritugami(n), one who approaches a woman sexually at the fit time i.e., after her courses, 136

Ritvij(as), a priest (usually four are named viz., Hotri, Adhvaryu, Brahman and Udgatri), 131fn.

Rudra, name of the god of tempest and father and ruler of Rudras and Maruts; in the Vedas he is closely connected with Indra and still more with Agni, the God of fire, which as a destroying agent, rages and crackles like the roaring storm, and also with kala or time, the all-consumer, 7fn.

Rudras, Rudra is supposed to have sprung from Brahma's forehead and to have afterwards separated himself into a figure half-male and half-female. The eleven Rudras, whose names differ, sprang from the former half. In another version the Rudras are represented as children of Kashyapa and Surabhi or of Brahma and Surabhi or of Bhuta and Surupa, 10, 13, 98, 105fn., 119, 135, 160, 162, 166, 170, 174, 256, 275fn., 292, 296, 308, 341, 354, 406

Saamni Anushtup Chhand, sixteen syllabic metre, 98fn.

Saamni Gayatri, twelve syllabic metre, 97fn.

Saamni Ushnik Chhand, fourteen syllabic metre, 98fn.

Sabha—Dharma, assembly of the religious, 261, 277fn.;—Rajya, assembly of the state, 261, 277fn.;—Vidya, academy of the learned 74fn., 261, 277fn.

Sailor, 216

samaddhi, intense contemplation on any object with a view to merge one's identity with the object meditated upon, 139fn.

Sama hymns, 259

Saman, Samana, one of the five vital airs (that which circulates about the naval and is essential for digestion); it is personified as a son of Sadhya, 10fn., 66fn., 89fn., 91fn., 105fn., 164, 174fn., 204fn., 214fn., 229fn., 374fn.

Samaveda, 'Veda of chants,' one of the three principal vedas; it contains a number of hymns, mostly borrowed from Rigveda; these are chanted by Udgatri priests at Soma sacrifices; it is said to have a special reference to the deceased, 19fn., 31, 57, 78, 81fn., 104, 105, 174, 175, 176, 227, 228, 229, 234, 241, 256, 287, 339fn., 373. 399, 401, 414, 425

Sambhuti, one from which all things have their origin i.e., the earth, 438fn.

Samudra, a very great number; one with fourteen zeros viz., $(10)^{14}$, 200

Samvatsar, a full year, 368

Sanjaya, a companion of Dhritarashtra, 368fn.

Sanshey, uncertainty, doubt, 98fn.

Sanyas Ashram, the fourth stage in the Hindu's religious life, 98fn., 163fn., 248, 427

Sanyasi, one who gives up worldly affairs and devotes himself to asceticism, 192, 197, 202

Saptdasha Stoma, a collection of seventeen hymns in the Atharvaveda, 274

Sarasvati, speech or the power of speech, eloquence, 85fn., 336, 342, 354, 359, 400fn; the goddess of eloquence and learning; she is considered the wife of Brahma, 308, 310

satan, 56

Satva, the quality of pure goodness regarded as the highest of the three Gunas, 43, 170, 173fn., 233fn., 277fn., 364, 375

sauce, 224

Savita, the Sun, 307, 310

Sayana, 208fn., 216fn., 365fn., 372fn., 397fn.

science of agriculture, 237

science of air, 194

science of archery, 68

science of clouds, 194

science of Electricity, 3, 194, 427

science of fire, 311

science of foam, 194

science of lightning, 239

science of medicine, 276, 283

science of water, 258

science of yoga, 68, 74

Sea, 318, 388

sea-boats, 106

seven breaths, 214

seven coverings, 375

seven domestic animals, 97fn.

seven flames, 214

seven forces, 148, 407

seven organs, 214

seven priests, 214

seven regions, 227

seven Rishis, 403

seven rivers, 403

seventeenfold praise song, 105

Shabd, the right word, correct expression, the sacred syllable OM, 105fn.

Shakvari metre, a metre of 7×8 or 4×14 syllables, 176

Shanda, an asura priest, son of sukra, 65fn.

Shankha, a very great number said to be a hundred billions or 100,000 crores, 200

Sharva, name of the god siva, 434

Sharyati, 71fn.

Shiksha, the science which teaches proper articulation and pronounciation of vedic texts, 98fn.

ships, 198, 368

Shodashi, sixteen parts, 83fn.

shooting weapons, 72

Shradha, faith, 82fn.

Shravan, hearing, listening, 98fn.

Shravan, month viz., mid. July to mid-August, 164

Shudra, lowest of the four original Hindu classes or castes, 72fn., 98fn., 131fn., 163, 192, 193fn., 230, 257, 300, 321, 327, 329fn., 365, 371, 374.

Shukra, the son of Bhrigu and the preceptor of Daityas, also the regent of the planet venus, 377

Siddhanta, principle, 98fn.

sin, 14, 257, 325, 334, 384, 393, 411, 435

Sita, a furrow, the track or line of a ploughshare, 140fn.

six Angas, 98fn.

six seasons, 17fn., 97fn., 305

sixteen qualities, 83

sixteen traits, 82, 83

Sky, 10, 19, 37, 44, 186, 292, 303, 318, 389

snake, 313

solstice, 224

Soma, a medicinal plant *Sarcostema Viminalis* or *Asclepias Acida*, 38, 100fn., 144, 231fn., 237, 242, 269, 306; juice; the stalks

GLOSSARY AND INDEX 449

of the soma plant were pressed between stones by the priests, then sprinkled with water, purified with a strainer and collected in large jars, 224, 236, 241, 247, 249, 253, 266, 267, 279, 337, 338; personified as one of the most important of Vedic gods, 106fn., 307, 309, 402

Soma yajna, the soma juice was mixed with ghee, flour &c., allowed to ferment and then offered in libations to the gods, 240

soul, 66fn., 89fn., 105fn., 204fn., 258fn., 277fn., 297, 335, 342, 358, 379, 387, 410, 433, 434

Soul-force, 45, 69

Space, 66fn., 91fn., 303, 321fn., 345

Sparsh, touch, 105fn.

Speaker, 109, 266

Sphulingini, one of the seven tongues of Agni or fire, 214fn.

Spleen, 318

Spring, 10, 309

Sravana, month i.e., mid july to mid August, 70, 293

Statesman, 5

steward, 368

Streams, 318

Sudhumravarna, one of the seven tongues of Agni or fire, 214fn.

Sulohita, one of the seven tongues of Agni, 214fn.

Sumanta, counsellor of Dasaratha, 368fn.

Summer, 309

Sun, 2, 3, 4, 5, 6, 7, 8, 66fn., 73, 89fn., 166, 177, 296, 303, 305, 306, 317, 325, 327, 346, 355, 356, 362, 363, 370, 381, 383, 403, 405, 409, 427, 428, 430

Sun and Moon, 2, 6, 12fn., 54fn., 60, 63, 96, 100fn., 105, 109, 241, 275, 276, 277, 280, 307, 308, 376fn., 377fn., 403

Supreme Spirit, 249

Surya, the Sun, 106fn., 257fn.

Sushumna, a vein of the body, lying between those called *ida* or *pingala*, and supposed to be the passage for the dormant *kundalini*, 139fn., 252fn.

sushupti, complete unconsciousness, 322

Sustenance, 378

swan, 249, 314

swapan, dream, drowsiness, 322

sword, 193

system of education, 7

Tamas, one of the three qualities or Gunas responsible for ignorance, illusion, lust and other passions, 43, 170, 173fn., 233fn., 277fn., 364, 375fn.

tanks, 193

Tarka, speculation; reasoning, 98fn.

tax collector, 368

Teja, shining with lustre, 433

telescope, 224

Ten Pranas, 98fn.

Things—animate, 292; crawling, 292; creeping, 292; inanimate, 292

Thirteenfold objects, 98

Thirty-four threads, 89

Thirty-three Gods, 105, 256, 275, 407

Thirty-threefold praise, 105, 176

Three bonds, 355

Three duties, 131

Three life winds, 25

Three lustres, 83

Three regions, 403

Three stages, 74, 131

Three steps, 379

Three worlds, 97

transmigration of souls, 133

trees—fig. 297; shalmali, 297

Trinava, a hymn having $3 \times 9 = 27$ verses, 274

triple light, 234, 430

Trishtup metre, a metre of 4×11 syllables, 7, 16, 36, 40, 86fn., 111, 128, 158, 273, 296, 301, 309, 348, 364, 426, 429

Trishtup verses, 120, 121, 123, 350

Triyambaka, 'three eyed' god, Rudra, Siva, 29fn.

Twashta, sun, 308, 313

twelve Adityas, 89fn.

twelve months, 15, 43, 70, 89, 162, 169, 275fn., 389

Twentyonefold praise-song, 105

twenty-sevenfold praise, 176

two physicians, 264, 265

two sleepless Gods, 408

Ubbat, 9fn., 13fn., 14fn., 15fn., 17fn., 19fn., 20fn., 22fn., 24fn., 26fn., 29fn., 38fn., 45fn., 298fn., 374fn.

Udan, one of the five vital airs in the human body (that which is in the throat and moves upwards), 10fn., 13, 57, 64, 66fn., 89fn., 91fn., 105fn., 156, 164, 169, 174fn., 204fn., 214fn., 223, 229fn., 271, 307, 309, 318, 347, 354, 364, 374fn., 387, 389, 426.

Udgata (Udgatri), one of the four chief-priests; he chants the hymns of the Sama Veda, 11fn., 68fn., 69fn., 259fn., 272fn.

Ukha, a vessel, 212fn.

Upabhrit, a sacrificial vessel or ladle made of wood, 11fn.

Upapati, a paramour, 367fn.

Upasana, Worship, adoration, 78fn., 158, 163fn.

Upvedas, writings subordinate to the Vedas; *Ayurveda* or the science of medicine; *Dhanurveda* or science of archery; *Gandharvaveda* or science of music; *Sthapatyaveda* or the science of architecture, 98fn., 144

Ushik, mother of Rishi Kakshivant; wife of Rishi Dirghatama, 24fn.

Ushniha, a vedic metre consisting of twentyeight syllabic instants, viz., two padas with eight instants and one with twelve; the varieties depend on the place of the twelfth syllabled pada, 272, 301, 309, 346, 349, 364

Uttarayan, sun's progress towards north of the Equator, the summer solstice, 224fn.

Vada, controversy, discussion, 98fn.

Vaishya, the third caste whose members were engaged in trade and also in agriculture, 7fn., 19fn., 36fn., 72fn., 98fn., 163, 179, 192, 193fn., 230, 257, 321, 327, 329fn., 365, 374

Vak, speech, 308, 433

Vamdevya, descended from the Rishi Vama deva, author of many hymns in the fourth mandala of Rigveda; name of various hymns in Samaveda, 127

Vanaprastha, the third stage in the Hindu's life when the stage of a householder is given up for practising asceticism in the forest, 30fn., 98fn., 130fn., 163fn.

Vanaspati, a stem, trunk, beam, 93fn.; lord of plants viz., the Soma, 345

Varuna, 'All enveloping sky', 9fn., 433; connected with water, 25fn.; as one of the oldest Vedic Gods and Supreme Deity, 307, 310; as possessing extraordinary power and wisdom, 64fn.; as presiding over the night, 388fn.

Vasishtha, a renowned vedic sage, the archetype of a Brahmanical Rishi; came into conflict with the legendary Visvamitra, who raised himself by indomitable will and herculean efforts from the Kshatriya (warrior) to the Brahmanical (priestly) caste or class, 158

Vasu, excellent, good, 7fn.

Vasus, a particular class of Gods who number eight; Indra, Agni and Vishnu are assigned the leadership of these gods in different texts; their names are variously given; the Vishnu Purana gives (1) Apa (2) Dhruva (3) Soma (4) Dhava (5) Anila (6) Anala or Pavaka (7) Pratiusha and (8) Prabhasa, 10, 13, 98, 105fn., 119, 135, 160, 161, 162, 166, 170, 174, 256, 275fn., 292, 296, 308, 315, 341, 354, 406, 426

Vayu, the god of the winds is assigned an equal rank with Indra; he is described as very handsome; he moves noisily in a resplendent drawn a pair of red or purple horses; occasionally the number of horses are increased upto thousand, 10fn., 82fn.

Vedas, originally these were three in number, called Rigveda, Yajurveda and Samaveda, collectively known as *Trayi* 'threefold knowledge.' Later a fourth called Atharvaveda was added; each Veda consists of two main parts, mantra and Brahmana. The former is a collection of hymns and the latter is a manual of instructions for performing sacrifices. Attached to each Brahmana is an Upanishad, mystic or secret doctrine, 6fn., 20, 24, 43, 44, 47, 54, 65fn., 74, 77, 85, 98fn., 135, 144, 162

vedic marriage, 139fn.

Vedic Samsthan, Lucknow, 271fn., 338fn.

Vedic Samsthan, Mathura, 97fn.

velocity of mind, 356

Vidura, the younger brother of Dhritarashtra and Pandu; all the three were sons of Vyasa, the former two by the widows of Vicitra-virya and the latter by the servant-maid of the elder widow. Vidura is described as one of the wisest men of the age of Mahabharata, 368

Vidyalankar, Jaidev, 6fn., 16fn., 36fn., 79fn., 81fn., 97fn., 174fn., 177fn., 231fn., 271fn., 316, 335fn., 339fn., 351fn., 364fn., 414fn.

Vidya Sabha, assembly for the spread of knowledge, 74fn.

viper, 313

Virat metre, a vedic metre of thirty three syllables, 310, 348, 364

GLOSSARY AND INDEX

Virat verses, name of some hymns of the Samaveda in Virat metre, 274fn.
virtues of a commander, 114
Virya, manly vigour, virility, 82fn.
Vishnu, the second deity of the Hindu triad, Brahma the creator, Vishnu the preserver and Siva the destroyer; in the vedic period he did not occupy the supreme position he enjoys today, 16fn., 303fn., 304, 307, 314
Vishruti, flowing forth, issuing from, 85fn.
Vishvakarma, the divine creative artist and architect; in the vedic period he was identified with Brahma as the creator of all things and architect of the universe, 176, 310
Vishvarupi, one of the seven tongues of Agni, 214fn.
Vishvavasu, being benevolent to all, Vishnu is called by this name; name of a Gandharva, 9fn.
Visikha, a posture in shooting, 209
vishvedevas, a particular class of gods; they are the sons of visva, daughter of Daksha; they are usually invoked at the time of *sraddhas*, 15fn., 397fn.
Viswakarma, name of a seer, 159
vital breaths, 15, 34, 52, 64, 164, 198, 199, 255, 257, 287, 292, 297, 301, 316, 321, 323, 374, 388, 401
vital parts, 174, 209
Vitanda, frivolous argument, 98fn.
Vyakarna, grammar, 98fn.
Vyan, one of the five vital airs which circulates through the body, 7fn., 25, 66fn., 89fn., 91fn., 105fn., 162, 164, 165, 169, 174fn., 185, 204fn., 214fn., 219, 223, 229fn., 252, 374fn.

War, 8
Washing basin, 224
Water, 66fn., 89fn., 91fn., 372fn.
Water animals—crocodile, 314; fish, 311; frog, 311, 314, 315; porpoise, 311; tortoise, 314
water-fall, 193
Waters—flowing, 291; healing, 291; moving, 291; ocean, 291; ordinary, 291; rain, 291; rising, 291; sea, 291; standing, 291; tank, 291
weapon, 177, 198, 361, 366
Weber, 365fn.
well, 193

white ant, 312
Wilson (Professor), 216fn., 365fn., 372fn.
wind, 166
Winter, 309

Yajman, one who promotes a sacrifice and employs a priest for performing it, 14fn., 79fn., 88fn., 266fn., 277fn.
Yajna(s), sacrifice, 1, 3, 4, 5, 6, 9, 10, 11, 12, 13, 16, 21fn., 27fn., 33, 39, 55, 79, 80, 250, 256, 259fn., 275fn., 279fn., 281fn., 298, 330, 331, 335fn., 338, 342, 343, 346, 347, 351, 352, 354; 375fn., 382, 401, 402, 409, 419, 421, 423fn., 427, 429
Yajnapati, lord of sacrifice i.e., the one defrays the expenses for the sacrifice, 12fn.
yajnashala, hall where the sacrifice is performed, 338
Yajnopavit, the investiture of the boys of the Brahmana, Kshatriya and Vaisya castes with the sacred thread; also the sacred thread itself, 54fn., 189, 241
Yajurveda, the collection of sacred mantras or hymns in prose in the form of a sacrificial prayer book for use of the *Adhvaryu* priests; the Yajurveda has two main divisions, Krishna or black and Shukla or white; in the former the samhita and Brahmana portions are not clear while in the latter it is not so, 19fn., 31, 33, 57, 78, 81fn., 127, 210fn., 227, 233, 234, 241, 256, 339fn., 373, 375fn., 399, 414, 425, 427
Yajushi Anushtup Chhand, eight syllabic metre, 97fn.
Yajushi Brihati Chhand, metre of nine syllables, 97fn.
Yajushi Pankti Chhand, metre of ten syllables, 97fn.
Yama, twin, one of a pair; name of the God who rules over the spirits of the dead; he is the son of Vivasvat (the sun) and Saranyu, the daughter of Tvastri; his twin sister is Yami, 138
Yama(s), self-control as one of the first eight angas in yoga for attaining mental concentration; any major moral rule or duty as opposed to *niyama*, a minor observance, 62, 63, 237, 296, 328
Yami, the twin sister of Yama; she is regarded as the first of women, while her brother as the first of men born to Viva-

svat (the sun) and Saranyu, before Saranyu had become afraid of her glorious husband; Yami entreated her brother Yama to become her husband, as there were no others to perpetuate the human race. But Yama refused and died. Her sorrow at his loss was so great that to assuage her the Gods created night, 138 year, 166fn., 167

yoga, 19fn., 62, 63, 64, 65, 103, 131fn., 212, 213, 226, 252, 295, 325, 327, 330, 383

yogi, 65, 202fn., 203, 205, 213, 214, 253, 437

NBD
2588
26/4/18